Core Curriculum for Transplant Nurses

Core Curriculum for Transplant Nurses

Edited by:

Linda Ohler, RN, MSN, CCTC, FAAN
Editor, *Progress in Transplantation*
Program Manager, CHF and Heart Transplant
Virginia Commonwealth University
Richmond, Virginia
Assistant Professor of Nursing
Marymount University
Arlington, Virginia

Sandra A. Cupples, RN, PhD
Heart Transplant Coordinator
Washington Hospital Center
Washington, DC

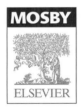

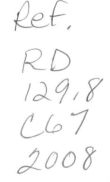

INTERNATIONAL
TRANSPLANT
NURSES
SOCIETY

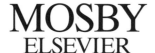

11830 Westline Industrial Drive
St. Louis, Missouri 63146

Core Curriculum for Transplant Nurses

ISBN-13: 978-0-323-04411-0
ISBN-10: 0-323-04411-5

Notice

Knowledge and best practice in this field are constantly changing. As new research and experience broaden our knowledge, changes in practice, treatment and drug therapy may become necessary or appropriate. Readers are advised to check the most current information provided (i) on procedures featured or (ii) by the manufacturer of each product to be administered, to verify the recommended dose or formula, the method and duration of administration, and contraindications. It is the responsibility of the practitioner, relying on their own experience and knowledge of the patient, to make diagnoses, to determine dosages and the best treatment for each individual patient, and to take all appropriate safety precautions. To the fullest extent of the law, neither the Publisher nor the Editors assumes any liability for any injury and/or damage to persons or property arising out or related to any use of the material contained in this book.

The Publisher

ISBN-13: 978-0-323-04411-0
ISBN-10: 0-323-04411-5

Executive Publisher: Barbara Nelson Cullen
Managing Editor: Maureen Iannuzzi
Senior Developmental Editor: Jennifer Ehlers
Publishing Services Manager: Jeff Patterson
Cover Design: Margaret Reid

Printed in the United States of America.
Last digit is the print number: 9   8   7   6   5   4   3   2   1

Working together to grow
libraries in developing countries

www.elsevier.com | www.bookaid.org | www.sabre.org

ELSEVIER   BOOK AID International   Sabre Foundation

This book is dedicated to

transplant nurses around the world, whose critical thinking and professional skil!s optimize outcomes of this complex patient population,

transplant recipients and their families, who remind us about love, life, and commitment,

and organ donors and their families, who create an enduring legacy of life.

Contributors

Terri Achanzar, RN, MS
Johns Hopkins Comprehensive Transplant Center
Kidney / Pancreas Transplant Program
Baltimore, Maryland
Pancreas and Kidney-Pancreas Transplantation

Greg Armstrong, RN, BSN
Brisbane, Queensland, Australia
Kidney Transplantation

Maria Angela Barone, RN
ISMETT
Palermo, Italy
Transplant Complications: Noninfectious Diseases

Michele D. Blakely, RN, MSN, CCTC
Post Transplant Coordinator
Wake Forest University Baptist Medical Center
Winston-Salem, North Carolina
Pancreas and Kidney-Pancreas Transplantation

Sally Bufton, RN, MSc
Liver Recipient Transplant Coordinator
University Hospital Birmingham NHS Foundation Trust
Queen Elizabeth Hospital
Birmingham, England, United Kingdom
Liver Transplantation

Lisa Burnapp, RN, MA
Renal Offices
Guy's Hospital
London, England, United Kingdom
Transplant Complications: Infectious Diseases

Anne-Marie Byerly, RN, BSN, CCTN
Primary Nurse Care Coordinator
Abdominal Transplant Unit
Thomas E. Starzl Transplantation Institute
University of Pittsburgh Medical Center
Pittsburgh, Pennsylvania
Liver Transplantation

Marcello Castellese, RN, CCTC
ISMETT
Palermo, Italy
Transplant Complications: Noninfectious Diseases

Agnes Costello, PharmD, MS
Genzyme Pharmaceuticals
Cambridge, Massachusetts
Transplant Pharmacology

Sandra A. Cupples, RN, PhD
Heart Transplant Coordinator
Washington Hospital Center
Washington, DC
Transplant Complications: Infectious Diseases; Transplant Complications: Noninfectious Diseases; Professional Issues in Transplantation; Heart Transplantation

Cheryl Dale, MS, RegN, NP/CNS
Hepatology and Liver Transplant
London Health Sciences Centre
London, Ontario, Canada
Solid Organ Transplantation: The Evaluation Process

Maria DeAngelis, RN, BsCN, MsCN, ACNP
Pediatric Transplantation
Hospital for Sick Children
Toronto, Ontario, Canada
IntestineTransplantation

Debi H. Dumas-Hicks RN, BS,CCTC
Senior Heart Transplant Clinical Coordinator
Cardiomyopathy and Heart Transplant Center
Heart and Vascular Institute
Ochsner Clinic Foundation
New Orleans, Louisiana
Transplant Complications: Infectious Diseases

Karen Emmett, RN, BSN, CCTN
Primary Nurse Care Coordinator
Abdominal Transplant Unit
Thomas E. Starzl Transplantation Institute
University of Pittsburgh Medical Center
Pittsburgh, Pennsylvania
Liver Transplantation

Grant Fisher, MScN, RN
Transplant Recipient Coordinator
Multi-Organ Transplant Program
London Health Sciences Centre
London, Ontario, Canada
Heart Transplantation

Maureen P. Flattery, RN, MS, NP
Heart and Lung Transplant Coordinator
Virginia Commonwealth University Health
System
Richmond, Virginia
*Solid Organ Transplantation: The Evaluation
Process*

Elizabeth Ann Sparks Ford, BSN, RN
Transplant Coordinator
National Institutes of Health
Bethesda, Maryland
Patient Education of the Transplant Recipient

Sandy Giammona, RN
ISMETT
Palermo, Italy
*Transplant Complications: Noninfectious
Diseases*

Donna Gwinn, RN, MSN, PhDc
Mayo Clinic
Jacksonville, Florida
Care of Living Donors

Christine Hartley RN, MS
Heart and Lung Transplant Coordinator
Department of Cardiothoracic Surgery
Stanford Hospital and Clinics
Stanford, California
Heart Transplantation

Mary Jo Holechek, MS, CRNP, CNN
Lead Transplant Nurse Practitioner
Abdominal Organ Transplant Service
Johns Hopkins Hospital
Baltimore, Maryland
Kidney Transplantation

Elizabeth V. John RN, MN
Liver Transplant Coordinator/EPN
South Australian Liver Transplant Unit
Flinders Medical Centre
Bedford Park, South Australia
Patient Education of the Transplant Recipient

Kay Kendall, MSW, LISW, ACSW
Department of Social Work
Cleveland Clinic Foundation
Cleveland, Ohio
Psychosocial Issues in Transplantation

Beverly Kosmach-Park, MSN, CRNP
Children's Hospital of Pittsburgh
Intestinal Transplant Program
Pittsburgh, Pennsylvania
Intestine Transplantation

Christiane Kugler, MScN, RN, PhD(c)
Hannover Thoracic Transplant Program
Division of Thoracic and Cardiovascular
Surgery
Hannover Medical School
Hannover, Germany
Lung and Heart-Lung Transplantation

Diane Lepley, RN, MPH
Johns Hopkins Comprehensive Transplant
Center
Kidney/Pancreas Transplant Program
Baltimore, Maryland
Pancreas and Kidney-Pancreas Transplantation

Jen Lumsdaine, PhD
Transplant Unit
Royal Infirmary
Edinburgh, Scotland, United Kingdom
Care of Living Donors

Maureen I. O'Dell, MSW, RSW
Multi-organ Transplant Program
Toronto General Hospital
Toronto, Ontario, Canada
Psychosocial Issues in Transplantation

Linda Ohler, RN, MSN, CCTC, FAAN
Editor, *Progress in Transplantation*
Program Manager, CHF and Heart
Transplant
Virginia Commonwealth University
Richmond, Virginia
Assistant Professor of Nursing
Marymount University
Arlington, Virginia
Basics in Transplant Immunology

Glen J. Pearson, PharmD, FCSHP
Assistant Professor of Medicine
Co-Director, Cardiac Transplant Clinic
Department of Medicine
Division of Cardiology
University of Alberta Hospital
Edmonton, Alberta, Canada
Transplant Pharmacology

Giovanni Scianna, RN
ISMETT
Palermo, Italy
*Transplant Complications: Noninfectious
Diseases*

Nancy Stitt, RN, BSN
University of Pittsburgh Medical Center
Liver Transplantation
Pittsburgh, Pennsylvania
*Transplant Complications: Noninfectious
Diseases*

Frank E.L. Van Gelder, RN, BSN, ECTC
Senior Transplant Coordinator
Department of Transplant Coordination
University Hospital–Leuven
Leuven, Belgium
Basics in Transplant Immunology

Grainne Walsh, BSc, RN, RSCN
Pediatric Transplant Sister
Children's Hospital
Guy's & St. Thomas' NHS Foundation
Trust
London, England, United Kingdom
Pediatric Solid Organ Transplantation

Connie White-Williams, MSN, RN, FAAN
Cardiothoracic Transplant Coordinator
Heart and Lung Transplantation
University of Alabama Medical Center at
Birmingham
Birmingham, Alabama
Lung and Heart-Lung Transplantation

Brian Widmar, MSN, RN, APRN, BC, CCRN
Acute Care Nurse Practitioner
Departments of Cardiac and Thoracic
Surgery
Cardiovascular and Inpatient Medicine
Patient Care Center
Vanderbilt University Medical Center
Nashville, Tennessee
Lung and Heart-Lung Transplantation

Rebecca Winsett, PhD, RN
Professor
University of Tennessee
Memphis, Tennessee
Professional Issues in Transplantation

Barbara V. Wise, PhD, RN, CPNP
Pediatric Nurse Practitioner
National Institutes of Health
Bethesda, Maryland
Pediatric Solid Organ Transplantation

Janelle Yorke, MRes, Grad. Dip. CertEdu, RGN
Lecturer
Faculty of Health and Social Care
School of Nursing
University of Salford
Greater Manchester, England, United
Kingdom
Professional Issues in Transplantation

Mariella Ziino, RN
ISMETT
Palermo, Italy
Transplant Complications: Noninfectious Diseases

Reviewers

Sharon Beer, RN, RM, MSc, Cert Coun
Lead Nurse Recipient Coordinator
Heart and Lung Transplantation
University Hospital of Birmingham, NHS
Trust
Birmingham, United Kingdom

Robert Bray, PhD
Histocompatibility
Emory University
Atlanta, Georgia

Brian D. Carlos, MD
Associate Medical Director
Heart Transplantation Service
Washington Hospital Center
Washington, DC

Jennifer Cross, RN, MScN, ANP
Nurse Practitioner
Renal Transplant and Living Donation
Program
London Health Sciences Centre
London, Ontario, Canada

Clare Curran, MSN, RN, CCRN
Clinical Nurse II
Surgical Intensive Care Unit
University of North Carolina Hospitals
Chapel Hill, North Carolina
Clinical Instructor
Duke University
Durham, North Carolina

Judy Currey, RN, BN, PhD
Senior Lecturer
Coordinator, Postgraduate Critical Care
and Perioperative Programs
Faculty of Health, Medicine, Nursing and
Behavioural Sciences
Deakin University
Burwood, Victoria, Australia

Bernadette Dodd, RN, BScN
Recipient Transplant Coordinator
University of Alberta Hospital
Edmonton, Alberta, Canada

Kathleen Falkenstein, PhD, CPNP
Assistant Professor
Drexel University
Philadelphia, Pennsylvania

Gayle Frohloff, RN, RM
Princess Alexandra Hospital
Woolloongabba, Brisbane, Australia

Steve Gabardi, PharmD
Brigham and Women's Hospital
Boston, Massachusetts

Anne Griffiths, RN, RM, FRCNA
The Alfred Hospital
Melbourne, Victoria, Australia

Monica Horn, RN, CCRN, CCTC
Children's Hospital of Los Angeles
Los Angeles, California

Annemarie Kaan, RN, MCN, CCN(c), CCTN
Adjunct Professor
University of British Columbia
Clinical Nurse Specialist
Heart Failure Transplantation
St. Paul's Hospital
Vancouver, British Columbia, Canada

Tammy Leatherdale, BSCN, BA
University of Alberta Hospital
Edmonton, Alberta, Canada

Jan D. Manzetti, RN, PhD
University of Pittsburgh
Pittsburgh, Pennsylvania

Catherine Martin, BSW, MBioeth
Princess Alexandra Hospital
Brisbane, Queensland, Australia

Jacques Pirenne, MD, PhD
Abdominal Transplant Surgeon
Head, Laboratory of Transplant
Immunology
University Hospital Leuven
Leuven, Belgium

Jorge Reyes, MD
University of Washington
Seattle, Washington

Cynthia L. Russell, RN, PhD
Assistant Professor
University of Missouri–Columbia
Sinclair School of Nursing
Columbia, Missouri

Shmuel Shoham, MD
Director, Transplant Infectious Diseases
Washington Hospital Center
Washington, DC

Prof Dr. Takaaki Koshiba
Kyoto University
Kyoto, Japan

Charlie Thomas, LCSW, ACSW
Transplant Services
Banner Good Samaritan Medical Center
Phoenix, Arizona

Marc Waer, MD, PhD
Transplant Immunologist
Head, Department of Experimental
Transplantation
University Hospital Leuven
Leuven, Belgium

Preface

Professional licensure indicates that a clinician has met the basic requirements of a generalist within a field of practice. Certification, however, provides validation that a nurse has obtained requisite knowledge and expertise within a specialized area. With both education and practice requirements, certification assures the public that a specialist meets consistent standards of quality established by a professional association.

Certification has become a key measure of professional competencies in nursing. The Institute of Medicine (IOM) has issued several reports on patient safety in its *Quality Chasm Series*. In its evaluation of education for health care professionals, the IOM states that professional organizations that grant certification to clinicians are ensuring that those individuals have met the highest professional standards within a given area of specialization.[1]

Recognizing the value and importance of certification for the highly specialized field of transplant nursing, the American Board of Transplant Certification in collaboration with the International Transplant Nurses Society (ITNS), developed a standardized credentialing examination for transplant nurses: the Certified Clinical Transplant Nurse (CCTN) examination.

The purpose of *Core Curriculum for Transplant Nurses* is to articulate the knowledge base relative to the art and science of transplant nursing practice—and thus serve as a comprehensive resource for all transplant clinicians, and particularly for nurses preparing for the CCTN examination. The text uses the CCTN examination blueprint as a basis for determining relevant content. Information is presented in an embellished outline format so that the text can be used as an easy reference guide.

Information pertinent to the pre- and post-transplant care of each type of abdominal and thoracic transplant recipient is presented in six organ-specific chapters. Other chapters address key elements that are common to all types of solid organ transplantation: the transplant evaluation process, immunology, pharmacology, psychosocial aspects of transplantation, patient education, and infectious and noninfectious complications. Three chapters focus on professional issues in transplantation, care of living donors, and pediatric transplantation. More than 160 sample test questions are included to assist readers with evaluating their comprehension of the material presented. Tables, figures, and graphs complement the information presented in the text. Two appendices provide readers with information regarding laboratory values and electrolyte abnormalities.

Consistent with the international focus of the ITNS, the chapters of *Core Curriculum for Transplant Nurses* are authored by experts in transplantation from several continents. Information included in the appendices is presented in both conventional units and the System of International Units. This unique international dimension is also symbolized by the flags depicted on the cover.

Transplant patients are one of the most complex and challenging of all patient populations. Recognizing the value of certification, and committed to enhancing patient safety and quality care, we and ITNS hope that this text will not only contribute to a nurse's success on the CCTN examination, but also serve as a comprehensive resource for transplant nurses around the globe.

We wish to thank ITNS for providing us with this opportunity and to extend our sincere gratitude to our expert contributors and reviewers. Without their willingness to share their knowledge, expertise, time, and talents, this book would not have been possible.

Linda Ohler, RN, MSN, CCTC, FAAN
Sandra A. Cupples, RN, PhD

Editors

---

[1]Institute of Medicine: *Patient Safety: Achieving a New Standard of Care*. Washington, DC: National Academies Press, 2004.

Contents

1 Solid Organ Transplantation: The Evaluation Process

MAUREEN P. FLATTERY

CHERYL DALE

INTRODUCTION

I. Introduction
   A. Solid organ transplantation is a viable treatment option for end-stage disease. Post-transplant care requires compliance with a complex medical regimen for a successful outcome.
   B. In addition, the immunosuppressant regimen can exacerbate pre-existing conditions that can adversely affect both quality of life and survival.
II. Purpose of transplant evaluation process
   A. Most candidates referred for transplantation have one or more chronic illnesses that may affect their candidacy for transplantation.
      1. Therefore, it is paramount that candidates be thoroughly evaluated to determine the appropriateness of proceeding with transplantation.
      2. Additionally, the transplant evaluation may reveal problems amenable to other interventions besides transplantation.
III. This chapter will outline the transplant evaluation process for solid organ transplantation.
   A. General procedures for all organs as well as organ-specific requirements will be presented.
   B. Additionally, waiting list criteria for specific organs will be addressed.
IV. Coordination of the transplant evaluation and patient education
   A. The role of the transplant coordinator includes overseeing the transplant process and providing education to patients and their families.
      1. Often, the coordinator is the first contact that the patient may have with the transplant team.
         a. Providing an overview of the transplant evaluation process will provide the patient and family an opportunity to ask appropriate questions of the transplant team members as they proceed through evaluation.
         b. Patients and families should be given information about each test and consult so they know what to expect and how to prepare.
      2. History and other valuable information may be obtained over the phone, prior to the patient's initial appointment.

3. During the assessment process, the coordinator consults with the patient and family to obtain history and provide education concerning the transplant process.
4. This information includes what the patient should expect during the evaluation, the time line for team decision-making, issues concerning the waiting period for transplant, the organ allocation process, and what to expect after transplantation.
5. The stress of the situation may interfere with the ability of the patient and his or her family to retain information.
   a. Expect to repeat information.
   b. Refer to Chapter 3 for more detailed information on patient education.
6. Most patients and families are unaware of the United Network for Organ Sharing (UNOS) listing criteria, the length of time it may take to receive a suitable donor organ, and follow-up at the transplant center during the waiting period.
   a. Transplant center–specific information should be provided regarding the expected waiting time.
   b. Many transplant centers have monthly support groups for individuals and families awaiting a transplant. These support groups often include educational programs.

B. General evaluation process
   1. All candidates referred for organ transplantation will undergo a general evaluation process prior to more specific and invasive testing.
   2. This process begins with a thorough history and physical examination of the candidate.
   3. Following this, baseline lab work and consultations will be performed as outlined below.

V. Lab work
   A. Candidates referred for solid organ transplantation undergo a battery of lab assessments to determine suitability for transplantation and to assess for the presence of comorbid conditions.
   B. General lab work includes basic metabolic panel, hepatic panel, lipid profile, complete blood count, thyroid panel, RPR (rapid plasma reagin), urinalysis, and creatinine clearance assessment (extra renal transplant candidates only).
   C. In addition, transplant-specific lab work is performed. This includes the following:
      1. ABO blood typing. It is a requirement of UNOS that prospective recipients have their blood typing done on two separate occasions.[1]
         a. Both results should be recorded in the medical record.
         b. At the time of listing, a second member of the transplant team will confirm the blood type in the UNET[sm] system.
         c. Eurotransplant currently has no written policy determining or confirming blood types for recipients at the time of listing.[2]
         d. Canada also has no written policy.
      2. Panel reactive antibody (PRA). In order to determine the likelihood of developing acute and/or chronic rejection following solid organ transplantation, the serum of a prospective recipient is tested against a panel of lymphocytes for the presence of circulating antibodies reactive against HLA antigens.

    a. This result is generally expressed as a percent of panel reactivity (the number of wells with positive reactivity over the total number of wells tested × 100)[3].

    b. Different laboratory techniques are employed in different centers and may include flow cytometry, enzyme-linked immunosorbent assay (ELISA), or complement-dependent cytotoxic assay.

    c. A prospective cross match may be indicated at the time of transplantation based on center- and organ-specific determination of elevation of the PRA.

    d. Additionally, specific therapies may be attempted to desensitize the recipient prior to transplantation. This, too, is center- and organ-specific.

3. Human leukocyte antigen. Human leukocyte antigen (HLA) is the term that describes six separate polymorphic genetic loci clustered together in a single area of the human genome, and expressed on the lymphocyte, that can predict rejection.[4]

    a. HLA is assessed preoperatively and is used in the allocation of cadaveric kidneys. It is a requirement of UNOS and the European transplant registries when listing patients as candidates.

    b. In other organs it is considered useful information to predict rejection, and is a necessary step in determining cross match positivity, but is often assessed following transplantation.

    c. The increased use of molecular testing to determine HLA can lead to confusion in the setting of recent blood transfusions.

        i. The sensitivity of this method can identify antigens from the transfusion and obscure the HLA.

        ii. For that reason, it is best to avoid HLA testing within 72 hours of a blood transfusion.

4. Virology screening. Virology screening is performed both to determine a recipient's suitability for transplantation and to determine the recipient's post-transplant infection risk. Assessment includes:

    a. Human immunodeficiency virus (HIV). The initial test for HIV is done by enzyme immunoassay.

        i. Equivocal or positive results are confirmed by Western blot.

        ii. Currently, most centers consider the presence of HIV a contraindication to transplantation.

        iii. However, with the advent of highly active antiretroviral therapy and the improved survival of HIV infected individuals, some centers are performing kidney and liver transplants on patients who are HIV+.[5]

        iv. In thoracic organ transplantation, there is one anecdotal report of an HIV+ patient receiving a heart transplant[6] and no reports of lung transplantation in HIV infected patients.

    b. Hepatitis screening. Hepatitis screening is performed both to determine previous exposure to hepatitis and to determine the need for further testing or treatment of those who may have had a known exposure.

        i. Hepatitis is an indication for liver transplantation.

        ii. However, active hepatitis infection is typically a contraindication to the transplantation of other solid organs.

        iii. Initial hepatitis screening consists of the convalescent battery (Table 1-1).

TABLE 1-1

■ **Convalescent Hepatitis Battery for Screening**

Test:	Positive results indicate:
Anti-HCV (Hepatitis C antibody)	Exposure to hepatitis C
HBsAg (Hepatitis B surface antigen)	Infection with hepatitis B
HBsAb (Hepatitis B surface antibody)	Immunity to hepatitis B
HBcAb IgG (Hepatitis B core antibody)	Previous hepatitis B infection/exposure

      iv. Further testing will be determined by the results of initial testing (Table 1-2) (Figure 1-1).

   c. Herpes virus screening. As a result of their immunosuppressive status, organ transplant recipients are at greater risk of developing more severe viral infections than healthy individuals.

      i. The herpes family of viruses has been implicated in 25% to 30% of all post-transplant infections.[7]

      ii. Knowledge of a transplant recipient's previous exposure and immune status may direct the acceptance of donor organs as well as determine the need for prophylactic therapy.

      iii. Preoperative screening includes assessment of the following:

   d. Cytomegalovirus (CMV) screening. CMV is a member of the Betaherpesvirinae family.

      i. Approximately 80% of adults are exposed to CMV during the first two decades of life either as an asymptomatic infection or as a benign infectious mononucleosis-like syndrome.[8]

      ii. At the time of infection, cell-mediated immune responses develop but do not completely eradicate the virus.

      iii. CMV establishes latency and may therefore reactivate later in life.

      iv. Historically, up to 85% of solid organ transplant recipients who are seronegative but receive a seropositive donor organ will develop CMV disease.[9]

      v. CMV status is established by testing the recipient's blood for the presence of CMV antibodies, specifically IgG.

   e. Epstein Barr virus (EBV) screening. EBV is a member of the Gammaherpesvirinae family and is acquired in adolescence or early adulthood.

      i. EBV is responsible for the infectious mononucleosis syndrome.

      ii. EBV is classified as a group 1 carcinogen and is strongly associated with Burkitt's lymphoma, nasopharyngeal carcinoma, Hodgkin's disease, and immunosuppression-related lymphoproliferative disease.[10]

TABLE 1-2

■ **Hepatitis BsAg Positive—Further Testing***

HBeAg-

HBeAb-

HBV DNA-

HBcAb IgM-positive = acute hepatitis B or reactivation of virus

*Suggest referral to a hepatologist for further assessment and management of hepatitis.

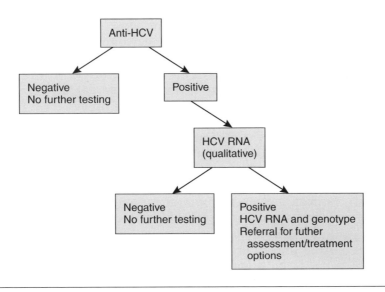

Figure 1-1. Hepatitis C evaluation process.

      iii. Post-transplant lymphoproliferative disease (PTLD) can affect both graft and patient survival.

      iv. EBV status is established by testing the recipient's blood for the presence of EBV antibodies, specifically IgG.

   f. Herpes simplex type-1 (HSV) screening. HSV is an Alphaherpesvirinae which is also acquired in childhood or young adulthood.

      i. Impairment of the immune response as a result of immunosuppression predisposes transplant recipients to reactivation infection.

      ii. HSV status is established by testing the recipient's blood for the presence of HSV antibodies, specifically IgG.

5. Toxoplasma screening. *Toxoplasma gondii* is a coccidian parasite of the cat population for which humans are intermediate hosts.[11]

   a. Although a large proportion of the population is infected by toxoplasma, it is an uncommon cause of disease.

   b. In immunocompromised individuals it can be life-threatening.

        c.   Those recipients with prior exposure, or who receive an organ from an individual with a prior exposure, are at risk for developing reactivation disease following transplantation.

        d.   Toxoplasma status is established by testing the recipient's blood for the presence of toxoplasma antibodies, specifically IgG.

   6. Tuberculosis (TB) testing. All candidates should be tested for TB.

        a.   The most commonly performed test is the PPD, an intradermal skin test.

        b.   Those candidates with prior exposure or those who have been vaccinated with bacille Calmette-Guérin (BCG) may test positive.

           i.   Chest x-ray will then be indicated.

        c.   Candidates who are extremely ill may be anergic, meaning they cannot respond appropriately to immune stimuli.

           i.   Therefore, it is best to apply a control test at the same time as the PPD to determine response.

           ii.   Candida and mumps are two commonly used PPD controls since most people have been exposed to these two organisms.

   7. Cancer screening. Transplant recipients are at increased risk of developing cancer because of their immunosuppressive regimen.

        a.   Any undetected, pre-existing cancer, in the setting of immunosuppressive medications, may become untreatable and lead to the recipient's death.

        b.   Candidates should be screened based on past medical history (e.g., history of colon polyps, family history of cancer) as well as age- and gender-appropriate screening as outlined by the American Cancer Society.[12] This includes:

           i.   Cervical cancer screening for women older than 21, mammography for women older than 40, colonoscopy for men and women older than 50.

           ii.   Prostate-specific antigen (PSA) blood test and digital rectal examination for men over 50.

        c.   All candidates should have a chest x-ray performed, although this is a poor method for detecting lung cancer.

   8. Osteoporosis screening. All post-menopausal women, as well as all candidates with a smoking history, chronic corticosteroid use, or cholestatic liver disease, should be assessed for the presence of osteopenia or osteoporosis by bone densitometry.

        a.   Solid organ transplant recipients are at increased risk of developing bone loss as a result of the immunosuppressive regimen.[13]

        b.   All abnormal findings should be treated appropriately.

  D. In addition to laboratory testing and procedures, patients referred for transplantation undergo evaluation and consultation with several specialists.

VI. Psychosocial evaluation.

  A. This is an integral part of the pre-transplant evaluation process.

  B. The evaluation is done to assess a candidate's appropriateness for transplantation, ability to comply with a complex post-operative regimen, and social support structure.

  C. Any current and past history of substance abuse is carefully screened during the psychosocial evaluation. Additional laboratory screening may be required to determine if the potential candidate is currently using drugs or alcohol.

VII. Financial evaluation.

   A. Unfortunately, pre-, peri-, and post-operative transplant care is expensive. Post-transplant medications cost in excess of $1200 (U.S.) monthly.

   B. Commercial insurance companies have different requirements for eligibility which may include referral to designated transplant centers.

   C. In the U.S., Medicare, the federally funded program that provides medical insurance for the elderly and disabled, funds transplants at designated centers only.

   D. Medicaid requirements and provisions vary from state to state. Requirements in other countries will also vary depending on the requirements of each payment system.

   E. The purpose of the evaluation is to determine if the candidate has sufficient access to financial resources to ensure a positive outcome following transplantation.

VIII. Nutritional evaluation.

   A. All candidates for solid organ transplantation should undergo nutritional assessment with a registered dietitian.

      1. This is especially important for candidates who are either overweight or underweight or who may have impaired digestion.

      2. Obesity is considered a comorbidity and if severe, may be a contraindication to transplantation.[14, 15, 16]

      3. Cachexia can adversely affect surgical outcome and these candidates may require nutritional intervention in the form of supplements or enteral or parenteral nutrition.

      4. In addition, immunosuppressant medications can cause hyperlipidemia.

      5. Candidates should be aware of the need to follow a heart-healthy diet following transplantation.

IX. Surgical evaluation.

   A. In addition to determining if transplantation is the appropriate procedure for the candidate, it must also be determined if the transplant is surgically feasible.

      1. Patients may be poor surgical candidates for a variety of reasons that may include the findings of testing and consultations, as well as anatomic barriers to transplantation, most notably from previous surgeries.

      2. The transplanting surgeon must determine if the intended procedure can be done safely.

X. Additional testing and consultations may be indicated for transplant candidates, based on the results of the initial testing and the medical history. As well, candidates may require further testing because of their age. This may include:

   A. Cardiac evaluation. All candidates for transplantation, regardless of age, should have an electrocardiogram.

      1. More extensive testing should be done based on medical history and age.

   B. An echocardiogram should be performed on any candidate for extra cardiac transplantation who complains of shortness of breath or who has a murmur by physical examination.

      C. Candidates with a previous history of coronary artery disease, hypertension, diabetes, or with a history of smoking will require a cardiac stress test to evaluate myocardial perfusion.
1. Exercise stress testing is the most accurate; however, many patients with end-stage organ disease are unable to walk on a treadmill.
2. In those cases, dipyridamole or dobutamine stress testing is appropriate.
3. Those patients with a positive stress test should proceed to cardiac catheterization.
4. Any candidate with abnormal findings should be referred to a cardiologist for complete evaluation.

XI. Pulmonary evaluation.
- A. All candidates for transplantation should have a chest x-ray and an oxygen saturation evaluated by pulse oximetry.
- B. In addition, candidates with a smoking history or a history of chronic obstructive lung disease should undergo pulmonary function testing.
- C. Any candidate with abnormal findings should be referred to a pulmonologist for further evaluation.

XII. Vascular evaluation.
- A. All candidates with a history of diabetes, coronary artery disease, claudication, or cerebrovascular accident should undergo Doppler imaging.
  1. This should include at least bilateral lower extremity and bilateral carotid artery imaging.
  2. Angiography and/or referral to a vascular surgeon may be warranted by abnormal results.
  3. Candidates for specific organs may require more extensive testing.

Candidates for solid organ transplantation may require additional consultations with medical specialists based on clinical findings, test results, and comorbid conditions.

ORGAN-SPECIFIC EVALUATION

In this section we will discuss additional tests necessary to evaluate candidates for specific organ transplants. Heart, lung, heart/lung, liver, kidney, kidney/pancreas, pancreas, and intestinal transplantation will be discussed in detail.

    I. Heart. Cardiac transplantation is indicated for patients with advanced congestive heart failure (New York Heart Association Class III-IV) for whom there are no other medical or surgical options to improve quality of life and survival.
- A. The primary indications for heart transplantation are equally distributed between ischemic and nonischemic cardiomyopathy, both of which comprise 45% of those referred for transplantation.[17]
- B. Additional indications include valvular disease, congenital heart disease, and retransplantation.
- C. Candidates referred for cardiac transplantation will have a thorough evaluation of cardiac function and anatomy to determine if another procedure, such as coronary artery bypass grafting or valve repair/replacement will relieve symptoms and improve quality of life. Candidates will also undergo testing to determine the severity of their illness and the urgency for transplantation. These tests include:

1. Cardiac catheterization: Patients referred for cardiac transplantation will require both a right and left heart catheterization.
   a. The right heart catheterization is performed to determine right heart function and degree of pulmonary hypertension.
      i. Severe, fixed pulmonary hypertension is a contraindication to heart transplantation; therefore, those patients with pulmonary hypertension may require additional procedures to determine if the hypertension is amenable to medical manipulation.
      ii. This may include the use of vasodilators, such as oxygen, nitroglycerin, milrinone, nesiritide, or prostaglandin.
      iii. Once a patient is listed for heart transplantation, the right heart pressures will be evaluated at regular intervals to determine changes in the patient's condition as well as to direct therapy.
   b. Coronary angiography, or left heart catheterization, is performed to determine if there are any lesions amenable to intervention that would relieve the patient's symptoms. Angiography need not be repeated unless changes in the candidate's symptoms warrant additional investigation.
2. Cardiopulmonary exercise testing (CPET) with direct measurement of ventilatory gas exchange provides the most reliable determination of functional capacity in patients with congestive heart failure.[18]
   a. The test is performed by exercising the patient on either a treadmill or bicycle ergometer using a standard protocol of increasing workload.
   b. During exercise, the candidate will breathe through a mouthpiece which allows for the continuous measurement of gas exchange to determine the patient's aerobic capacity.
   c. CPET is used to assess progression of disease and help determine timing for transplantation as well as to provide an exercise prescription for cardiopulmonary rehabilitation.
3. Cardiac MRI or PET scan: Candidates who are being considered for revascularization or ventricular aneurysectomy may require more extensive testing to determine myocardial viability. Both tests are limited by patient's suitability for the procedure (presence of MRI contraindications such as a pacemaker) and availability of procedures.

D. Waiting list criteria for cardiac transplantation vary from country to country.
1. These criteria play an instrumental role in organ allocation, regardless of location.
2. The systems have been devised in an attempt to allocate organs as justly as possible. Ideally, patients at the greatest risk of dying receive organs first.
3. Allocation systems are frequently reviewed and amended in order to ensure that the systems are just.
4. In the U.S. and Canada, hearts are allocated based on severity of disease as well as medical urgency. Table 1-3 outlines the information criteria required at the time of listing and Table 1-4 outlines medical urgency categories.

TABLE 1-3

■ **Listing Criteria for Heart Transplant Candidates**

Demographics
- date of birth
- ethnicity
- gender
- state or province of residence

ABO blood typing (confirmed by second person in UNET^sm system)

Height and weight

Diagnosis

Medical urgency

Donor information
- weight range
- age range
- distance to transplant center
- need for prospective cross match

TABLE 1-4

■ **Medical Urgency for Heart Transplant**

U.S.	Canada	Medical Urgency for Heart Transplant
7	0	On hold; not currently accumulating time on the list
2	1	Waiting at home
2	2	In hospital, stable
1B	3A	On VAD or IV inotropes in hospital or at home. In U.S., VAD> 30 days without complication.
1A	3B	In ICU on high dose inotropic therapy, invasive monitoring, VAD <30 days or VAD malfunction.
	4	In ICU and ventilated

II. Lung. Lung transplantation is indicated for patients with end-stage pulmonary disease who are sick enough to need a transplant, but well enough to survive a transplant.
   A. As with heart transplantation, there are patients who may benefit from a different surgical procedure.
   B. Some patients with emphysema may be suitable candidates for lung volume reduction surgery (LVRS).[19]
      1. The decision to perform this surgery is based on the results of pulmonary function testing, functional capacity as determined by a six-minute walk test, and oxygen requirements.
      2. Unfortunately, this procedure is limited to a few candidates.

a. There is no alternative surgical therapy for patients with pulmonary fibrosis, cystic fibrosis, pulmonary hypertension, or connective tissue disorders; thus lung transplantation may be indicated in such cases.

C. Candidates for lung transplantation will undergo additional testing. This includes:

1. Computerized axial tomography (CT) scan: CT scanning (with contrast) is performed to define the anatomy of the thorax to identify any barriers to surgery. Additionally, it may help define the pulmonary pathology.

2. Ventilation/perfusion (V/Q) scan: V/Q scanning is performed to determine if a difference in lung function exists in the event that a single lung transplant is the intended surgery.

   a. The percent of ventilation by each lung is determined as well as the perfusion to each lung.

   b. A significant mismatch or inequality will help determine which lung to replace.

3. Six-minute walk: A six-minute walk test is performed to determine degree of functional impairment as well as determine rehabilitation potential.

   a. The candidate is asked to walk for six minutes at his or her own pace.

   b. The candidate is allowed to stop as often as needed. The distance is then determined at the end of the six minutes.

   c. Oxygen saturation is monitored and degree of dyspnea is evaluated at intervals during the six minutes.

4. Arterial blood gas: The results of an arterial blood gas may be useful in determining the need for supplemental oxygen, progression of disease, and overall prognosis.

5. Continuous pH testing: Severe gastric reflux disease can contribute to infectious complications in the transplanted lung. Ambulatory continuous monitoring may be performed to determine the need for either medical or surgical intervention to correct reflux.

D. In 2005, UNOS implemented the Lung Allocation Score as an attempt to equitably allocate donor organs. Prior to this system, organs were allocated by seniority on the list. This algorithm attempts to assign urgency to patients listed for transplant. Refer to Table 1-5 for the variables required for listing. Testing is updated every six months.

III. Heart/lung. Heart and lung transplantation is indicated for those candidates with either concurrent end-stage heart and lung disease or those with severe, fixed pulmonary hypertension.

A. The procedure is most commonly performed in adult candidates with congenital cardiac anomalies who have developed pulmonary hypertension as a result of long-standing cyanosis or shunting (Eisenmenger syndrome).

B. Primary pulmonary hypertension and cystic fibrosis have also been reported as indications for surgery.[20]

TABLE 1-5

■ **Criteria for Lung Allocation Score**

Demographics
- date of birth
- height and weight
- gender
- ethnicity
- state or province of residence

Donor information
- desired height range
- desired age range
- distance from transplanting center
- requested organs: right, left, either, both lungs

NYHA Heart Failure Classification

Diabetes (yes/no)

Assisted ventilation (yes/no)

Requires supplemental oxygen (yes/no)

Pulmonary function test (date)
- Forced vital capacity (in liters)
- Percent predicted forced vital capacity

Most recent heart catheterization results (date)
- Pulmonary artery systolic pressure (mm Hg)
- Pulmonary artery pressure mean (mm Hg)
- Pulmonary capillary wedge pressure (mm Hg)

Six-minute walk distance (feet) (date)

Serum creatinine (mg/dl) (date)

    C. The number of centers performing the procedure has significantly decreased in the last decade. This decline has been related to an increase in the use of bilateral lung transplantation for some indications as well as increasing competition for organs.
    D. The evaluation process for candidates for this procedure includes those procedures outlined in the sections on heart and lung transplantation.
    E. Candidates for heart/lung transplantation are listed for both heart and lung transplantation. The listing center must provide the same information as outlined in the sections on heart and lung transplantation.
  IV. Liver. Liver transplantation is indicated for patients with either acute or chronic liver failure.
    A. Occasionally, liver transplantation is done as a curative measure for certain metabolic disorders which do not directly provoke liver failure (e.g., primary hyperoxaluria, familial amyloidosis polyneuropathy).
    B. A list of the more common etiologies for liver disease is included in Table 1-6.
    C. The nature of the disease and the degree of failure will determine the elements included in the evaluation as well as the urgency of the timing for evaluation.

D. In addition to the general transplant evaluation, the following tests should be included:

1. Lab work. Additional blood tests are performed in these candidates to evaluate the etiology of their chronic liver disease (Table 1-7).

   a. In addition, patients at risk for the development of cancer are tested for alpha-fetoprotein (AFP), a tumor marker for hepatocellular carcinoma (HCC), and CA 19-9, a tumor marker for cholangiocarcinoma. Cholangiocarcinoma is a contraindication to liver transplantation.

   b. Additional evaluation may be warranted depending upon the etiology of liver failure (hypercoaguable screening for patients with Budd-Chiari syndrome).

2. Pathologic assessment. A liver biopsy is not routinely performed; however, in some cases it may be warranted for staging or presence of disease (domino transplant candidates, or rarely, to ascertain diagnosis of the underlying liver disorder).

TABLE 1-6

■ **Common Etiologies for Acute and Chronic Liver Disease/Failure**

Common Etiologies for Chronic Liver Disease/Failure

Alcoholic cirrhosis	Metabolic disorders
Alpha-1 antitrypsin deficiency	Non-alcoholic steatohepatitis
Autoimmune hepatitis	Primary biliary cirrhosis
Biliary atresia	Primary sclerosing cholangitis
Budd-Chiari syndrome	Viral hepatitis
Hemochromatosis	Wilson's disease
Hepatocellular carcinoma	

Common Etiologies of Acute Liver Failure

Autoimmune hepatitis
Toxin/drug-induced
Wilson's disease
Viral hepatitis

TABLE 1-7

■ **Additional Lab Work for Chronic Liver Diseases**

- Viral hepatitis—HBsAg, anti-HCV
- Autoimmune hepatitis—immunoglobulins, anti-nuclear antibody, anti-smooth muscle antibody
- PBC—anti-mitochondrial antibody
- Wilson's disease—ceruloplasmin, 24-hour urine for copper
- Hemochromatosis—C282Y, ferritin
- Alpha-1 antitrypsin disease—alpha-1 antitrypsin level
- Budd-Chiari syndrome—hypercoagulation screen
- Hepatocellular carcinoma—alpha-fetoprotein
- Cholangiocarcinoma—CA19-9

3. Abdominal imaging. An abdominal ultrasound is performed to assess the liver contour and other abdominal organs, as well as to look for anatomical changes associated with portal hypertension.
   a. Focal liver lesions suggestive of HCC may be identified and lead to further imaging.
   b. Some centers will perform routine CT scans to assess for liver lesions, whereas others perform it in a step-wise manner to assess for HCC once suspicion arises.
   c. As MRI becomes more readily available and techniques improve, it will be used more frequently for detection and clarification of liver lesions.
   d. For candidates with primary or secondary sclerosing cholangitis, endoscopic retrograde cholaniopancreaticography (ERCP) or magnetic resonance cholaniopancreaticography (MRCP) may be warranted for further visualization of the biliary tree.
   e. A portal vein Doppler is done to assess patency of the portal venous system and hepatic vasculature.
   f. If thromboses are identified in vessels, angiography may be necessary to determine the adequacy of these vessels for surgical anastamoses.
4. Gastrointestinal evaluation. Upper endoscopy is routinely undertaken to survey for portal hypertension and provide therapeutic intervention if necessary.
   a. Additionally, it can prove beneficial for screening for peptic ulcer disease, *Helicobacter pylori,* and Barrett's esophagus.
   b. All patients with inflammatory bowel disease require colonoscopy with biopsy to rule out dysplasia prior to transplantation.
5. Alcohol screening. Alcohol ingestion can worsen liver function. It is imperative that all candidates for liver transplantation remain abstinent.
   a. Criteria for assessment of abstinence vary from center to center.
   b. Most centers require a six-month period of abstinence prior to listing.
   c. Alcohol-related cirrhosis remains an indication for transplantation.[21]
   d. Some centers require attendance in a formal rehabilitation program or attendance at Alcoholics Anonymous for individuals diagnosed with alcohol-related disease.
   e. Centers may also require the patient to sign a contract of alcohol abstinence and perform random toxicology screening to confirm ongoing abstinence.
E. Additional evaluation. Candidates with liver failure may also have concurrent dysfunction of other organ systems, most notably the renal and pulmonary systems, as a direct result of chronic liver failure.
   1. Both hepatorenal syndrome (HRS) and hepatopulmonary syndrome (HPS) are reversible with transplantation, and are not contraindications, but indications to proceed with transplantation.
   2. Mild to moderate portopulmonary hypertension may also be amenable to transplantation.[22]
   3. The evaluation for HPS includes standing and supine arterial blood gas analysis performed on room air and 100% oxygen.

a. A macro aggregated albumin scan is performed to assess for a shunt.
b. Bubble echocardiography can be performed to assess for the presence of a right to left atrial shunt.
c. For patients with HRS, a nephrology consult is indicated for assessment and provision of dialysis as a bridge to transplantation.

F. Ongoing assessment. Since waiting times can be prolonged for liver transplant candidates, ongoing assessment is required.
1. All listed candidates require surveillance for HCC with ultrasound and AFP every 3 to 12 months depending upon the underlying diagnosis.
2. If the candidate is at risk for cholangiocarcinoma, a CA 19-9 should also be performed routinely.
3. The liver synthetic function (hepatic panel) should be monitored every 3 months. Changes in function may impact the candidate's listing status in some jurisdictions.
4. Surveillance and therapeutic endoscopies are performed as indicated.
5. Review of other organ systems and updating of tests is usually done as indicated by patient condition.

G. Organ allocation. The allocation of organs remains difficult. Systems have been devised in order to allocate the organs justly, with an attempt to give the organs to those patients in the greatest need.
1. Different countries have different systems that are based not only on specific criteria but also on sharing agreements.
2. The Canadian system is outlined in Table 1-8.

TABLE 1-8
■ Medical Urgency for Liver Transplant (Canada)

Canada	Medical Urgency for Liver Transplant
0	On hold, not currently accumulating time on list
1	Waiting at home
1T	Patient with tumor
2	Stable in hospital *or* Awaiting combined liver/bowel
3	In ICU or equivalent care due to liver disease, but not intubated, with one or more of the following: - Serum creatinine consistently > 200 µmol/L or rising > 50 µmol/L (adults) - Grade III hepatic encephalopathy despite optimal therapy - Serum creatinine > twice normal for age (pediatrics)
3F	ICU or equivalent care due to fulminant hepatic failure, but not intubated - must fulfill King's College criteria for high mortality risk without transplant
4	In ICU and intubated due to severe liver disease, but not fulfilling King's College criteria
4F	In ICU and intubated due to fulminant hepatic failure. May include primary allograft non-function
*	Pediatric patients <12 years are given an additional status

3. In the U.S., the status system for non-acute liver failure was changed to a scoring system in 2002.
   a. The model for end-stage liver disease/pediatric model for end-stage liver disease (MELD/PELD) determines how urgently a patient requires liver transplantation within a 3 month window.
   b. The calculation is based upon total bilirubin, creatinine, INR, and etiology of disease.
   c. Scores range from 8 to 34, with higher scores indicating advanced disease.
   d. Scores must be updated at regular intervals (Table 1-9).

V. Kidney. Kidney transplantation is indicated for patients with end-stage renal disease (ESRD).
   A. Early referral has proven beneficial to transplant outcomes.
   B. Discussion and preparation for transplant assessment ideally begins early in the work-up of ESRD, even prior to dialysis.
   C. Preemptive transplantation may also be offered.
   D. In addition to the general transplant evaluation, the following tests are performed:
      1. Specific laboratory evaluation. Further testing is done to assess other metabolic parameters and organ systems (Table 1-10).

TABLE 1-9[23, 24]

■ **Model for End-Stage Liver Disease/Pediatric Model for End-Stage Liver Disease**

MELD: 10 x [.957 x log e(serum creatinine mg/dl) + .378 x log e(total bilirubin mg/dl) + 1.12 x log e(INR) + .643]

PELD: [0.436(age <1 yr)] − 0.678 x log e(albumin g/dl) + 0.480 x log e(total bilirubin mg/dl) + 1.87 x log e(INR) +0.067 [growth failure (<2 standard deviations present)]

*Patients with hepatocellular carcinoma are given a MELD score based upon where the tumor fits into the Milan criteria.

MELD Score	Frequency of Recalculation
>25	Every 7 days
19-24	Every 30 days
11-18	Every 90 days
<10	Yearly

TABLE 1-10

■ **Additional Lab Tests for Kidney, Kidney/Pancreas, and Pancreas Assessment**

Electrolytes including Ca, Mg, PO
Fasting blood glucose, HgbA1c
Pancreatic profile—amylase, lipase
Lipid profile
INR/PT
Urinalysis/culture and sensitivity
24-hour urine protein
Creatinine clearance

   a. Specific urine tests are performed. Urine volume, protein, microscopy, and culture and sensitivity are assessed to provide a preoperative baseline.
   b. Any candidate with a history of grafts or shunt thrombosis should be screened for hypercoaguability.
      i. This includes testing for activated protein C resistance, factor V and prothrombin gene mutations, anticardiolipin antibody, lupus anticoagulant, protein C and S, antithrombin III, and homocystiene levels
2. Abdominal imaging.
   a. Ultrasound to assess the kidneys should be performed.
   b. CT scanning may be necessary to further delineate anatomic abnormalities.
   c. In some cases, renal vessel angiography is indicated.
   d. Candidates with a history of bladder dysfunction or urinary tract disease may require a kidney-ureter-bladder (KUB) x-ray as well as a voiding cystourethrogram.
      i. These candidates should be referred to an urologist to determine if existing, uncorrected urinary tract disease may lead to post-transplant morbidity.[25]
      ii. Other tests which may be done if concerns arise with the urinary tract are listed in Table 1-11.
   e. Men, especially those over 50 who exhibit symptoms of urinary retention or who have an enlarged prostate by digital rectal examination may require a transrectal biopsy of the prostate to rule out malignancy.
   E. Organ allocation. Allocation of kidneys is a complicated algorithm with variations in different countries.
      1. Tissue typing, in addition to ABO blood type, is an important criteria for the allocation of cadaveric organs.
      2. Kidneys can remain outside of the body for 24 hours. Therefore, it is possible to allocate kidneys across greater distances than other solid organs.
VI. Kidney-pancreas/pancreas. The evaluation process for kidney/pancreas (K/P) or pancreas transplantation is the same as for isolated kidney.
   A. Candidates for K/P and pancreas transplantation have diabetes mellitus which increases the risk of post-operative morbidity and mortality.
      1. Candidates with diabetes have higher rates of cardiovascular and peripheral vascular disease.
      2. It is essential that these candidates undergo careful and extensive evaluation, as outlined in the sections on cardiovascular and vascular evaluation.[21]

TABLE 1-11
■ Urological Assessment

Uroflometry and residual urine
Pressure flow urodynamic studies
Video urodynamics
Retrograde pyelogram
Cystoscopy
Uteroscopy

    B. Those candidates for pancreas transplantation who are not on dialysis require the same renal assessment as all other candidates for extra renal transplantation.

    C. Additional evaluation for the candidate with diabetes. Candidates with diabetes are at risk for post-operative infections from skin ulcers related to diabetic neuropathy, impaired wound healing, osteomyelitis, and peritonitis.

        1. Preoperative assessments by infectious disease specialists or plastic surgeons may be indicated to determine post-operative risk as well as for management of existing problems.[26]

            a. Diabetic gastric paresis in itself is not a contraindication to transplantation.

                i. Should be evaluated in order to effectively manage it in the peri- and post-operative phase.

                ii. Often, diagnosis may be made based upon symptomotology; however, a gastric emptying study may be necessary.

                iii. Diabetic patients waiting for prolonged periods will require reassessment of their cardiac and vascular status at 1-2 year intervals.[26]

VII. Intestinal and multi-visceral transplantation. Intestinal transplantation is a recognized therapy for both children and adults with life-threatening complications from intestinal failure.

    A. Candidate selection and early referral are important factors in successful outcomes.[27]

    B. The assessment process is key to candidate selection and helps to determine if ongoing medical therapies are sufficient or if transplantation is warranted.[28]

    C. Dependent upon underlying disease process and other coexistent organ failure, three transplant options exist for candidates with intestinal failure:

        1. Isolated intestinal transplant.

        2. Liver/small bowel transplant.

        3. Multi-visceral transplant.

    D. Two broad classifications of intestinal failure exist: structural and functional failure (Table 1-12).

        1. Structural problems are the result of massive surgical resection or anatomical loss.

        2. Functional problems are characterized by disease processes that impair gut motility or absorption.[29]

        3. They affect both children and adults.

        4. To warrant intestinal transplantation, organ failure in conjunction with one or more life-threatening complications or failure of parenteral nutritional therapy must exist. These complications include:

            a. Loss of vascular access preventing fluid and nutritional maintenance.

            b. Frequent episodes of severe sepsis or dehydration.

            c. Presence of or impending liver failure.[29]

    E. Other important consults include review by a dietitian for nutritional assessment and ongoing management (Table 1-13).

    F. In addition to the general transplant evaluation, the following tests are performed:

TABLE 1-12
■ Structural and Functional Causes of Intestinal Failure

Structural	Functional
Adult	*Adult*
• Crohn's disease	• Radiation damage
• Ischemia	• Pseudo-obstruction
• Familial adenamotous polyposis	
• Trauma	*Pediatric*
	• Hirschsprung disease
Pediatric	• Microvillus inclusion disease
• Necrotizing enterocolitis	• Pseudo-obstruction
• Gastroschisis	
• Malformation/volvulus	
• Atresia and stenosis	
• Trauma	

TABLE 1-13
■ Nutritional Assessment

Thorough history
• Nutrition history
• Height and weight including recent weight loss or gain
• Oral or enteral intake and formula
• TPN and formula
• Elimination patterns/stormy output
• Diet and eating history
• Medication history
• Eating behaviors/aversions

Diagnostics
• Calorie counts
• Fecal fat measurement
• Bone density measurement
• Serial anthropometries

1. Additional lab testing. Lab work to obtain baseline parameters of nutritional state and renal and hepatic function are performed (Table 1-14).
2. Abdominal imaging. Candidates will require imaging of the intestinal tract to assess for structure and functional abnormalities.
   a. If motility issues are a concern, gastric emptying studies and other motility testing may be warranted.
   b. Candidates may require visualization of their gastrointestinal tract with upper endoscopy and/or colonoscopy.
   c. Refer to Table 1-15 for a list of possible tests.
3. Liver evaluation. If the patient has liver dysfunction, a thorough work-up of the liver is required to ascertain the need for concurrent liver transplantation.

TABLE 1-14

■ **Lab Tests for Intestinal/Multi-visceral Assessment**

Electrolytes including Ca, Mg, PO
BUN, creatinine
CBC
INR/PTT
Liver function—bilirubin total and direct, albumin, INR
Liver enzymes—AST, ALT, alkaline phosphatase
Viral serology
Urinalysis and microscopy
Blood cultures (if sepsis a concern)

TABLE 1-15

■ **Imaging and Diagnostic Evaluation for Intestinal/Multi-visceral Transplant**

- Upper GI series
- Small bowel follow-through
- Barium enema
- Upper endoscopy
- Colonoscopy
- Gastric emptying study
- Esophageal motility and pH studies
- Abdominal CT scan
- Abdominal ultrasound and portal vein Doppler
- Doppler ultrasound of vessels

    a. An examination of the patient may reveal hepato- or splenomegaly, or stigmata of chronic liver disease, which may be suggestive of hepatic failure.

    b. An abdominal ultrasound and portal vein Doppler may assist in further diagnosis.

    c. Liver biopsy may be necessary to determine the degree of fibrosis or presence of cirrhosis.

    d. While candidates are awaiting transplantation, they require ongoing assessment for complications of intestinal failure and malnutrition.

    e. As with all candidates for solid organ transplantation, candidates awaiting intestinal or multi-organ transplantation should be evaluated for changes in status on a regular basis. This may include:

        i. Abdominal imaging for the development of HCC.

        ii. Endoscopy for changes or the development of varices.

        iii. Lab evaluation for changes in organ function.

PRETRANSPLANT CARE

    I. Adult candidates awaiting transplantation should be vaccinated for hepatitis A and hepatitis B. *S. pneumoniae*, tetanus, varicella, and annual influenza vaccines are recommended for most transplant candidates during the waiting period.[30]

II. Candidates enrolled in colleges or universities may also consider the meningitis vaccine [30.]

III. Family members, close contacts, and health care workers should also be vaccinated against influenza annually.[30]

IV. Periodic reevaluation during the waiting period.
  A. Most candidates are followed by transplant centers with physical exams, and updates on any pertinent laboratory testing.
  B. Kidney candidates.
    1. Follow-up lab tests are requested on a regular basis from dialysis centers for patients awaiting kidney transplantation.
    2. High-risk kidney candidates are defined as those with comorbid conditions such as diabetes, coronary heart disease, obesity, or advanced age.[31]
    3. Tests used at the majority of kidney transplant centers in managing candidate risk factor include:[31]
      a. Annual PSA for males.
      b. Annual mammogram and gynecologic exams for females.
      c. Dobutamine echocardiogram.
      d. Angiography.
      e. Exercise thallium.
      f. Nuclear perfusion scans.
      g. Candidates with an elevated PRA have this test updated at least monthly at many transplant centers.
  C. Heart candidates.
    1. Heart candidates on left ventricular assist devices are followed according to transplant center protocols. Most are followed weekly.
    2. Most heart candidates are followed at transplant centers to evaluate their status.
    3. The following tests are followed as necessary by most transplant centers:
      a. Right heart catheterization to evaluate pulmonary pressures.
      b. Echocardiogram or MUGA to evaluate ejection fraction and ventricular contractility.[32]
      c. MVO_2.
      d. Creatinine is evaluated to ensure adequate perfusion of the kidneys with increasing pump failure.
    4. High-risk patients are evaluated frequently based on their comorbidities such as obesity, diabetes, and pulmonary congestion.
  D. Lung candidates.
    1. Candidates for lung transplantation are usually required to participate in a pulmonary therapy program several times a week.
    2. Lung candidates are followed closely at most transplant centers.
      a. Each center may have different requirements for follow-up based on diagnosis, severity of illness, comorbidities, and distance from transplant center.
    3. The Lung Allocation System (LAS) requires information updates every six months on:
      a. FVC.
      b. Six-minute walk distance.
      c. Serum creatinine.

        d.   Other changes (see Table 1-5) as necessary.

   E. Liver candidates.

      1.   Most transplant centers follow liver candidates closely due to their cirrhosis. Tests are done every 3 months for:

         a.   Alpha-fetoprotein (AFP) to evaluate for hepatocellular carcinoma.

         b.   CBC, Chem 24 and INR, Protime.

      2.   Annual MRI of the abdomen.

      3.   Cardiovascular testing is done on an annual basis:

         a.   Dobutamine stress echocardiogram.

CONCLUSION

   I. The success of solid organ transplantation is based on the appropriate referral and thorough evaluation of transplant candidates.

  II. In this chapter, we have attempted to outline the evaluation process for each solid organ.

 III. The information contained here is general to the transplant process and may not include center-specific criteria.

REFERENCES

1.   United Network for Organ Sharing. Organ blood typing policy. Available at: www.unos.org/policies. Accessed May 19, 2005.

2.   Eurotransplant. Blood typing policy. Available at: http://www.eurotransplant.org/. Accessed June 3, 2005.

3.   Betkowski AS, Graff R, Chen JJ & Hauptman PJ. Panel-reactive antibody screening practices prior to heart transplantation. *J Heart Lung Transplant*, 2002, 21: 644-650.

4.   Abbas AK, Lichtman AH & Pober JS. *Cellular and Molecular Immunology*. Philadelphia: WB Saunders, 1994. p. 102.

5.   Roland ME & Stock PG. Review of solid organ transplantation in HIV infected patients. *Transplantation*, 2003, 75: 425-429.

6.   Calabrese LH, Albrecht M, Young J, et al. Successful cardiac transplantation in an HIV-1-infected patient with advanced disease. *N Engl J Med*, 2003, 348: 2323-2328.

7.   Gnann JW. Herpes simplex and varicella zoster virus infection after hemopoietic stem cell or solid organ transplantation. In RA Bowden, P Ljungman & CV Paya (eds). *Transplant Infections* (2nd ed.). Philadelphia: Lippincott, Williams & Wilkins, 2003. p. 350.

8.   Paya CV & Razonable RR. Cytomegalovirus infection after solid organ transplantation. In RA Bowden, P Ljungman & CV Paya (eds). *Transplant Infections* (2nd ed.). Philadelphia: Lippincott, Williams & Wilkins, 2003. p. 298.

9.   Preiksaitis JK, Sandhu J, & Strautman M. The risk of transfusion acquired CMV infection in seronegative solid-organ transplant recipients receiving non-WBC-reduced blood components not screened for CMV antibody (1984 to 1996): Experience at a single Canadian center. *Transfusion*, 2002, 42: 396-402.

10.   Crawford DH. Biology and disease associations of Epstein-Barr virus. *Phil Trans R Soc Lond B*, 2001, 356: 461-473.

11.   Lumbrebas C & Aguado JM. Toxoplasmosis after solid organ transplantation. In RA Bowden, P Ljungman & CV Paya (eds). *Transplant Infections* (2nd ed.). Philadelphia: Lippincott, Williams & Wilkins, 2003. p. 541.

12.   American Cancer Society. Cancer detection guidelines. Available at: http://www.cancer.org/docroot/PED/content/PED_2_3X_ACS_Cancer_Detection_Guidelines_36.asp/. Accessed June 6, 2005.

13. Maalouf NM & Shane E. Osteoporosis after solid organ transplantation. *J Clin Endocrinol Metab*, 2005, 90: 2456-2465.

14. Cimato TR & Jessup M. Recipient selection in cardiac transplantation: Contraindications and risk factors for mortality. *J Heart Lung Transplant*, 2002, 21: 1161-1173.

15. Hade AM, Shine AM, Kennedy NP & McCormick PA. Both under-nutrition and obesity increase morbidity following liver transplantation. *Ir Med J*, 2003, 96: 140-142.

16. Singh D, Lawen J & Alkhudair W. Does pretransplant obesity affect the outcome in kidney transplant recipients? *Transplant Proc*, 2005, 37: 717-720.

17. Taylor DO, Edwards LB, Boucek MM, Trulock EP, et al. The Registry of the International Society for Heart and Lung Transplantation: Twenty-first official adult heart transplant report—2004. *J Heart Lung Transplant*, 2004, 23: 796-803.

18. Hanson P. Exercise testing and training in patients with chronic heart failure. *Med Sci in Sports Exerc*, 1994, 26: 527-537.

19. Ciccone AM, Meyers BF, Guthrie TJ, Davis GE, et al. Long-term outcome of bilateral lung volume reduction in 250 consecutive patients with emphysema. *J Thorac Cardiovasc Surg*, 2003, 125: 513-525.

20. Trulock EP, Edwards LB, Taylor DO, Boucek MM, et al. The registry of the International Society for Heart and Lung Transplantation: Twenty-first official adult lung and heart-lung transplant report—2004. *J Heart Lung Transplant*, 2004, 23: 804-815.

21. Burra P & Lucey MR. Liver transplantation in alcoholic patients. *Transpl Int*, 2005, 18: 491-498.

22. Murray KF & Carithers RL. AASLD Practice Guidelines: Evaluation of the patient for liver transplantation. *Hepatology*, 2005, 41: 1407-1432.

23. Edwards E & Harper A. Does MELD work for relisted candidates? *Liver Transplantation*, 2004, 10, Suppl 2: S10-16.

24. McDiarmid SV, Merion RM, Dysstra DM & Harper AM. Selection of pediatric candidates under the PELD system. *Liver Transplantation*, 2004, 10, Suppl 2: S23-30.

25. Power RE, Hickey DP & Little DM. Urological evaluation prior to renal transplantation. *Transplant Proc*, 2004, 36: 2962-2967.

26. Pirsch JD, Sollinger HW & Smith C. Kidney and pancreas transplantation in diabetic patients. In G. Danovitch (Ed.) *Handbook of Kidney Transplantation* (4th ed.). Philadelphia: Lippincott, Williams & Wilkins, 2005. p. 390.

27. Kosmach-Park B. Intestine Transplantation. Organ Transplant. Available at: http://www.medscape.com/viewarticle/436543. Accessed on May 5, 2005.

28. Robinson J. Intestinal transplantation: the evaluation process. *Prog Transplant*, 2005, 15: 43-53.

29. Buchman AL, Scolapio J & Fryer J. AGA technical review on short bowel syndrome and intestinal transplantation. *Gastroenterology*, 2003, 124: 1111-1134.

30. Guidelines for vaccination of solid organ transplant candidates and recipients. *Am J Transplant*, 2004, 4 (supp 10): 160-163.

31. Danovitch GM, Hariharan S, Pirsch JD, et al. Management of the waiting list for cadaveric kidney transplants: Report of a survey and recommendation by the clinical practice guidelines committee of the American Society of Transplantation. *J Am Soc Nephrol*, 2002, 13(2): 528-535.

32. Costanza M, Augustine S, Bourge R, et al. Selection and treatment of candidates for heart transplantation. *Circulation*, 1995, 92: 3593-3612.

REVIEW QUESTIONS

1. The purpose for evaluating candidates for solid organ transplantation includes which of the following?
   a. To determine if there are other options for managing the current disease
   b. To determine if there are comorbidities contraindicated for transplantation
   c. To evaluate the patient's ability to comply with long-term follow-up requirements
   d. All of the above
   e. a and b only

2. Most candidates will have a PPD and intradermal skin test for TB, but due to the severity of their illness, may be anergic. In such cases the patient will have controls placed. The two most commonly used skin test controls used are:
   a. BCG and HTLVI.
   b. Candida and mumps.
   c. Measles and influenza.
   d. Mumps and BCG.

3. HIV testing is done by enzyme immunoassay at many centers. Equivocal or positive results are confirmed by which of the following methods?
   a. ELISA
   b. Complement dependent cytotoxic assay
   c. Flow cytometry
   d. Western blot

4. There are no surgical alternatives other than transplantation for which of the following diseases?
   a. Pulmonary hypertension
   b. Cystic fibrosis
   c. Pulmonary fibrosis
   d. Emphysema
   e. All of the above
   f. a, b, and c only

5. A V/Q scan is ordered on patients being considered for lung transplantation to determine:
   a. The lung with the best ventilation and perfusion.
   b. A mismatch between ventilation and perfusion.
   c. To determine which lung to replace.
   d. Difference in lung function between right and left lungs.
   e. All of the above.
   f. b and c.

6. Cholangiocarcinoma is a contraindication to liver transplantation. A test/tumor marker to detect the presence of cholangiocarcinoma is:
   a. AFP (alpha-fetoprotein).
   b. BRCA 1 and 2.
   c. CA 151.
   d. CA 19-9.
   e. CA 125-2.

7. Potential liver transplant candidates with a history of alcohol abuse may require which of the following prior to listing for transplantation at most centers?
   a. 2 years abstinence from alcohol
   b. 6 months abstinence from alcohol
   c. A signed contract stating the patient will submit to random toxicology screening
   d. Attendance at regular alcoholic anonymous meetings
   e. All of the above
   f. b, c, and d

8. The Lung Allocation Score requires updates every 6 months on which of the following tests?
   a. FVC
   b. Serum creatinine
   c. 6-minute walk
   d. All of the above
   e. a and c

9. High-risk kidney transplant candidates include which of the following?
   a. Those of advanced age
   b. Obese individuals
   c. Kidney patients with diabetes as a comorbidity
   d. Candidates with mild coronary disease
   e. All of the above
   f. b and c

10. Tests most commonly used to evaluate potential heart candidates include which of the following?
    a. MUGA or ECHO to determine ejection fraction
    b. MVO_2 to determine functional capacity
    c. Right heart catheterization to determine pulmonary pressures
    d. Left heart catheterization to determine pulmonary pressures
    e. a, b, and c
    f. a, b, and d

Correct answers:

1. d	4. f	7. f
2. b	5. e	8. d
3. d	6. d	9. e
		10. e

2 Basics in Transplant Immunology

FRANK E. L. VAN GELDER

LINDA OHLER

INTRODUCTION

I. Introduction to the human immune system.
  A. Functions of the immune system.
    1. The human body is attacked daily by millions of exogenous and endogenous factors that can cause physiological harm.
      a. We possess a unique defense system, called the immune system, that protects us on different levels and by different mechanisms.
      b. It consists of highly mobile complex cell systems that travel throughout the body to detect foreign molecules and provide protection by producing immunogenic reactions.
      c. A key characteristic of the immune system is its ability to protect us by distinguishing self molecules from non-self.
    2. The immune system provides protection by different mechanisms (1-6) (Figure 2-1):
      a. Surveillance: recognition of foreign antigens present on membranes of cells or microorganisms.
      b. Defense: a non-specific mechanism that destroys foreign intruders and a specific mechanism that targets particular foreign intruders to which there has been previous exposure.
      c. Homeostasis: capacity of keeping the balance between protection and destruction within the system.
    3. The immune response is composed of two different components: humoral and cellular immune responses.
      a. The humoral immune reaction involves the production of immunoglobulins (antibodies) by plasma cells.
      b. The cellular immune reaction is based on communication signals between cells such as lymphocytes and antigen presenting cells (dendritic cells, macrophages).
        i. Antigen presenting cells alert T-helper lymphocytes of non-self antigens.
        ii. This action leads to intracellular destruction of foreign cells.

iii. The different mechanisms function on strategic places in the body (airways, gastrointestinal system, spleen, lymph nodes) in order to ensure adequate attack.

iv. These strategic places are determined by the reticuloendothelial system (RES) (Figure 2-2).

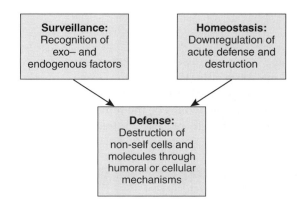

Figure 2-1. The immune system: mechanics.

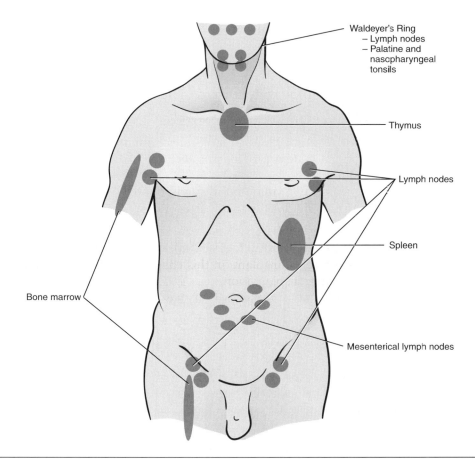

Figure 2-2. Strategic places of the immune system (reticuloendothelial system).

4. Although the immune system's protective nature is invaluable, that same system can produce some undesirable effects.
    a. In addition to responding to non-self antigens, the immune system can also destroy self antigens and produce an autoimmune disease.
    b. This same immune system that serves to protect us can also cause rejection of newly transplanted organs because it recognizes antigens in the new organ as non-self.
    c. This chapter is designed to provide readers with an understanding of how the immune system functions in transplantation.
B. Defining the various types of transplants that can be performed between donors and recipients (Figure 2-3).
    1. Auto-transplantation is transplantation of self tissue.
        a. An example would be the removal of bone marrow from an individual prior to potentially toxic chemotherapy and the reinfusing of the same marrow back into the individual following the medical intervention.
        b. Some patients will also give a pint of their own blood prior to an elective surgery.
            i. This blood is then auto-transfused into the same patient during the procedure.
            ii. The transplanted tissue is not considered "foreign;" therefore, risk of rejection is absent.
    2. Iso-transplantation refers to the transplantation of tissue or organs between genetically identical individuals, such as identical twins, and does not activate an immune response.
        a. This is also known as syngeneic transplantation.
    3. Allotransplantation occurs in the genetically different donor and recipient where the allo-antigens will be seen as foreign or non-self and will trigger an immune response.
        a. This is the type of transplant we will be discussing in this chapter.
        b. Whether the donor is living or deceased, solid organ transplants are allogeneic.
            i. The term allograft is used in transplantation when clinicians are describing rejection or function of the graft.
            ii. Allograft simply refers to a transplanted organ.
            iii. While the term allograft could refer to a bone marrow or stem cell transplant, in this chapter we will focus on solid organ transplantation.
    4. Xenotransplantation involves transplantation between biologically different species and poses the greatest risk for rejection.
        a. This procedure is being studied by researchers as an option to help alleviate the organ shortage.
        b. The use of animal organs, mostly pigs or baboons, has been very controversial for a number of reasons.
            i. While risks of rejection pose the greatest challenge in xenotransplantation, the risks of infection carry an even greater concern.
                a) Currently in allogeneic organ transplantation, the greatest morbidity and mortality arise from infections.

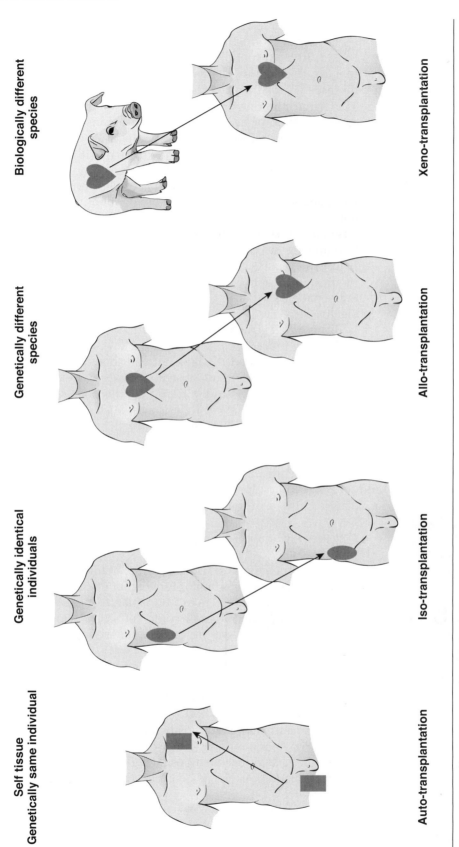

Figure 2-3. Different types of transplantation.

b) The majority of newly emerging infectious diseases have been linked to animals: SARS, Cruetzfeld-Jacob Disease (mad cow disease), West Nile virus, monkeypox, and H5N1 (bird flu).

    ii. We may be even more challenged to control infectious diseases in patients receiving xenotransplants.

II. Antigen recognition mechanism of the immune system.

  A. The major histocompatibility complex (MHC).

    1. The system that drives rejection in allotransplantation is identified as the histocompatibility system.

    2. In humans, this is called human leukocyte antigen system (HLA).

      a. HLA-antigens define the immunologic identity of an individual.

      b. Based on the presentation of these HLA molecules to cells of the immune system, the immune system of an individual does not react against self, but reacts strongly against non-self HLA-antigens

      c. After recognition of the foreign antigens, the immune system produces a specific cascade of responses to destroy the foreign tissue.

      d. With the development of clinical transplantation, this system has been closely examined and analyzed over the last decades.

    3. HLA antigens are protein markers present on the surface of most of our cells and act as a genetic identification label (Figure 2-4).

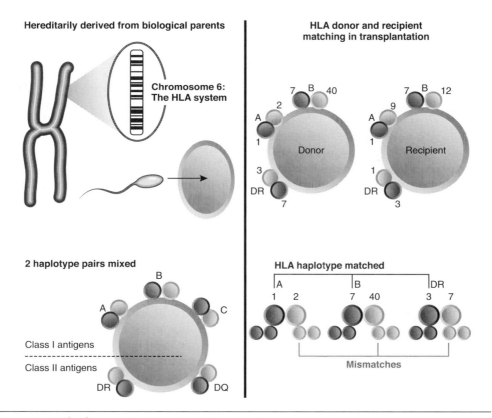

Figure 2-4. The human leukocyte antigen system.

a. The antigens are determined genetically by two haplotypes.

b. Haplotypes are derived hereditarily from the biological parents.

    i. One set comes from the biological father and one set from the biological mother of an individual.

    ii. These haplotypes are coded on the short arm of chromosome 6.

c. The diversity of antigens results in immense combination possibilities; thus, the probability of finding a perfect HLA match within a population is often difficult.

    i. Calculated within a Caucasian population, the chance of an identical HLA match is 1 out of 50,000.

d. HLA antigens are not found on erythrocytes; this accounts for our not considering HLA antigens for blood transfusions.

    i. In contrast, the Rh (rhesus) antigens are not present on tissue cells, explaining why they are not taken into account for organ transplantation.

    ii. As ABO antigens are present on all cells, we ensure that the blood types are compatible between donors and recipients, but we need not be concerned with whether the Rh is positive or negative.

    iii. Nevertheless, recently, clinical protocols were developed to allow ABO incompatibility between donor and recipient.

e. HLA-antigens are divided into two different classes, class I and class II.[1,7,8]

    i. Class I consists of HLA-A, HLA-B, and HLA-C antigen loci, while class II consists of HLA-DR, HLA-DQ, and HLA-DP antigen loci.

        a) Class I HLA-antigens are expressed on plasma membranes of all nucleated cells of the human body.

            1) Class I antigens are strongly associated with cellular aspects of rejection (see below).

        b) Class II HLA-antigens are expressed on activated cells of the immune system.

            1) They trigger the immune reaction through expression of small peptide elements of the HLA class II system.

            2) Class II antigens are strongly associated with humoral rejection (see below).

    ii. For each locus (A, B, C, DR, DQ), there are two antigens.

        a) During immunologic matching of organs for transplantation, a match is created based mainly on the antigens expressed on three loci, -A, -B, and -DR antigens.

        b) Every antigen on its own is called a broad antigen; within the broad antigen split, antigens can be identified and, within the group of split antigens, allele antigens can be seen.

        c) Thus six antigens in total (three loci with two antigens each) are matched.

        d) The antigen matching goes to the level of split antigens.

        e) Currently, only kidney and bone marrow transplantation are considering HLA antigens matching.

1) Kidneys are preferentially matched on HLA-A, -B, and -DR antigens (HLA specific antibodies in the recipient oblige HLA matching).
2) This chapter will also address testing for preformed antibodies, cross matching, and specificities.

iii. It is not the presence of these antigens, but the degree of expression on the cell membrane, that triggers the immune reaction and consequently rejection.

a) With repeated and prolonged exposure to "foreign" HLA antigens, the immune system produces specific HLA-antibodies against these antigens, resulting in memory.
b) The presence of preformed HLA-antibodies in transplant recipients leads to a higher incidence and risk of rejection.

1) Hence, screening for HLA-antibodies and identifying the HLA-antigens of the individual through HLA-typing is important in potential organ transplant recipients.
2) A complete immune profile of the recipient can influence the allocation of a more compatible organ for that individual, ultimately impacting the long-term success of the transplant.
3) Components of this individualized immune profile should include:

i) HLA tissue typing results.
ii) Panel of reactive antibodies (PRA): a test revealing any preformed antibodies.
iii) Identification of any specific antigens to which a potential recipient may have developed antibodies.

B. HLA tissue typing.
1. In years past, this test was done with serology testing and often required 6 to 8 tubes of blood.
2. Today, this test can be performed using DNA technology and can be accomplished with a drop of blood, a hair follicle, or a swab from mucous membrane.
3. HLA tissue typing identifies an individual's antigens at each of the major six loci.
   a. In bone marrow or stem cell transplantation, clinicians evaluate additional alleles identified at loci -C, -CW, -DP, -DQ, and beyond.[8]
   b. They have found that precise matching improves outcomes.
4. In solid organ transplantation, matching is assessed prospectively in renal transplantation.
5. Thoracic and liver transplant clinicians evaluate HLA matching retrospectively for several reasons.
   a. With thoracic transplantation, time constraints enforce review of donor and recipient HLA retrospectively.
   b. With a 4-5 hour window of cold ischemic time, the ability to match organs has not been feasible.

       c. Livers, however, seem to have a protective immune quality for which HLA matching has not been determined to be necessary.[9, 10]

    6. Retrospective data analysis by Dr. Gerhard Opelz (Collaborative Transplant Study) in Germany has demonstrated improved outcomes of solid organ transplantation in many cases with matching, especially at the class II DR levels.[11]

C. Panel of reactive antibodies.

    1. This test identifies any antibodies which have formed against specific HLA-antigens and are poised to destroy them.[12]

       a. Preformed antibodies in a recipient put a newly transplanted organ at risk for rejection.

          i. Transplanting an individual with an elevated PRA may result in a hyperacute rejection and subsequent destruction of the organ.

          ii. Hyperacute rejection (described below) seldom occurs when results of an elevated PRA have been reported and treated.

    2. A PRA is performed on potential candidates for solid organ transplantation.[12]

       a. Test results are reported as a percentage and serve as an index of probabilities.

       b. Serum from a potential candidate is mixed with lymphocytes from a selected group of panel donors.

       c. If the candidate does not possess antibodies against any of the donors, the test result is reported as 0%.

       d. If, however, the candidate reacts against a quarter of the donors, the PRA is reported as 25%.

          i. Here is where probabilities enter the equation.

          ii. The recipient now has a 25% chance of possessing antibodies against a donor.

          iii. If the PRA is 75%, the recipient has a risk of developing a positive cross match against 75% of all donors.

          iv. Having preformed antibodies may result in longer waiting times for a donor organ.

       e. Preformed antibodies develop in individuals who have had multiple blood transfusions, previous transplants, and in women who have had multiple pregnancies.

       f. It has been reported that individuals requiring support from a ventricular assist device (VAD) have developed preformed antibodies within a few weeks after device implantation.[13, 14]

       g. All patients who have preformed antibodies greater than 10% are usually retested on a regular basis, according to the transplant center's protocol.

          i. This could be monthly and, in the case of patients on VADs, it may be done weekly.

       h. Additional testing involving cross matching and identifying HLA specificities has significantly improved our ability to identify high-risk transplants and prevent hyperacute rejections.

D. Specificities.

    1. Immunology laboratories are now able to identify HLA-antigens to which an individual has developed preformed antibodies.

2. Clinicians list the specific antibody in the organ allocation computer system system [United Network for Organ Sharing (UNOS), Eurotransplant].
   a. When a donor becomes available, the donor's HLA is entered into the system.
   b. If a candidate has a specific antibody against this donor's HLA, the recipient is excluded from the match run since the likelihood of having a positive cross match is very high, resulting in acute rejection of the allograft.
   c. Since immunologists developed a method for determining specificities, the need to perform a cross match in significant large groups of potential recipients has decreased.[15, 16]

E. Cross-match[15, 16]
   1. This test is usually performed prospectively just prior to kidney transplantation.
   2. A cross match is performed on thoracic patients with a PRA > 10%.
   3. In most cases of liver and thoracic transplantation, the cross match is reviewed retrospectively.
      a. The cross match is performed by mixing donor lymphocytes (or tissue from the spleen or a lymph node) with serum (white blood cells) from the potential recipient.
      b. If the recipient has antibodies against donor antigens, the recipient antibodies on the cell membrane will bind to the donor cells and destroy them.
      c. This would be a positive cross match and would demonstrate a contraindication against transplantation of this donor organ into this recipient.
      d. Recently, protocols have been developed where recipients are treated preoperatively with plasmapheresis and intravenous immunoglobulins (IVIG) to decrease the levels of HLA antibodies and, hence, the risks associated with transplanting across a positive cross match.
      e. Long-term results are not available, but reports of success with this protocol have been encouraging and more transplant centers have adopted this protocol.

F. Minor histocompatibility antigens (Mi HC).
   1. Besides the MHC antigens, another still incompletely identified antigen mechanism may provoke rejection.
   2. In general, these Mi HC are peptides that are presented through the MHC (HLA) antigens.
   3. They are coded by genes located on chromosomes other than the HLA genes.
   4. These Mi HC may explain why HLA identical donor grafts can still be rejected.

III. Components of the immune system.
   A. Lymphocytes play a key role in the recognition of the transplanted organ as a foreign protein.[1, 3, 4]
      1. Their specific role is seen in mounting a response to the foreign antigens (mostly microbial antigens, but also foreign HLA antigens).

B. Antigen presenting cells (APCs) are derived from the bone marrow and are present in lymphoid tissues, organs, and circulating blood.[1, 3, 17-19]

1. APCs are:
    a. Dendritic cells.
    b. Monocytes.
    c. Macrophages.
2. APCs serve as scavengers because they engulf the debris of dead cells.[3]
3. When cells die a programmed death, the process is called apoptosis.
    a. Macrophages do not notify or alert the lymphocytes of any danger when cells die a programmed death.
    b. Apoptotic deaths are anticipated and the macrophages just ensure the area is kept clear.
        i.   An example of apoptotic cell death is the red blood cell which usually dies after a life expectancy of about 120 days.
        ii. Once the cell membrane weakens and the red blood cell dies, the macrophages clear the debris.
4. While macrophages are doing their day-to-day job, they are basically inactivated for their role in the immune response.[3]
    a. Once they recognize a dangerous microbe, they engulf the foreign antigens, and express them on their cell surface linked with HLA class I and II molecules.
    b. They do this by connecting with the T-cell receptor molecules and delivering the antigen to the activated T-cell.
    c. The activation is based on a three-signal (see below) activation pathway to stimulate and activate T-cell proliferation and activation of effector cells of the immune system.
    d. Once this process occurs, T-helper cells become activated to begin the proliferation of other cells, a phenomenon that we call the immune response.
        i.   Without APCs, there will be no immune response as they have to initiate it.
        ii.   Without activated T-cells and their subgroups, there will be no body defense against dangerous foreign antigens.
        iii. A good example of this is the HIV virus that must be eliminated by the immune system.
            a) Unfortunately, the HIV virus attacks the CD 4+ T-lymphocytes themselves, preventing the body from initiating an adequate response to itself or dangerous, foreign microbes.
            b) HIV also attacks macrophages, which further diminishes the body's ability to identify and destroy dangerous microbes or antigens, both HIV or other.
5. Two types of APCs can stimulate activated T-cells in allotransplantation.
    a. Donor APCs or passenger leukocytes directly stimulate recipient T-cells (direct pathway).
    b. Recipient APCs can absorb and present foreign donor antigens and subsequently present them to recipient CD4+ T-helper cells (indirect pathway).

C. T cells are pivotal in graft rejection, and, based on their specific coreceptor molecules and their function, they can be divided into subgroups.

D. The T-helper CD4+.[1, 3, 4, 6]

    1. Can be indirectly activated by APCs that have taken up foreign antigens shed from the transplanted organ.

    2. CD4+ cells, referring to a type of coreceptor molecule that usually is present on the T-helper cell membrane.

    3. T-helper cells directly communicate with other cells by means of cytokines.

    4. Within the T-helper cell population, two different subtypes exist.

        a. The T-helper 1 cell (TH1) is responsible for the cellular immune response, while the T-helper 2 cell (TH2) is responsible for the humoral immune response.

            i. TH1 mechanism: Receptors on the membrane of TH1 cells bind with HLA class II antigens present on the cell surface of the APC (antigen presenting cell), resulting in the release of IL2, an interferon γ, stimulating effector T-cells (mostly CD8+) or macrophages.

            ii. Activated T-cytotoxic CD8+ cells then directly attack donor cells and destroy them.

        b. TH2 cells secrete IL-4, IL-5 and IL-6 which stimulate clonal proliferation of B-lymphocytes and induce them to differentiate into plasma cells.

            i. The primary function of plasma cells is antibody production.

E. CD 8+ cytotoxic cells.[1, 3, 4, 6]

    1. Activated by stimulation signals from T-cells through IL-2 release.

    2. When activated, this subpopulation of T-lymphocytes can directly kill cells, including those of the transplanted organ, by adhering to foreign antigens expressed on the cell surface membrane in association with class I molecules.

    3. CD8+ refers to the coreceptor molecule present on its cell membrane.

F. B-lymphocytes.[1, 3, 4, 6]

    1. Derived from the bone marrow, their main function is to produce antibodies, also known as immune globulins.

    2. The antibodies may be freely circulating or bound to the membrane of B-lymphocytes.

    3. The binding of antigens with antibodies is an important step in the immune reaction that leads to the destruction of foreign cells and pathogens.

        a. Antibodies or immune globulins can attach to antigens resulting in a reinforced immune reaction.

        b. IgM and IgD antibodies mainly sit on the surface of B-lymphocytes and function mainly as receptor molecules.

        c. IgG antibodies provide specific immunity against foreign antigens and are the most abundant of all immune globulins.

    4. All immune globulins have the same basic structure: Two light chains bound to two heavy chains.

        a. The variable region of immune globulins locates where the two light chains pair with parts of the heavy chain.

        b.   This area is also referred to as the Fab region, and the variability in this area allows for the ability of immune globulins to bind different antigens.

        c.   The constant region, the Fc region, is made up of two heavy polypeptide chains and binds to activated immune cells or to the complement system.

G. Antigens.[1, 3, 4, 6, 7]

    1.   Exist as small entities or more complex protein structures made up of different molecules.

    2.   Can be directly recognized, or indirectly recognized through presentation by the complex HLA antigen system.

    3.   The entire antigen molecule can fit into the receptor, as in the case of the large foreign HLA protein complexes, or only parts of the antigen, the epitopes, can fit into the "peptide binding groove" of the HLA receptor molecules.

H. Cytokines.[1, 2, 4, 6]

    1.   Cytokines are messenger proteins that communicate with cells of the immune system.

        a.   Cytokines tell cells to proliferate or to become activated in response to received danger signals after connecting through specific cytokine receptor molecules.

    2.   Cytokines are named for the cell type that produces them.

        a.   Lymphokines are produced by lymphocytes.

            i.   Lymphokines play a crucial role in the stimulation and augmentation of various components of the immune system.

           ii.   This group of proteins interacts on multiple levels and pathways.

        b.   Interferons were initially named for their role in "interfering" with viral replication.

            i.   Interferons (IFN): IFN-α, IFN-β, and IFN-γ play an important role in eradicating viral infections.

           ii.   IFN-γ, which is produced by T-helper cells, also functions to stimulate on various levels the proliferation of B-lymphocytes and cytotoxic T-cells during immune recognition in organ transplantation.

        c.   Interleukins (IL) are mediators of the inflammatory response.

            i.   They initiate fever.

           ii.   They stimulate the production of leukocytes such as neutrophils.

          iii.   IL-1 through IL-23 are cytokines which perform a wide range of functions within the immune system.

          iv.   Il-2 is exclusively produced by activated T-lymphocytes and promotes T-cell proliferation and amplifies T-cell activation and is seen as the pivotal interleukin in allograft transplantation.

              a)   Cytokines produced by activated T-cells stimulate a number of other immune cells, resulting in the activation of the rejection cascade at all levels.

              b)   Therefore, IL-2 has a central role within transplant rejection.

        d.   Colony stimulating factors are cytokines that stimulate the production of stem cells in the bone marrow.

e.   Tumor necrosis factor (TNF) and lymphotoxin are cytokines that are important in supporting general reactions within the immune system.

I. Complement.[1, 2, 4, 6]

1. A complex system of about 20 proteolytic enzymes and proteins found in plasma.

2. These proteins and enzymes reinforce the immune response by lysing certain cells, stimulating chemotaxis, and facilitating phagocytosis.

3. Direct complement activation stimulates APCs to bind with foreign antigens.

4. When activated, the complement system results in an increase in phagocytosis with lysis of foreign cells.

5. A major function of complement activation is known as opsonization.[1, 3]

   a.   When antigens are coated with complement, the antigen-antibody complexes are more easily digested by macrophages and are more efficiently cleared.

   b.   Making cells more attractive for phagocytosis is called opsonization.

   c.   There is also a chemotactic aspect to the complement system.

      i.   Chemotaxis is a process whereby specific cells are attracted to an area.

      ii. In this case, an influx of leukocytes is triggered through the chemotactic abilities of complement.

      iii. With more leukocytes, such as neutrophils, the inflammatory response heightens.

      iv. The attraction of neutrophils to a site creates greater lysis due to their phagocytic functions.

6. Complement activation may occur through:

   a.   The alternative pathway: The pathogen surface directly stimulates complement activation resulting in immediate cleanup of the pathogen.

   b.   The classical pathway: Stimulation of complement occurs through the antigen-antibody complex and results in the same outcome: removal of pathogens.

   c.   The lectin binding pathway: A third, more recently discovered complement pathway that actually plays an important role.

      i.   Mannose binding lectin (MBL) is a protein manufactured by the liver.

      ii. Lectin binds to carbohydrates and mannose is a carbohydrate found on the surface of many pathogens.

      iii. It has been shown to bind with yeasts such as *Candida albicans*, to viruses such as HIV, and to influenza A, but does not bind to healthy human cells and tissues.

      iv. This process results in the removal of pathogens.

   d.   The cleanup process of pathogens can be divided into three different mechanisms:

      i.   Phagocytosis.

      ii. Opsonization.

      iii. Lysis .

   e.   No matter which reaction takes places, the result is the same.

      f.   The liver and spleen also produce complement inactivators to down regulate the complement cascade to avoid damage to normal tissue.

IV. Synthesis of the immune reaction: Rejection in organ transplantation.[2, 4, 20]

  A. When an organ is transplanted between two genetically different individuals, an immense number of foreign cells and antigens are exposed to the immune system of the recipient.

  B. The circumstance surrounding the donor before, during, and after organ retrieval activates the expression of antigens on the cell membranes of the organ, increasing the immune challenges associated with organ transplantation.

  C. Brain death and cell ischemia reinforce antigen expression through extensive and massive cytokine release while tissue reperfusion injury results in immense antigen release and triggering of the host immune system.

  D. The combination of the difference between the HLA-antigens of the donor and the recipient and the physiologic impact of cell ischemia and reperfusion injury causes a strong immune response and contributes significantly to rejection.

  E. This is the reason we see similar optimal results in both living donor, non-HLA–matched kidneys and good HLA-matched deceased donor kidneys.

    1. In the first group, the cell ischemia is less and the quality is optimal.

    2. In the second group, the allogeneic difference is smaller.

V. Building up the immune response: Rejection (Figure 2-5).[2, 5, 21, 22]

  A. The immune response is a cascade of various reactions activated after the immune system of the host has identified "foreign" cells.

  B. Although the timing is not really clear, there are essential steps that occur within the immune system to prepare the best possible defense.

  C. Rejection is an immunologic response involving the HLA recognition of exposed antigens on the donor endothelial cells by recipient-derived lymphocytes or circulating antibodies.

  D. T-cell activation occurs through APCs stimulation and costimulation.

    1. This step is essential for proliferation of T-cells and B-cells.

    2. T-cell activation occurs through a cascade of three signals in connection and costimulation with APCs.

      a. Current studies have shown that blockage of the three signals can result in better graft survival and avoidance of allograft rejection. The three signals involve the following:

        i. APCs connect through HLA-peptide complexes with CD3+ T-cell receptor molecules on the activated T-cell.

        ii. A second signal occurs and is based on costimulation through a CD80-CD 28 connection between APCs and CD28+ receptor molecules on activated T-cells.

        iii. The third signal occurs after IL-2 has been produced to facilitate further cell proliferation through IL2-CD25 receptor molecule stimulation.

  E. Receptor or host APCs engulf and decode the antigens (phagolysosomy) and express them on their cell surface.

    1. This step is essential in order for CD4+ T-helper cells to recognize and bind foreign HLA-class II antigens.

    2. Once activated, T-helper cells produce interleukins, which will activate additional APC cells and lymphocytes.

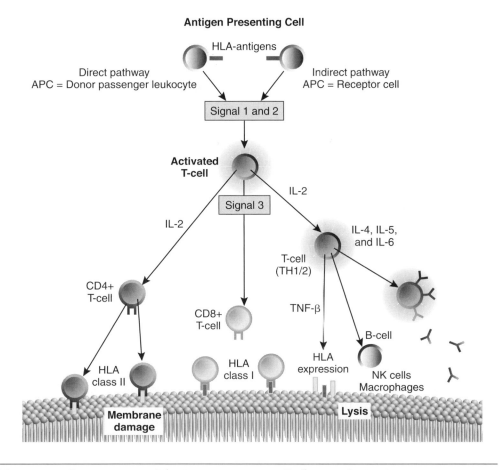

Figure 2-5. Components of the immune system: Pathway of rejection.

3. Within the T-helper cell, activation and proliferation are based on a three-signal model of stimulation and costimulation.

F. Immune globulins located on the cell membrane of B-lymphocytes enable them to bind foreign antigens.

1. Foreign antigens bound in this manner will also activate T-helper cells to produce interleukins.

2. IL-2 and IFN-γ produced by activated T-cells trigger T-cytotoxic CD8+ cells to bind foreign antigens through their CD8+ receptor and destroy foreign cells.

3. IL-2, IL-4, and IL-5, produced by activated T-cells, stimulate B-lymphocyte proliferation, differentiation, and production of specific immune globulins.

4. IL-2 is one of the most important cytokines, as it functions to:
   a. Activate cytotoxic T-cells.
   b. Stimulate HLA antigen expression.
   c. Up-regulate APC activation.
      i. INF-γ induces vascular endothelial and parenchymal cells of the donor organ to increase expression of their class I and II HLA antibodies and through activation of macrophages, produce lytic enzymes.

  ii. Therefore, not all cells in the donor organ need to be targeted to trigger rejection.

  iii. Vascular occlusion can damage the organ, causing the function to be lost.

 d. Rejection of the allograft can be divided into three different levels and time periods.

  i. Antigen presentation and T-cell activation.

  ii. Clonal proliferation of the different effector cells associated with multiple cytokine release.

  iii. Graft destruction based on lysis of target graft cells, antibody production, and reactions to the allograft.

G. Tempo of rejection: Types and mechanisms.[5, 21-23]

 1. The rate and timing of rejection after transplantation depends entirely on the underlying effector mechanism.

 2. In order to devise methods to prevent rejection, it is necessary to understand the underlying mechanism as well as the time frame in which it can occur.

  a. Hyperacute rejection occurs minutes to a few hours after recirculation of the vascularized organ.

   i. It occurs in patients who have pre-existing antibodies against the transplanted graft, based on earlier exposure to HLA antigens of the same type as the donor antigens.

   ii. Anti-HLA antigens can occur in patients with numerous blood transfusions, multiple pregnancies, and previous organ transplants.

   iii. ABO incompatibility and xenotransplantation also lead to hyperacute rejection, due to natural antibodies in our immune system against the ABO type and other animal species.

   iv. Hyperacute rejection can be avoided by prospective cross match and optimal ABO matching.

  b. Acute rejection occurs after a few days to a few weeks, and the underlying mechanism is based on primary activation of the T-cells.

   i. When a host is presensitized to antigens of the graft, a secondary, more rapid activation of T-cells takes place and causes a faster rejection process.

  c. Chronic rejection occurs after months and even years and is based on a slow buildup of the immune reaction.

   i. Factors such as donor and recipient HLA matching and immunosuppressive (IS) regimens can influence chronic rejection.

   ii. Other factors, such as noncompliance with IS drug regimens and sensitivity to IS drugs, can strongly influence the time frame with which chronic rejection takes place.

   iii. In organ transplantation, persistent, untreated rejection will lead to graft loss.

   iv. During rejection, there is intimal hyperplasia of graft blood vessels, which eventually interrupts circulation and causes progressive decline in graft function.

   v. Chronic rejection remains the greatest challenge in long-term graft survival.

a) Significant reduction in the rate of hyperacute and acute rejection has had minimal effect on long-term graft survival.
b) Therefore, control of the chronic rejection process will determine the time frame in which the organ finally is rejected.

VI. Immunosuppressive therapy: Decreasing the risk of rejection.[4, 5, 21-23]
   A. Downregulation of the host immune system after allotransplantation is absolutely necessary to guarantee success.
   B. However, the function of the immune system should stay intact at a level to maintain protection against infections and malignancies.
   C. The greatest challenge in immunosuppressive therapy (IST) is to find the ideal balance, considering three key factors:
      1. IST must be sufficient to protect the graft against allogeneic response.
      2. IST must be low enough to maintain protection against infection and tumors.
      3. Combination IST increases efficacy while minimizing possibility of drug toxicity.
   D. Immunosuppressive therapy can be grouped into two categories:
      1. Antigen specific agents.
         a. Antigen-specific therapy will only suppress activity of target cells associated with specific donor alloantigens, leaving all the other systems intact.
      2. Antigen non-specific agents.
         a. Antigen non-specific agents are most frequently used.
         b. They abolish the activity of the immune system regardless of the specific antigen.
         c. Current IST is still based on this principle, resulting in infections and other side effects.

VII. Non-specific immunosuppressive agents actually in use.[4, 5, 21, 24]
   A. Over the last 30 years, the number of immunosuppressive drugs available to combat rejection has steadily increased, with the greatest surge occurring in the last 5 years.
   B. Most immunosuppressive drugs, with the exception of prednisone, interfere with T-cell and B-cell function and proliferation.
   C. All immunosuppressive therapy regimens are based on a combination of agents to maintain a balance between efficacy in avoiding allograft rejection and safety in order to prevent various side effects, acutely and long-term.
   D. One difficulty with immunosuppressive drugs is the wide variability in patient response to the same regimen.
      1. Finding a balance between therapeutic and toxic doses is very individual thus making IST unique in its setting.
      2. Using different immunosuppressive agents in the most ideal cocktail while preserving quality of life continues to be the challenge.
   E. The action of the agents currently in use is based on three principles:
      1. Depleting of lymphocytes.
      2. Diverting lymphocyte traffic.
      3. Blocking lymphocyte response pathways.
   F. These agents can be divided into seven categories based on the different mechanisms of action of the immune system.

1. Glucocorticosteroids
   a. Prednisone, methylprednisolone.
   b. These agents have an anti-inflammatory effect.
   c. They suppress, at different levels, activated immune cells such as macrophages and antigen-presenting cells.
   d. Glucocorticosteriods also the suppress expression of HLA antigens and reverse the effect of IFN-γ.
   e. At high doses, they suppress many genes involved in T-cell activation.
2. Calcineurin-inhibitors.
   a. Tacrolimus and cyclosporine.
   b. These agents inhibit transcription of the cytokine (IL-2) gene involved in T-cell activation and suppress the expression of IL-2 receptor molecules.
3. mTOR-inhibitors.
   a. Sirolimus, erolimus, and everolimus.
   b. These agents inhibit T-lymphocyte proliferation directly or through inhibiting IL-2, -7, and -15 signaling.
   c. They are an overall T-cell growth factor signal transduction inhibitor.
4. Antimetabolites and nucleotide synthesis inhibitors.
   a. Azathioprine, mycophenolate mofetil, brecuinar, malononitrilamides, leflunomide, FK778, mizoribine.
   b. These agents inhibit nucleotide synthesis and, therefore, hinder proliferation.
   c. They interfere with purine or the pyrimidine biosynthesis on which T- and B-lymphocytes are selectively dependent.
5. Polyclonal antibodies.
   a. rATG, ALG.
   b. These agents are antibodies with multiple distinct antigen combining sites.
      i. Result in functional inhibition and suppression of T-cell mediated immune responses.
      ii. Block the different T-cell receptor molecules or deplete T-cells
6. Monoclonal antibodies.
   a. Basiliximab, daclizumab, and alemtuzumab.
   b. These agents are humanized or chimeric antibodies that block IL-2 receptors which are up-regulated on activated T-lymphocytes.
   c. By blocking the receptor, the action of IL-2 is impeded.
7. Immunomodulators.
   a. FTY720
   b. These are agents that decrease responsiveness of lymphocytes to cytokines by inhibiting T-cell infiltration into inflammatory tissue and the transplanted organ.
   c. They provoke a transient migration of lymphocytes from the peripheral blood to secondary lymphoid organs.

VIII. Future perspectives: Chimerism and tolerance.[2, 4, 22, 23]
   A. Chimerism.
      1. Chimerism is the presence of donor and host hemopoietic cells in transplant recipients.

      a.   This was first noted in liver transplant patients who stopped their immunosuppressive agents unbeknownst to the medical team.

      b.   Research in these patients showed a greater number of two different cell types which were not recognized by their own system as foreign.

      c.   The evidence indicated that a greater number of donor hemapoietic cells present in the liver graft migrated to the host thymus and, as such, were seen as acceptable by the developing host immune system under the unique condition of immune suppression.

      d.   After stopping the medication, the graft was no longer recognizable by the immune system of the host.

B.   Tolerance.[2, 23, 22]

   1.   Research into solutions to prevent chronic rejection without the need for immunosuppressive drugs is tending to focus more and more on the induction of tolerance of the host to the donor graft.

   2.   Functional or clinical tolerance is seen as long-term survival of primary grafts in the absence of/or with very low doses of immunosuppressive drugs, where the graft is tolerated by the host.

   3.   Immunological tolerance is seen as the absence of detectable immune response, or T-cell hyporesponsiveness to specific donor alloantigens in a immunosuppressive-free regimen.

   4.   How to induce such tolerance is a difficult task.

   5.   Tolerance can be created in neonates because the central immune system can be modulated early enough to foreign cells.

   6.   However, in transplantation, peripheral tolerance is the goal, and the mechanisms to induce this are currently under research.

   7.   Different protocols have already been investigated and implemented such as stem cell transplantation of donor cells together with the donor organ.

   8.   Therefore, the tolerance induction in transplantation has to be seen in a setting of paralyzing and desensitizing T-cell populations.

      a.   Up-regulating apoptosis of allogenic T-cells.

      b.   Stimulating anergy by deactivating the T-cell in contact with the alloantigen.

      c.   Blocking cell trafficking of activated T-cells in allotransplantation.

   9.   Recent research has strongly focused on an important subgroup of T-cells that may induce tolerance.

  10. The primary objective of the immune system is to defend against invading foreign cells.

  11. Due to the potential risk that those effector cells may also attack the host itself, the immune system possesses different strategies to keep these effector cells under control.

  12. One of the mechanisms is activation of T-regulatory cells, down-regulating the immune answer.

  13. This self-tolerance mechanism, induced predominantly by T CD4+-CD25+ cells, has become of great interest for researchers to examine the potential of self-tolerance in allograft transplantation.

IX. Conclusion
   A. An overview of the normal functions of an intact immune system shows how complex this system really is.
   B. It is a proof that selective actions undertaken to block certain mechanisms within the system can affect a lot of other systems.
   C. Organ transplantation has created a specific domain in immunology, flirting with all basic principles of resistance against foreign intruders of the human body.
   D. The main goal of organ transplantation focuses on the life-saving treatment of patients while preserving a high quality of life, long-term.
   E. The desire to preserve optimal organ function after allotransplantation drives the work of all clinical professionals working in the field of organ transplantation.
   F. Transplant nurses.
      1. Witness first-hand the adverse effects of immunosuppressive drugs.
      2. Play a key role in motivating patients to comply with therapy.
   G. Knowledge of the immune system will guide our understanding of the complexity and importance of immunosuppression and its effect on long-term outcomes in organ transplantation.
   H. Today, it is necessary to guide and educate patients in their daily immunosuppressive therapy.
   I. It is a central task of the transplant nurse to clinically manage issues relating to the care of the transplant patient.

REFERENCES

1. Rote N. Immunity. In K McCance & S Huether (eds.). *Understanding Pathophysiology*, 3rd ed. Mosby: St. Louis, 2006.
2. Kirk A.D. Immunosuppression without immunosuppression? How to be a tolerant individual in a dangerous world. *Transplant Infectious Disease* 1999; 1 (1): 65-75.
3. Sompayrac L. *How the Immune System Works*, 2nd ed. Malden, MA: Blackwell Publishing, 2003.
4. Martinez O & Rosen HR. Basic concepts in transplant immunology. *Liver Transplantation*, 2005; 11(4): 370-381.
5. Kirk AD. Immunology of transplantation. In JA Norton, et al. (eds.). *Surgery: Basic Science and Clinical Evidence*. New York: Springer-Verlag, 2001.
6. Understanding the Immune System: How it Works. NIH Publication No. 03.5423, 2003, at www.niaid.nih.gov/publications/immune/the_immune_system.pdf. Accessed March 23, 2006.
7. Duquesnoy RJ. Histocompatibility in Organ Transplantation, at http://tpis.upmc.edu/tpis/immuno/wwwHLAtyping.htm. Accessed September 25, 2005.
8. Petersdorf EW, Kollman C, Hurley CK, et al. Effect of HLA Class II gene disparity on outcome of unrelated donor hematopoietic stem cell transplantation for chronic myeloid leukemia: The U. S. National Marrow Donor Program experience. *Blood*, 2001; 98(10): 2922-2929.
9. Pirenne J & Kawai M. The protective effect of the liver: Does it apply to the small bowel too? *Transplantation*, 2006; 81(7): 978-979.
10. Navarro V, Herrine S, Katopes C, et al. The effect of HLA Class I and Class II compatibility on liver transplantation outcomes: An analysis of the OPTN database. *Liver Transplantation*, 2006; 12(4): 652-658.
11. Opelz G, Wujciak T, Dohler B, et al. HLA compatibility and organ transplant survival: Collaborative Transplant Study. *Rev Immunogenet*, 1999; 1(3): 334-342.

12. Wahrmann M, Exner M, Haidbauer B, et al. Flow PRA screening—a specific assay for selective detection of complement activating anti-HLA alloantibodies. *Human Immunology,* 2005; 66(5): 526-534.

13. Pamboukian SV, Costanzo MR, Dunlap S, et al. Relationship between bridging with ventricular assist device on rejection after heart transplantation. *J Heart Lung Transplant,* 2005 Mar; 24(3): 310-315.

14. Tsau PH, Arabia FA, Toporoff B, et al. Positive panel reactive antibody titers in patients bridged to transplantation with a mechanical assist device: Risk factors and treatment. *ASAIO J,* 1998 Sep-Oct; 44(5): M634-637.

15. Bray R, Nickerson PW, Kerman RH, et al. Evolution of HLA antibody detection: Technology emulating biology. *Immunol Res,* 2004; 29(1-3): 41-54. Review.

16. Lobo PI, Isaacs R, Spencer CE, et al. Improved specificity and sensitivity when using pronase-digested lymphocytes to perform flow-cytometric crossmatch prior to renal transplantation. *Transpl Int,* 2002 Nov; 15(11): 563-569.

17. Orosz CG & Pober JS. Antigen presentation. *Graft,* 1999; 2(1): 29-30, 43-47.

18. Suciu-Foca N, Cortesini R. Antigen presentation, *Graft,* 1999; 2(1): 28, 31-33.

19. Morelli AE & Thompson AW. Antigen presentation, *Graft,* 1999; 2(1): 28, 34-42.

20. Nomura M, Plain KM, Verma N, et al. The cellular basis of cardiac allograft rejection. Ratio of naive CD4+CD25+ Tcells/CD4+CD25- T-cells determines rejection or tolerance. *Transpl Immunol,* 2006 Apr; 15(4): 311-318.

21. Bruno DA, Dhanireddy KK, et al. Challenges in therapeutic strategies for transplantation, where now from here? *Transpl Immunol,* 2005 Dec; 15(2): 149-155.

22. Aki A, Luo S, Wood KJ, et al. Induction of transplantation tolerance – the potential of regulatory T-cells. *Transpl Immunol,* 2005 Aug; 14(3-4): 225-230.

23. Ciriaco A, Piccirilo CA, Rthan M, et al. Cutting edge: Control of CD8+ T-cell activation by CD4+CD25+ immunoregulator cells. *J Immunol,* 2001; 167: 1137-1140.

24. Roitt I, Brostoff J, Male D. *Immunology* (6th ed.). St. Louis: Mosby, 2001.

REVIEW QUESTIONS

1. An example of autotransplantation is:
   a. Transplanting the organs from one species to another.
   b. Transplanting organs from one human to another human.
   c. Transplanting a kidney from one identical twin to another.
   d. Transfusing a pint of a patient's blood back into the same patient.

2. Messengers of the immune system that tell cells to proliferate in response to foreign cells are called:
   a. CD8+ cells.
   b. Cytokines.
   c. CD4+ cells.
   d. Signal one.

3. Examples of antigen presenting cells include:
   a. Macrophages, monocytes, and erythrocytes.
   b. Dendritic cells, macrophages, and monocytes.
   c. Erythrocytes, lymphocytes, and platelets.
   d. Mitochondria, macrocytes, and thrombocytes.

4. The T-cell lymphocyte that can be directly activated by an antigen presenting cell is called:
   a. CD4+ T-helper cell.
   b. CD8+ cytotoxic T-cell.
   c. CD25+ toleragenic T-cell.
   d. CD40+ antigenic T-cell.

5. The test performed on all candidates that detects antibodies formed against a patient's HLA is called:
   a. Final cross match.
   b. Tissue typing.
   c. Panel of reactive antibodies.
   d. FAB lymphocyte testing.

6. When we down-regulate the immune system with immunosuppressive agents, the greatest risk of morbidity and mortality in transplant recipients is:
   a. Acute and chronic rejection.
   b. Osteoporosis.
   c. Renal failure.
   d. Infection.

7. Immunosuppressive agents that are humanized or chimeric antibodies that block IL-2 receptors are classified as:
   a. Calcineurin inhibitors.
   b. M-Tor inhibitors.
   c. Polyclonal antibodies.
   d. Monoclonal antibodies.

8. In transplantation, we consider blood type when allocating organs but not the Rh factor. Thus a person with B negative blood can receive a donor organ from someone with B+ blood. This is true because of which of the following statements?
   a. There are insufficient organs to go around so patients cannot be identically matched.
   b. The epithelial cells of organs do not recognize erythrocytes as foreign.
   c. HLA antigens are not found on erythrocytes.
   d. Rh antigens are not present on lymphocytes.
   e. C and D
   f. B and D

9. The test performed by mixing donor lymphocytes or tissue from the donor spleen with white blood cells from the recipient is called:
   a. PRA.
   b. HLA tissue typing.
   c. Trough level.
   d. Cross match.

10. Until the mid 1990s, HLA tissue typing was performed using serology testing and required 6-8 tubes of blood. Today, the test can be performed without blood and can be determined with a hair follicle or a swab of mucous membranes using which of the following methods?
    a. MHC molecular technology.
    b. DNA technology.
    c. PCR technology.
    d. ELISA technology.

3 Patient Education for the Transplant Recipient

ELIZABETH ANN SPARKS FORD

ELIZABETH V. JOHN

INTRODUCTION

I. Introduction.
   A. Education in organ transplantation is multifaceted, brings together a number of medical disciplines, and requires the patient to learn concepts relevant to past, present, and future health.
   B. Topics a patient needs to understand:
      1. End-stage disease.
      2. Health and wellness while waiting for a suitable donor organ.
      3. Health management after transplant.
      4. New medications.
      5. Changes in lifestyle and employment status.
   C. Education of a transplant patient is a continuous process.
      1. It begins almost as soon as the patient is told to consider transplantation and continues for the life of the organ.
      2. Patient education can be defined as imparting information, skills, or knowledge with the aim of bringing about a change in behavior or attitude.[1,2]
      3. It is also a means of assisting patients and their families in developing coping mechanisms to deal with alterations in their health and lifestyle patterns.[3]
      4. Education provides patients and families with tools for:[3]
         a. Making informed decisions.
         b. Changing behavior for a healthier lifestyle.
         c. Placing emphasis on wellness.
   D. For the purposes of this chapter, the pre-transplant period begins when the patient is referred to the transplant center and continues until the point of surgery.
   E. The post-transplant period begins when the patient returns from the operating room and continues through the discharge period.
II. Learning theory and effective patient education strategies: The Health Belief Model.
   A. When applied to the nursing process, educational models can serve as an important part of the nursing assessment in determining whether the patient is ready to move to the next stage of learning.

1. Educational models can help the nurse plan, design, and employ an appropriate educational intervention.
2. Based on behavioral theory, the Health Belief Model (HBM) is one of many educational models developed to explain, predict, and influence patient health-related behavior. [2, 4-6]
   a. Originally, it was developed to predict the likelihood of a person participating in health promotion activities.
   b. It has been successfully adapted to patients with acute and chronic illnesses.
   c. This model has generated more research than any other theoretical approach in attempting to explain an individual's health-related behavior.
   d. It proposes that health-related behavior is a function of both patient knowledge and motivation determined by the following factors: [2, 4-6]
      i. Perceived susceptibility to illness.
      ii. Perceived severity of illness.
      iii. Value of treatment benefits in reducing the susceptibility and severity of the illness.
      iv. Barriers to treatment.
      v. Costs of treatment (physical and emotional), or modifying factors such as demographic variables and social influences.
      vi. Cues that motivate a patient to take action toward treatment of illness.
   e. The major assumption of this model is that there has to exist sufficient motivation to make the health issue relevant to the patient before a modification in his or her health-related behavior takes place. [5, 6]
      i. The patient must believe that he or she is vulnerable to the health problem or to the sequela of that health problem.
      ii. Recommendations of the health care team must be beneficial in reducing the vulnerability without too much cost or sacrifice to the patient. [5, 6]
      iii. The HBM seeks to determine:
         a) The patient's individual perceptions.
         b) Influences impacting that patient's life—what one has to risk or gain.
         c) Likelihood of the patient taking action to alter behavior.
      iv. The nurse should determine:
         a) What motivates this patient to seek out health care or health care service?
         b) What makes this patient compliant?
         c) What does the patient understand and believe to be true about the severity of the disease?
         d) What does the patient find to be an acceptable approach to its resolution? [2, 4, 5]
   f. The HBM is a way to make an education needs assessment.
      i. Aids the nurse in determining where to start education, and then based on the patient, where to go next.
      ii. Example 1: A patient who already has a realistic view of end-stage disease.

a) May not need reinforcement of the current medical regimen.
b) Can proceed directly to education about transplantation.

iii. Example 2: A patient who shows up for a transplant evaluation only because the spouse or doctor set up the appointment.

a) In this case, the patient may believe the end-stage disease will reverse itself and, therefore, may not be ready to hear about transplantation.
b) This is when the patient needs reinforcement education about end-stage disease.
c) The patient must be ready to believe he or she needs a transplant before transplant education can be effective.

III. Effective patient education strategies.
  A. Successful patient education depends on the following:
    1. The skills and characteristics of a good educator.
       a. A good educator will possess:
          i. A nonjudgmental and respectful attitude.
          ii. An empathetic and caring approach to the patient.
    2. Knowledge of appropriate teaching processes.
       a. The nurse should proceed with the patient's education in a non-threatening and friendly environment to facilitate the open exchange of information.
       b. Nurses must assess patients for:
          i. Motivation to learn.[7]
             a) Motivation can be enhanced by recognizing accomplishments and building on strengths, rather than focusing on weaknesses.[8]
          ii. Learning needs.
          iii. Readiness to learn.
          iv. Learning style.
             a) Younger patients may prefer interactive learning as opposed to books or slide presentations.
             b) Many born after 1985 have grown up with computers and will prefer to learn by accessing information on the web or in podcasts.
          v. Barriers to learning.[9]
             a) Lack of time or scheduling problems
             b) Although transplant recipients are hospitalized and may be a "captive audience," shorter lengths of stay have greatly affected time available for formal education programs prior to discharge.
             c) Most transplant programs require patient and family education prior to discharge; therefore, nurses should schedule time each day for patient education.
          vi. Lack of interest.
          vii. Level of education.
          viii. Language problems.
          ix. Cultural issues.
          x. Intellectual disability.
          xi. Physical disability (such as sight or hearing deficits).

          xii. Impaired cognition (related to medication side effects, pain, or effects of disease processes).

          xiii. Fatigue or pain.

          xiv. Noisy or disruptive environment.

          xv. Level of anxiety related to medical condition and treatment. [10]

          xvi. Significant learning barriers may prevent the patient from participating actively in the education process, and in some instances the primary learner may be the patient's support person.[9]

             a) Appropriate involvement of the family and support persons in the teaching process may relieve anxiety, and improve their ability to cope with the patient's health status.[11]

          xvii. The nurse should also assess the patient's existing transplant knowledge to ensure relevant learning goals and teaching outcomes are developed.[9, 12]

  B. Teaching methods and materials may include the following:

    1. Written material.

      a. Content should be presented at a grade six educational level and in "lay language" to ensure understanding by those with a basic educational background.[8]

    2. Individual patient and family teaching sessions.

    3. Group education sessions.

    4. Video and audio material.

    5. Computer-based learning packages.

    6. Slides, pictures, and diagrams.

    7. Interactive computer programs.

    8. Role playing.

    9. Case studies/examples.

    10. Demonstrations with return demonstrations from patients.

    11. Educational podcasts.

  C. Multidisciplinary approach.

    1. Utilization of expert resources provided by other health care team members will help consolidate learning outcomes for the patient.

    2. When incorporating a multidisciplinary approach to education, it is important to document the patient's teaching plan.

      a. By recording the education completed with the patient, all team members involved in the transplant process can establish what information the patient has been given, and determine the patient's current level of understanding.

      b. Documentation also provides evidence that education has been completed for accreditation purposes.[9]

  D. Creating an environment for learning.[13]

    1. Patients need to have an environment where it is safe to ask questions about complex self-care post-transplantation.

    2. Successful learning environments include active participation.

      a. Patients and families feel safe in demonstrating and applying new information and skills.

    3. Effective learning environments include programs where patients and families collaborate with transplant team members to determine learning needs.

4. Respectful learning environments build confidence and self-esteem for applying the new skills and information.
5. Ongoing evaluation is crucial to assess whether teaching outcomes are being met.
    a. Patient knowledge and competency should be assessed regularly, and educational interventions revised accordingly.
    b. The educator must be aware that transplant education is not a finite process.
        i. The main educational concepts will require long-term reinforcement and review.

IV. Pre-transplant phase.
   A. Pre-transplant education must cover a large volume of content.
      1. Should include planned education employing a variety of techniques as outlined in the previous section.
      2. Begins with the referral and evaluation of the transplant candidate, and concludes when the transplant candidate is transplanted.
      3. The content to be covered will vary widely based on the following:
         a. The organ to be transplanted.
         b. Requirements of the transplant center.
   B. Education in the pre-transplant phase helps patients understand the evaluation process.
      1. The first contact the patient has with the transplant center is the referral.
         a. Education about transplantation should begin here.
         b. Provides patients with information to make an informed decision about available options.
      2. A baseline assessment of a patient's level of understanding about disease status should be obtained with this initial phone contact.
         a. Past medical history.
         b. Etiology of end-stage organ failure.
         c. Can the patient tell you what caused the end-stage disease?
         d. Can the patient tell you what medications he or she is taking, and why?
         e. Natural history of the disease process.
         f. Knowledge about the transplant process.
            i. Provides a launching point for patient-specific education during the evaluation.
            ii. Why is the patient interested in receiving a transplant?
            iii. What does getting a transplant mean to the patient?
            iv. Has the patient done any research about transplantation?
            v. What perceptions is the patient bringing into this process?
               a) Are they accurate perceptions?
            vi. For some patients, it may be appropriate to discuss the role and importance of the immune system, and introduce some basic terms like *immunosuppression* and *rejection.*
            vii. Explain the next steps in the transplant evaluation, and explain the process of becoming a transplant candidate.
               a) Follow up this conversation by sending the patient reading material to review prior to the evaluation.
               b) For patients that have access, it may be beneficial to direct them to appropriate educational websites.

V. The evaluation.
   A. Testing and planned educational sessions are carried out during the evaluation process.
   B. Both the transplant center and the transplant patient are being evaluated.
      1. The patient is assessed by the transplant team to determine suitability for transplantation.
      2. At the same time, the patient is evaluating the transplant process.
         a. The center, the team, and distance from home.
         b. Whether to pursue the option of transplantation.
         c. Comparing risks and benefits.
   C. Based on the needs of the transplant team and the patient, we can identify three major educational goals for the patient:
      1. To understand transplant candidate evaluation requirements.
      2. To identify the risks and benefits of transplantation.
      3. To develop an understanding of transplant-related processes.
   D. So that the patient can understand what is required for the transplant team to make an assessment and determination of transplant suitability, explain to the patient:
      1. What to expect from the transplant team during the evaluation process.
      2. What will be expected of the patient during the evaluation process.
      3. The laboratory tests and consultations required for the evaluation.
         a. The transplant team will use results of tests and consults to make an assessment and determination of transplant suitability.
      4. Requirements must be completed in order to be fully considered for transplant.
   E. So that the patient can understand the risks and benefits of transplantation, explain that:
      1. Transplantation is a treatment option and not a cure.
      2. Life with a transplant is often a trade-off.
         a. Renal failure: transplantation versus life on dialysis.
         b. Brittle diabetes: transplantation versus life with diabetes.
         c. End-stage heart, lung, or liver disease: transplantation versus death.
         d. The patient should have an awareness of what life will be like after a transplant in order to establish realistic goals.
   F. So that the patient can develop an understanding of transplant-related processes, explain the following:
      1. Sending panel reactive antibody (PRA) samples for cross match purposes as per center policy and frequency.
      2. Regular visits to the transplant center for routine monitoring.
      3. Requirements for remaining on the transplant waiting list, the expectations of the postoperative period, and the need for follow-up visits.
      4. A complete list of topics to cover during the evaluation is shown in Table 3-1.
VI. Educational goal 1: Understand transplant candidate evaluation requirements.
   A. Testing.

TABLE 3-1

■ **Topics to Cover During Candidate Evaluation**

Topics to Cover[12]	Related Educational Goal: The Patient Will Understand
Evaluation Requirements • Tests • Consults • Blood work	Transplant Candidate Evaluation Requirements
Overview of Specific Organ Transplantation	Risks and Benefits of Transplantation
Surgery and Hospitalization	
Post-transplant Medications • Anti-rejection • Anti-infective	
Post-transplant Complications • Infections • Rejection • Malignancies	
Quality of Life After Transplant	
Waiting for a New Organ • Staying healthy while waiting • Diet and exercise • When to call the transplant center	Transplant Processes
The Organ Allocation System	
Follow-up Visits to the Transplant Center • Pre • Post	

"Topics to Cover" adapted from Cupples SA & Ohler L. *Transplantation Nursing Secrets*. Philadelphia: Hanley & Belfus, 2003. p. 306.

1. For patients completing all of the evaluation at the transplant center, it is helpful for the patient to have a written schedule of where and when to report, along with written instructions of how to prepare for the test. Patients also appreciate having a contact name and number on the schedule in the event assistance is required, or if questions arise.
2. This schedule can also serve as a contact for other health care providers such as radiology technicians or hospital staff that require clarity on orders.
3. For a patient that must arrange for testing to be completed outside of the transplant center, it is helpful to provide a written list of the required tests so it can be shared with the practitioner who will be arranging the testing for the patient.
4. The patient should be told what testing will be carried out, how it will be performed, and why it is necessary.
   a. Routine radiologic tests required for surgery.

      b.   Laboratory tests.

      c.   Required cancer screening tests and infectious disease testing should be discussed in the context of the patient's immune system. Patients should understand that identification of cancers and infectious diseases in the pre-transplant period is necessary to ensure patients with active diseases and cancers are not immunosuppressed.

          i.   Patients should understand that cancer and infectious diseases that are detected in the pre-transplant period may halt the evaluation.

         ii.   It is necessary for patients to understand that post-transplant immunosuppression will worsen any preexisting malignancy or infection.

B. Consults.

    1.   Care of the transplant recipient is ultimately the responsibility of the multidisciplinary team.

    2.   The potential transplant candidate will meet a number of consultants during the evaluation:

      a.   Transplant physician.

      b.   Transplant surgeon.

      c.   Transplant coordinator.

      d.   Social worker.

      e.   Financial coordinator.

      f.   Dietitian.

      g.   Pharmacist.

      h.   Others as indicated.

C. Roles of transplant team members.

    1.   Transplant surgeon.

      a.   Implants organ into the recipient.

      b.   Often manages immediate postoperative care.

    2.   Medical physicians.

      a.   Collaborate with the surgeons.

      b.   Guide the medical care of the patient pre- and post-transplant

    3.   Transplant coordinator.

      a.   Facilitates, assesses, and coordinates the multidisciplinary care of the patient referred to the transplant center.

      b.   Educates patients and families as they move through the phases of transplantation, while communicating with the rest of the transplant multidisciplinary team.

      c.   The patient can arrange testing, follow-up appointments, and communicate with consultants through the transplant coordinator.[14]

    4.   Social worker.

      a.   Establishes an alliance with the patient.

      b.   Completes a psychosocial assessment during the pre-transplant evaluation.

      c.   Helps determine the potential impact a transplant will have on a patient's life.

      d.   Assesses patient's emotional support, tangible support (e.g., transportation resources), coping skills, social habits, compliance, educational level, and financial issues.

        e.   Identifies the patient's access to health care and medications.[15, 16, 17]

           i.   This is relevant to current and future health care needs, as these issues can affect survival and have an impact on the ability of the patient and family to cope pre- and post-transplant.[18]

          ii.   Through awareness of these issues, the patient and family may identify potential stressors, risks, benefits, and expectations throughout the transplant period, such as:

              a)   The anticipated cost of medications in the post-transplant period.

              b)   Potential "out of pocket" costs.

              c)   Transportation requirements for follow-up visits.

              d)   Potential loss of disability income.

              e)   Ability to provide for the family after the transplant.

              f)   Fear of becoming a financial and emotional burden on his or her family.

    5.   Dietitian.

        a.   May review pre-transplant dietary practices for dietary restrictions relevant to the patient's disease process and also for weight optimization purposes.

    6.   Pharmacist.

        a.   Assists with patient education regarding medication regimens.

           i.   Scheduling medications.

          ii.   Drug interactions.

         iii.   Side effects.

         iv.   Trough levels.

D. Blood work.

    1.   Patients can be easily overwhelmed when they see the number of tubes that need to be drawn for the purposes of being evaluated for a transplant.

    2.   It is important to educate the patient about the approximate number of tubes to be drawn, as well as the reason for the large number (what tests are to be done).

        a.   General clinical labs.

        b.   Labs specific to the organ to be transplanted.

        c.   Cancer screening labs.

        d.   Infectious disease history.

        e.   Panel reactive antibody (PRA).

        f.   Human leukocyte antigen (HLA).

VII. Educational goal 2: Identify the risks and benefits of transplantation.

  A. Immune system and immunosuppression.

    1.   When presenting the risks and benefits of transplantation to the patient, discuss the role and function of the immune system.

    2.   Discuss how the immune system will be altered in the post-transplant period.

        a.   This is fundamental to many of the postoperative risks to be weighed, as well as the rationale for postoperative care and follow-up measures.

B.   The surgery and hospitalization.
1.   Depending upon the medical history and experiences of the patient, this may be his or her first major surgery.
2.   Education about the surgical process.
a.   For kidney recipients, describe where the organ is to be placed and what happens to the organ remaining in place.
b.   For heart, lung, and liver recipients, describe what will happen to the organ being removed.
c.   Describe the surgical incision (immediately postoperative and beyond).
i.   Show pictures of the incision as it will look in the immediate postoperative period.
ii. Show pictures of the same incision 1 year later as an example of what to expect the incision and resulting scar to look like in the postoperative period.
d.   Discuss care of the incision in the immediate postoperative period to prevent infection.
e.   Describe what the dressing will look like, and tell the patient how long to expect to have the dressing in place.
f.   Discuss activity restrictions as related to avoiding postoperative complications:
i.   Lifting restrictions to avoid hernias or sternal complications.
ii. Driving after discharge.
g.   Describe any tubes that may be used for drainage and the difference between normal and abnormal drainage.
h.   Describe potential surgical complications related to the organ being transplanted.
C.   Education about postoperative care.
1.   Patients and families should know before the surgery what medical devices will be present when the patient returns from the operating room.
2.   Discuss the use of a ventilator and potential time for post-transplant extubation.
3.   Describe the use of central, peripheral, or arterial lines the patient will have in the immediate postoperative period.
4.   Explain the purposes of these medical devices.
5.   Discuss the placement and purpose of the Foley catheter post-transplantation.
6.   For those patients requiring chest tubes, explain the rationale for their use and the placement of the tubes.
7.   Describe the possible location of drainage tubes in the immediate postoperative period.
8.   Each patient learns differently, and each patient will want to know more, or less, about things like medical devices depending upon his or her level of readiness at the time.
9.   Describe the postoperative routine such as:
a.   Getting out of bed.
b.   Employment of deep diaphragmatic breathing.
c.   Use of the incentive spirometer.
d.   Leg exercises.
e.   Use of sequential compression devices.[19]

10. Explain where the patient will go after surgery; e.g., to the postanes-thesia care unit, the intesive care unit, or the transplant unit.
11. For elective surgeries, it is the practice of some centers to have patients visit the unit prior to transplant surgery.
12. Pain management strategies should be discussed preoperatively.
    a. This discussion can begin during the patient evaluation.
    b. Discussion should be reviewed immediately prior to surgery.
    c. The patient and the nurse should develop a plan to assess pain in the postoperative period.
    d. A review of pain medication.
        i. The type and delivery of pain medication.
        ii. Potential use of patient-controlled analgesia (PCA).
        iii. How long it takes to start working and how long the effects last.
            a) To clarify any misperceptions about pain, the patient should have a realistic expectation about the relief from pain and pain management.
            b) The patient must be assured that although pain may not be completely eliminated, it will be controlled.[19]
        iv. Side effects.
        v. It is important to identify expectations regarding pain man-agement in the post-transplant period.
D. Postoperative period.
    1. One of the first questions often asked is "How long am I going to be in the hospital?"
        a. In 2000, the average length of stay for heart, lung, and heart-lung transplant recipients was between 19 and 32.1 days.
        b. Kidney transplant recipients were only hospitalized for an aver-age of 8.6 days.[20]
    2. The patient may be given an approximate number of days to expect to be in the hospital.
        a. It will be important to reinforce with the patient that this esti-mate is approximate and can depend upon what happens dur-ing the hospitalization.
        b. The estimate is formulated not just in terms of what happens to the patient clinically, but whether the appropriate patient educa-tion is complete.
E. Post-transplant medications and complications.
    1. An introduction to the possible medications taken after transplanta-tion may begin as part of education during the evaluation.
    2. Medications, particularly the anti-rejection and anti-infective medi-cations, should be covered.
    3. An introduction to the drug indications and side effects may be dis-cussed at this time.
        a. Post-transplant complications including infections, rejection, and malignancy can be incorporated into the discussion of med-ications because the use of the post-transplant medications has serious implications for post-transplant complications.
        b. Patients and families should understand the relationship among infection, malignancies, and immunosuppression as well as the relationship between rejection and immunosuppression.

    c.   If the perceived physical and emotional costs of these medications and their side effects are too great in the eyes of the patient, it is possible the patient may not be amenable to taking these medications postoperatively.

    d.   Remember, in the health belief model, patients have to weigh the risks of treatment in terms of physical *and* emotional costs.[4-6]

    e.   In order for the patient to be compliant with the medication regimen, the patient's perception of the benefits of transplantation must outweigh the perceived costs.

4.   Quality of life after transplantation.

    a.   The patient must know what his or her expected quality of life will be after transplantation.

        i.   The patient may have to redefine what "normal" means.

        ii.   For many, the prospect of receiving a transplant initially means a freedom from illness and a return to the life one had before becoming ill.

        iii.   The reality of transplantation, however, is not the return to the life and health experienced prior to needing a transplant, but a return to a different state of health.

    b.   Encourage the patient to define what quality of life is expected after transplant.

        i.   Give the patient a realistic view of what health in the post-transplant period will be like.

    c.   Discuss follow-up visits to the transplant center, frequent lab draws, and the self-monitoring required at home in the post-transplant phase.

VIII.   Educational goal 3: Develop an understanding of transplant-related processes.

    A.   Waiting for a new organ.

        1.   Patients waiting for a deceased donor organ will have to be aware of the requirements of the transplant center while waiting for their transplant.

        2.   Patients identified to be malnourished or morbidly obese are at a higher risk for perioperative complications.

           a.   Patients should be encouraged to reach their optimal weight, whether overweight or underweight, and exercise as much as their medical condition and physician will allow.[21]

        3.   Patients should be instructed to communicate with the transplant team on a regular/prescribed basis.

           a.   Changes in contact information (including vacation plans or planned moves) must be communicated for the purposes of finding patients during organ-offer situations, and contact for re-evaluations.

           b.   Changes in their health status, including hospitalizations, need to be communicated to the transplant team in a timely manner, as medical problems discovered at the time of an organ offer can ultimately cancel the surgery.

    B.   The organ allocation system.

        1.   Most patients will not require a complete, in-depth explanation about the organ allocation system.

a. Patients will, however, want to know a little about how the organ allocation system works and how long to expect to wait for their transplant.

b. The nurse should keep in mind that certain patients may want additional information and know how to appropriately direct the patient to obtain the most useful information.

c. Patients should be aware that waiting times and organ allocation will vary by blood group, age of patient (pediatric versus adult), and type of transplant (life-saving versus non-life-saving).

C. Follow-up visits to the transplant center.

1. Follow-up visits and lists of requirements during the pre- and post-transplant periods should be identified during the evaluation.

a. Timing of visits depends on the condition of the patient and the organ being transplanted.

b. Identify the frequency of lab tests for clinical care in the pre- and post-transplant period.

c. Describe the frequency of clinic visits to the transplant center.

d. Identify other studies that will be required by the transplant center in the post-transplant phase.

e. Identify the clinical care that can take place with local or primary care physicians versus that which must take place at the transplant center.

   i. Some patients may be required to live near the transplant center for a period of time in the initial post-transplant period.

   ii. Others may be required to move closer to the center while awaiting transplantation.

f. While discussing follow-up care and visits to the transplant center, identify patient specific barriers to postoperative follow-up and devise a plan for preventing or overcoming such barriers.

   i. Can the patient and family realistically meet the requirements of the follow-up plan of care both pre- and post-transplantation?

D. Post-transplant phase.

1. Goals of patient education after transplantation are to:

a. Consolidate the educational preparation that has begun during the pre-transplant phase.

b. Equip the patient and family with the knowledge and skills to actively participate in the patient's long-term health care management.

c. Prepare for impending discharge and outpatient follow-up.

2. To achieve these goals, post-transplant education must address a wide range of topics such as those outlined in Table 3-2.

E. Potential complications.

1. Infection.

a. Infection is one of the most common causes of morbidity and mortality post-transplant.[22]

b. The patient should therefore be aware of:

   i. The need for constant observation for infectious complications.

TABLE 3-2

■ **Topics to be Covered with Patients in Preparation for Discharge Post-transplant**

Potential complications
- Infection
- Rejection
- Renal dysfunction
- Long-term complications and surveillance

Medication management

Lifestyle issues
- Nutrition
- Activity limitations
- Sexual activity and pregnancy
- Travel

Patient self-care practices
- Vital signs
- Weight
- Fluid balance,
- Blood glucose levels
- Self-medication
- Wound care
- Catheter and drain care
- Ostomy care

Follow-up care post-discharge

When to call the transplant team

    ii.   The relationship between immunosuppression and susceptibility to infection.
  c.   The risk of infection is often greatest in the first 6 months posttransplant;[23] however, the patient should also be aware that this risk is present for as long as he or she is immunocompromised.
  d.   There are many pathogens that may cause infection in transplant recipients (see Chapter 5).
    i.   Patients should have a basic understanding of the most common sources and manifestations of infections as outlined in Table 3-3.
    ii.   It should be noted that the risk of infection by a particular pathogen may vary in different geographic regions.
  e.   Preventing infection post-transplantation.
    i.   The clinical manifestations of infection are varied, depending on the type and site of infection.
    ii.   Some typical signs and symptoms associated with infection (such as fever) may be absent or masked due to corticosteroid use.
    iii.   The patient and family or significant others should be educated to recognize and report the following signs and symptoms which may indicate infection (Table 3-4):
      a)   Fever.
      b)   Rigors/shaking chills.
      c)   Rash.
      d)   Muscle aches.
      e)   Nausea, vomiting.
      f)   Diarrhea.
    iv.   When returning to the home environment, the risk of infection may cause some anxiety for the transplant recipient.
      a)   The patient should be reassured that most transplant patients successfully incorporate infection control measures into their lifestyle with minimal disruption.
    v.   Family or significant others who will be supporting the recipient at home should also be educated regarding these measures.

TABLE 3-3

■ **Common Infectious Pathogens Post-transplant**

Infection	Pathogen[23]	Patient education points
Bacterial	*Staphylococcus aureus* (including multi-resistant *Staphylococcus aureus*) Vancomycin-resistant Enterococcus *Clostridium difficile* *Pseudomonas aeruginosa* Legionella *Nocardia asteroides* *Listeria monocytogenes* Salmonella *Mycobacterium tuberculosis*	Bacterial infections account for approximately 50% of infections post-transplant.[23] Potential sites for all bacterial infections may include surgical wounds, in-dwelling lines and catheters, lungs, abdominal cavity/biliary tree, kidneys and urinary tract, gastrointestinal tract, bloodstream, and the central nervous system.
Viral	Influenza virus	If cold or flu symptoms appear with fever, the patient should contact the transplant team.
	Herpes simplex virus	Usually causes oral or genital mucocutaneous sores/blisters, but can affect other viscera.[22]
	Cytomegalovirus	Predilection to involve allograft, can cause febrile "flu-like" illness.[22]
	Epstein-Barr virus	Can cause mononucleosis-like illness, is a risk factor for post-transplant lymphoproliferative disease.[22]
	Varicella zoster virus	Dermatomal blistering rash is the usual symptom, disseminated disease can be fatal,[22] requires urgent medical treatment.
	Hepatitis B virus Hepatitis C virus	Risk of acquisition via allograft or blood transfusion for all organ recipients, (re-infection may occur in liver transplant recipients if primary disease).[22]
Fungal	Candida	Commonly occurs in mouth, throat, peri-anal region, and vagina. May also infect urinary tract, wound, and rarely, bloodstream.[11]
	Aspergillus	Likely to occur early in post-transplant period, with lungs the most common site of infection.[23]
	Pneumocystis carinii	Likely to occur within 6 months post-transplant, and causes pneumonia. Occurrence rare if on an appropriate prophylactic agent.[22]
	Histoplasma	Spread by airborne spores from contaminated soil.
Protozoal	*Toxoplasma gondii*	Most commonly infects cardiac tissue in heart recipients, symptoms may mimic rejection.[22]
	Cryptosporidium	Parasitic infection that causes severe, watery diarrhea.[23]
	Strongyloides	Intestinal nematode that may cause severe hemorrhagic enterocolitis, or if disseminated, hemorrhagic pneumonia.[23]

TABLE 3-4

■ **Signs and Symptoms of Infection** [24, 25 (p. 157)]

- Fever (over 37.8° Celsius)
- Persistent chills or "hot flushes"
- Cough (persistent or productive of coloured sputum)
- Shortness of breath
- Changes in urination (increased frequency, burning, pain, hematuria)
- Nausea, vomiting, or diarrhea lasting more than 24 hours
- Anorexia/weight loss
- Persistent fatigue

- Joint pain or muscle ache
- Swollen glands
- Persistent or severe sore throat
- Persistent "head cold " symptoms such as nasal discharge, sinus pain, and/or headache
- Persistent headache, with or without alteration in level of consciousness
- Skin rash or lesions
- Vaginal discharge or burning
- Redness, swelling, pain, odor, or discharge at wound, drain, or stoma site

    f. General precautions for all organ recipients may include the following measures:

       i. Hand washing. Good hand washing practice is a key component to infection prevention.

         a) Hands should be washed often with soap, especially:

           1) After using the bathroom.

           2) After petting animals.

           3) Before preparing food.

           4) Before eating.

         b) Family or friends coming into contact with the patient should be advised to do the same.

         c) Antibacterial hand gel is a useful alternative if soap and fresh water are not available.

       ii. Dietary precautions. Due to the risk of food-borne pathogens, provide patients with guidelines about safe eating and food preparation practices.

         a) Raw or partially cooked meat or seafood should be avoided.

         b) Fruits and vegetables should be washed thoroughly.

         c) Unpasteurized milk products should not be consumed.

         d) Cross-contamination between raw and cooked foods should be prevented by ensuring countertops, cutting surfaces, utensils, and dishcloths are cleaned carefully.

         e) Care must be taken to ensure drinking water is safe, and if uncertain, the water should be boiled.

      iii. Visitor and family restrictions. The patient must feel confident to ask friends and family who are unwell not to visit.

         a) Household members with illnesses should avoid close contact with the patient while unwell.

         b) They should be advised:

           1) Not to share intimate items.

           2) To cover mouth and nose when coughing or sneezing.

           3) To wash their hands frequently.

         c) The patient exposed to a communicable disease such as measles or chickenpox should contact his or her transplant team immediately.

        1) Prophylactic treatment or close observation may be necessary in some circumstances.

    d) Patients should be instructed to try to avoid common community-acquired infections.

  iv. Care of pets. While there is no doubt that pets can have a therapeutic effect on a patient's well-being, one needs to be aware of the potential for infection that arises when caring for animals.

    a) Animal waste can harbor microorganisms that can infect the immunocompromised patient.

    b) Cat litter, bird cages, and fish tanks should be cleaned by other members of the household.

        1) If these tasks must be carried out by the patient, he or she should be instructed to wear gloves and a facemask when appropriate and thoroughly wash hands when complete.

  v. Vaccinations. Some vaccines may not be effective in the immunosuppressed individual, so it is preferable that vaccinations are updated pre-transplant when possible.

    a) Post-transplant, the transplant team may recommend certain immunizations such as:

        1) Influenza vaccination.

        2) Pneumococcal vaccine.

        3) Tetanus boosters.[23]

    b) It should be noted that boosters may be required more frequently in an immunocompromised patient.

    c) Live attenuated viruses should not be administered to the immunocompromised patient due to the risk of viral replication.[26]

    d) The patient should be instructed to check with the transplant team before receiving any vaccinations.

  vi. Dental care. The patient should employ good oral hygiene practices.

    a) Regular visits to the dentist are recommended.

    b) Invasive dental procedures may disrupt the integrity of the oral mucosa, resulting in a risk of systemic infection from oral pathogens.

        1) Antibiotic prophylaxis is recommended before any dental procedure.

        2) Patients should inform their dentist of their immunocompromised state and the need for antibiotic prophylaxis.

        3) Most transplant centers prescribe dental antibiotic prophylaxis in accordance with the American Heart Association (AHA) Guidelines for the prevention of endocarditis.

        4) The AHA recommends prescribing amoxicillin 2 grams orally, 1 hour prior to procedure; or if the patient is allergic to penicillin, clindamycin 600 milligrams orally, 1 hour prior to procedure.[27]

vii. Other general precautions against infection should be highlighted to the patient as appropriate.
   a) The patient should wear gloves when gardening, and a facemask if using potting soil or compost due to the risk of airborne soil pathogens.
   b) Due to the risk of water-borne pathogens, the patient should always ensure the cleanliness of swimming pools, lakes, or hot tubs before entering.
   c) Patients should be counseled regarding the risk of acquiring HIV and other infections through intravenous drug use.

2. Rejection
   a. The patient should be aware that strict compliance with immunosuppressive therapy is necessary to prevent rejection episodes.
      i. However, the patient should also be aware that rejection may occur despite careful adherence to medication regimens.
   b. In most instances, rejection can be treated successfully with high-dose steroids and adjustment of immunosuppressant medications.
      i. Early diagnosis and treatment is crucial for successful management of rejection.
   c. Patients should be aware of potential signs and symptoms of rejection as outlined in Table 3-5.

TABLE 3-5
■ Signs of Rejection

Liver[24, 25]	Kidney[25]	Heart[28, 25]	Lung[29, 22]	Pancreas[30]	Intestine[31, 32]
Raised liver enzymes	Raised urea and creatinine	Irregular heartbeat	Shortness of breath	High blood glucose levels	Change in stool output
Tenderness over liver	Decreased urine output	Very fast or very slow heartbeat	Tiredness		Tiredness
Yellow color to eyes or skin	Weight gain	Low blood pressure	Productive cough		Abdominal pain or distention
Dark urine	Pain at site of kidney	Shortness of breath	Change in color of sputum		Nausea and vomiting
Tiredness	Tiredness	Leg swelling	Decrease in spirometry readings		Dusky stoma
Ascites	Leg swelling	Weight gain	Fever		Weight loss
Fever	Fever	Tiredness			Bleeding
		Fever			Fever

    d. Biopsy.
        i. Biopsies may be required for routine surveillance and/or urgent clinical indications.
        ii. Tissue biopsy of the transplanted organ is usually required if an episode of rejection or graft dysfunction is suspected.
        iii. On discharge from the hospital, patients must be prepared for the likelihood that they may be required to return for a biopsy if clinically indicated.
        iv. Protocols determining the frequency of routine surveillance biopsies will depend upon the organ transplanted and the policy of the transplant center.
            a) Patients should be informed of any routinely scheduled biopsies.
            b) Admission for a biopsy may require an overnight stay in the hospital, or longer if certain treatment options are initiated.
            c) A follow-up biopsy may be required to assess response to rejection treatment.
        v. Tissue biopsy is an invasive procedure and patients should be informed of the risks and complications associated with the procedure.

3. Renal dysfunction.
    a. Renal dysfunction is not uncommon in the transplant recipient.[33]
    b. Renal dysfunction may be precipitated by pre-existing renal disease, hypovolemia post-surgery, infection, or the use of nephrotoxic agents such as calcineurin inhibitors.
    c. In the event of renal failure or dysfunction post-transplant, renal replacement therapy (dialysis) may be required.
        i. The patient should be prepared for this possibility and have a basic understanding of the dialysis process.
        ii. Dialysis can be explained as a therapy that removes waste products and excess fluid from the body when the kidneys are no longer working sufficiently.[34]
        iii. There are two types of dialysis therapies that should be outlined to the patient.
            a) Hemodialysis is a process in which blood is pumped from the body, through a fistula or catheter, into a machine that removes waste products and excess water from the blood.
               1) The blood is returned to the body through the same fistula or catheter.
            b) Peritoneal dialysis involves dialysis fluid being drained into the abdomen via an abdominal catheter.
               1) This fluid allows waste products and excess water to pass from the blood into the abdomen.
               2) The fluid containing the waste products and excess water is then drained out of the abdomen via the same catheter a few hours later.[34, 35]
        iv. If dialysis is to continue after discharge, the patient should have an understanding of how to care for the fistula or catheter to ensure it does not become infected or blocked.[36]

      v. The frequency of dialysis will depend upon the severity of the renal dysfunction.

     vi. Patients can be reassured that the dialysis procedure is usually well-tolerated, but should be informed of possible complications or side effects.[35]

4. Long-term complications and surveillance (see Chapter 5).

   a. The long-term use of immunosuppressive agents means the patient has a lifetime risk of complications related to these medications.

   b. The patient should be aware of these risks, and the need for ongoing surveillance for these complications.

   c. Common complications include the following:

      i. Hypertension, hyperlipidemia, and diabetes.[37]

        a) These conditions can predispose the patient to renal dysfunction and cardiovascular disease.

     ii. Osteoporosis is also a significant problem in transplant patients, due to:

        a) Chronic pretransplant illness.

        b) Post-transplant immunosuppressive medications.[37]

    iii. Malignancy is another major risk for the immunosuppressed patient.

        a) Cancer may develop anywhere in the body, although lymphomas and skin cancers are most common.

        b) The importance of cancer surveillance and preventive measures should be impressed upon the patient.

        c) General guidelines for skin cancer prevention and screening should be available.

        d) Women should understand the importance of having regular Pap smears, breast self-examinations, and mammograms as appropriate.

        e) Men must be educated regarding regular prostate and testicular examinations.

        f) Bowel cancer surveillance guidelines recommend regular sigmoidoscopy or colonoscopy screening for patients:

          1) Greater than 50 years of age.

          2) With inflammatory bowel disease.

          3) With a familial history of bowel cancer.

        g) All transplant patients should be counseled regarding the risks of smoking and lung cancer.[37]

F. Medication management.

   1. Medication counseling for the transplant recipient has been acknowledged as an important factor in ensuring adherence to medication regimens.[38]

2. Medication counseling aims to improve the patient's knowledge of his or her post-transplant drug therapy and empowers the patient to safely assume responsibility for medication administration at the time of discharge.

3. When educating the patient about post-transplant medications, information must be provided to the patient in a clear and concise manner.

   a. Medical terminology should be simplified when possible.

   b. The "four Rs" of medication administration, as outlined below, are a useful guide with which to teach safe transplant medication management.[39]

      i. Right medication.

         a) The patient should know the names of each medication (including generic and brand names) and be able to identify the medication correctly.

         b) Medication education should include the purpose of the drug and its main side effects. See Table 3-6 as a sample of a medication chart.

         c) Patients should be instructed how to maintain a list of all current prescribed and over-the-counter medications.

         d) Patients should be encouraged to question any medication changes that do not appear to be correct.

         e) Use of medication identification stickers or the Organ Transplant Visual Med Scheduler (OTVMS) are excellent sources of educational resources for transplant recipients. These tools are available at www.itns.org.

      ii. Right dose.

         a) The correct dose should be clearly identified to the patient.

         b) The patient should be made aware that some drug doses, particularly the antirejection medication, will vary over time.

            1) Explain why these doses may change as the team aims for therapeutic drug levels that achieve a balance between preventing rejection and minimizing side effects.

         c) Different drug strengths should be identified to the patient with the understanding that a combination of strengths may be required to obtain the right dose.

TABLE 3-6

■ **Sample Patient Medication Chart**

Name & picture (insert sticker or tape actual drug)	Purpose	Dose and Time				Common side effects	Patient education points
		9am	12pm	6pm	9pm		
Cyclosporine *(include brand or generic names)*	Anti-rejection					Headaches, tremors, hypertension, excess hair growth, gum overgrowth, high cholesterol levels, kidney problems[11, 40, 41]	Take twice a day, 12 hours apart, with or without food (as long as consistent). Drug levels are required – **on blood test days do not take morning dose until after blood test.**
Tacrolimus *(include brand or generic names)*	Anti-rejection					Headaches, tremors, numbness or tingling in hands/feet, high blood sugar levels, nausea, diarrhea, hair loss, kidney problems[11, 40, 41]	Take twice a day, 12 hours apart, with or without food (as long as consistent). Drug levels are required – **on blood test days do not take morning dose until after blood test.**
Mycophenolate mofetil *(include brand or generic names)*	Anti-rejection					Nausea, vomiting, diarrhea, low white blood cell count[11, 40, 41]	Swallow capsule whole.
Sirolimus *(include brand or generic names)*	Anti-rejection					High cholesterol levels; nausea; vomiting; diarrhea; low red cell, white cell, and platelet counts[11,40,41]	Daily dose. Drug levels are required – **on blood test days do not take morning dose until after blood test.**
Azathioprine *(include brand or generic names)*	Anti-rejection					Low red and white blood cell and platelet counts, nausea, hair loss, inflamed pancreas[11,40,41]	May be taken with food to avoid nausea.
Corticosteroid *(include brand or generic names)*	Anti-rejection					Weight gain, increased appetite, mood swings, insomnia, high blood sugar levels, gastric irritation, acne, bruising, bone loss[11, 40, 41]	Take with food, preferably in the morning. Blood glucose levels may need to be monitored while on steroids.
Anti-viral agents *(include brand or generic names)*	Prevent viral infection					Low red and white cells, low platelets, may cause birth defects[42]	Take with food. Swallow whole – do not break or crush tablet. Use effective birth control methods.
Trimethoprim/ Sulpha-methoxazole *(include brand or generic names)*	Prevent lung infection					Nausea, rash and itching, may lower blood cell counts[42]	Do not take if allergic to sulfur.
Anti-fungal agents *(include brand or generic names)*	Prevent oral thrush					Nausea, vomiting, diarrhea[42]	Take after meals and other medications.
Proton pump inhibitors *(include brand or generic names)*	Prevent gastric symptoms					Side effects uncommon[42]	Usually a daily dose

      d)   Patients should be instructed what to do in the event that a dose is missed, or if prolonged diarrhea or vomiting occurs.

   iii. Right time.

      a)   For medications that require therapeutic levels, timing of drug administration is crucial.

      b)   The patient should be aware of the need to take medications at the same time every day.

      c)   The patient should be aware of when to take medication on days that drug levels are to be tested.

      d)   To assist the patient with correct medication administration, the nurse may consider recommending the use of:

         1)   Pre-filled pillboxes.

         2)   Reminder systems such as wrist watches with alarms.

         3)   Organization of medication times around meals.

      e)   Patients must be encouraged to take responsibility for having an adequate supply of medication at all times.

         1)   This includes giving the transplant team sufficient time to provide refill prescriptions when required.

   iv. Right way.

      a)   Information should be supplied as to whether a drug is to be taken with or without food and whether it can be safely mixed, crushed, or broken.

      b)   The patient should be counseled regarding the risk of drug and food interactions, because many may interact with calcineurin inhibitors.[11, 39]

         1)   Other drugs.

           •   Anti-inflammatory medications can have an additive nephrotoxic effect when taken with calcineurin inhibitors.[40]

           •   Patients should be advised to check with the transplant team before taking any drugs prescribed by another provider, over-the-counter medications, dietary vitamin or mineral supplements, herbal remedies, or Chinese medicines.

         2)   Herbal preparations.

         3)   Foods.

           •   For example: grapefruit and grapefruit juice must not be taken with cyclosporine, tacrolimus, or sirolimus as it will increase the therapeutic drug levels.[39, 40]

      c)   Information regarding the safe storage of medications should be reviewed as indicated, including special instructions such as refrigeration or protection from light, heat, or moisture.

G. Lifestyle issues.

   1. Before discharge, the nurse must provide the transplant recipient with the required knowledge to successfully implement any necessary lifestyle changes.

   2. The patient and family may need reassurance that post-transplant routines should not be all-consuming or restrictive.

3. Post-transplant lifestyle issues that may be discussed with the patient and family are outlined below.
    a. Nutrition.
        i.   The patient should be given clear instructions regarding dietary and fluid requirements at home.
        ii. A healthy diet that encompasses foods low in fat, sugar, and salt should be encouraged.
        iii. Adequate fluids should be consumed, preferably water, unless a fluid restriction is indicated.
        iv. Drinking alcohol may be contraindicated in some patients, and information about abstinence or safe levels of alcohol consumption should be discussed.
        v.   A high calorie diet may be prescribed in the early post-transplant period if the patient is malnourished.
        vi. Weight gain can be a long-term complication of transplant medication, and dietary and exercise advice may be required in the future to help avoid this.
        vii. Diabetes, hyperlipidemia, and electrolyte imbalances may require specific dietary intervention, and appropriate information and dietitian consultation should be provided.
    b. Activity limitations.
        i.   Exercise is an important part of post-transplant recovery, helping to improve fitness, control weight, and improve general well-being.
        ii. Participation in exercise will vary depending upon the clinical condition of the patient and the transplant physician's discretion.
        iii. The physical therapy department should be consulted regarding a safe exercise program.
        iv. Care should be taken by heart transplant patients when exercising due to the physiological effects of cardiac denervation.[28]
             a) Because the donor heart is denervated, it must rely on circulating catecholamines and increased venous return to increase heart rate in response to exercise.
             b) As a result, heart transplant recipients require a 10-15 minute warm-up period prior to exercise.
             c) Similarly, heart transplant recipients require a 10-15 minute cool-down period after exercise.
        v.   General guidelines for post-transplant exercise include regular, gentle (low-impact) exercise such as walking or cycling.
        vi. Fitness levels should be improved by gradually increasing the time and intensity of the exercise activity.
        vii. Contact sports should be avoided, and water activities such as swimming should be discussed with the transplant team first, due to the potential for infection.
        viii. Recipients of a heart or lung transplant will usually have a lifting restriction of approximately 4 kilograms over a 6-8 week period while their sternum heals.[11]
        ix. Recipients of abdominal organs should avoid lifting anything heavier than approximately 4-5 kilograms for 2-3 months due to the risk of incisional hernias.[24]

x. Before driving, transplant patients should check local regulations regarding any restrictions that may apply to people who have undergone general anesthesia and organ transplantation.

    a) Patients should also be aware of any physical limitations that may make it unsafe for them to drive.

xi. Returning to a previously held job, seeking new employment, or returning to school is an important goal for many transplant patients.

    a) It is generally advised that patients wait for 3 months before returning to work or school, as it is during this time that the risk of infection is greatest.

    b) This time is also a period of close medical monitoring.

    c) The patient may need to return to work or school on a part-time basis initially, and gradually increase attendance as energy levels improve.

    d) Occupational hazards such as heavy lifting or exposure to toxic or infectious agents should be identified and appropriate precautions taken.

    e) Some patients may not be able to return to their former employment due to unacceptable work requirements or hazards; these patients should be referred to vocational rehabilitation as indicated.

c. Sexual activity and pregnancy.

    i. In most instances, sexual activity can be resumed as soon as the patient feels comfortable.

    ii. It is not uncommon for the recipient to experience a loss of libido or varying degrees of sexual dysfunction, both of which may be related to certain medications.

    iii. The patient should be reassured that these problems can usually be resolved and should feel comfortable to discuss these issues with the transplant team.

    iv. Patients should be advised to follow safe sex practices to prevent the transmission of sexually transmitted diseases.[43]

    v. Female recipients who ceased menstruation before transplant may find that their menstrual cycle resumes after transplant.

    vi. Women should be aware that corticosteroid use can stop menstrual flow; however, ovulation still occurs and pregnancy is possible.[43]

    vii. Effective contraceptive measures should be discussed with the patient before discharge.

        a) Condoms, diaphragms, and spermicidal jellies are safe methods of contraception.

        b) Use of the oral contraceptive pill may be allowed in some female recipients; however, this should be discussed with the transplant team first.

        c) Due to the risk of drug interactions with immunosuppression, alteration in liver functions, and an increased risk of clotting disorders, the contraceptive pill may not be suitable for all recipients.

        d) Intrauterine devices (IUDs) are not recommended due to the risk of pelvic inflammatory disease.[44]

    viii. Successful pregnancy can occur following transplantation.

        a) Pregnancy is not advised unless the function of the transplanted organ is stable, and there are no other health related contraindications.

        b) A one-year waiting period between transplant and pregnancy is recommended.

        c) Patients should be strongly advised to discuss plans for pregnancy with the transplant team in order to consider the safety of the patient, the child, and the transplanted organ.

        d) It is important for the transplant team and the patient to discuss:

           1) The appropriate timing of pregnancy.

           2) The risk of fetal damage due to transplant medications.

           3) The risk of rejection.

           4) The physiological effects of pregnancy in the transplant patient.

           5) Ethical issues related to the recipient's lifespan and potentially limited ability to care for a child.[44]

        e) Male recipients can successfully father children post-transplant.

  d. Travel.

    i. Following successful transplantation, patients often regain a new enthusiasm for life which may include travel.

    ii. Information should be provided to patients so they may plan travel safely.

    iii. Destinations should be chosen carefully, taking into consideration:

        a) The current health of the patient.

        b) The risk of infection.

        c) Any physical limitations.

        d) Any endemic infections reported in the area being visited.

    iv. Travel insurance is recommended, as is the purchase of a Medic Alert tag.

    v. The patient should carry documentation from the transplant team outlining the medical history and current medication regimen of the patient.

    vi. Maintaining medication regimens is important, and, if traveling across time zones, medication should be taken at the same time as they would be taken at home.

    vii. The patient should pack more medication than is needed, stored in the original labeled containers and sealed in an airtight package.

    viii. All medication supplies should be carried in hand luggage to ensure that they are not lost or exposed to extreme temperatures.

ix. Some transplant centers give their patients a supply of broad-spectrum antibiotics to take in the event that they develop a bacterial illness, particularly if patients are traveling to remote areas with limited access to medical care.

x. A basic medical kit should be taken that contains a thermometer, antiseptic, and other medicines to treat cuts, bruises, nausea, and diarrhea.

xi. Vaccination requirements should be discussed with the transplant team well in advance of departure.[43]

e. Patient self-care practices.

i. Patients should be empowered to share the responsibility for their health, and develop the confidence to engage in self-care practices.

ii. Following discharge, the transplant team will rely on the patient to monitor and report significant changes in his or her health.

iii. The patient should be encouraged to maintain a post-transplant log and should be taught how to accurately assess and record relevant clinical signs.

iv. Clinical signs to be recorded may include vital signs, weight, fluid balance, blood glucose levels, and spirometry readings.

v. Validate the competence of the patient in performing self-care practices through the use of return demonstration.

   a) Demonstration is a technique that is useful for teaching procedural skills that must be independently and accurately performed by the patient.

   b) Demonstration by the teacher should be followed by return demonstration, which involves the patient attempting to duplicate the task.

vi. This learning by imitation relies on the teacher following some general principles of good demonstration technique.

   a) The patient should be given a clear, concise picture of what is about to be taught.

   b) Complex procedures should be broken down into steps that can be mastered one at a time and then imitated by the patient with a minimum of delay.

   c) Give the patient short, verbal cues for easy recall, and avoid unnecessary explanations that may cause confusion.

   d) Provide written instructions using simple terminology as a backup.

   e) The patient should be given constant feedback and deemed competent when able to accurately perform the task without verbal cues.[45]

vii. Home nursing services may be required in some instances to assist the patient with self-care tasks.

viii. The following examples of self-care practices may be taught to the patient using the concepts of effective patient teaching as outlined previously.

a) Vital signs.
   1) The patient should demonstrate accurate measurement and recording of oral and axillary temperature readings, and be aware of what body temperature constitutes a fever.
   2) Ideally, the patient should learn how to use the thermometer by using the same type of thermometer to be used at home.
   3) The correct identification of both systolic and diastolic blood pressure measurements should be demonstrated.
   4) The patient should use the same type of blood pressure monitoring device to be used at home.
   5) The patient should be able to identify the upper and lower limits of normal blood pressure measurements.
   6) The correct identification of radial and carotid pulses should be demonstrated.
   7) The patient should be able to distinguish between regular and irregular heartbeat and be aware of the upper and lower limits of the pulse rate.
b) Weight.
   1) The patient should understand the importance of monitoring weight daily.
   2) The patient should be instructed to weigh in at the same time each day.
   3) Weighing is best done in the morning (after going to the bathroom and before eating) with the same amount of clothes on each day.
   4) The patient should use the same scale each day.
   5) The home scale should be reliable and calibrated regularly if possible.
c) Fluid balance.
   1) The patient should demonstrate the ability to accurately measure or estimate fluid intake and urinary output (or stool output, if the patient has diarrhea).
   2) Intake and output should be recorded over a 24-hour period and calculated as a negative or positive balance.
   3) The patient should be aware of acceptable parameters and when to notify the transplant team.
d) Capillary blood glucose levels—The patient should be able to demonstrate:
   1) Knowledge of the correct time to check BGLs.
   2) Knowledge of the correct technique for finger pricking.
   3) The ability to troubleshoot simple glucometer problems.
   4) The ability to record BGL readings.
   5) Knowledge of the limits for hypoglycemia and hyperglycemia.

6) The ability to verbalize the appropriate action to take in the event of a hypoglycemic or hyperglycemic episode.

f. Self-administration of medications.
   i. The patient should be observed administering medications in a competent and safe fashion.
   ii. The patient should be able to verbalize the name, the administration time, dosage, purpose, possible side effect(s), and interactions of each medication.
   iii. The patient should identify which medications require blood work (serum drug levels) to be drawn prior to administration.

g. Wound care.
   i. Surgical wounds should be kept clean and dry.
   ii. If a wound is poorly healed, the patient or caregiver should be able to demonstrate appropriate wound care practices using good aseptic technique.
   iii. If staples or sutures are still in place at the time of discharge, the nurse should ensure the patient has a follow-up appointment to have the staples removed.
   iv. The patient should know to report to the transplant team any wound dehiscence, redness, heat, swelling, pain, odor, new discharge or change in color of discharge.

h. Catheter and drain care.
   i. Indwelling urinary catheters, wound drains, or intravenous catheters may remain in place at the time of discharge.
   ii. The patient or caregiver should be taught the principles of aseptic technique in order to avoid infection.
   iii. Accurate measurement of output should be recorded.
   iv. The patient should be aware of basic care techniques such as safely securing loose dressings or managing leakage from tube.
   v. The patient should be able to identify possible signs of infection such as redness, pain, swelling at insertion site, and any change in color or volume of drainage.
   vi. The patient should also be familiar with the emergency management of a catheter that becomes disconnected or dislodged.

i. Ostomy care.
   i. If an ostomy is required, the patient should be able to manage the ostomy independently.
   ii. The patient should verbalize and demonstrate how to effectively empty, measure, and record ostomy output.
   iii. The patient should be able to change appliances with a correct fit and seal, and have an understanding of techniques to manage high output.
   iv. The patient should know when to notify the transplant team regarding changes in output, signs of stomal bleeding, infection, or ischemia.[32]

H. Follow-up care post-discharge.
1. Follow-up care after discharge will depend upon the transplant center's protocol and the clinical status of the patient.
2. Most transplant patients will have frequent contact with their transplant team for at least the first 3 months post-transplant
    a. Thoracic transplant recipients are usually managed for life by the transplant center.
3. If the patient lives a long distance from the transplant center, future care may be shared with a local physician, and coordinated via the transplant coordinator.
4. The patient should understand the importance of post-transplant surveillance and compliance with follow-up routines.
5. Written information advising of all outpatient appointments and tests should be given to the patient on discharge.
6. Clinic visits to the transplant center are usually weekly for the first 1-2 months.
7. Fortnightly (every 2 weeks), monthly, and quarterly visits are subsequently initiated as the patient's clinical status stabilizes.
8. Patients may be evaluated in the transplant clinic by the surgeon, physician, transplant coordinator, or nurse practitioner.
9. Blood tests are generally done once or twice a week initially after discharge, with the frequency decreasing as the patient's condition stabilizes.
10. All transplant patients must have immunosuppressant drug levels monitored closely, as well as electrolytes, renal and liver function tests, and hematology counts.
11. Cytomegalovirus surveillance, lipid profiles, and blood glucose levels should also be monitored.

I. How and when to contact the transplant team.
1. Written guidelines on how and when to contact the transplant team should be given to the patient and his or her support person at the time of discharge.
2. It should be made clear to the patient that assistance from the transplant team is always available for urgent matters; however, routine matters should be addressed during working hours.
3. Guidelines for contacting the transplant team are outlined in Table 3-7.

IX. Barriers to postoperative follow-up.
A. Medication noncompliance.

TABLE 3-7

■ **When the Patient Should Contact the Transplant Team**[11, 25]

- Questions about appointments, medication refills, or insurance matters
- Questions regarding medication regimen
- Signs or symptoms of infection
- Signs or symptoms of rejection
- Unable to take medication due to nausea, vomiting, or diarrhea
- Experiencing shortness of breath, difficulty breathing, productive cough, changes in sputum color
- Experiencing pain, tightness, or pressure in chest, neck, or arms

- Noticing a change in urine color
- Experiencing severe headache or vision disturbances
- Increasing tiredness
- Severe or unmanageable side effects of medication
- Exposure to mumps, measles, chickenpox, or shingles
- Emergency room or hospital admission

1. Medication noncompliance can be defined as the discontinuation of one immunosuppressive drug or missing drug doses frequently or occasionally.[46]
2. Rates of noncompliance with immunosuppressive therapy vary from 2-68% in this patient group.[47]
3. Failure to take medications as prescribed can be voluntary or involuntary, each requiring a different intervention.
4. Voluntary reasons for not taking medications can include:
   a. Fear of side effects such as weight gain and the subsequent body image changes associated with weight gain.[16]
   b. Frustration with the number of medications and the frequency of dosing.
   c. A belief, over time, that immunosuppression is no longer needed.[46]
5. Reasons for involuntary noncompliance can include:
   a. Lack of knowledge of the medications and dosing schedule.
   b. Cost of medications.
   c. Forgetfulness.[46]
   d. Physical/mental learning disability.[10]
6. In one study, Talas and Bayraktar[48] observed that more than half of patients sometimes skipped doses of their drugs; 56.3% of these patients blamed forgetfulness.
7. Not every patient misses doses or voluntarily discontinues medications; therefore it is important that the entire multidisciplinary transplant team has an understanding of what to look for and how to improve compliance.
8. Interventions to foster patient medication compliance include:
   a. Simplifying the medication regimen where possible.
   b. Delivering medication education that is tailored to the individual patient's learning needs.[12, 49]
   c. Utilizing a variety of teaching tools such as:
      i. Computer learning modules.

        ii.   Audiovisual aids.

        iii. Verbal counseling.

        iv Written materials.

9. Education should include information on the administration, purpose, action, and side effects of the medication, as well as advice on drug levels and drug interactions.

10. Many centers construct medication charts for their patients (see Table 3-6) provide pillboxes, and give pre- and post-counseling tests as part of their medication education sessions.[38, 50, 51]

11. The health care team should be available to answer patient questions or concerns and deliver the information in a format that is appropriate for the patient's educational level, language, and culture.

B. Noncompliance with postoperative therapies and follow-up.

1. Along with effective education and teamwork, patient compliance is a crucial factor in ensuring optimal long-term outcomes post-transplant.

2. Noncompliance with the medical regimen and follow-up has been identified in the literature as a significant problem among all types of transplant patients.[52]

3. Factors that have been associated with noncompliance among transplant recipients include gender, race, socioeconomic status, and level of social support.

4. The patient's perception of the level of control he or she has over health care outcomes is also thought to affect compliance.

   a. Patients with an internal locus of control (a belief that it is possible to undertake the required behavior to achieve a successful outcome) are more likely to comply with professional advice.[6, 52]

5. Effective discharge preparation promotes compliance by reinforcing the patient's belief that he or she can be proactive in his or her own recovery.

6. Lack of compliance with the entire medical regimen, including follow-up visits to the transplant center and frequent lab draws, as well as medication noncompliance, can be in direct conflict with returning to a normal life.

   a. Normalcy can be defined as age- and socially appropriate activities for that patient.[53]

   b. Patients are encouraged to return to work, and to resume roles previously put on hold during the pre-transplant illness. However, the frequency of clinic visits and multiple interactions with the transplant team may reinforce a continuation of the sick role.[54]

      i. In combating this phenomenon, Schneider and colleagues[54] empowered patients in the active review and assessment of their health status following transplantation.

      ii. As a result, face-to-face clinic visits were decreased, patients felt more confident in talking about changes in their health status, and the health care professional was provided with information from the patient significant to the delivery of the patients' care.[54]

REFERENCES

1. Luker K & Caress A. Rethinking patient education. *J Adv Nurs,* 1989; 14: 711-718.
2. Rankin S & Stallings K. *Patient Education Principles and Practice,* 4th ed. Philadelphia: Lippincott Williams & Wilkins; 2001: 4-50, 78-107.
3. Speers A. Patient education: Theory and practice. *J Nurs Staff Devel,* 1989; 5(3): 121-126.
4. Maiman L, Becker M, Kirscht J, Haefner D, et al. Scales for measuring health belief model dimensions: A test of predictive value, internal consistency and relationships among beliefs. *Health Education Monographs,* 1977; 5(3): 215-230.
5. Bellamy R. An introduction to patient education: Theory and practice. *Medical Teacher,* 2004; 26(4): 359-365.
6. Rosenstock I, Strecher V & Becker M. Social learning theory and the health belief model. *Health Education Q,* 1988; 15(2): 175-183.
7. Knowles MS. *Self-directed learning: A guide for learners and teachers.* Chicago: Follett Publishing Co., 1975.
8. Klug-Redman B. *The practice of patient education.* St. Louis: Mosby, 2001, 37-71.
9. Messina CJ, Russell CL, Ewigman MA, Ward C, et al. Teaching patients about kidney transplantation: Documentation. *Prog Transplant,* 2000; 10(3): 169-176.
10. Bass M, Galley-Reilley J, Twiss DE, & Whitaker D. A diversified patient education program for transplant recipients. *ANNA J,* 1999; 26(4): 287-292, 343.
11. Bahruth, AJ. What every patient should know: Pretransplantation and posttransplantation. *Crit Care Nurs Q,* 2004; 27: 31-61.
12. Ohler L. Patient education. In SA Cupples & L Ohler. *Transplantation Nursing Secrets.* Philadelphia: Hanley & Belfus, 2003: 305-311.
13. Billington DD. Seven characteristics of highly effective adult learning programs. www.newhorizons.org/lifelong/workplace/billington.htm. Accessed March 8, 2006.
14. Donaldson, TA. The role of the transplant coordinator. In SA Cupples & L Ohler. *Transplantation Nursing Secrets.* Philadelphia: Hanley & Belfus, 2003: 17-26.
15. Corsini JM, White-Williams C, & Cupples SA. Evaluation of patients for solid organ transplantation. In SA Cupples & L Ohler. *Transplantation Nursing Secrets.* Philadelphia: Hanley & Belfus, 2003: 27-44.
16. Cochran C, Callahan M, & Atkins C. Hoping and planning: A multidisciplinary look at the pretransplant phase. *Nephrology Nursing Journal,* 2003; 30: 334-335.
17. Cupples SA. Overview of solid organ transplantation. In SA Cupples & L Ohler. *Solid organ transplantation: A handbook for primary health care providers.* New York: Springer Publishing Company, 2002: 1-17.
18. Harrison JD & Cupples SA. Psychosocial issues in transplantation. In SA Cupples & L Ohler. *Transplantation Nursing Secrets.* Philadelphia: Hanley & Belfus, 2003: 45-59.
19. Ford EAS, Leshko ME, & Corsini JM. Nursing care of the living renal donor. In SA Cupples & L Ohler. *Transplantation Nursing Secrets.* Philadelphia: Hanley & Belfus, 2003: 201-211.
20. Ortner NJ. Milliman Research Report: 2005 organ and tissue transplant costs and discussion. Available at: http://www.milliman.com/pubs/Healthcare/content/research_reports/US-Organ-Tissue-Transplant-2005-RR.pdf. Accessed April 13, 2007.
21. Hasse J. Nutritional issues in adult organ transplantation. In SA Cupples & L Ohler. *Solid organ transplantation: A handbook for primary health care providers.* New York: Springer Publishing Company, 2002: 64-87.
22. Singh N. Infections in solid organ transplant recipients. *Am J Infect Control,* 1997; 25(5): 409-417.
23. Cupples SA. Infectious disease. In SA Cupples & L Ohler. *Transplantation Nursing Secrets.* Philadelphia: Hanley & Belfus, 2003: 247-270.
24. Flynn BM. Liver transplantation. In SA Cupples & L Ohler. *Transplantation Nursing Secrets.* Philadelphia: Hanley & Belfus, 2003: 151-171.

25. Randolph S, Scholz K. Self care guidelines: Finding a common ground. *J Transplant Coordination*, 1999; 9(3): 156-160.

26. Australian Technical Advisory Group on Immunisation (for National Health and Medical Research Council). *The Australian Immunisation Handbook*, 8th Edition, 2003. Available at: http://www.immunise.health.gov.au/internet/immunise/publishing.nsf/Content/handbook03. Accessed June 17, 2005.

27. American Heart Association. Endocarditis prophylaxis information. Available at: http://www.americanheart.org/presenter.jhtml?identifier=11086. Accessed June 17, 2005.

28. Cupples SA. Heart transplantation. In SA Cupples & L Ohler. *Transplantation Nursing Secrets*. Philadelphia: Hanley & Belfus, 2003: 85-105.

29. Manzetti JD & Lee A. Lung transplantation. In SA Cupples & L Ohler. *Transplantation Nursing Secrets*. Philadelphia: Hanley & Belfus, 2003: 75-83.

30. Mize JB. Pancreas and simultaneous pancreas-kidney transplantation. In SA Cupples & L Ohler. *Transplantation Nursing Secrets*. Philadelphia: Hanley & Belfus, 2003: 143-149.

31. Kosmach-Park B. Intestinal transplantation. In SA Cupples & L Ohler. *Transplantation Nursing Secrets*. Philadelphia: Hanley & Belfus, 2003: 173-190.

32. Augustine SM & Nicholson-Macdonald A. *Transplantation nursing: Acute and long-term management*. Norwalk, CT: Appleton and Lange, 1995; 334-359.

33. Ojo AO, Held PJ, & Port FK. Chronic renal failure after transplantation of a non renal organ. *N Engl J Med*, 2003; 349: 931-940.

34. The National Kidney Foundation (UK). Patient information: Dialysis. *Nurs Stand*, 2002; 16(33): page n/a.

35. Rose BD & Post TW. Patient information: Haemodialysis. Available at: http://patients.uptodate.com/topic.asp?file=kidn_dis/4967&title+Dialysis. Accessed June 17, 2005.

36. National Kidney Foundation. Haemodialysis access. Available at: http://www.kidney.org/atoz/atozItem.cfm?id=71. Accessed June 17, 2005.

37. Augustine SM & Flattery MP. Long-term complications of solid organ transplantation. In SA Cupples & L Ohler. *Transplantation Nursing Secrets*. Philadelphia: Hanley & Belfus, 2003: 271-278.

38. Partovi N, Chan W & Reesor-Nimmo C. Evaluation of a patient education program for solid organ transplant patients. *Can J Hosp Pharm*, 1995; 48(2): 72-78.

39. Cupples S. Transplant medications part 2: Top 20 tips. *Prog Transplant*, 2002; 12(3): 231-232.

40. Dumas-Hicks DH. Immunosuppression. In SA Cupples & L Ohler. *Transplantation Nursing Secrets*. Philadelphia: Hanley & Belfus, 2003: 67-74.

41. Cupples S. Transplant medications part 1: An overview. *Progress in Transplantation*, 2002; 12(1): 71-72.

42. AMH Pty Ltd. *Australian Medicines Handbook*. Electronic version January 2005. Available at: http://intra.fmc.sa.gov.au/fido/Clinresources/Clintools/Handbooks/AMH_HTML/index.html. Accessed June 17, 2005.

43. John L (ed.). Transplant diary: *A patient self management tool*. Roche Products and Transplant Nurses' Association. Sydney, Australia, 2004.

44. Blazek JD. Pregnancy after transplantation. In SA Cupples & L Ohler. *Transplantation Nursing Secrets*. Philadelphia: Hanley & Belfus, 2003: 279-288.

45. Watts NT. *Handbook of clinical teaching*. Edinburgh, U.K.: Churchill Livingstone, 1990; 135-142.

46. Pruna A & Fornairon S. European multicenter survey on noncompliance after solid organ transplantation. *Transplant Proc*, 2000; 32: 393-395.

47. Non adherence to immunosuppressive therapy is a significant problem after solid organ transplantation. *Drugs Therapy Perspectives*, 2002; 18(12): 19-21.

48. Talas M & Bayraktar N. Kidney transplantation: Determination of the problems encountered by Turkish patients and their knowledge and practices on healthy living. *J Clin Nurs*, 2004; 13: 580-588.

49. Logham-Adham M. Medication noncompliance in patients with chronic disease: Issues in dialysis and renal transplantation. *Am J Managed Care*, 2003; 9(2): 155-171.

50. Kmietowicz Z. Post-transplant challenge. *Nurs Stand*, 2004; 18(23): 21.

51. Russell CL, Conn VS, & Ashbaugh C. Medication taking beliefs of adult renal transplant recipients. *Clin Nurse Specialist*, 2002; 17(4): 200-2008.

52. Teichman BJ, Burker EJ, Weiner M, & Egan TM. Factors associated with adherence to treatment regimens after lung transplantation. *Prog Transplant*, 2000; 10(2): 113-121.

53. Wilkins F, Bozik K, & Bennet K. The impact of patient education and psychosocial supports on return to normalcy 36 months post-kidney transplant. *Clin Transplant*, 2003; 17: 78-80.

54. Schneider S, Winsett RP, Reed L, & Hathaway DK. Use of structured self-monitoring in transplant education. *Prog Transplant*, 2001; 11: 133-136.

REVIEW QUESTIONS

1. Patient and family education on transplantation begins with the first interaction with a nurse, whether it is on the phone or face to face. Patients and families need to learn about the transplant process early in the evaluation phase to provide them with tools for which of the following?
   a. Making informed decisions.
   b. Understanding the steps in the evaluation process.
   c. Selecting healthy lifestyles while awaiting transplantation.
   d. All of the above.

2. Prior to initiating educational sessions for a patient, the nurse first assesses which of the following?
   a. Motivation to learn
   b. Learning style
   c. Learning needs
   d. All of the above

3. Teens and younger children may respond to a different learning style since computers are an integral part of their lives. Strategies for educating these populations may include:
   a. Books and pamphlets about transplantation with frequently asked questions.
   b. Interactive computer games about medications and transplant-related issues.
   c. Podcasting information to the patient's computer or iPod.
   d. All of the above.
   e. B and C.

4. Educational content during the evaluation phase should include information about transplantation including:
   a. Risks and benefits of transplantation.
   b. Tests and consults required during the evaluation.
   c. Organ allocation system in your country.
   d. All of the above.
   e. A and B.

5. Education about transplantation should include the surgical procedure as well as estimated time for hospitalization post-transplantation. Additional topics about the transplant should also include medications required post-transplantation as well as topics on preventing infection and rejection. These topics are presented early to ensure the patient has a realistic understanding of:
   a. The need for compliance with post-transplant medications.
   b. Long-term follow-up care after transplantation.
   c. Risks and benefits.
   d. All of the above.

6. In explaining the surgical procedures it is important to provide patients and families with information and diagrams or photos about which of the following?
   a. The surgical incision
   b. The implanted new organ
   c. How stitches and staples are removed
   d. The various tubes and invasive monitoring that may be used
   e. All of the above

7. Prior to transplantation, patients should receive information about self-care management that includes:
   a. Signs and symptoms of rejection and infection.
   b. Wound care management.
   c. Activity limitations.
   d. Return to work.
   e. All of the above.

8. Patients and families should be educated about immediate post-op care that addresses the following:
   a. What medical devices will be used postoperatively.
   b. What invasive lines, Foley catheters, and spirometers will be used postoperatively.
   c. Length of time to be intubated.
   d. Visiting hours and any limitations on foods, flowers.
   e. All of the above.

9. Patients should be aware of potential complications in the immediate post-transplant period. Complications that should be discussed with patients prior to surgery include:
   a. Possible need for dialysis for kidney recipients.
   b. Potential prolonged ventilation for patients following heart or lung transplantation.
   c. Bleeding and the need to return for corrective surgery following liver, heart, or lung transplantation.
   d. Osteoporosis.
   e. A, B, and C only.

10. Teaching the patient about post-operative routines should include which of the following?
    a. Need for coughing, deep-breathing, and leg exercises
    b. Rationale for use of sequential compression devices
    c. Which venipuncture sites will be used for each IV
    d. All of the above
    e. A and B

11. Prior to discharge, patients should be able to demonstrate which of the following?
    a. Self-administration of medications
    b. Taking and recording blood pressure, pulse, weight, and temperature
    c. How to contact the individual on call at the transplant center
    d. Incision care, management of any drains, intake and output
    e. All of the above

12. The most challenging learning for patients involves their multitude of medications post-transplantation. A pharmacist or nurse should work with the patient and family to ensure their understanding of:
    a. Drug-drug or food-drug interactions.
    b. When to hold medications prior to testing trough levels of drugs.
    c. Side effects of medications.
    d. Scheduling medications.
    e. All of the above.

Correct answers:

1. D	5. D	9. E
2. D	6. E	10. E
3. D	7. E	11. E
4. D	8. E	12. E

4 Transplant Pharmacology

AGNES COSTELLO

GLEN J. PEARSON

INTRODUCTION

I. Introduction
  A. The introduction of potent immunosuppressive agents dramatically reduced the incidence and severity of acute rejection which resulted in improvements in patient and graft survival.
    1. Development of these immunosuppressive agents often parallels the understanding of transplant immunology.
    2. Immunosuppressive agents:
      a. Target specific areas of the immune activation cascade.
      b. Have unique pharmacological and toxicity profiles.
        i. Used synergistically to produce an intense state of immuno-suppression.
        ii. Used in combination to minimize short-term and long-term toxicity.
      c. Can be classified under two major categories:
        i. Antibody preparations.
          a) Monoclonal and polyclonal antibodies.
          b) Used to either prevent acute rejection (induction) or to treat acute rejection.
        ii. Small molecule preparations.
          a) Can be further classified based on their mechanism of actions into:
            1) Calcineurin inhibitors.
            2) Antiproliferative agents.
            3) mTOR inhibitors.
            4) Corticosteroids.
    3. Calcineurin inhibitors (CNI).
      a. Cyclosporine (CsA).
        i. The first CNI used in transplantation.
        ii. Introduced to the market in the early 1980s.
        iii. Revolutionized transplant medicine and contributed to transforming organ transplantation from an experimental procedure into routine clinical practice.

       iv. Dramatically decreased the incidence of acute graft rejection in the absence of myelotoxicity.

         a) Through selective immunosuppressive actions.

       v. Quickly became the standard for primary immunosuppression.

       vi. There are two formulations of CsA:

         a) Sandimmune.

         b) Neoral (microemulsion).

         c) There are generic equivalents for both formulations of CsA.

    b. Tacrolimus (TAC).

       i. The other CNI.

       ii. A macrolide lactone antibiotic isolated from the fungus *Streptomyces tsukubaensis.*

       iii. Introduced in 1994.

       iv. Differs structurally from CsA.

         a) More potent CNI than CsA.

    c. Results of randomized, multicenter trials comparing TAC and CsA.

       i. Demonstrated TAC to be more effective in preventing acute rejection than CsA in kidney, liver, and pancreas rejection[1-8]

       ii. However, recent analyses showed no differences in efficacy between CsA and TAC with the current dosing strategies and the use the microemulsion formulation of CsA.

       iii. Both CNIs provide excellent rejection prophylaxis.

         a) Use is limited by their long-term side effects, specifically nephrotoxicity.

           1) Contributes to chronic allograft nephropathy (CAN).

           2) Recent clinical trials have focused on identifying immunosuppressive regimens that avoid or minimize side effects of CNIs.

             i) Withdrawal of CsA at 3 months post-transplant and initiating rapamycin in selected patients resulted in the prevention of chronic allograft nephropathy.[9, 10]

             ii) Complete avoidance of CNIs at the time of transplant using a combination of sirolimus (SRL) and mycophenolate mofetil (MMF) with antibody induction.[11-14]

             iii) Further studies with longer follow-up are needed to determine the long-term safety and efficacy of CNI sparing and avoidance regimens.

    d. Mechanism of action.

       i. CNIs primarily suppress the activation of T lymphocytes.

         a) Inhibit the production of cytokines, specifically interleukin-2 (IL-2).

         b) Interfere with the IL-2 gene transcription essential for activation and proliferation of cytotoxic T-cells in response to alloantigens.

    ii. CsA inhibits calcineurin by binding to an intracellular protein cyclophilin.[15]

       a) CsA reversibly inhibits immunocompetent lymphocytes in certain phases of the cell cycle.

       b) Leads to preferential inhibition of T lymphocytes.

    iii. TAC inhibits calcineurin by binding to the intracellular cytosolic protein called FKBP-12 (FK binding protein).

       a) Prevents gene transcription and the formation of lymphokines such as IL-2 and gamma interferon.[16]

       b) The net effect is inhibition of T-cell activation resulting in immunosuppression.

e. Dosing and administration of cyclosporine.[15]

    i. Recommended starting oral dose:

       a) Kidney transplant patients is 9 ± 3 mg/kg/day in 2 divided doses.

       b) Liver transplant patients is 8 ± 4 mg/kg/day in 2 divided doses.

       c) Heart transplant patients is 7 ± 3 mg/kg/day in 2 divided doses.

    ii. The intravenous dose is usually one-third the oral dose and is administered as an intermittent IV infusion over 4 to 6 hours.

f. Dosing and administration of tacrolimus.[16]

    i. Recommended starting oral dose:

       a) Kidney transplant patients is 0.2 mg/kg/day in 2 divided doses.

       b) Liver transplant patients is 0.10-0.15 mg/kg/day in 2 divided doses.

       c) Heart transplant patients is 0.075 mg/kg/day in 2 divided doses.

       d) Pediatric liver transplant patients is 0.15-0.20 mg/kg/day in 2 divided doses.[16]

    ii. The usual intravenous dose is 0.03-0.05 mg/kg/day as a continuous infusion.

g. The decision on the initial dose and the time to initiate CNIs is dependent on:

    i. Initial allograft function.

    ii. Other medical conditions.

    iii. Use of concurrent immunosuppressive agents.

    iv. Subsequently, the dose of CNI is adjusted based on blood concentrations.

h. Therapeutic drug monitoring.

    i. Due to the inter-individual variability in CsA and TAC pharmacokinetics, individualization of dosing regimen is necessary for optimal therapy.

       a) Cyclosporine.

         1) The reported therapeutic range for 12-hour trough levels (C_0) appears to be between 100 and 400 ng/mL.[15]

         2) Results from recent studies suggested that monitoring peak CsA levels 2 hours after administration

(C_2) may be better reflective of drug exposure than trough levels.

3) The therapeutic range for C_2 is much higher than C_0 and appears to be between 800 and 1200 ng/mL.[17]

b) Tacrolimus.

1) Reported therapeutic range for 12-hour trough levels from whole blood appears to be between 5 and 20 ng/mL.[16]

ii. The target therapeutic range for CNIs varies depending on:

a) Type of organ transplanted.

b) Functional status of the allograft.

c) Medical conditions of the patient.

d) Concurrent immunosuppressive agents used.

i. Drug interactions (Table 4-1).

i. Any drugs that either inhibit or induce cytochrome P450 3A4 will alter the metabolism of CsA and TAC leading to:

a) Toxicity (inhibits metabolism).

b) Increased risk of rejection (induces metabolism).[15, 16]

ii. A list of the drugs that commonly interact with CsA and TAC is provided in Table 4-1.[15, 16]

a) Please note that this list is not comprehensive.

b) Drugs that are nephrotoxic such as gentamicin and amphotericin B may potentiate the nephrotoxic effects of CNI.

1) Concurrent administration of these agents should be avoided or they should be carefully administered with dose considerations.

j. Adverse effects.

i. Cyclosporine.

a) The most common side effects of CsA are:[1-8, 15]

1) Hypertension.

TABLE 4-1

■ **Drugs that Commonly Interact with CsA and TAC**

Increases CsA or TAC Concentrations	Decreases CsA or TAC Concentrations

Antifungal agents
   clotrimazole, fluconazole, itraconazole, ketoconazole
Calcium channel blockers
   diltiazem, nicardipine, nifedipine, verapamil
Macrolide antibiotics
   clarithromycin, erythromycin, telithromycin, troleandomycin
HMG-CoA reductase inhibitors
   atorvastatin, cerivastatin, lovastatin, simvastatin
Others
   bromocriptine, danazol, fluvoxamine, grapefruit juice, metoclopramide, omeprazole, protease inhibitors
	Antibiotics
	   nafcillin, rifabutin, rifampin
	Anti-epileptic agents
	   carbamazepine, phencbarbital, phenytoin, rifabutin, rifampin
	Others
	   St. John's wort, octreotide, orlistat

        2) Hyperlipidemia.

        3) Cosmetic (hirsutism, gingival hyperplasia).

        4) Nephrotoxicity.

        5) Diabetes mellitus.

        6) Tremor.

        7) Gastrointestinal.

        8) Rarely, it can cause seizures and hepatotoxicity.

ii. Tacrolimus.

    a) The most common side effects of TAC are:[1-8, 16]

        1) Hypertension.

        2) Hyperkalemia.

        3) Hypophosphatemia.

        4) Hypomagnesemia.

        5) Nephrotoxicity.

        6) Diabetes mellitus.

        7) Tremor.

        8) Diarrhea.

iii. Adverse events are very similar between CsA and TAC.

    a) TAC is less likely to cause hyperlipidemia, hypertension, and cosmetic problems than CsA.

    b) TAC is more likely to induce new onset of diabetes mellitus.

    c) Recently, TAC has been suspected of inducing polyoma viral nephropathy.[18]

iv. As with all immunosuppressive agents, long-term use of CNI is associated with an increased risk of opportunistic infection and malignancy.

k. Role of CNIs in solid organ transplantation.

    i. Used in solid organ transplantation as the foundation of maintenance regimens to prevent allograft rejection.

    ii. Initiated at the time of transplantation and usually are continued for the life of the allograft.

    iii. Used in combination with other immunosuppressants including:

        a) Corticosteroids.

        b) CellCept® (mycophenolate mofetil, MMF).

        c) Myfortic® (mycophenolate sodium).

        d) Imuran® (azathioprine, AZA).

        e) Rapamune® (rapamycin) in either double or triple drug therapy protocols.

    iv. Clinical studies have compared the relative safety and efficacy of these combinations with corticosteroids (CS), such as CsA and MMF, CsA and AZA, TAC and MMF, and TAC and AZA.

    v. The results from these clinical studies suggested that the TAC and MMF combination appeared to be the most effective in preventing acute rejection and the best tolerated regimen in renal transplant recipients.[19-22]

    vi. With the exception of heart and intestinal transplant recipients, the combination of TAC, MMF, and CS is the most frequently used regimen for solid organ transplant recipients in the U.S.[23]

4. Antiproliferative agents.
   a. Sometimes referred to as antimetabolites.
      i. First used in transplantation in the early 1960s after the development of azathioprine (AZA).
         a) AZA, which suppresses B- and T-cell proliferation, became the first immunosuppressive agent to achieve widespread use in organ transplantation.
         b) Use of AZA has declined significantly since the approval of MMF.
      ii. Since its introduction in 1995, mycophenolate mofetil (MMF) has rapidly replaced AZA as the primary antiproliferative agent used in clinical transplantation.
         a) MMF is utilized in combination with CsA or TAC plus corticosteroids (CS) and recently has been used in combination with sirolimus (SRL) to avoid CNIs.
         b) Myfortic, an enteric-coated formulation of mycophenolate sodium, has been introduced into the market recently.
            1) Enteric-coated mycophenolate sodium was developed to help circumvent the upper gastrointestinal (GI) effects by facilitating release in the small intestine rather than the stomach.
            2) However, two clinical trials failed to demonstrate any statistically significant difference in overall GI symptoms when patients were given equivalent doses of MMF or Myfortic.[24, 25]
         c) Both Myfortic and MMF are converted to mycophenolic acid (MPA) in the liver.
   b. Mechanism of action.
      i. Antiproliferative agents inhibit synthesis of guanosine monophosphate nucleotides by blocking purine synthesis and preventing B- and T-cell proliferation.
         a) Structurally, these resemble cell metabolites.
         b) The most frequently used antiproliferative agents include purine, pyrimidine, and folic acid analogues.
         c) Antiproliferative agents.
            1) May inhibit enzymes of critical metabolic pathways.
            2) May be incorporated during synthesis to produce faulty molecules.
         d) Antiproliferative agents are most effective against cells undergoing proliferation or differentiation.
      ii. Azathioprine is a purine analog antimetabolite.[26]
         a) Incorporates into cellular deoxyribonucleic acid (DNA) and ribonucleic acid (RNA).
         b) Inhibits purine synthesis.[26]
      iii. Mycophenolate mofetil and mycophenolate sodium both inhibit inosine monophosphate dehydrogenase, a key enzyme in purine synthesis.[27]
         a) Interferes with the de novo pathway of purine synthesis and DNA replication.
         b) Produces cytostatic effects on B- and T-cells.

iv. Both CellCept and Myfortic are converted to the same active compound, mycophenolate acid (MPA), which may undergo enterohepatic recirculation.

c. Dosing and administration.

  i. Azathioprine.

   a) The recommended initial oral dose is 3 to 5 mg/kg once daily.

    1) Dose is usually further reduced to a maintenance dose of 1 to 3 mg/kg/day depending on the allograft function and the patient's medical conditions.[26]

  ii. CellCept.[27]

   a) The recommended oral starting dose, given in two to four divided doses, is:

    1) 2 g/day in kidney transplant patients.
    2) 3 g/day in liver transplant patients.
    3) 2 g/day in heart transplant patients.

   b) The starting dose in pediatric kidney transplant patients is 1.2g/m^2.[27]

   c) The recommended intravenous dose, given twice daily, is:

    1) 1 g in kidney transplant patients.
    2) 1 g in liver transplant patients.
    3) 1.5 g in heart transplant patients.
    4) Usually infused no less than 2 hours.
    5) Dosing adjustment is necessary in patients with renal dysfunction due to accumulation of MMF metabolites.

  iii. Myfortic.[28]

   a) The recommended starting dose is 720 mg twice daily.

   b) Dosing adjustment is necessary for patients with renal dysfunction.[28]

d. Therapeutic drug monitoring.

  i. Azathioprine.

   a) Complete blood counts, including platelets, should be monitored frequently during the early post-transplant period, and at least every 3 months thereafter.

  ii. Cellcept and Myfortic.[29]

   a) Both CellCept and Myfortic are metabolized to MPA.

   b) The clinical utility of MPA monitoring is controversial and is currently being investigated.

   c) Frequent monitoring of white blood cell counts is recommended.

e. Drug interactions.

  i. Azathioprine.

   a) Any thiopurine S methyltransferase (TPMT) enzyme inhibitor may increase AZA concentration.

   b) Significant drug interaction has been reported to occur with allopurinol, aminosalicylates, and warfarin.[26]

  ii. CellCept and Myfortic.

   a) Antacids with magnesium and aluminum hydroxides can decrease the absorption of CellCept and Myfortic.

b) Drugs that are myleosuppressive, such as ganciclovir, may exaggerate the bone marrow toxicity of CellCept and Myfortic.[27, 28]
f. Adverse effects.
   i. Azathioprine.[27]
      a) Bone marrow depression, resulting in leukopenia, pancytopenia, thrombocytopenia, and/or macrocytic anemia, occurs to varying degree in >50% of patients.
      b) Other side effects included nausea, vomiting, hepatotoxicity, and pancreatitis.
   ii. CellCept and Myfortic.
      a) The most common side effects of MMF are:
         1) Gastrointestinal (diarrhea, constipation, nausea, vomiting).
         2) Bone marrow suppression (leukopenia, thrombocytopenia, anemia).
      b) MMF has also been associated with increase risk of CMV infection.
g. Role in solid organ transplantation.
   i. Antiproliferative agents are used in conjunction with other maintenance immunosuppressive agents in solid organ transplantation to prevent graft rejection.
   ii. They are most effective when given at the time of transplantation and are usually continued for the life of the allograft.
   iii. MMF is the most frequently used antiproliferative agent.
      a) Clinical trials have demonstrated that MMF is superior to either placebo or AZA in prevention of acute rejection in kidney, pancreas, liver, heart, and lung transplantation.[30-40]
      b) MMF does not appear to be nephrotoxic or to adversely effect glucose and lipid metabolism.
      c) MMF has become an integral component of low toxicity regimens that aim to minimize patient exposure to the nephrotoxic effects of CNI and the metabolic complications of CS.
5. Mammilian target of rapamycin (mTOR).
   a. A key regulatory kinase in the process of cell division.
   b. The term "mTOR inhibitor" refers to immunosuppressant drugs whose mode of action is closely linked to inhibition of this kinase.
   c. In 1999, the FDA approved Rapamune® (sirolimus, SRL), the first mTOR inhibitor, for use in adult kidney transplant recipients.
      i. A series of clinical trials demonstrated that, when used in combination with CsA and CS, SRL produced a significant reduction in the incidence of acute rejection (AR) episodes in the early post-transplant period.[41, 42]
      ii. SRL is a macrolide antibiotic isolated from *Streptomyces hygroscopicus* that is structurally similar to TAC but mechanistically different.
      iii. SRL is only FDA approved for use in kidney transplantation.

   a) SRL has a black box warning for use in liver transplantation.
      1) States the use of SRL in combination with CsA or TAC was associated with an increased rate of hepatic artery thrombosis.[43]
   d. Certican® (everolimus) is another mTOR inhibitor that has been used in Europe and is under review by the FDA for prevention of acute rejection in kidney and in heart transplant recipients.
      i. Everolimus is very similar to sirolimus in terms of mechanism of action and side effect profile.
   e. mTOR inhibitors were developed for use with CsA.
      i. The combination increased nephrotoxicity, hemolytic-uremic syndrome, and hypertension.[41, 42]
         a) Because of this, SRL has been used in combination with TAC to avoid the toxicity of SRL/CsA combinations.[44]
         b) Clinical trials in renal transplantation showed that SRL plus TAC produced more renal dysfunction and hypertension than did MMF plus TAC.
            1) Indicates that SRL may potentiate TAC nephrotoxicity, especially at higher doses.[44, 45, 46]
         c) Other studies are experimenting with withdrawing CNIs in patients receiving mTOR inhibitors.
            1) Early data indicate that withdrawing CsA in these patients reduces renal dysfunction and hypertension.
               i) There is a small increase in rejection episodes, which suggests a strategy for avoiding the long-term toxic effects of CNIs.[47-49]
   f. Mechanism of action.
      i. SRL is a macrocyclic lactone isolated from *Streptomyces hygroscopicus*.[43]
         a) Modulates the immune response by inhibiting the activity of a regulatory protein critical to the coordination of events required for cells to move from G_1 to the S phase of the cell cycle.
         b) SRL inhibits IL-2- dependent T lymphocyte proliferation and stimulation caused by cross-linkage of CD28.
            1) Possibly by blocking activation of mTOR.
            2) Has no effect on calcineurin activity.
         c) SRL also has antineoplastic effects.
   g. Dosing and administration.
      i. Sirolimus.[46]
         a) The recommended loading dose is 6 mg/day followed by a maintenance dose of 2 mg/day.[46]
            1) After withdrawal of CsA, SRL dose should be adjusted to obtain whole blood trough concentrations between 12 and 24 ng/mL.
            2) SRL has been reported to be associated with impaired wound healing and delay in renal allograft recovery.

i) Delaying the initiation of SRL may be warranted in these clinical situations.[50, 51, 52]

    ii. Everolimus.
       a) The dose used in clinical studies was either 0.75 mg orally twice daily or 1.5 mg orally twice daily.

h. Therapeutic drug monitoring.
    i. Sirolimus.[53]
       a) Routine monitoring of SRL trough level is recommended.
       b) Therapeutic target is usually between 4 and 12 ng/mL dependent on concurrent immunosuppression.
       c) During and following CsA withdrawal, it is recommended that the dose of SRL be adjusted to maintain a therapeutic target between 12 and 24 ng/mL.
       d) Optimally, trough levels should be obtained at least 4 to 5 days after a dose change to ensure that the trough level is at steady state before any further dosing adjustment is made.
    ii. Everolimus.
       a) Routine whole blood therapeutic drug monitoring (TDM) is recommended.
       b) Based on exposure efficacy and exposure-safety analysis, patients achieving everolimus whole blood levels ≥3.0 ng/mL have been found to have a lower incidence of acute rejection in both renal and cardiac transplantation compared with the patients whose trough levels are below 3.0 ng/mL.
       c) The upper limit to the therapeutic range is recommended at 8 ng/mL.
       d) Optimally, dose adjustments of everolimus should be based on trough levels obtained more than 4-5 days after previous dosing change.

i. Drug interactions.
    i. Since both SRL and everolimus are metabolized by P450 enzyme system, its drug interaction profile is very similar to that of CsA and TAC.

j. Adverse effects.[43]
    i. The adverse effects of SRL and everolimus are very similar.
    ii. The most common side effects are:
       a) Hypertension.
       b) Hypercholesterolemia.
       c) Hypertriglyceridemia.
       d) Hyperlipidemia.
       e) Thrombocytopenia.
       f) Anemia.
       g) Diarrhea.
       h) Acne.
       i) Rash.
    iii. Sirolimus has also been associated with pneumonitis.[54]
    iv. Renal dysfunction has been reported with both SRL and everolimus.

         a) Especially when they are used in combination with CsA.

         b) Recently, SRL has been reported to be associated with proteinuria.[55]

     v. SRL has also been associated with delayed wound healing and wound complications and delayed renal allograft recovery.

  k. Role in solid organ transplantation.

     i. mTOR inhibitors are used in solid organ transplantation as part of a maintenance regimen with other maintenance immunosuppressive agents to prevent AR.

     ii. mTORs are promising as part of various CNI minimization and withdrawal regimens to improve:

         a) Renal function in renal transplant recipients.

         b) Renal function in other solid organ transplant recipients.

         c) Recent reports of renal toxicities of SRL, such as delayed renal allograft recovery and proteinuria, have questioned the best approach to utilize mTOR in transplantation.

6. Corticosteroids.

  a. Mechanism of action.

     i. The mechanism of corticosteroids (CS) is complex and multifaceted.

     ii. CS are produced by the adrenal gland and are part of the normal endocrine system of animals and humans.

         a) Have a wide spectrum of effects.

         b) Diffuse effects of CS on the body reflect the fact that most mammalian tissues have glucocorticoid receptors within the cell cytoplasm that serve as targets for the effects of CS.

         c) Bind to receptors where they alter RNA and DNA synthesis.

         d) Inhibit secretion of interleukin-1 (IL-1) from macrophages and interleukin-2 (IL-2) secretion from T-cells.

            a) Inhibit the generation of cytotoxic T-cells.

  b. Dosing and administration.

     i. The dose of CS varies depending on:

         a) Type of preparation.

         b) Type of transplant.

         c) Timing of transplantation (induction versus maintenance).

         d) Indication (prevention or treatment of rejection).

     ii. Methyprednisolone is the most frequently used CS during the early post-transplant period.

         a) Used as an induction agent.

         b) Doses range from 250 to 1000 mg given intra-operatively with a subsequent tapering regimen.

         c) Prednisone is the most frequently used CS during the maintenance phase.

            1) Doses ranges from 0 to 10 mg/day.

2) Dose used to treat acute rejection also varies depending on:
   i)   Type of transplant.
   ii) Severity of the rejection.
   iii) The typical treatment regimen is methylprednisolone 250 to 1000 mg intravenously daily for 3 to 5 days.

c. Adverse effects.
   i.   CS side effects depend on the dose and the duration of exposure.
   ii. Short courses of CS are usually well-tolerated with fewer and milder side effects than longer courses of CS.
   iii. Side effects of CS are well-known and well-described.
      a) Range from mild annoyances to serious irreversible bodily damages and include:
         1) Glucose intolerance.
         2) Weight gain.
         3) Bone growth inhibition in children.
         4) Osteoporosis.
         5) Osteonecrosis.
         6) Hypertension.
         7) Hyperlipidemia.
         8) Cataracts.
         9) Suppression of the hypothalamic- pituitary-adrenal axis.
         10) Fluid retention.
         11) Potassium loss.
         12) Headache.
         13) Muscle weakness.
         14) Puffiness of and hair growth on the face.
         15) Thinning and easy bruising of the skin.
         16) Glaucoma, cataracts.
         17) Peptic ulceration.
         18) Worsening of diabetes.
         19) Irregular menses.
         20) Convulsions.
         21) Psychic disturbances.

d. Role in solid organ transplantation.
   i.   CS were the first immunosuppressive drugs used in transplantation.
      a) Not FDA approved for use in organ transplantation.
         1) Highly effective.
         2) Have anchored maintenance immunosuppressive regimens since the early 1960s.
         3) CS are utilized in organ transplant for both the treatment of acute organ rejection and maintenance immunosuppression.
         4) Typically used as part of a combination immunosuppressive regimen including CNIs and an antiproliferative agent.
         5) Used as a first line agent to treat acute cellular rejection.

b) CS have numerous side effects, especially when used in combination with CNIs.

1) Either directly or in part, the use of CS has been responsible for:

i) Post-transplant hypertension.

ii) Bone loss.

iii) Diabetes.

iv) Increased incidence of infection.

2) The safety profile associated with CS use, along with the cost of therapy for treatment of its adverse events, has motivated increased efforts to reduce or eliminate CS as a component of immunosuppressive therapies.

3) Earlier CS withdrawal studies reported high incidence of acute rejection and graft loss, despite significant reduction of CS-associated adverse effects.

4) The introduction of antibody induction, TAC, MMF, and SRL has led to renewal interest in CS withdrawal and avoidance regimens.

5) CS withdrawal generally implies the discontinuation of CS administration.

i) May begin as early as several weeks post-transplant to several months after transplantation.

ii) Early CS withdrawal, or rapid discontinuation, needs to be differentiated from CS avoidance.

- In CS avoidance, the medication is either administered for a very short period of time (up to 7 days) or not administered at all.

- There is evidence that CS avoidance or early withdrawal may be safer than later CS withdrawal.

- Because the side effects of CS are a cumulative result of the high doses that are given in the early postoperative period and the small maintenance doses given for long-term therapy, there is good reason to focus efforts on avoiding their administration altogether.

7. Monoclonal antibodies.[56]

a. There have been several monoclonal antibodies (mAbs) developed for use in transplantation over the last two decades.

i. Two of these, OKT3 and alemtuzumab (Campath), are depleting mAbs.

a) OKT3 is a murine (mouse) mAb that recognizes and binds the CD3 receptor present on all mature T-cells.

1) The resulting antibody-CD3 receptor complex leads to the depletion of CD3-expressing T lymphocytes.

2) Humans produce neutralizing antibodies against muromonab-CD3 because it is a foreign protein originated from the mouse.

         i)   These human anti-mouse antibodies are anti-idiotypic.
- Result in a loss of efficacy with repeated administration due to blocking the active portion of the monoclonal antibody.

        ii) OKT3 therapy is associated with a cytokine release syndrome that typically occurs during the first two days of therapy and consists mainly of high fever, chills, and pulmonary edema.

3) Alemtuzumab.

        i)   A humanized mAb directed against the CD52 receptor.

        ii) Present on most B and T lymphocytes, natural killer (NK) cells, monocytes, macrophages, and tissues of the male reproductive system.

        iii) Utilized for induction therapy in solid organ transplantation.

        iv) Induces a profound pancytopenia.
- Lymphopenia is the basis of its immunosuppressive action.
- Alemtuzumab is FDA approved only for treating refractory B-cell chronic lymphocytic leukemia.
  — Carries a black box warning for this indication that states increased risk of severe hematologic toxicities, infusion reactions, infection, and opportunistic infections.
- Alemtuzumab is not approved for immunosuppressive therapy in solid organ transplantation; it is currently being used off-label for induction therapy in a limited number of transplant centers.

4) Two non-depleting mAbs, both interleukin-2 (IL-2) receptor antagonists, are currently approved as induction therapy to prevent rejection in patients who have a low-to-moderate risk of rejection.

        i)   Daclizumab (DAC), a humanized IgG mAb produced by recombinant DNA technology, is a composite or chimeric antibody of human (90%) and murine (10%) antibody sequences.

        ii) Basiliximab (BAS) is also a chimeric (murine/human) mAb that contains more mouse protein and is also produced by recombinant DNA technology.

        iii) Both drugs bind to the alpha subunit of the IL-2 receptor expressed only on activated T-cells and inhibit their proliferation.

        iv) Both DAC and BAS are used as induction therapy and have been shown to reduce AR rates.

  ii. Mechanism of action.

a) Monoclonal antibodies (mAb) were originally developed against specific targets such as antigens or receptors on the surface of the cell membrane.

b) Currently, mAbs against B and T lymphocytes are being used in solid organ transplantation.

c) Two types of mAbs are generally recognized based on the overall mechanism of action.

    1) The first type leads to the destruction of the lymphocytes, and hence, are called depleting mAbs, which include:

        i) OKT3.

        ii) Alemtuzumab.

    2) The second type of mAbs is directed to block a specific pathway in the immune response, but does not cause destruction of lymphocytes; these are considered non-depleting mAbs, which include:

        i) DAC.

        ii) BAS.

d) OKT3.

    1) OKT3 is a murine monoclonal antibody that binds to the CD3 receptor of the T lymphocyte.

        i) Blocks the recognition of foreign antigens.

e) Alemtuzumab.

    1) Alemtuzumab is a recombinant DNA-derived humanized mAb (Campath).

        i) Directed against the 21-28 kD cell surface glycoprotein CD52.

        ii) CD52 is expressed on the surface of normal and malignant B and T lymphocytes, NK cells, monocytes, macrophages and tissues of the male reproductive system.

f) Daclizumab and basiliximab.

    1) Both DAC and BAS function as an IL-2 receptor antagonist by binding to the alpha subunit of the human high-affinity IL-2 receptor.

        i) Expressed on the surface of activated but not resting lymphocytes.

        ii) Inhibits IL-2 binding; inhibits IL-2-mediated activation of lymphocytes, a critical pathway in the cellular immune response involved in allograft rejection.

g) Dosing and administration.

    1) OKT3.

        i) For the treatment of rejection:

          • Recommended dose is 5 mg/day in a single injection for 10 to 14 days in adults.

          • 2.5 mg/day in pediatric patients weighing less than or equal to 30 kg.

        ii) Due to the formation of antibodies against OKT3, daily increases of dose by 2.5 mg increments may be necessary to achieve the desired suppression of CD3 cell counts.

         iii) The maximal dose is usually about 10 to 12.5 mg/day. Routine monitoring of CD3 cell counts is recommended.

    2) Campath.

      i) Given in two to four divided doses; clinical trials using Campath for induction have used doses ranging from 20–40 mg/day for one to two days.

      ii) Information on the proper dosing and administration of Campath in solid organ transplant recipients is lacking.

    3) Daclizumab.

      i) Daclizumab is given 1 mg/kg intravenous over 15 to 30 minutes every 14 days for a total of 5 doses.

      ii) Recent studies have reported that alternative dosing strategy of daclizumab (e.g., 2 mg/kg on day 0 and day 7) may be as effective as the approved 5 dose regimen.

    4) Basiliximab.

      i) Basiliximab is given 20 mg intravenously over 15 to 30 minutes on day 0 and day 4 post-transplant.

h) Therapeutic drug monitoring.

    1) OKT3.

      i) Monitoring of CD3 count and anti-OKT3 antibodies should be performed during and after OKT3 therapy.

        • To evaluate the efficacy of treatment.

        • To assess whether retreatment with OKT3 is possible.

      ii) It is particularly important that monitoring of peripheral CD3 positive cells be performed during therapy to achieve circulating target numbers of <25 to 50 cells/mm^3.

    2) Campath.

      i) Complete blood counts and platelet counts should be monitored routinely.

    3) Daclizumab and basiliximab.

      i) Currently, routine therapeutic monitoring of daclizumab and basliximab is not warranted.

i) Drug interactions.

    1) No formal drug-drug interactions have been reported to date.

j) Adverse effects.

    1) OKT3.

      i) Cytokine release syndrome is common during the first 2 days of treatment.

      ii) Most patients experienced pyrexia (90%).

        a. 19% had temperature $\geq 40.0°$ C (104° F).

        b. Chills (59%).

        iii) Other adverse effects included dyspnea, nausea, vomiting, chest pain, diarrhea, tremor, wheezing, headache, tachycardia, rigor, and hypertension.

        iv) In acute renal allograft rejection, potentially fatal edema has been reported in less than 2% of patients.

        v) Other side effects included aseptic meningitis, hypertension, hypotension, tachycardia, diarrhea, nausea, and vomiting.

        vi) OKT3 is associated with an increased risk of opportunistic infection and post-transplant lymphoproliferative disorder.

    2) Campath.

        i) Infusion-related side effects of Campath are common including fever, chills, hypertension, and hypotension.

        ii) The side effects of Campath in solid organ transplant patients are different than oncology patients because of the differences in dosage used.

        iii) The use of Campath has been associated with increased risk of opportunistic infection and autoimmune disorders.

    3) Daclizumab and basiliximab.

        i) Both daclizumab and basiliximab are well-tolerated.

        ii) Occasionally infusion-related side effects such as fever and chills have been reported.

        iii) Rarely, anaphylaxis has been reported to occur with basiliximab.

k) Role of mAbs in solid organ transplantation.[56]

    1) mAbs are used in solid organ transplantation for short and predefined periods in combination with other long-term maintenance immunosuppressive agents.

        i) Used in transplantation for two main purposes:

           • Prevention of acute rejection.

               — Induction therapy is the utilization of a specific immunosuppressive agent during the peri-operative period and for a relatively short and predefined duration post-transplant.

               — Induction agents are used as rejection prophylaxis therapy with the following goals:

                   - Decreasing the overall rate of AR in the early post-operative period.

                   - Minimizing maintenance immunosuppressive agents.

           • Treatment of acute rejection.

— Treatment for acute cellular rejection is usually a course of high-dose CS.
— In patients with either severe rejection (defined histologically) or with CS-resistant rejection, lymphocyte depleting mAbs are used to reverse the rejection process.
— Due to the redundancy of the immune system, IL-2 receptor blocker (DAC and BAS) is not effective in treatment of acute rejection.

8. Polyclonal antilymphocyte globulins.[56]
   a. Polyclonal antilymphocyte globulins are a group of antibodies targeting multiple antigens on the cell membrane of lymphocytes.
      i. Produced by immunizing animals such as horses and rabbits with human lymphoid cells.
      ii. Results in the production of multiple and different antibodies, including antibodies to CD2, CD3, CD4, CD8, CD11a, and CD18; thus the term polyclonal.
      iii. These antibodies are removed from the animal and processed for IV administration in humans.
      iv. Anti-thymocyte antibody binds to lymphocytes that display the specific surface antigen.
         a) Leads to the elimination of the lymphocytes from the circulation.
         b) Depletes peripheral lymphocytes in a process that is sustained for at least several weeks.
         c) This lymphopenia is the basis for the immunosuppressive action of polyclonal antibodies.
         d) Thymoglobulin® (anti-thymocyte globulin, rabbit; Genzyme Corporation) is generated by immunizing rabbits with human thymocytes, a waste product of pediatric cardiac surgery.
         e) In the U.S., Thymoglobulin is approved for the treatment of AR in kidney transplant recipients.
         f) It is widely used as an induction agent in many types of solid organ transplantation.
      v. Atgam® (anti-thymocyte globulin, equine; Pfizer Inc.) is produced in horses immunized with human thymus lymphocytes.
         a) Atgam is FDA approved for the treatment of AR in transplant recipients.
         b) Additional uses include:
            1) Induction therapy in solid organ transplantation.
            2) Treatment of hematologic disorders.
      vi. ATG Fresenius® (anti-thymocyte globulin, rabbit; Fresenius Biotech), like Thymoglobulin, is produced in rabbits.
         a) Jurkat cells, an immortalized T-cell lymphoma cell line, serve as the immunogen for this polyclonal antibody.
         b) ATG Fresenius is currently approved only outside the U.S. for the treatment and prevention of AR.

b. Mechanism of action.
   i. Thymoglobulin.
      a) The mechanism of action by which polyclonal antilymphocyte preparations suppress immune responses is not fully understood.
      b) Possible mechanisms that may induce immunosuppression include:
         1) T-cell clearance from the circulation.
         2) Modulation of T-cell activation.
         3) Homing and cytotoxic activities.
      c) Thymoglobulin is thought to induce T-cell depletion and modulation by a variety of methods:
         1) Receptor-mediated complement-dependent lysis.
         2) Opsonization and phagocytosis by macrophages.
         3) Immunomodulation leading to long-term depletion via antibody dependent cell-mediated cytotoxicity.
         4) Activation-induced cell death.
      d) Thymoglobulin has also been shown to prevent B-cell proliferation and differentiation.
         1) Prevents ischemia-reperfusion injury through its interaction with adhesion molecules and the endothelium.
   ii. Atgam.
      a) Atgam promotes the depletion of T-cells from the circulation through opsonization and complement-assisted, antibody-dependent cell-mediated cytotoxicity.
   iii. ATG Fresenius.
      a) ATG Fresenius binds to activated T lymphocytes and other immune-competent cells such as endothelial cells.
         1) Binds to lymphocytes and induces apoptosis, cytolysis, and opsonization of the target cells.
         2) Blocks the interactions between lymphocytes and endothelial cells.
            i) Because the immunogen used is an immortalized T-cell line (Jurkat cell line), it will have minimal binding to B-cell specific antigens.
c. Dosage and administration.
   i. Thymoglobulin.
      a) For treatment of acute rejection, the recommended dose is 1.5 mg/kg/day for 7 to 14 days.
      b) For induction therapy, the dose used in clinical trials is usually 1.5 mg/kg/day for 3 to 7 days.
      c) A reduction in dosage must be considered if:
         1) The platelet count is between 50,000 and 75,000 cells/mm^3.
         2) The white cell count is between 2,000 and 3,000 cells/mm^3.
      d) Discontinuation of Thymoglobulin treatment should be considered if:
         1) Persistent and severe thrombocytopenia (<50,000 cells/mm^3) occurs.
         2) Leukopenia (<2,000 cells/mm^3) develops.

    e) To prevent infusion-related side effects, it is recommended that the patient receive premedication with corticosteroids, acetaminophen, and antihistamine an hour prior to the infusion.

      1) Thymoglobulin should be administered through a high flow vein.

      2) The first dose of Thymoglobulin should be infused over at least 6 hours and subsequent doses should be infused over at least 4 hours.

      3) Peripheral administration of Thymoglobulin.

        i) Mix with heparin and hydrocortisone in a 0.9% sodium chloride infusion solution.

          • Minimizes the potential for local adverse events and the possible risk of thrombotic events.

    f) Following administration of Thymoglobulin, appropriate anti-viral prophylaxis is recommended to reduce the risk of CMV infection and PTLD.

  ii. Atgam.

    a) For prevention of acute rejection, the recommended dose is 15 mg/kg/day for 14 days, then every other day for 14 days for a total of 21 doses in 28 days.

    b) For treatment of acute rejection, the recommended dose is 10 to 20 mg/kg/day for 8 to 14 days.

      1) An additional alternate day therapy up to a total of 21 doses can be given.

    c) Atgam should be administered through an in-line 0.22 μm filter and infused over 4 to 6 hours.

      1) To prevent infusion-related side effects, it is recommended that the patient receive premedication with corticosteroids, acetaminophen, and antihistamine an hour prior to the infusion.

  iii. ATG Fresenius.

    a) The recommended dose is 2 to 5 mg/kg for 5 to 14 days; however, recent studies used 9 mg/kg in a single dose.

d. Therapeutic drug monitoring.

  i. White blood cell and platelet counts should be monitored during and following the end of treatment with any polyclonal antibody preparation.

    a) Due to the formation of anti-horse antibodies and the batch to batch variations with Atgam, routine monitoring of CD3 counts may be necessary to ensure adequate depletion of T cells.

    b) This does not occur with Thymoglobulin and ATG Fresenius.

e. Drug interactions.

  i. No formal drug-drug interactions have been reported to date.

f. Adverse effects.

  i. Thymoglobulin.

    a) The most common side effects are infusion-related (fever, chills, headache), leukopenia, and thrombocytopenia.

b) Other side effects include hypertension, tachycardia, dyspnea, abdominal pain, and diarrhea.

c) Thymoglobulin has also been associated with increase risk of CMV infection and PTLD.

ii. Atgam.

a) The most common side effects are infusion-related (fever, chills, headache), leukopenia, thrombocytopenia, rash, nausea, vomiting, diarrhea, and increased risk of infection.

b) Serum sickness has also been reported.

iii. ATG Fresenius.

a) The most common side effects are fever, chest pain, headache, nausea, vomiting, dyspnea, and myalgias.

    1) Other side effects that have been seen in clinical trials include thrombocytopenia, leukopenia, hypotension, hypertension, tremor, and serum sickness.

g. Role of polyclonal antibodies in solid organ transplantation.

i. Polyclonal antibodies are used in transplantation primarily for induction therapy and treatment of acute rejection.

a) Due to their potent and immediate immunosuppressive effects, polyclonal antibodies allow for postponement in the initiation of CNIs in the setting of delayed graft function.

b) When given intra-operatively, prior to reperfusion, Thymoglobulin has been shown to reduce the incidence of delayed graft function.

c) Often used as part of corticosteroids minimization and CNIs minimization regimens.

9. Adjuvant pharmacotherapy in solid organ transplant recipients.

a. Antimicrobials.

i. Infections continue to represent an important cause of morbidity and mortality after solid-organ transplantation.

ii. This population is at risk for:

a) Post-operative infections.

b) Nosocomial or hospital-associated infections.

c) Community-acquired infections.

d) Opportunistic infections.

e) Reactivation of latent infections as a consequence of immunosuppressive therapy.

iii. Predicting infectious complications is often a function of the timing since the transplant surgery (Figure 4-1).

a) Post-transplant infectious complications are generally classified as occurring:

    1) Early (first month).

    2) Mid (months 2 to 6).

    3) Late (>6 months) post-transplant period.

b) Classification scheme is somewhat arbitrary.

    1) Helps us to understand most of the relevant reasons for infections to develop.

    2) Serves to guide diagnostic and therapeutic strategies for managing infectious complications in this population.[57]

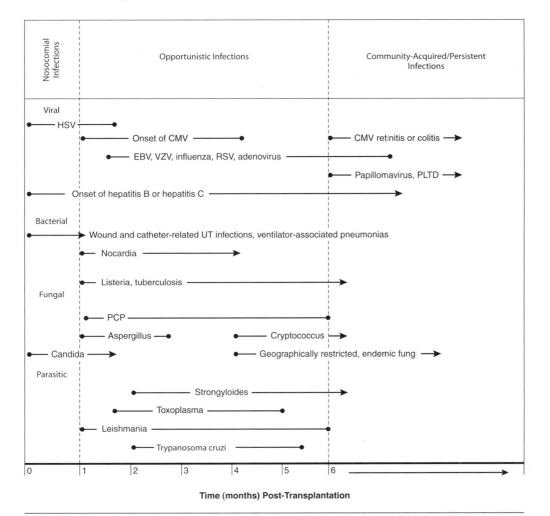

Figure 4-1. Timetable for infectious complications following solid-organ transplantation. Adapted from Fishman JA, Rubin RH. *New J Med,* 1998; 338(24): 1741-1751. HSV= herpes simplex virus; CMV = cytomegalovirus; EBV = Epstein-Barr virus; VZV = varicella zoster virus; RSV = respiratory syncytial virus; PTLD = posttransplant lymphoproliferative disease; UT = urinary tract; PCP = *Pneumocystis carinii* pneumonia.

    c) It is common practice in most organ transplant centers to administer antibiotics to patients on-call to the operating room to prevent surgical site infections.[58]

    d) Most transplant programs routinely administer antibiotic prophylaxis with trimethoprim/sulfamethoxazole to prevent *Pneumocystis carinii* (*jiroveci*) pneumonitis (PCP).

        1) Also effective for preventing infections with *Toxoplasma gondii, Nocardia sp.,* and *Listeria monocytogenes.*[58,59]

    e) Detailed pharmacologic information regarding selected antibiotics that are more commonly used in transplant patients is provided in Table 4-2.

f) Opportunistic fungal and viral infections are another major concern in the first months after transplantation.

1) Viral infections with cytomegalovirus (CMV) are a major cause of morbidity and mortality in solid organ transplant recipients.[59-63]

2) In high-risk patients (the CMV sero-negative recipient of a sero-positive donor organ).

   i) Prophylactic use of intravenous ganciclovir or oral valganciclovir in is common practice to prevent CMV infections.[58,59]

   ii) If both the patient and donor are CMV negative, no prophylaxis is required.[58,59]

   iii) Sero-positive recipients of sero-negative donor.

     • Closely assess for CMV through serologic monitoring.

     • Administer pre-emptive therapy with intravenous ganciclovir or oral valganciclovir, as necessary.[58,59]

g) Antiviral therapies which are commonly employed in the treatment and prophylaxis of viral complications in immunosuppressed transplant patients are summarized in Table 4-3.

h) Aspergillosis and *Candida* species are common fungal infections after transplantation.[61]

1) Prophylaxis of oropharyngeal candidiasis with nystatin oral solution or clotrimazole troches is standard for 6-12 months after surgery in most transplant centers.

2) Prevention of oral candidiasis with nystatin or clotrimazole should also be considered during periods of enhanced immunosuppression.

i) Systemic fungal infections are treated with more potent antifungal agents. Table 4-4 reviews the pharmacology of these agents.

b. Analgesics.

i. Acute pain management in the post-operative period for solid organ transplant recipients is managed with routine opioid agents (narcotics), such as morphine sulfate, codeine, and fentanyl.

a) Post-surgical principles of good pain management apply to this population.

1) Readers interested in a comprehensive review of the pharmacologic approach to pain management or detailed information about the pharmacology of opioid and non-opioid analgesics should refer to Baumann[64] or another medical reference.

2) The use of some non-narcotic analgesics for intermittent pain management is generally safe.

3) Salicylates and nonsteroidal anti-inflammatory drugs (including COX-2 inhibitors) should generally be avoided because of their increased risk of toxicities, especially renal dysfunction.[60]

TABLE 4-2

■ **Selected Antibacterial Agents[57,58,68-70]**

Drug	Mechanism of Action	Indication	Dosage	Common Side Effects	Common Drug Interactions
Cefazolin Sodium	First generation cephalosporin; Bactericidal; Interferes with cell wall synthesis of bacteria	Prophylaxis of surgical site infections. Has a broad spectrum of activity that includes gm (+) and gm (-) organisms, such as: methicillin – susceptible Staph aureus, PCN susceptible strep pneumoniae, group B streptococci, and viridans streptococci	Prophylaxis: 1 gm IV on call to operating room Treatment of skin and soft tissue infections: 1 gm IV Q8h *renal dose adjustments required	Fever, chills, joint pain, rash, urticaria, or pruritus or manifestation of allergic reaction, diarrhea, clostridium – difficile – associated diarrhea and colitis, and headache	May ↓ efficacy of mycophenolate mofetil due to a ↓ in enterohepatic recirculation.
Vancomycin HCl	Bactericidal against gm (+) bacteria through the inhibition of cell-wall synthesis; also selectively inhibits RNA synthesis and alters the permeability of the cell membrane in susceptible bacteria	Prophylaxis of surgical site infections in patients unable to take penicillin or cephalosporin or in settings with a high prevalence of MRSA; Severe or life-threatening infections (staphylococcal species)	Prophylaxis: 1 gm IV on-call to the operating room Treatment: 500 mg – 1gm IV Q12 hrs for systemic infections; 125 mg po Q12 x 10-14 days for Clostridium difficile colitis *renal dose adjustment required	Infusion reactions histamine – mediated (nausea, chills, fever, wheezing, dyspnea, pruritus, urticaria, and rash), nephrotoxicity, neutropenia, and thrombocytopenia	May ↓ efficacy of mycophenolate mofetil due to a ↓ in enterohepatic recirculation. Potential ↑ risk of nephrotoxicity when combined with other nephrotoxic drugs such as tacrolimus and cyclosporine. May ↑ valacyclovir and acyclovir levels.
Metronidazole	Amebicidal, trichomonacidal and bactericidal through the inhibition of DNA replication; -Active against both anaerobic gm (-) bacilli and anaerobic gm (+) cocci	First-line therapy for clostridium difficile colitis	250-500 mg po TID or QID for 10-14 day for clostridium difficile	Nausea, diarrhea, vomiting, metabolic taste disturbance, dyspepsia, dysuria, and darkening of urine (no clinical significance), transient eosinophilia or leukopenia	May ↓ efficacy of mycophenolate mofetil due to a ↓ in enterohepatic recirculation. May ↑ tacrolimus and cyclosporine levels (weak CYP P450 3A4 inhibitor).
Trimethoprim (TMP)/ Sulfamethoxazole (SMX) [Cotrimoxazole]	Synergistic, bactericidal combination of antibacterial agents which act sequentially in 2 successive steps to inhibit the biosynthesis of nucleic acids	Prevention and treatment of: Pneumocystis Carinii (jiroveci) pneumonitis (PCP), Toxoplasma gondii, Nocardia sp., and Listeria monocytogenes	Prophylaxis: 80 mg TMP/400 mg SMZ or 160 mg TMP/800 mg SMZ once daily or three times/ week for 3 to 12 months post-transplant; also, reinstituted during periods of augmented immunosuppression treatment of rejection)	Hyperkalemia, anorexia, headache, GI disturbances, neutropenia, leukopenia, thrombocytopenia, (bone marrow suppression), allergic rash, and photosensitivity	May ↓ efficacy of mycophenolate mofetil due to a ↓ in enterohepatic recirculation. May ↑ voriconazole levels since SMZ is a CYP P450 2C9 inhibitor. *Sulfa-allergic patient alternatives: Pentamidine 300 mg inhalation monthly; Dapsone 50-100 mg po daily; Atovaquone 1500 mg po daily with food (PCP only).

TABLE 4-3

■ **Antiviral Agents**[59-63,68-70]

Drug	Mechanism of Action	Indication	Dosage	Common Side-Effects	Common Drug Interactions
Acyclovir	Intracellular conversion to active form—acyclovir triphosphate—which selectively inhibits DNA synthesis & viral replication through competition with deoxyguanosine triphosphate for DNA polymerase & integration into viral DNA. Active in vitro against: herpes simplex virus types 1 and 2 (HSV-1 & HSV-2), varicella-zoster virus (VZV), Epstein-Barr virus (EBV), herpesvirus simiae (B- virus), & cytomegalovirus (CMV).	Treatment and suppression of the following infections: herpes zoster (shingles), varicella (chickenpox), and herpes simplex.	*Varies by indication:* Herpes zoster: 800 mg orally 5x/day x 7-10 days *(initiate therapy within 48 hrs of symptom onset). Varicella: 800 mg orally 4-5x/day x 5-7 days HSV infections: 200 mg orally 5x/day x 10 days or 400 mg orally TID x 7-10 days; *Chronic suppressive therapy* 400 mg orally BID x up to 12 months IV Dosing: 5-20 mg/kg IV every 8 hrs x 5-10 day *renal dose adjustment required	Nephrotoxicity, ↑ liver enzymes, headaches, gastrointestinal symptoms (nausea, vomiting, diarrhea, abdominal pain), dizziness, paresthesia	Probenecid and cimetidine ↑ the area under the curve (AUC) of acyclovir by competitively inhibiting active renal tubular secretion. An ↑ in plasma AUC of acyclovir & the inactive metabolite of mycophenolate mofetil occur when coadministered -- no dosage adjustment is necessary because of the wide therapeutic index of acyclovir. Increased risk of nephrotoxicity when administered with cyclosporine or tacrolimus or other nephrotoxic drugs.
Valcyclovir	The L valyl ester prodrug of acyclovir; rapidly & extensively converted to acyclovir. Oral bioavailability is significantly greater than acyclovir.	Treatment and suppression of the following infections: herpes labialis (cold sores); herpes zoster (shingles); genital herpes.	*Varies by indication:* Herpes labialis: 2000 mg orally q12 hrs x 2 doses *(initiate therapy at earliest symptom). Herpes zoster: 1000 mg orally TID x 7 days *(initiate therapy within 48 hrs of symptom onset). Genital herpes: 1000 mg orally BID x 7-10 days for 1st episode; 500 mg BID x 3-5 days if recurrent *renal dose adjustment required		

(Continued next page.)

Drug	Mechanism of Action	Indication	Dosage	Common Side-Effects	Common Drug Interactions
Ganciclovir	Intracellular conversion to active form –ganciclovir triphosphate -- which inhibits DNA synthesis & viral replication through competition with deoxyguanosine triphosphate for DNA polymerase & integration into viral DNA.	The prevention and treatment of cytomegalovirus (CMV) disease.	*Varies by indication:* CMV disease: Induction: 5 mg/kg 12 hrs x 14-21 days, given as an IV infusion over 1 hr. Maintenance: 5 mg/kg given as an IV infusion over 1 hr once/day x 7 days/ week, or 6 mg/kg once/day x 5 days/week; or 1000 mg orally TID CMV retinitis: Induction: 5 mg/ kg 12 hrs x 14-21 days, given as an IV infusion over 1 hr. Maintenance: 5 mg/kg given as an IV infusion over 1 hr once/day x 7 days/ week; or 1000 mg orally TID CMV prevention: 1000 mg orally TID *orally administered with food *renal dose adjustment required	Nephrotoxicity, ↑ liver enzymes, neurotoxicity (confusion agitation, seizures, peripheral neuropathy), hematologic toxicity (neutropenia, anemia, leucopenia thrombocytopenia,) gastrointestinal symptoms (anorexia, nausea, vomiting, diarrhea, abdominal pain), fever, chills, confusion, pruritus, phlebitis.	Probenecid ↑ the area under the curve (AUC) of ganciclovir by competitively inhibiting active renal tubular secretion An ↑ in plasma AUC of ganciclovir & the metabolites of mycophenolate mofetil may occur when coadministered -- carefully follow renal dosing guidelines for ganciclovir when used with mycophenolate. ↑ risk of nephrotoxicity when administered with cyclosporine or tacrolimus or other nephrotoxic drugs. ↑ risk of hematologic toxicity when administered with or other bone marrow suppressive agents nephrotoxic drugs. ↑ risk of generalized seizures when coadministered with imipenem-cilastatin -- these drugs should not be used together.
Valganciclovir	The L-valyl ester prodrug of ganciclovir; rapidly & extensively converted to ganciclovir. Oral bioavailability is significantly greater than ganciclovir.	The prevention and treatment of cytomegalovirus (CMV) disease.	*Varies by indication:* CMV disease and CMV retinitis: Induction: 900 mg orally BID x 21 days Maintenance: 900 mg orally once daily CMV prevention: 900 mg orally once daily *administered with food *renal dose adjustment required		

Drug	Mechanism of Action	Indication	Dosage	Common Side-Effects	Common Drug Interactions
Famciclovir	Oral prodrug which is rapidly transformed to penciclovir. The active form, penciclovir triphosphate inhibits viral DNA polymerase competitively with deoxyguanosine triphosphate and is incorporated into the extending DNA.	Treatment and suppression of the following infections: herpes labialis (cold sores); herpes zoster (shingles); genital herpes.	*Varies by indication:* Genital herpes: 250 mg orally TID x 7-10 days for 1st episode; 125 mg BID x 5 days if recurrent Herpes labialis: 125-250 mg orally BID x 5 days *(initiate therapy at earliest symptom). Herpes zoster: 500 mg orally TID x 7 days *renal dose adjustment required	Fatigue, headache, dizziness, fever, nausea, vomiting, diarrhea, abdominal pain, flatulence, pruritus.	May ↑ serum digoxin concentrations and ↑ risk of toxicity – renal excretion ↓ by competition for active tubular transport.
Lamivudine	A synthetic nucleoside (dideoxynucleoside analogue) whose antiviral activity is related to its conversion intracellularly to lamivudine triphosphate. Once incorporated into viral DNA by hepatitis B polymerase results in DNA chain termination.	For the treatment of patients with chronic hepatitis B and evidence of hepatitis B virus (HBV) replication.	100 mg orally once daily *renal dose adjustment required	malaise and fatigue, respiratory tract infections, headache, abdominal discomfort and pain, nausea, vomiting and diarrhea	Coadministration with trimethoprim/sulfamethoxazole ↑ lamivudine exposure by about 40% -- no dosage adjustment of lamivudine is necessary, unless the patient has renal impairment. ↑ risk of lactic acidosis when used in combination with nucleoside analogue therapy (adefovir, didanosine) in patients with HIV.

TABLE 4-4

■ **Antifungal Agents**[61, 68-70]

Drug	Mechanism of Action	Indication	Dosage	Common Side-Effects	Common Drug Interactions
Fluconazole	Highly selective inhibitor of fungal cytochrome P450 sterol C-14-α-demethylation in the cell membrane of fungi; an essential step in ergosterol biosynthesis	Candidiasis; cryptococcal meningitis	100-400 mg po or IV daily * renal dose adjustment required	Hepatotoxicity (↑ liver enzymes) GI disturbances (nausea, vomiting, diarrhea, abdominal pain, dyspepsia), rash, and headache	↑ toxicity of CYP P450 3A4 metabolized drugs: cyclosporine, tacrolimus, sirolimus, statins, erythromycin, phenytoin, warfarin. Rifampin ↓ effect of fluconazole by ↑ hepatic metabolism.
Itraconazole	Highly selective inhibitor of fungal cytochrome P450 sterol C-14-a-demethylation in the cell membrane of fungi; an essential step in ergosterol biosynthesis	Invasive/non-invasive aspergillosis; Candidiasis; Histoplasmosis; Sporotrichosis; Para-coccidioidomycosis; Chromomycosis; Blastomycosis; Dermatomycosis; Onychomycosis	100-400 mg po or 200 mg IV per day Administered OD or BID -Systemic mycoses required 3 to 6 months of treatment *renal dose adjustments required	Hepatotoxicity (↑ liver enzymes) GI disturbances (nausea, vomiting, diarrhea, abdominal pain, dyspepsia), rash, headache, hypertension, and hypertriglyceridemia	↑ toxicity of CYP P450 3A4 metabolized drugs: cyclosporine, tacrolimus, sirolimus, statins, erythromycin, phenytoin, warfarin. Efficacy of itraconazole ↓ by carbamazepine, isoniazid, phenobarbital, phenytoin, and rifampin (inducers of hepatic enzyme metabolism) Oral drug absorption ↓ by antacids, H$_2$-antagonisits, proton-pump inhibitors, and sulcrate
Voriconazole	Highly selective inhibitor of fungal cytochrome P450 sterol C-14-a-demethylation in the cell membrane of fungi; an essential step in ergosterol biosynthesis	Invasive aspergillosis	Intravenous: 6 mg/kg x 2 doses 12 hrs apart for loading dose (LD) followed by maintenance dose (MD) of 4 mg 1kg Q12hrs. Oral: 400 mg Q12 hrs x 2 doses (LD) followed by MD of 200 mg/d (100 mg/d if pt < 20 kg) *renal dose adjustments required	Hepatotoxicity (↑ liver enzymes) visual disturbances, fever, rash, nausea, vomiting, diarrhea, headache, and abdominal pain	Voriconazole inhibits CYP P450 isoenzymes (2C19, 2C9, 3A4) therefore, potential to ↑ plasma concentrations of drugs metabolized by these isoenzymes and ↑ risk of toxicity. Significant ↑ in cyclosporine and tacrolimus levels; sirolimus in contraindicated with voriconazole Efficacy ↓ with enzyme inducers.

Drug	Mechanism of Action	Indication	Dosage	Common Side-Effects	Common Drug Interactions
Clotrimazole	Clotrimazole and nystatin appear to inhibit the enzymatic conversion of 2,4-methyl-enedihydrol-anosterol to demethylsterol, the precursor to ergosterol which is an essential building block of the cytoplasmic membrane of the fungi.	Treatment or prophylaxis of oropharyngeal candidiasis	Treatment: 10 mg 5x/day dissolved orally x 14 days Prophylaxis: 10 mg TID dissolved orally x 3–6 months *patients should be instructed not to chew or swallow troches whole.	Hepatotoxicity (↑ liver enzymes), nausea vomiting, abdominal cramps	None.
Nystatin Oral Suspension		Treatment or prophylaxis of oropharyngeal candidiasis	Treatment: 4–6 mL (400,000 to 600,000 units) QID swish & swallow x 14 days or at least 48 hrs after perioral symptoms have resolved Prophylaxis: 1–4 mL (100,000 to 400,000 units) BID to QID swish & swallow x 3–6 months	Nausea, vomiting, diarrhea abdominal pain	None.
Amphotericin B Deoxycholate Fungizone®	-Derived from Streptomyces nodosus -Birds sterols present in the cytoplasmic membrane of fungi; resulting in increased membrane permeability and loss of fungal integrity	Candidiasis; blastomycosis; aspergillosis' coccidioidomycosis; cryptococcosis; leishmaniasis; and sporotrichosis.	0.3 to 1.5 mg1kg/day IV *renal dose adjustment required.	Nephrotoxicity, hypokalemia, hypomagnesemia, anemia, anorexia, nausea, vomiting, diarrhea, and hepatotoxicity (↑ liver enzymes)	Potential ↑ risk of nephrotoxicity when combined with other nephrotoxic drugs such as cyclosporine or tacrolimus. May ↑ valacyclovir and acyclovir levels. ↑ risk of hypokalemia and other electrolyte abnormalities with diuretics.
Amphotericin B Lipid Complex Abelcet®		Aspergillosis; candidiasis; cryptococcia meningitis	5 mg1kg/day IV *renal Dose adjustment required	Infusion – related reactions (chills, rigors, fever, and phlebitis)	
Liposomal Amphotericin B (AmBisome®)		Aspergillosis; candidiasis; cryptococcia meningitis	3 to 5 mg1kg/day IV *renal dose adjustment required	Nephrotoxicity and infusion-related reactions less frequent with Amphotericin B lipid Complex and liposomal Amphotericin B	
Caspofungin	Inhibits the synthesis of B (1,3) – D-glucan which is an integral component of the fungal cell wall	Invasive aspergillosis and Candidiasis	70 mg IV or day 1(LD); then 50 mg IV daily (MD) *dose adjustment required for patients with hepatic impairment – 35 mg IV daily (MD) for Child – Pugh Class B	Fever, headaches, hepatotoxicity (↑liver enzymes), infusion reactions, pruritus, nausea, vomiting, and skin rash	May ↓ tacrolimus and sirolimus levels – monitor carefully. Cyclosporine may ↑ caspofungin levels and ↑ liver enzymes (ALT, AST). Combination with carbamazepine, phenytoin, rifampin, and dexamethasonc may ↓ caspofungin levels and efficacy (↑ clearance).

        i) An exception to this rule is the use of low-dose aspirin for the prevention of cardiovascular and/or cerebrovascular events, which is generally considered safe.

        ii) The non-prescription analgesic of choice for transplant patients is acetaminophen, based upon its proven safety profile.
- It is also the antipyretic of choice for this group.
- This agent is not without toxicities:
  — Liver dysfunction with acute or chronic excessive consumption.
  — Careful patient monitoring is recommended.

c. Drugs to manage post-transplant diabetes mellitus (PTDM).
  i. Diabetes mellitus is a well-known complication of transplantation.
   a) Decreases patients' quality of life.
   b) Worsens long-term outcomes.[60, 66, 67]
  ii. New-onset post-transplant diabetes mellitus (PTDM) occurs in up to 50% of solid organ transplant recipients within the first 3 months.[58, 60]
   a) High-dose corticosteroid use in many immunosuppressive protocols is implicated as a major cause of PTDM.
   b) Calcineurin inhibitors also contribute to the development of PTDM.[58, 60]
  iii. Management of PTDM is essentially the same as in the non-transplant population and includes:
   a) Dietary and lifestyle modifications.
   b) Pharmacotherapy.
  iv. Table 4-5 succinctly delineates the pharmacology of the major categories of insulin and oral-hypoglycemic medications used in the management of diabetes.
d. Gastrointestinal symptoms.
  i. Gastrointestinal issues such as peptic ulcers and gastroesophageal reflux disease (GERD) symptoms are very common in the transplant population, especially in the early post-operative period.
   a) The increased rates of peptic ulceration have been attributed to the use of steroids for immunosuppression.[58]
   b) Other medications used in treatment or prophylaxis of transplant patients are associated with significant gastrointestinal toxicities.
   c) Prophylactic therapy is commonly prescribed to patients post-transplantation.
  ii. In Table 4-6, the pharmacology of the common anti-ulcer medication classes is summarized.
e. Cardiovascular complications.
  i. Hypertension is the most common medical problem in the post-transplant population.[58, 60]
   a) Cyclosporine is considered to be the primary cause of this problem.

TABLE 4-5

■ **Anti-hyperglycemic Agents**[66-70]

Drug	Mechanism of Action	Indication	Dosage	Common Side-Effects	Common Drug Interactions
Insulin various formulations): Rapid Acting: Humalog® (insulin lispro); Novolog® (insulin aspart) Short Acting: Humulin R®; Novolin R® Intermediate Acting: NPH; Humulin N®; Novolin N®; Lente; Humulin L®; Novolin L® Long Acting: Humulin U® (ultra-lente); Lantus® (insulin glargine)	The primary activity of insulin is the regulation of glucose metabolism. In addition, all insulins have several anabolic and anticatabolic actions on many tissues in the body. In muscle and other tissues (except the brain), insulin causes rapid transport of glucose and amino acids intracellularly, promotes anabolism, and inhibits protein catabolism. In the liver, insulin promotes the uptake and storage of glucose in the form of glycogen, inhibits gluconeogenesis and promotes the conversion of excess glucose into fat. Insulin preparations differ in onset, peak and duration of action.	For the treatment of hyperglycemia in insulin-requiring or insulin-dependent diabetic patients.	The dosage of insulin is individually determined in accordance with the requirements of the patient.	Hypoglycemia; prolonged administration of insulin subcutaneously can result in lipoatrophy (depression in the skin) or lipohypertrophy (enlargement or thickening of tissue) in rare cases.	Insulin requirements may be increased by medications with hyperglycemic activity such as corticosteroids, isoniazid, certain lipid lowering drugs (e.g., niacin), estrogens, oral contraceptives, phenothiazines, and thyroid replacement therapy. Insulin requirements can be increased, decreased, or unchanged in patients receiving diuretics.

(Continued next page.)

Drug	Mechanism of Action	Indication	Dosage	Common Side-Effects	Common Drug Interactions
Sulfonylureas Glimepirimide Glyburide Glipizide	Stimulates an ↑ in insulin release from functional β-cells in the pancreas. Binds to an ATP-dependent K⁺ channel in the β-cell plasma membrane which causes a depolarization of the membrane and opening of the voltage-dependent Ca⁺ channels – it is the ↑ in intracellular Ca⁺ that produces the insulin secretion.	Control of hyperglycemia in Type 2 diabetics.	Glimepirimide 1-8 mg orally daily; taken with first main meal Glyburide 1.25-20 mg/day given once daily or BID; taken with first main meal Glipizide 2.5-40 mg/day given once daily or BID; taken 30 minutes before meals *renal dose adjustment required	Hypoglycemia, dizziness, asthenia, headache, nausea	Intolerance to alcohol (disulfiram-like reaction: flushing, sensation of warmth, giddiness, nausea and occasionally tachycardia) may occur in patients treated with a sulfonylurea. This reaction can be prevented by avoiding the use of alcohol. Hypoglycemia may be potentiated when a sulfonylurea is used concurrently with agents such as: insulin and other oral antidiabetics, anabolic steroids and androgens, cyclophosphamide, disopyramide, fibrates, fluoxetine, miconazole, monoamine oxidase inhibitors, propranolol, quinolones, sympatholytic agents (e.g., beta-blockers), & tetracyclines. Certain drugs tend to produce hyperglycemia and may lead to loss of blood sugar control; these include: barbiturates, corticosteroids, diuretics (thiazides, furosemide), glucagon, nicotinic acid (in pharmacologic doses), oral contraceptives (estrogen plus progestogen), phenytoin, rifampin, sympathomimetic agents (e.g., epinephrine) and thyroid hormones.
Insulin secretagogues Nateglinide Repaglinide	Chemically unrelated to oral sulphonylureas, but similar mechanism of action (see above). Insulin release with these agents is glucose dependent and diminishes at low blood glucose concentrations.	Control of hyperglycemia in Type 2 diabetics	Nateglinide 120 mg orally TID with meals Repaglinide 0.5-4 mg orally TID with meals	Hypoglycemia, nausea, vomiting, diarrhea, constipation, dyspepsia, headache, arthralgia, back pain, chest pain.	

Drug	Mechanism of Action	Indication	Dosage	Common Side-Effects	Common Drug Interactions
Biguanides Metformin	The biguanide derivatives only produce an antihyperglycemic effect in the diabetic when there is insulin secretion. They have no effects on the pancreatic β-cells. While the MOA of this class is not fully understood, it has been postulated that they might potentiate the effect of insulin or enhance the effect of insulin on the peripheral receptor site—this increased sensitivity seems to follow an increase in the number of insulin receptors on cell surface membranes.	Control of hyperglycemia in Type 2 diabetics	Metformin 500–850 mg orally BID *contraindicated in moderate to sever renal impairment	Gastrointestinal symptoms (diarrhea, nausea, vomiting, abdominal bloating, flatulence, and anorexia) which are dose-related. Lactic acidosis is a rare, but serious, metabolic complication that may occur due to drug accumulation during treatment with metformin. The risk of metformin accumulation and lactic acidosis increases with the degree of impairment of renal function (substantial renal excretion of the drug).	As above, for hypoglycemic and hyperglycemic drugs, plus the following additions: Cationic drugs (e.g., amiloride, digoxin, morphine, procainamide, quinidine, quinine, cimetidine, ranitidine, triamterene, trimethoprim, and vancomycin) that are eliminated by renal tubular secretion, theoretically have the potential for interaction with metformin by competing for common renal tubular transport systems.
α-Glucosidase inhibitors Acarbose Miglitol	The antihyperglycemic action of these agents results from a competitive, reversible inhibition of pancreatic α-amylase and membrane bound intestinal α-glucoside hydrolase enzymes. In diabetic patients, this enzyme inhibition results in a delayed glucose absorption and a smoothing and lowering of postprandial hyperglycemia, resulting in improved glycemic control.	Control of hyperglycemia in Type 2 diabetics	Acarbose 50–100 mg orally TID, taken at the start of each meal Miglitol 50–100 mg orally TID, taken at the start of each meal	Gastrointestinal symptoms (flatulence, diarrhea and abdominal pain) which can be minimized by starting on a low dose and titrating slowly; rash; ↑liver transaminases.	As above, for hypoglycemic and hyperglycemic drugs.

(Continued next page.)

Drug	Mechanism of Action	Indication	Dosage	Common Side-Effects	Common Drug Interactions
Thiazolidinediones Pioglitazone Rosiglitazone	Potent and highly selective agonist for peroxisome proliferator-activated receptor-gamma (PPARγ) which are found in tissues important for insulin action such as adipose tissue, skeletal muscle, and liver. Activation of PPARγ nuclear receptors modulates the transcription of numerous insulin responsive genes involved in the control of glucose and lipid metabolism, and in the maturation of pre-adipocytes. These agents ↓ insulin resistance in the periphery and liver, resulting in ↑ insulin-dependent glucose disposal and ↓ hepatic glucose output respectively.	Control of hyperglycemia in Type 2 diabetics	Pioglitazone 15-45 mg orally once daily Rosiglitazone 4-8 mg/day orally given once daily or BID	Hypoglycemia, headache, sinusitis, pharyngitis, myalgias, fluid retention, edema, weight gain, abnormal liver function tests. Contraindicated in patients with known congestive heart failure (CHF), as well as those with ↑ ALT >2.5 times the upper limit of normal.	As above, for hypoglycemic and hyperglycemic drugs. The CYP P450 isoform 3A4 is partially responsible for the metabolism of these agents. Specific formal pharmacokinetic interaction studies have not been conducted with the thiazolidinediones and other drugs metabolized by this enzyme; therefore, monitor carefully when used together.

TABLE 4-6

■ **Anti-ulcer Agents**[67-69]

Drug	Mechanism of Action	Indication	Dosage	Common Side-Effects	Common Drug Interactions
H₂-antagonists Cimetidine Famotidine Nizatidine Ranitidine	Antagonists of histamine at gastric H$_2$-receptor sites – results in the inhibition of both basal gastric secretion and gastric acid secretion induced by histamine, pentagastrin and other secretagogues.	Treatment of NSAID-induced lesions (ulcers, erosions) and their gastrointestinal symptoms and prevention of their recurrence; the prophylaxis of gastrointestinal hemorrhage from stress ulceration in seriously ill patients; the prophylaxis of recurrent hemorrhage from bleeding ulcer; prophylaxis and maintenance treatment of duodenal or benign gastric ulcer in patients with a history of recurrent ulceration	Cimetidine 300 mg QID or 400 mg BID or 800 mg QHS orally Famotidine 20-40 mg BID or 40 mg QHS orally; 20 mg q12 hrs IV Nizatidine 150 mg BID or 150-300 mg QHS Ranitidine 150 mg BID or 300 mg QHS orally; 50 mg q6-8 hrs IV *renal dose adjustment required	Headache, fatigue, malaise; dizziness; somnolence; insomnia, constipation, diarrhea, nausea, vomiting, abdominal discomfort/pain, dry mouth, dry skin, rash.	May ↓ the bioavailability of itraconazole and ketoconazole by a pH-dependent ↓ on absorption or a change in volume of distribution. Cimetidine inhibits CYP450 1A2, 2C9, 2D6, 2C19 and 3A4. Coadministration of cimetidine may ↑ amiodarone, β-blockers (propranolol, metoprolol, labetolol, pindolol), carbamazepine, lidocaine, nifedipine, phenytoin, quinidine, and warfarin.
Proton Pump Inhibitors Esomeprazole Lansoprazole Omeprazole Pantoprazole	Inhibits the gastric enzyme H$^+$,K$^+$-ATPase (the proton pump) which catalyzes the exchange of H$^+$ and K$^+$, which inhibits both basal acid secretion and stimulates acid secretion in a dose-dependent manner.	Treatment of conditions where a reduction of gastric acid secretion is required, such as: duodenal ulcer, gastric ulcer; NSAID-associated gastric and duodenal ulcers; reflux esophagitis; symptomatic gastroesophageal reflux disease (GERD), Zollinger-Ellison syndrome (pathological hypersecretory condition); and eradication of *Helicobacter pylori*.	Esomeprazole 20-40 mg daily or BID orally Lansoprazole 15-30 mg daily orally;30 mg/day IV infusion over 30 mins Omeprazole 20 mg daily or 20 mg BID orally Pantoprazole 20 mg BID or 40 mg daily orally; 8 mg/hr IV x 72 hrs for upper GI bleed *renal dose adjustment required	Diarrhea, headache, flatulence, abdominal pain, constipation, nausea, vomiting, dry mouth and dizziness/vertigo.	Extensive liver metabolism; CYP P450: 2C19inhibitor and 3A4 substrate; therefore, other drugs metabolized through these cytochrome P450 isoenzymes should be carefully monitored when co-administered. May ↑ the absorption of digoxin and ↑risk of toxicity. May ↑ the INR in patients on warfarin – mechanism unknown. ↓ the absorption of ketoconazole and itraconazole.
Cytoprotective Agent Sulcrate (Sulcrafate)	Exerts a generalized gastric cytoprotective effect by enhancing natural mucosal defense mechanisms.	Treatment of duodenal and non-malignant gastric ulcer; prophylaxis of duodenal ulcer recurrence; treatment of duodenal ulcer and for the prophylaxis of gastrointestinal hemorrhage due to stress ulceration in critically ill patients.	1000 mg QID orally or 10 mL QID of suspension	Constipation	Concomitant administration ↓ bioavailability of digoxin and ↓ extent of absorption of phenytoin, warfarin & fluoroquinolone antibiotics (ciprofloxacin and norfloxacin, etc). Avoid by separating administration of sucralfate from that of the other agent by 2 hours.

1) Has the propensity to cause vasoconstriction.
2) Postulated mechanisms:
   i) Decreased prostacyclin and nitric oxide production.
   ii) Promotes sodium water retention by increasing sodium retention in the proximal tubule.
3) Drugs of choice for cyclosporine associated hypertension include:
   i) Calcium channel blockers such as diltiazem.
   ii) Angiotensin-converting enzyme (ACE) inhibitors.
   iii) Angiotensin II AT$_1$ receptor blockers (ARB).
4) These and other antihypertensive mediation classes are reviewed in more detail in Table 4-7.
5) Many hypertensive transplant patients will require multiple drugs to achieve control of their blood pressure.

  ii. Hyperlipidemia is another post-transplant cardiovascular complication.[58, 60]

    a) Immunosuppressive agents known to increase cholesterol and triglyceride levels include the following:
1) Cyclosporine.
2) Steroids.
3) Sirolimus.

    b) Management of dyslipidemia is common in transplant patients, with the 3-hydroxy-3methylglutaryl coenzyme A (HMG-CoA) reductase inhibitors (statins) serving as the primary pharmacotherapeutic approach.[58, 60]

    c) The pharmacologic details of this class of medications are also reviewed in Table 4-7.

10. Conclusions.
   a. Immunosuppression has evolved over the past few decades, from single agent to multiple agents.
      i. More options are now available:
         a) To individualize therapies.
         b) To achieve the fine balance between adequate immunosuppression.
         c) To prevent short- and long-term toxicities of immunosuppression.
   b. Medical complications are common in transplant patients.
      i. Understanding the mechanism of these complications helps guide the appropriate selection of medications which are likely to be most effective.
      ii. Clinicians must understand the complexities of post transplant care including:
         a) Additive medication toxicities.
         b) Drug-drug interactions between the immunosuppressive agents.
         c) Adjuvant medications prescribed to manage medical complications.
         d) Potential opportunistic infections.

TABLE 4-7

■ Cardiovascular Medications[57,59,67-69]

Drug	Mechanism of Action	Indication	Dosage	Common Side-Effects	Common Drug Interactions
		β-Adrenoreceptor Blockers			
Cardio-selective agents (β₁-selective) Atenolol Metoprolol Bisoprolol	Competitive ability to selectively antagonize catecholamine-induced tachycardia at β₁-adrenoreceptors sites in the heart, thus ↓ heart rate, cardiac contractility and cardiac output.	Used in the treatment of hypertension, angina pectoris and to reduce mortality in patients with myocardial infarction; selected agents also used in the treatment of left-ventricular systolic dysfunction (carvedilol) and cardiac arrhythmias (including supraventricular and ventricular tachycardias). Propranolol used for the treatment of essential tremors.	Atenolol 50-200 mg/day orally 5-10 mg IV bolus Metoprolol 50-400 mg/day orally given OD or BID Bisoprolol 10-20 mg/day	Exertional tiredness, gastrointestinal disorders (diarrhea, constipation, flatulence, nausea and vomiting), disturbance of sleep patterns, syncope, vertigo, light-headedness, postural hypotension; 2ⁿᵈ and 3ʳᵈ degree AV block; may mask the symptoms of hypoglycemia in insulin-dependent diabetics Contraindicated in patients with: (a)bronchospasm (including asthma and COPD); (b) sinus bradycardia; and (3) 2ⁿᵈ or 3ʳᵈ degree AV block	Negative inotropic, dromotropic and chronotropic effects may occur when metoprolol is given together with calcium antagonists. Verapamil and diltiazem ↓ metoprolol clearance. β-blockers may enhance the negative inotropic and negative dromotropic effect of antiarrhythmic agents such as quinidine and amiodarone.
Non-Selective Agents (β₁ and β₂ activity) Propranolol Nadolol	Same as above for β₁-blockade; however, blockade of β₂-adrenoreceptors causes smooth muscle contraction.		Propranolol 20-320 mg/day orally given BID-QID 0.1 mg/kg IV Nadolol 40-320 mg/day		
Vasodilatory β-Blocker Carvedilol Labetalol HCl	Nonselective β-adrenoceptor blocker [activity present in the S(-) enantiomer] and alpha₁-adrenoceptor blocker [equal potency activity present in R(+) & S(-) enantiomers]. β-blocker effects greater than α-blocker effects: β:α ratio is 10:1 for carvedilol and 4:1 for labetalol.		Carvedilol 3.125-25 mg orally BID Labetalol 100-600 mg orally BID 40-80 mg IV q10 mins (for hypertensive emergency)		

(Continued next page.)

Drug	Mechanism of Action	Indication	Dosage	Common Side-Effects	Common Drug Interactions
Calcium Channel Blockers (CCB)					
Non-dihydropyridine type Diltiazem Verapamil	Selectively inhibits the influx of calcium ions at the voltage-gated (or slow) calcium channels of the plasma membrane into cardiac muscle and vascular smooth muscle. This results in a ↓ of free calcium ions in the muscle tissue, leading to a depression of mechanical contraction of myocardial and smooth muscle and depression of both impulse formation (automaticity) and conduction velocity in the CV system. The non-dihydropyridines have an ↑ effect on AV nodal conduction and weaker vasodilatory effects. Dihydropyridines are strong vasodilators, acting via relaxation of vascular smooth muscle cells, with little direct effect on myocardial contractility or SA/AV nodal conduction.	Hypertension; chronic stable angina; coronary artery disease due to vasospasm; atrial fibrillation/flutter	Diltiazem 120-360 mg/day orally given once daily to QID; 0.25-0.35 mg/kg IV bolus over 2 mins; then 5-15 mg/hr infusion. Verapamil 188-480 mg/day orally given once daily to QID; 2.5-10 mg IV over 2 mins; may repeat 5-10 mg dose after 15-30 mins.	nausea, swelling/edema, arrhythmia (AV block, bradycardia, tachycardia and sinus arrest), headache, dizziness, lightheadedness, rash, anorexia, constipation, diarrhea, dyspepsia, vomiting.	May ↑ cyclosporine, tacrolimus and sirolimus levels – CYP P450 3A4 inhibitors [an exploitable drug interaction]. When combined with a β-blockers, amiodarone, or other anti-arrhythmic agents ↑ risk of hypotension, bradycardia and AV block. Toxicity ↑ with 3A4 isoenzyme inhibitors (azole antifungals, erythromycin grapefruit juice) and efficacy ↓ with 3A4 isoenzyme inducers (phenobarbital, phenytoin, rifampin).
Dihydropyridine type Amlodipine Felodipine		Hypertension; chronic stable angina.	Amlodipine 5-10 mg orally once daily Felodipine 2.5-10 mg orally once daily	Pedal edema, flushing, palpitations, headache, dizziness, lightheadedness, nausea, diarrhea, constipation (verapamil), vomiting, and gingival hyperplasia.	These agents under-go biotransformation by the CYP P450 system, mainly via CYP 3A4 isoenzyme. Co-administration of these drugs with others that follow the same route of biotransformation may result in altered bioavailability of one or the other. Toxicity ↑ with 3A4 isoenzyme inhibitors (azole antifungals, erythromycin grapefruit juice) and efficacy ↓ with 3A4 isoenzyme inducers (phenobarbital, phenytoin, rifampin).

Drug	Mechanism of Action	Indication	Dosage	Common Side-Effects	Common Drug Interactions
Angiotensin Converting Enzyme Inhibitors (ACE-inhibitors)					
Enalapril Lisinopril Quinapril Ramipril	Angiotensin converting enzyme (ACE) catalyzes the conversion of angiotensin I to angiotensin II. ACE-inhibitors suppress the production of angiotensin II, which is the most vasoactive product of the renin-angiotensin system. ACE-inhibition leads to ↓ systemic arteriolar resistance and mean diastolic and systolic blood pressure. In patients with CHF, inhibition of ACE results in ↓ afterload and heart rate as well as ↑ cardiac output, stroke volume and stroke work.	Hypertension (1st line); congestive heart failure and left-ventricular dysfunction; post-myocardial infarction; prevention of CV events; diabetic nephropathy.	Enalapril 5-40 mg/day orally given once daily or BID Lisinopril 10-80 mg once daily Quinapril 10-40 mg once daily Ramipril 2.5-20 mg once daily	Impaired renal function (↑ serum creatinine), hypotension, dizziness, hyperkalemia, maculopapular rash, nausea, vomiting, and angioedema. Persistent, dry cough attributed to the accumulation of kinins in the respiratory tract due to inhibition of Kinase II.	When combined with agents such as potassium-sparing diuretics, potassium supplements or potassium-containing salt substitutes, severe hyperkalemia may occur. Antihypertensive effect of ACE-inhibitors is augmented by antihypertensive agents which cause renin release, such as thiazide diuretics. Lithium toxicity, with co-administration due to ↓ renal elimination of lithium due to ↓ aldosterone secretion or ↓ renal function.
Angiotensin II AT₁ Receptor Blockers (ARB)					
Atacand Losartan Telmisartan Valsartan	Antagonizes angiotensin II by blocking the angiotensin type 1 (AT₁) receptor. Angiotensin II AT₁ receptor blockers act selectively on AT₁, the receptor subtype that mediates the known cardiovascular actions of angiotensin II, the primary vaso-active hormone of the renin-angiotensin-system.	Hypertension; congestive heart failure, left-ventricular dysfunction and post-myocardial infarction (in ACE-inhibitor intolerant patients); diabetic nephropathy.	Atacand 8-32 mg/day orally given once daily or BID Losartan 25-100 mg/day orally given once daily or BID Telmisartan 20-80 mg/day orally given once daily or BID Valsartan 80-320 mg/day orally given once daily	Similar to ACE-inhibitors. No drug-induced cough.	Similar to ACE-inhibitors.

(Continued next page.)

Drug	Mechanism of Action	Indication	Dosage	Common Side-Effects	Common Drug Interactions
3-hydroxy-3methylglutaryl Coenzyme A (HMG-CoA) Reductase Inhibitors (Statins)					
Atorvastatin Pravastatin Rosuvastatin Simvastatin	Blocks hepatic synthesis of cholesterol by inhibiting HMG CoA reductase-mediated conversion of HMG CoA to mevalonic acid, an early precursor of cholesterol. This leads to a compensatory ↑ in the number of low-density lipoprotein (LDL) receptors, principally in the liver, that play a role in clearance of LDL from plasma and reduction of VLDL assembly and secretion, leading to a ↓ in LDL production.	Management of dyslipidemias; CV event risk reduction	Atorvastatin 10-80 mg orally once daily Pravastatin 10-40 mg orally once daily Rosuvastatin 5-40 mg orally once daily *(5 mg/d max. dose recommended in U.S. product monograph for patients on cyclosporine; contraindicated with cyclosporine in Canada) Simvastatin 10-80 mg orally once daily *(10 mg/d max. dose recommended in U.S. product monograph for patients on cyclosporine)	Gastrointestinal problems (abdominal pain/cramps, constipation, diarrhea, flatulence, nausea vomiting, heartburn), headache, dizziness, rash, pruritus, arthralgias, myalgias, ↑ creatine kinase (CK), ↑ liver transaminases.	CYP3A4 inhibitors and substrates (amiodarone, clarithromycin, cyclosporine, diltiazem, erythromycin, grapefruit juice, itraconazole, ketoconazole) lead to ↑ plasma concentrations of atorvastatin and simvastatin due to ↓ metabolism potentially resulting in ↑ myopathy. Rifampin ↓ plasma levels of statins secondary to induction of CYP2C9 and CYP3A4. Additive pharmacodynamic interaction with drugs that possess inherent myotoxic potential such as fibric acid derivatives and niacin.

e) predictable metabolic, gastrointestinal and cardiovascular complications associated with immunosuppressive therapy

f) appropriate prophylactic and treatment pharmacotherapeutic strategies for each transplant organ program

REFERENCES

1. Pirsch JD, Miller J, Deierhoi MH, Vincenti F, et al. for the FK506 Kidney Transplant Study Group. A comparison of tacrolimus (FK506) and cyclosporine for immunosuppression after cadaveric renal transplantation. *Transplantation*, 1997; 63: 977-983.

2. Vincenti F, and the Tacrolimus Kidney Transplant Study Group. Tacrolimus (FK506) in kidney transplantation: Five-year survival results of the U.S. multicenter, randomized, comparative trial. *Transplant Proc*, 2001; 33: 1019-1020.

3. Mayer AD, Dmitrewski J, Squifflet JP, et al. for the European Tacrolimus Multicenter Renal Study Group. Multicenter randomized trial comparing tacrolimus (FK506) and cyclosporine in the prevention of renal allograft rejection. *Transplantation*, 1997; 64: 436-443.

4. Mayer AD for the European Tacrolimus Multicentre Renal Study Group. Four-year follow-up of the European tacrolimus multicenter renal study. *Transplant Proc*, 1999; 31(Suppl 7A): 27S-28S.

5. U.S. Multicenter FK506 Liver Study Group. A comparison of tacrolimus (FK506) and cyclosporine for immunosuppression in liver transplantation. *N Engl J Med*, 1994; 331: 1110.

6. Wiesner RH for the U.S. FK506 Liver Study Group. A long-term comparison of tacrolimus (FK506) versus cyclosporine in liver transplantation. *Transplantation*, 1998; 66: 493-499.

7. Gruessner RW. Tacrolimus in pancreas transplantation: A multicenter analysis. Tacrolimus Pancreas Transplant Study Group. *Clin Transplant*, 1997; 11: 299-312.

8. Bechstein WO, Malaise J, Saudek F, et al. for the EuroSPK Study Group. Efficacy and safety of tacrolimus compared with cyclosporine microemulsion in primary simultaneous pancreas-kidney transplantation: 1-year results of a large multicenter trial. *Transplantation*, 2004; 77: 1221-1228.

9. Johnson RWG, Kreis H, Oberbauer R, et al. Sirolimus allows early cyclosporine withdrawal in renal transplantation resulting in improved renal function and lower blood pressure. *Transplantation*, 2001; 72: 777-786.

10. Oberbauer R, Kreis H, Johnson R, et al. Long-term improvement in renal function with sirolimus after early cyclosporine withdrawal in renal transplant recipients: 2-year results of the Rapamune maintenance regimen study. *Transplantation*, 2003; 76: 364-370.

11. Kreis H, Cisterne JM, Land W, et al. Sirolimus in association with mycophenolate mofetil induction for the prevention of acute graft reduction in renal allograft recipients. *Transplantation*, 2000; 69: 1252-1260.

12. Flechner SM, Goldfarb D, & Modlin C. Kidney transplantation without calcineurin inhibitor drugs: A prospective, randomized trial of sirolimus versus cyclosporine. *Transplantation*, 2002; 74: 1070-1076.

13. Flechner SM, Friend PJ, Brockmann J, et al. Alemtuzumab induction and sirolimus plus mycophenolate mofetil maintenance for CNI and steroid-free kidney transplant immunosuppression. *Am J Transplant*, 2005; 5: 3009-3014.

14. Grinyo JM, Gil-Vernet S, Cruzado JM, et al. Calcineurin inhibitor free immunosuppression based on antithymocyte globulin and mycophenolate mofetil in cadaveric kidney transplantation: Results after 5 years. *Transpl Int*, 2003; 16: 820-827.

15. Neoral® {Package Insert}. East Hanover, NJ: Novartis Pharmaceutical Corp.; 2004.

16. Prograf® (tacrolimus) in Heart Transplantation: Annotated PI. Deerfield, IL: Astellas Pharma U.S., Inc.; 2006.

17. Cole E, Maham N, Cardella C, et al. Clinical benefits of Neoral C2 monitoring in the long-term management of renal transplant recipients. *Transplantation*, 2003; 75: 2086-2090.

18. Nickeleit V, Hirshch HH, Zeiler M, et al. BK-virus nephropathy in renal transplants: Tubular necrosis, MHC-Class II expression and rejection in a puzzling game. *Nephrol Dial Transplant*, 2000; 15: 3324-3332.

19. Johnson C, Ahsan N, Gonwa T, et al. Randomzied trial of tacrolimus (Prograf) in combination with azathioprine or mycophenolate mofetil versus cyclosporine (Neoral) with mycophenolate mofetil after cadaveric renal transplantation. *Transplantation,* 2000; l69: 834-841.

20. Gonwa T, Johnson C, Ashan N, et al. Randomized trial of tacrolimus + mycophenolate mofetil or azathioprine versus cyclosporine + mycophenolate mofetil after cadaveric kidney transplantation: Results at three years. *Transplantation*, 2003; 75: 2048-5.

21. Ahsan N, Johnson C, Gonwa T, et al. Randomized trial of tacrolimus plus mycophenolate mofetil or azathioprine versus cyclosporine oral solution (modified) plus mycophenolate mofetil after cadaveric kidney transplantation: Results at 2 years. *Transplantation*, 2001; 72: 245-250.

22. Chan L, Gaston R, & Hariharan S. Evolution of immunosuppression and continued importance of acute rejection in renal transplantation. *Am J Kid Dis,* 2001; 38: S2-S9.

23. Meier-Kriesche HU, Li S, Gruessner RWG, et al. Immunosuppresson: Evolution in practice and trends, 1994-2004. *Am J Transplant*, 2006; 6: 1111-1131.

24. Salvadori M, Holzer H, de Mattos H, et al. Enteric-coated mycophenolate sodium is therapeutically equivalent to mycophenolate mofetil in de novo renal transplant patients. *Am J Transplant,* 2004; 4: 231-236.

25. Budde K, Curtis J, Knoll G, et al. Enteric-coated mycophenolate sodium can be safely administered in maintenance renal transplant patients: Results of a 1-year study. *Am J Transplant,* 2004; 4: 237-243.

26. *Imuran®* {Package Insert}. San Diego, CA: Prometheus Laboratories Inc.; 2003.

27. *Cellcept®* {Package Insert}. Nutley, NJ: Roche Pharmaceuticals; 2003.

28. *Myfortic®* {Package Insert}. East Hanover, NJ: Novartis Pharmaceutical Corp.; 2004.

29. van Gelder T, Shaw LM. The rationale for and limitations of therapeutic drug monitoring for mycophenolate mofetil in transplantation. *Transplantation*, 2005; 80: S244-S253.

30. Sollinger HW, for the U.S. renal transplant mycophenolate mofetil study group. Mycophenolate mofetil for the prevention of acute rejection in primary cadaveric renal allograft recipients. *Transplantation*, 1995; 60: 225-232.

31. Tomlanovich S, and the U.S. renal transplant mycophenolate mofetil study group. Mycophenolate mofetil in cadaveric renal transplantation. *Am J Kid Dis*, 1999; 34: 296-303.

32. Tricontinental Mycophenolate Mofetil Renal Transplantation Study Group. A blinded, randomized clinical trial of mycophenolate mofetil for the prevention of acute rejection in cadaveric renal transplantation. *Transplantation*, 1996; 61: 1029-1037.

33. Behrend M, and the European Mycophenolate Mofetil Cooperative Study Group. Mycophenolate mofetil in renal transplantation: 3-year results from the placebo-controlled trial. *Transplantation*, 1999; 68: 391-396.

34. European Mycophenolate Mofetil Cooperative Study Group. Placebo-controlled study of mycophenolate mofetil combined with cyclosporine and corticosteroids for prevention of acute rejection. *Lancet*, 1995; 1: 1321-1325.

35. Remuzzi G, Lesti M, Gotti E, et al. Mycophenolate mofetil versus azathioprine for the prevention of acute rejection in renal transplantation (MYSS): A randomized trial. *Lancet*, 2004; 364: 503-512.

36. Merion R, Henry M, Melzer J, et al. Randomized prospective trial of mycophenolate mofetil versus azathioprine for prevention of acute renal allograft rejection after simultaneous kidney-pancreas transplantation. *Transplantation*, 2000; 70: 105-111.

37. Kobashigawa J, Miller L, Renlund D, et al. A randomized active-controlled trial of mycophenolate mofetil in heart transplant recipients. *Transplantation*, 1998; 66: 507-515.

38. Palmer SM, Baz MA, Sanders L, et al. Results of a randomized, prospective, multicenter trial of mycophenolate mofetil versus azathioprine in the prevention of acute lung allograft rejection. *Transplantation*, 2001; 12: 1772-1776.

39. Wiesner R, Rabkin J, Klintmalm G, et al. Randomized double-blind comparative study of mycophenolate mofetil and azathioprine in combination with cyclosporine and corticosteroids in primary liver transplant recipients. *Liver Transplant*, 2001; 7: 442-450.

40. Jain A, Kashyap R, Kramer D, et al. Prospective, randomized trial of tacrolimus and prednisone versus tacrolimus, prednisone, and mycophenolate mofetil: A complete report on 350 primary adult liver transplantations. *Transplant Proc*, 2001; 33: 1342-1344.

41. Kahan B. Efficacy of sirolimus compared with azathioprine for reduction of acute renal allograft rejection: A randomized multicentre study. *Lancet*, 2000; 356: 194-202.

42. MacDonald AS. A worldwide, Phase III, randomized, controlled, safety and efficacy study of sirolimus/cyclosporine regimen for the prevention of acute rejection in recipients of primary mismatched renal allografts. *Transplantation*, 2001; 71: 271-280.

43. *Rapamune*® {Package Insert}. Philadelphia, PA: Wyeth Pharmaceutical Corp.; 2004.

44. Ciancio G, Burke GW, Gaynor JJ, et al. A randomized long-term trial of tacrolimus/sirolimus versus tacrolimus/mycophenolate versus cyclosporine/sirolimus in renal transplantation: Three-year analysis. *Transplantation*, 2006; 81: 845-852.

45. Larson TS, Dean PG, Stegall MD, et al. Complete avoidance of calcineurin inhibitors in renal transplantation: A randomized trial comparing sirolimus and tacrolimus. *Am J Transplant*, 2006; 6: 514.

46. Meier-Kriesche HU, Schold JD, Srinivas TR, Howard RJ, et al. Sirolimus in combination with tacrolimus is associated with worse renal allograft survival compared to mycophenolate mofetil combined with tacrolimus. *Am J Transplant*, 2005; 5(9): 2273-2280.

47. Johnson RWG, Kreis H, Oberbauer R, et al. Sirolimus allows early cyclosporine withdrawal in renal transplantation resulting in improved renal function and lower blood pressure. *Transplantation*, 2001; 72: 777-786.

48. Kreis H, Oberbauer R, Campistol J, et al. Long-term benefits with sirolimus-based therapy after early cyclosporine withdrawal. *J Am Soc Nephrol*, 2004; 15: 809-817.

49. Oberbauer R, Kreis H, Johnson R, et al. Long-term improvement in renal function with sirolimus after early cyclosporine withdrawal in renal transplant recipients: 2-year results of the Rapamune maintenance regimen study. *Transplantation*, 2003; 76: 364-370.

50. Dean PG, Lund WJ, Larson TS, et al. Wound-healing complications after kidney transplantation: A prospective, randomized comparison of sirolimus and tacrolimus. *Transplantation*, 2004; 77: 1555-1561.

51. McTaggart RA, Tomlanovich S, Bostrom A, Roberts JP, et al. Comparison of outcomes after delayed graft function: Sirolimus-based versus other calcineurin-inhibitor sparing induction immunosuppression regimens. *Transplantation*, 2004; 78: 475-480.

52. Stallone G, Di Paolo S, Schena A, et al. Addition of sirolimus to cyclosporine delays the recovery from delayed graft function but does not affect 1-year graft function. *Journal of the American Society of Nephrology*, 2004; 15: 228-233.

53. MacDonald AS, Scarola J, Burke JT, & Zimmermann JJ. Clinical pharmacokinetics and therapeutic drug monitoring of sirolimus. *Clinical Therapeutics*, 2000; 22: B101-B121.

54. Champion L, Stern M, Israel-Biet D, et al. Brief communication: Sirolimus-associated pneumonitis: 24 cases in renal transplant recipient. *Ann Intern Med*, 2006; 144: 505-509.

55. Straathof-Galema L, Wetzels JF, Dijkman HB, Steenbergen EJ, et al. Sirolimus-associated heavy proteinuria in a renal transplant recipient: Evidence for

a tubular mechanism. *Am J Transplant,* 2006; 6: 429-433.

56. Webster A, Pankhurst T, Rinaldi F, Chapman JR, et al. Polyclonal and monoclonal antibodies for treating acute rejection episodes in kidney transplant recipients: A systematic review of randomized trial data. *Transplantation,* 2006; 81(7): 953-965.

57. Fishman JA & Rubin RH. Infection in organ-transplant recipients. *New J Med,* 1998; 338(24): 1741-1751.

58. Ross H, Hendry P, Dipchand A, et al. 2001 Canadian Cardiovascular Society consensus conference on cardiac transplantation. *Can J Cardiol,* 2003; 19: 620-654.

59. Preiksaitis JK, Brennan DC, Fishman J, & Allen U. Canadian Society of Transplantation consensus workshop on cytomegalovirus managment in solid organ transplantation final report. *Am J Transplant,* 2005; 5: 218-227.

60. Lindenfeld J, Page RL, Zolty R, et al. Drug therapy in the heart transplant recipient: Part III: Common medical problems. *Circulation,* 2005; 111: 113-117.

61. Chiu LM, Domagal BM, & Park JM. Management of opportunistic infections in solid-organ transplantation. *Prog Transplant,* 2004; 14: 114-129.

62. Avery K. Prophylactic strategies before solid organ transplantation. *Curr Opin Infect Dis,* 2004; 17: 353-356.

63. Slifkin M, Doron S, & Snydman DR. Viral prophylaxis in organ transplant patients. *Drugs,* 2004; 64: 2763-2792.

64. Baumann TJ. Pain Management. In JT DiPiro, RL Talbert, GC Yee, GR Matzke, et al. *Pharmacotherapy: A Pathophysiologic Approach,* 5th Edition. Toronto, ON: McGraw-Hill Medical Publishing Division; 2002. 1103-1117.

65. Gabardi S & Luu L. Nonprescription analgesics and their use in solid-organ transplantation: A review. *Prog Transplant,* 2004; 14: 182-190.

66. Baltar J, Ortega T, Ortega F, et al. Post-transplantation diabetes mellitus: Prevalence and risk factors. *Transplantation Proc,* 2005; 37: 3817-3818.

67. Marchetti P. New-onset diabetes after liver transplantation: From pathogenesis to management. *Liver Transpl,* 2005; 11: 612-620.

68. Canadian Pharmacists Association. Compendium of Pharmaceuticals and Specialties. *The Canadian Drug Reference for Health Professionals.* Ottawa, ON: Canadian Pharmacists Association; 2005.

69. MICROMEDEX® Healthcare Series Vol. 129.

70. Page RL, Miller GG, & Lindenfeld J. Drug therapy in the heart transplant recipient: Part IV: Drug-drug interactions. *Circulation,* 2005; 111: 230-239.

REVIEW QUESTIONS

1. Immunosuppressive agents can be classified under two major categories: antibodies and small molecular preparations. An example of a monoclonal antibody used in solid organ transplantation to control allograft rejection is:
   a. Alemtuzemab.
   b. Rapamycin.
   c. Tacrolimus.
   d. Anti-thymocyte globulin.

2. Immunosuppressive agents can be classified under two major categories: antibodies and small molecular preparations. An example of a polyclonal antibody used in solid organ transplantation to control allograft rejection is:
   a. Alemtuzemab.
   b. Rapamycin.
   c. Tacrolimus.
   d. Anti-thymocyte globulin.

3. Immunosuppressive agents can be classified under two major categories: antibodies and small molecular preparations. An example of an mTOR inhibitor used in solid organ transplantation to control allograft rejection is:
   a. Alemtuzemab.
   b. Rapamycin.
   c. Tacrolimus.
   d. Anti-thymocyte globulin.

4. Immunosuppressive agents can be classified under two major categories: antibodies and small molecular preparations. An example of a calcineurin inhibitor used in solid organ transplantation to control allograft rejection is:
   a. Alemtuzemab.
   b. Rapamycin.
   c. Tacrolimus.
   d. Anti-thymocyte globulin.

5. When given intra-operatively, prior to reperfusion, anti-thymocyte globulin has been shown to reduce the incidence of:
   a. Chronic allograft rejection.
   b. Immediate post-operative atelectasis.
   c. Delayed graft function.
   d. Post-transplant infectious complications on days 3-5.

6. Hypertension is the most common medical problem post-transplantation. The apparent cause of this complication has been associated with which of the following drugs?
   a. Steroids/prednisone
   b. Mycophenolate mofetil
   c. Cyclosporine
   d. Calcium channel blockers

7. Common side effects associated with prednisone include which of the following?
   a. Glucose intolerance, weight gain
   b. Osteoporosis, hyperlipidemia
   c. Cataracts, headaches
   d. A and B
   e. All of the above

8. Leukopenia and GI disturbances are seen commonly with which antiproliferative agent?
   a. Azathioprine
   b. Rapamycin
   c. Mycophenolate mofetil
   d. Alemtuzemab

9. Fluconazole acts to inhibit cytochrome p 450 clearance and is also a highly selective inhibitor of fungal infections. Due to its action on cytochrome p 450, fluconazole may cause increased toxicity of which of the following immunosuppressive drugs?
   a. Tacrolimus
   b. Cyclosporine
   c. Sirolimus
   d. All of the above
   e. A and B

10. mTOR inhibitors were developed for use with cyclosporine or tacrolimus. However, studies have demonstrated an increase in which of the following with the combination of sirolumus plus cyclosporine or tacrolimus?
    a. Hepatotoxicity
    b. Nephrotoxicity
    c. Bone marrow suppression
    d. Hypertension

5 Transplant Complications: Infectious Diseases

SANDRA A. CUPPLES

DEBI H. DUMAS-HICKS

LISA BURNAPP

INTRODUCTION

I. Infection after solid organ transplantation (SOT) is a significant problem that affects not only morbidity and mortality but also quality of life.
  A. The development of novel and more potent immunosuppressive medications poses a challenge to managing the delicate balance between rejection and infection.
  B. Bacterial and viral post-transplant infections now exceed rejection as a cause of hospitalization in many solid organ transplant populations.[1]

PRETRANSPLANT INFECTIOUS DISEASE EVALUATION OF THE CANDIDATE

I. Purpose of pretransplant screening: to identify:[2]
  A. Presence and treatment of occult active infection
  B. Preexisting or concurrent infections that may constitute a contraindication to transplantation
  C. Post-transplant prophylactic strategies
II. Infection history
  A. Review consists of:[3]
    1. Childhood infections (for example, measles, mumps, chicken pox, infectious mononucleosis)
    2. Adult infections (for example, malaria, sexually transmitted diseases, hepatitis, endemic mycoses, recurrent infections)
    3. Travel history
    4. Immunization history
    5. Psychosocial history: incarceration; risky behavior such as alcohol/drug abuse, tattoos, body piercings, multiple sexual partners; hobbies (for example, gardening)
    6. Environmental exposure: previous and current geographic environments (domestic, occupational and recreational); (for example, southwestern United States and northern Mexico: exposure to *Coccidioides immitis*; Southeast Asia: exposure to *Strongyloides stercoralis*)

7. Exposure to pets and wild animals
8. Potential for post-transplant infections: nutritional status, home environment
9. Dietary habits: source of drinking water, consumption of meat that is raw or undercooked, unpasteurized dairy products, seafood
10. Allergies to antimicrobial agents

B. Infectious disease evaluation (Table 5-1)[3]
C. See Table 5-2 for major organ-specific pretransplant infections.

TABLE 5-1

■ **Infectious Disease Evaluation**[3]

Physical examination	Nutritional status: cachexia, obesity Integumentary (skin lesions) Eyes, ears, nose, throat Respiratory (rales, rhonchi, breath sounds) Cardiac (rub, murmur, endocarditis) Gastrointestinal (diarrhea, bleeding, ulcers) Genitourinary (prostate examination, Papanicolaou test)

Bloodwork	Complete blood cell count with differential leukocyte count
	Complete metabolic panel
	Cytomegalovirus IgG and IgM antibodies
	Toxoplasma gondii IgG and IgM antibodies
	Herpes simplex virus I and II IgG and IgM antibodies
	Varicella zoster titers
	Epstein Barr virus IgG and IgM antibodies
	Serologic screening for syphilis (rapid plasma reagin test)
	Human immunodeficiency virus (HIV) 1 and 2
	Hepatitis A, B, and C
	Fungal antibody screen
	Lyme titers (if indicated)
	Risk factors for increased susceptibility to infection:
	    Glycosylated hemoglobin (if indicated)
	    Hemoglobin A_1C (if indicated)

Other	Chest radiograph Computed tomography scan (if indicated) CT scan of paranasal sinuses (particularly for patients with cystic fibrosis or a history of recurrent sinus infections) Abdominal ultrasound Tuberculin skin test; anergy panel Urinalysis and urine culture Stool culture (if indicated) Stool for ova and parasites (if indicated) Dental screening
Organ-specific	Heart transplantation: *Toxoplasma gondii* IgG and IgM antibodies Lung transplantation: Sputum cultures to detect colonization of respiratory tract by *Aspergillus* species, *Burkholderia cepacia*

TABLE 5-2
■ Major Organ-Specific Pretransplant Infections

Organ	Infection
Kidney	Infection in native kidneys
	Occult abscesses
	Infections related to dialysis access devices or catheters
	Urinary tract infections
Pancreas	Urinary tract infections, particularly in women
Liver	Intra-abdominal infections (for example, bacterial peritonitis)
	Aspiration pneumonia
	Catheter-related infections
Heart	Catheter-related infections
	Infections related to ventricular assist devices
	Pneumonia
Lung	Pneumonia
	Pulmonary bacterial or fungal colonization

From Cupples, SA. Infectious disease. In SA Cupples & L Ohler (Eds). *Transplantation Nursing Secrets.* Philadelphia: Hanley & Belfus, 2003; pp. 247-270.

PRETRANSPLANT IMMUNIZATIONS

I. Transplant recipients may have a suboptimal response to vaccinations; therefore, it is critical to update immunizations prior to transplantation.
II. Vaccination should be done as soon as possible because the immune response is decreased in patients with end-stage organ disease.
III. Recommended vaccinations:[3]
   A. Inactivated polio virus
   B. Tetanus-diphtheria toxoid
   C. Influenza (yearly)
   D. Pneumococcal
   E. Varicella (if nonimmune)
   F. Hepatitis B
   G. Hepatitis A (if nonimmune)
   H. *Haemophilus influenzae* type B (pediatric candidates)
   I. Measles-mumps-rubella (pediatric candidates)
   J. Meningococcal vaccine (particularly for patients entering college within the next 1-2 years)

INFECTIONS IN POTENTIAL DONORS

I. Infections can be transmitted from the donor to the recipient.
II. The infectious disease evaluation of the potential organ donor is similar to that of the potential transplant candidate.
   A. Information about a deceased donor may be limited by the family's knowledge of the donor's medical history (prior infections, immunizations, and unusual exposures to infection) and psychosocial history (residence in or travel to endemic areas, drug abuse, risky sexual behavior, incarceration).
   B. Donors are also screened for nosocomial infections such as methicillin-resistant *Staphylococcus aureus* or vancomycin-resistant enterococci.
   C. Timing of serologic testing: Ideally, testing should be done before the administration of blood products; it is often done pre- and post-transfusion.
      1. If serologic testing is done after the donor is transfused, the number of units transfused should be recorded.
   D. Transplantation of organs from donors with infectious disease
      1. Some transplant centers may accept organs from hepatitis C virus (HCV)-positive or HIV-positive donors for certain patients (for example, HCV-positive or HIV-positive candidates).

SOURCES OF POST-TRANSPLANT INFECTION

I. Exogenous
   A. Allograft
   B. Blood transfusions
   C. Environment
      1. Hospital-associated
      2. Community-acquired
II. Endogenous
   A. Reactivation of latent infection in recipient

PERIODS OF INCREASED RISK

I. Early postoperative period when immunosuppression doses are highest.
II. Any time immunosuppressant therapy is increased to treat rejection.

FACTORS ASSOCIATED WITH RISK FOR INFECTION[4]

I. Epidemiologic exposure in the hospital or the community
II. Current antimicrobial therapy
III. Net state of immunosuppression: the combined effect of all of the factors that determine the patient's susceptibility to infection:[5]
   A. Current immunosuppressants
      1. Number of immunosuppressant medications
      2. Doses of immunosuppressant medications

B. Concurrent infection that is due to immune-modulating viruses such as cytomegalovirus (CMV), Epstein-Barr virus (EBV), hepatitis B virus (HBV), hepatitis C virus (HCV), or HIV

C. Concurrent metabolic disorders (for example, malnutrition, diabetes mellitus [DM])

D. Concurrent neutropenia or lymphopenia

E. Disruption of normal endothelial or epithelial barriers

F. Post-transplant sequelae (for example, undrained fluid collections)

EXPOSURE TO INFECTION

I. Types of exposure within the hospital environment[5]

   A. Domiciliary: occurs on patient's hospital unit

      1. May result from contamination of air or water, person-to-person contact, or contaminated equipment

      2. Examples of pathogens:

         i. *Pseudomonas aeruginosa*

         ii. Vancomycin-resistant *Enterococcus faecium*

         iii. Methicillin-resistant *Staphylococcus aureus*

         iv. *Clostridium difficile*

   B. Nondomiciliary: occurs when a patient is exposed to contaminated air outside of the unit (for example, during transport to other areas of hospital)

      1. Example: *Aspergillus* infection acquired when patient is transported through construction area within hospital

II. Types of exposure within the community

   A. Respiratory viruses

   B. Food-borne pathogens

   C. Geographically restricted mycoses

POST-TRANSPLANT INFECTION TIMELINE

I. For all types of solid organ transplantation procedures, certain infections are more likely to appear at certain post-transplant intervals (Table 5-3).

II. Timing of opportunistic infections[3, 4, 6]

   A. Opportunistic infections typically occur after the first post-transplant month because the development of these infections is a function of both the *type* and *intensity* of immunosuppressive agents and the *duration* of immunotherapy.

CLINICAL MANIFESTATIONS OF INFECTION—GENERAL

I. Important clinical manifestations of infection include:[4, 7]

   A. Fever without localizing findings

   B. Fever with headache

   C. Central nervous system (CNS) changes, including changes in level of consciousness

   D. Unexplained skin lesions

TABLE 5-3

■ **Post-transplant Intervals of Infection**

Time Period	Type of Infection	Example
First month	Continuation of recipient's pre-transplant infection	*Pseudomonas aeruginosa* infections in lung transplant candidates with cystic fibrosis
	Infections related to the surgical procedure, other iatrogenic procedures, and indwelling lines and catheters	Anastomotic leaks, obstructions Lymphoceles Infection related to invasive lines, catheters[1]
	Transmission of infection by the donor allograft	Staphylococcus, streptococcus, *Pseudomonas* spp., *Salmonella* spp., *Aspergillus* spp., *Candida* spp. CMV, EBV, HHV-6, HSV, VZV, HTLV 1 and 2, HIV, HBV, HCV, mycobacteria, West Nile virus, rabies, Chagas' disease, Leishmania, toxoplasmosis, respiratory viruses[1]
	Early reactivation of latent viruses	Reactivation of herpes viruses
Months 2-6	Infections caused by opportunistic organisms or immunomodulating viruses	Reactivation of latent viral infections: CMV, EBV, HSV, VZV, HBV, HCV, BK polyomavirus[1]
After 6 months	Community-acquired infections similar to those in immunocompetent individuals	Upper respiratory tract infections caused by influenza virus, adenoviruses, etc. Chronic viral infection (HBV, HCV, EBV, papillomavirus, BK virus nephropathy) Recurrent *Clostridium difficile* colitis Recipients with poor allograft function are at increased risk for opportunistic infections[1]

Adapted from Cupples, SA. Infectious disease. In SA Cupples & L Ohler (Eds). *Transplantation Nursing Secrets*. Philadelphia: Hanley & Belfus, 2003; pp. 247-270.

CMV = cytomegalovirus; EBV = Epstein-Barr virus; HHV-6 = human herpes virus-6; HSV = herpes simplex virus; VZV = varicella zoster virus; HTLV = human T-cell lymphotropic virus; HIV = human immunodeficiency virus; HBV = hepatitis B virus; HCV = hepatitis C virus

    E. Febrile pneumonitis
II. Important characteristics of CNS infections include the following:[5, 8, 9]
    A. The signs of meningeal irritation may be masked by immunosuppressants.
    B. Changes in level of consciousness may be subtle.
    C. The most reliable indication of a CNS infection is the simultaneous presence of unexplained fever and headache.

1. Patients presenting with these manifestations should have an immediate and complete neurologic workup (CT scan or MRI imaging of brain; lumbar puncture [unless otherwise contraindicated]).

ETIOLOGY OF FEVER

I. Time since transplantation[7, 8]
   A. First post-transplant month
      1. Technical complications related to the surgery, indwelling catheters, etc.
      2. Allograft rejection
      3. Antilymphocyte therapy
   B. Months 2 to 6
      1. Viral infections (particularly CMV)
      2. Antilymphocyte therapy
   C. After 6 months
      1. Opportunistic infections
      2. Antilymphocyte therapy
II. Fever of unknown origin[4, 9-11]
   A. Infectious agents
      1. Systemic disease due to CMV or EBV
      2. Disseminated tuberculosis
      3. Histoplasmosis
      4. Cryptococcosis
      5. Systemic toxoplasmosis
      6. *Pneumocystis carinii* infection (early)
   B. Noninfectious causes
      1. Rejection (particularly in liver, kidney, and lung recipients)
      2. Organ ischemia due to infarction or poor perfusion
      3. Pulmonary emboli
      4. Deep vein thrombosis
      5. Drug reactions (antilymphocyte therapy, antibiotics)
      6. Malignancy

DIAGNOSIS OF POST-TRANSPLANT INFECTIONS

I. The diagnosis of post-transplant infections is difficult because:[4, 11]
   A. Immunosuppressive agents (particularly corticosteroids) may decrease the inflammatory response, resulting in:
      1. Masking of fevers and white blood cell count elevations
      2. False-negative skin tests and circulating antibody tests
   B. Certain infections may not be associated with the development of a fever (for example, undisseminated herpes simplex and herpes zoster infections).
   C. Fever may be associated with other phenomena such as rejection, drug reactions, pulmonary embolism, deep vein thrombosis.
II. Because typical diagnostic tests may lack sensitivity, more precise and advanced diagnostic tests are often used immediately for symptoms that initially seem benign and/or vague:[4]

    A. DNA probes

    B. Polymerase chain reaction (PCR)

    C. Antigen detection by monoclonal antibodies

    D. Computed tomography (CT)

    E. Magnetic resonance imaging

    F. Biopsies

III. Factors to consider in the diagnosis of post-transplant infections are shown in Table 5-4.

IV. General principles in diagnosing infection:[8, 12]

    A. Immunuotherapy alters the inflammatory response and mutes the clinical manifestations of infection.

    B. The most important determinants of survival are how quickly the diagnosis is made and pathogen-specific therapy is initiated; therefore, more sensitive and precise diagnostic tests (for example, CT scans) are often done in lieu of traditional diagnostic tests (for example, conventional radiography).

    C. The post-transplant infection timeline is useful in making a differential diagnosis.

TABLE 5-4

■ **Factors to Consider in Diagnosis of Post-transplant Infection**

Factor	Example
Pretransplant host factors	Age, nutritional status, comorbidities (e.g., diabetes mellitus), medications (e.g., steroid use), infection history (particularly infections that further suppress the immune system, such as CMV, EBV, HBV, HCV)
Preoperative factors	Invasive devices (e.g., intra-aortic balloon pump, assist devices, mechanical ventilation, hemodialysis)
Type of organ transplanted	Risk of infection greater for lung transplant recipients
Perioperative factors	Ischemic time, blood loss, transfusions
Donor factors	Donor CMV-seropositive, recipient CMV-seronegative
Immunosuppression regimen	Maintenance therapy (medications, doses, frequency), use of antilymphocyte therapy
Rejection history	Severity, treatment, and response to treatment
Current antimicrobial regimen (if any)	Use of prophylactic antiviral therapy to prevent CMV infection
Post-transplant exposure to nosocomial, community, or geographic sources of infection	Any recent hospitalizations, community outbreaks of infection, exposure to endemic fungi
Onset of symptoms	Bacterial infections usually manifest over a 24-48 hour time period, but they can evolve over several (3-5) days

Adapted from Cupples, SA. Infectious disease. In SA Cupples & L Ohler (Eds). *Transplantation Nursing Secrets.* Philadelphia: Hanley & Belfus, 2003; pp. 247-270.

D. Information from the recipient's self-monitoring records provides important clues and aids in triage.
   1. Information regarding signs (for example, temperature, blood pressure, blood glucose levels)
   2. Information regarding symptoms (for example, headache, rash, vomiting, diarrhea)
E. Because of the difficulty in establishing a diagnosis and the need for prompt treatment, transplant recipients are often hospitalized when infection is suspected, particularly if:[8, 10]
   1. There are chest infiltrates on chest radiography or CT.
   2. The patient has persistent fevers of 101° F (38.5° C) or higher.
   3. The patient appears toxic.
   4. The patient cannot perform activities of daily living.

MAJOR TYPES OF INFECTION

I. The major pathogens that cause infections in transplant recipients are listed in Table 5-5.

TABLE 5-5

■ **Major Pathogens That Cause Infection in Transplant Recipients**

Bacterial	Viral	Fungal	Parasitic
Enteric gram-negative bacteria	Cytomegalovirus	*Candida* species	*Toxoplasma gondii*
Pseudomonas aeruginosa	Epstein-Barr virus	*Aspergillus* species	*Cryptosporidium*
Legionella species	Herpes simplex virus	*Cryptococcus neoformans*	*Strongyloides stercoralis*
Nocardia asteroides	Varicella zoster virus	*Pneumocystis carinii*	
Listeria monocytogenes	Hepatitis B virus	*Coccidioides immitis*	
Salmonella species	Hepatitis C virus	*Histoplasma capsulatum*	
Mycobacterium tuberculosis	Human herpesvirus-6	*Blastomyces dermatitidis*	
Nontuberculous mycobacteria	Papillomavirus		
	Adenoviruses		
	Respiratory syncytial virus		
	Influenza virus		
	Enterovirus		
	Papovavirus		

Adapted from Cupples, SA. Infectious disease. In SA Cupples & L Ohler (Eds). *Transplantation Nursing Secrets*. Philadelphia: Hanley & Belfus, 2003; pp. 247-270.

VIRAL INFECTIONS

I. Overview
   A. Most viral infections in transplant recipients are caused by:
      1. Herpes viruses (CMV, EBV, HSV 1 and 2, and varicella zoster)
      2. Hepatitis viruses
   B. Clinical sequelae
      1. Direct effects: Clinical syndrome associated with the virus (for example, pneumonia, hepatitis)
      2. Indirect effects:
         a. Alteration in the net state of immunosuppression and increased susceptibility to opportunistic infections
         b. Potential allograft injury
         c. Potential oncogenesis[13]
   C. Herpes viruses
      1. Characterized by latency: once the virus is present, the individual will always harbor the viral genome.
      2. Replication of latent herpes viruses can be triggered by immunosuppression.
      3. Herpes viruses: "infection" versus "disease"
         a. The term "infection" refers to the presence of viral replication as indicated by cultures or serological testing.
         b. The term "disease" indicates that the patient has specific symptoms that are caused by a herpes virus. Viremia and tissue invasion are evidence of disease.[4, 5]

II. Cytomegalovirus
   A. Overview
      1. CMV commonly occurs after the first post-transplant month[3] and is the most important pathogen that affects transplant recipients.
      2. Over the course of the first post-transplant year, over 50% of transplant recipients demonstrate evidence of CMV viral replication.[14]
      3. Most adults develop CMV infection at some time during their lifespan and the CMV virus persists in a latent stage following the acute phase of the infection.[3]
   B. Effects of CMV[3, 4]
      1. Direct effects: infection, tissue injury, and clinical disease
         a. Infection: "isolation of the CMV virus or detection of viral proteins or nucleic acid in any body fluid or tissue specimen"[15, p. 1094]
         b. CMV disease (Table 5-6)[15]
      2. Indirect effects: opportunistic infections, allograft injury, rejection
   C. Bidirectional relationship between CMV and rejection
      1. CMV can trigger rejection.
      2. Inflammation associated with rejection (and rejection therapy) can increase CMV viral replication.
   D. Organ-specific effects on allograft: The allograft is more likely to be affected by CMV than a native organ.
      1. Liver: vanishing bile duct syndrome
      2. Heart: coronary artery vasculopathy
      3. Lung: bronchiolitis obliterans
      4. Kidney: glomerulopathy

TABLE 5-6

■ **Types of CMV Disease**[15]

Type	Definition: Combination of
Pneumonia	Signs and/or symptoms of pulmonary disease and detection of CMV in fluid obtained from bronchoalveolar lavage or from tissue samples
Gastrointestinal disease	Clinical symptoms (upper or lower gastrointestinal tract) and endoscopy-detected macroscopic mucosal lesions and detection of CMV infection in tissue obtained from gastrointestinal tract biopsy
Hepatitis	↑ bilirubin and/or liver enzymes and absence of any other documented etiology of hepatitis and detection of CMV infection in tissue obtained from liver biopsy
Central nervous system	Central nervous system symptoms and detection of CMV in cerebrospinal fluid or in tissue obtained from brain biopsy
Nephritis	In patient with renal dysfunction: detection of CMV infection and histological identification of CMV in tissue obtained from kidney biopsy
Cystitis	In patient with cystitis: detection of CMV infection and histological identification of CMV in tissue obtained from bladder biopsy
Myocarditis	In patient with myocarditis: detection of CMV infection and histological identification of CMV in tissue obtained from heart biopsy
Pancreatitis	In patient with pancreatitis: detection of CMV infection and histological identification of CMV in tissue obtained from biopsy of pancreas tissue

E. Epidemiological patterns[3, 16]

1. Primary infection: CMV-seronegative recipient receives cells that are latently infected with CMV from a CMV-seropositive donor; viral replication ensues.
   a. Compared with reactivation infection and superinfection (below), primary CMV infections have:
      i. Higher rates of CMV infection, symptomatic disease, and recurrence
      ii. Higher mortality rates
      iii. Earlier onset post-transplant
      iv. Increased risk of disseminated disease[17]
2. Reactivation infection: Recipient is CMV-seropositive and endogenous latent virus reactivates.
   a. An inflammatory process or stress can promote reactivation (for example, rejection, antilymphocyte therapy, sepsis).[12]
3. Superinfection: CMV-seropositive recipient receives an allograft from a CMV-seropositive donor and the strain of CMV virus that reactivates is from the donor.

F. Risk factors for CMV disease
   1. CMV serology (Table 5-7)[3]
   2. Incidence of CMV by type of allograft is shown in Table 5-8.[3]
G. Recipients at highest risk for CMV infection
   1. CMV-seronegative recipients who received allografts from CMV-seropositive donors.
   2. CMV-seropositive recipients who are given antithymocyte globulin, antilymphocyte globulin, or muromonab-CD3 as rejection therapy.[14]
H. CMV prevention: prophylaxis versus preemptive therapy[18]
   1. Prophylaxis: administration of antiviral agent to *all* recipients
   2. Preemptive therapy: administration of antiviral agent to a select group of recipients who are at high risk for developing CMV as evidenced by microbiological markers.
      a. Preemptive therapy has been shown to reduce the risk of CMV disease.[19]
I. Ganciclovir-resistant CMV
   1. Often a late-onset complication of solid organ transplantation[20]
      a. Median onset, lung transplantation: 4.4 months[21]
      b. Median onset, non-lung transplantation: 10 months[22]
   2. Risk factors:
      a. Serostatus: recipient CMV-seronegative and donor CMV-seropositive[22]
      b. High CMV viral load[23]
      c. Potent immunosuppression[22]
      d. Multiple episodes of CMV disease[20]
      e. Prolonged CMV prophylaxis with oral ganciclovir[22, 23]
      f. Suboptimal antiviral drug concentration[20]

TABLE 5-7

■ **CMV Serology[3]**

Risk Level	Serology	Comment
High	Donor +, Recipient -	Up to 60% of recipients in this group will develop CMV infection.
	Patients who receive antilymphocyte therapy as induction or treatment for rejection	Increases the risk of CMV disease in CMV-seropositive recipients
Moderate	Donor +, Recipient + Donor -, Recipient +	Incidence of CMV disease in this group is 20% to 40%.
Low	Donor -, Recipient -	On rare occasions, recipients in this group may develop primary CMV infection from community exposure or after receiving blood products that have not been screened for CMV or properly administered.

TABLE 5-8

■ **Incidence of CMV[3]**

Level of Risk	Type of Allograft
High	Lung
	Small bowel
Intermediate	Liver
	Pancreas
	Heart
Low	Kidney

      g. Type of solid organ transplant procedure: in descending order (highest to lowest risk):[21, 24-26]
         i.   Kidney/pancreas
         ii. Lung
         iii. Heart and kidney
         iv. Liver
   3. Indications that CMV strain may be resistant:[26]
      a. Patient shows no significant improvement or resolution of symptoms after a 14-day course of full-dose IV ganciclovir.
      b. There is no decrease in viral load after a 14-day course of full-dose IV ganciclovir.
  J. See Table 5-9 for the clinical manifestations, prevention/prophylaxis, diagnosis, and treatment of CMV.
III. Epstein-Barr virus (EBV)
  A. Overview
    1. Because approximately 90% of adults are EBV-seropositive, the majority of EBV infections in transplant recipients are reactivation infections.[20]
      a. EBV latency occurs because the virus establishes a persistent infection in B-cells.
      b. In immunocompetent individuals, this persistent infection is optimally controlled by EBV-specific cytotoxic T-lymphocytes.
      c. In immunocompromised individuals, the cytotoxic T-lymphocyte response is impaired, thus increasing the potential for EBV-driven B-cell proliferation.
    2. EBV-seronegative recipients can acquire primary EBV infection from the:
      a. Community
      b. Allograft
      c. Blood transfusions
    3. Incidence:
      a. EBV replication occurs in approximately 20% to 30% of all solid organ transplant recipients and in 80% of recipients who receive antilymphocyte antibody therapy.[18]
      b. Reactivation infections occur in approximately 30% to 40% of EBV-seropositive recipients.[8]

TABLE 5-9

■ **Major Organisms Causing Post-transplant Infection: Clinical Manifestations, Prevention/Prophylaxis, Diagnostic Tests, and Treatment Options**

Organism	May Cause	Clinical Manifestations	Prophylaxis/Preemptive Therapy	Diagnostic Tests	Treatment Options
CMV	CMV syndrome Tissue invasive disease: Gastroenteritis Myocarditis Pneumonitis Retinitis (rare) Encephalitis (rare) Pancreatitis (rare)	CMV syndrome: Fever Fatigue Malaise Leukopenia Thrombocytopenia Elevated LFTs Gastroenteritis: Anorexia, dysphagia Abdominal cramping Nausea, vomiting, diarrhea Ulceration, bleeding Pneumonitis: Fever Dyspnea[10,70-72]	CMV-negative, filtered, or leukocyte-poor blood products Ganciclovir Acyclovir Valacyclovir CMV hyperimmune globulin Unselected immunoglobulin Preemptive therapy for patients at high risk (e.g., IV ganciclovir during anti-lymphocyte antibody therapy)[14,70,71] Most commonly used agents: Valganciclovir Ganciclovir[18] Duration of prophylaxis: Range: 3-12 months post-transplant[18]	Serologic: Complement fixing assay Immuno-fluorescence ELISA Latex agglutination systems Virologic: Antigenemia assay Quantitative polymerase chain reaction Tissue culture Biopsy[3,9,71] Definitions:[15] Viremia: isolation of CMV by culture (standard techniques or shell viral techniques) Antigenemia: CMV pp65 detected in leukocytes DNAemia: CMV DNA detected in plasma, whole blood, isolated peripheral blood leukocytes, or buffy-coat specimens RNAemia: CMV RNA detected in plasma, whole blood, isolated peripheral blood leukocytes, or buffy-coat specimens	IV Ganciclovir followed by oral ganciclovir CMV hyperimmune globulin for tissue-invasive disease[18] Immunoglobulin For ganciclovir-resistant organisms: Foscarnet Ganciclovir + Foscarnet Foscarnet followed by cidofivir Intravenous immune globulin (IVIG) CMV hyperimmune globulin[18,26,70,71]

Organism	May Cause	Clinical Manifestations	Prophylaxis/Preemptive Therapy	Diagnostic Tests	Treatment Options
Epstein-Barr	Mononucleosis PTLD: nodal or extranodal disease of CNS, GI tract, lungs or bone marrow[29]	Mononucleosis: Lymph node hyperplasia Splenomegaly Atypical mononuclear leukocytes Abnormal LFTs Fever Sore throat PTLD: Mononucleosis-like syndrome Weight loss Fever of unknown origin Abdominal pain Anorexia Jaundice Bowel perforation GI bleeding Renal and hepatic dysfunction Pneumothorax Pulmonary infiltrates CNS findings (seizures, altered LOC) Allograft involvement[9,28]	Preemptive therapy for patients at high risk (e.g., IV ganciclovir during antilymphocyte antibody therapy)[9]	Mononucleosis: CBC EBV antibody LFTs Heterophil agglutination antibody test PTLD: CT scan: Note: absence of adenopathy does not rule out PTLD; disease can be entirely extranodal[9] Tissue biopsy	Mononucleosis: Acyclovir PTLD: benign polyclonal polymorphic B-cell hyperplasia: Acyclovir Ganciclovir Decreased immunosuppression (possibly) PTLD: early malignant polyclonal polymorphic B-cell lymphoma: Acyclovir Ganciclovir Interferon-α Gamma globulin Anti-B-cell antibodies (anti-CD 20) Decreased immunosuppression (possibly) PTLD: monoclonal polymorphic B-cell lymphoma: Chemotherapy Radiation Resection Decreased immunosuppression[9,18,28]

(Continued next page.)

Organism	May Cause	Clinical Manifestations	Prophylaxis/Preemptive Therapy	Diagnostic Tests	Treatment Options
Herpes simplex 1 / Herpes simplex 2	Herpes labialis Herpetic esophagitis Anogenital lesions Visceral infection is rare[29]	HSV 1: Crusted ulcerations Verrucous lip lesions HSV-2: Coalescing ulcerations without clear-cut vesicles[9]	Acyclovir (low-dose) Ganciclovir (has low oral bioavailability) Valacyclovir Famciclovir[3, 18] Duration of prophylaxis: typically 30–90 days[18]	Viral culture Direct immunofluorescence studies Tzanck smear[3, 9, 28]	Acyclovir* Ganciclovir Valacyclovir Famciclovir Foscarnet for resistant strains *Adjust dose according to renal function[3, 18, 73]
Varicella zoster	Localized dermatomal zoster Disseminated infection	Localized dermatomal zoster that involves 2 or 3 adjoining dermatomes without visceral involvement (viral reactivation) Primary, disseminated infection: associated with hemorrhagic pneumonia, skin lesions, encephalitis, hepatitis, pancreatitis, and disseminated intravascular coagulation[9]	Seronegative recipients with significant exposure (same room contact with diagnosed case of chicken pox or direct contact with skin lesion of shingles)[74] Varicella zoster hyperimmune globulin within 72 hours of significant exposure IV acyclovir within 24 hours of eruption of skin rash	Characteristic unilateral vesicular lesions VZV antibody titer Tzanck smear Direct immunofluorescence studies	Localized infection: Acyclovir (oral) Famciclovir (oral) Valcyclovir (oral)[3, 73] Disseminated infection: Acyclovir (IV; high-dose) VZV immune globulin for VZV-seronegative recipients within 72 hours of exposure to VZV[18, 28, 29]
HHV-6	Bone marrow suppression Encephalitis Interstitial pneumonitis	Fever Malaise Rash Bone marrow dysfunction[9]	None at present	Serologic testing PCR assay	Ganciclovir Foscarnet[29]
Hepatitis viruses	Acute or chronic hepatitis Cirrhosis	Recurrent HBV infection: + HbsAg (typically 2 to 6 months post-transplant) Hepatocellular symptoms that can range from mild hepatitis to fulminant liver failure HCV: chronic hepatitis[28]	HBV vaccine for nonimmune transplant candidates Perioperative anti-HBV immune globulin for liver transplant candidates with HBV infection	HBV: Serologic testing HCV: Detection of HCV-RNA by reverse transcriptase PCR Liver biopsy	HBV: Immune globulin HCV: Interferon + ribavirin[12]

Organism	May Cause	Clinical Manifestations	Prophylaxis/Preemptive Therapy	Diagnostic Tests	Treatment Options
Polyoma-virus: BK virus	Tubulointerstitial nephritis Ureteral stenosis Obstructive nephropathy Progressive graft dysfunction Graft loss[3]	Fever Persistent hematuria Elevated serum creatinine level[34]		Plasma and urine assays: detection of virus DNA by PCR Urine cytology: detection of characteristic "decoy" cells Immunohistochemistry Tissue biopsy (gold standard) May be difficult to differentiate virus infection from rejection; definitive diagnosis requires visualization of polyomavirus inclusion bodies in biopsy specimen[34]	Decrease immunosuppression Agents under investigation:[35,75] Cidofovir Leflunomide Quinolone antibiotics IVIG Supportive care[3,34]
Polyoma-virus: JC virus	Multifocal demyelination in brain Progressive neurologic deficits	May involve cerebral cortex, brain stem, or cerebellum[38,76] Cortical syndromes: Visual deficits (hemianopsia) Hemiparesis Frontal lobe dementia Brain stem lesions: Contralateral hemiparesis or hemisensory deficits Unilateral lesions: Clumsiness Limb incoordination Midline lesions: Imbalance, falls Disequilibrium Gait disturbance Cerebellar lesions: Blurred vision Dysarthria Classic triad: dementia, hemiparesis, hemianopsia		MRI of head CT scan EEG PCR analysis of spinal blood and spinal fluid Biopsy of brain with *in situ* hybridization for JC virus[38,76]	Decrease immunosuppression Corticosteroid therapy Nucleoside analogs: interfere with DNA synthesis: Cytosine arabinoside Adenosine arabinoside Iododeoxyuridine Zidovudine Interferons: stimulate natural killer cells[38,76] Nucleoside analogs: interfere with DNA synthesis: Cytosine arabinoside Adenosiine arabinoside Iododeoxyuridine Zidovudine

(Continued next page.)

Organism	May Cause	Clinical Manifestations	Prophylaxis/Preemptive Therapy	Diagnostic Tests	Treatment Options
Respiratory syncytial virus	Upper respiratory infection Lower respiratory tract disease Organ rejection Bronchiolitis obliterans[42]	Rhinorrhea Sinus congestion Otalgia Nausea; abdominal pain Cough Dyspnea Fever > 100.4° F (38° C) Wheezing, rales, rhonchi Infiltrates on chest radiograph Sinusitis on sinus radiograph[43]	Aggressive infection control measures Aerosolized ribavirin IVIG[42]	Antigen detection by immunofluorescence assay Antigen detection by immunoassay RNA detection by reverse transcription PCR Serology: Demonstration of RSV-IgM antibody (acute infection) Significant increase in RSV-IgG antibody between acute- and convalescent-stage sera Culture: less sensitive and specific in adult population versus pediatric population[43]	Aerosolized ribavirin IVIG[42] RSV pneumonitis: Aerosolized ribavirin Palivizumab (RSV monoclonal antibody) plus aerosolized ribavirin
Influenza virus	Influenza syndrome Secondary bacterial complications	Fever Chills Rigors Cough (typically nonproductive) Sore throat Fatigue Headache Myalgia[77]	Aggressive infection control measures Annual vaccination of patients and household contacts (unless otherwise contraindicated) Annual vaccination of health care workers	History and clinical examination Detection of virus-infected cells (via nasopharyngeal washing or respiratory secretions) with specific fluorescent-labeled antibody probes[40]	Influenza A: Early administration of: Amantadine Rimantadine Influenza B: Olsetamivir* Zanamivir *If started within 36–48 hours of symptom onset[40]
Para-influenza virus	Can cause mild upper respiratory disease May progress to pneumonia[40]	May mimic influenza[40]	No definitive recommendations	Viral isolation Viral shell assays Rapid antigen detection	Ribavirin has been used for lower respiratory tract disease[42]

Organism	May Cause	Clinical Manifestations	Prophylaxis/Preemptive Therapy	Diagnostic Tests	Treatment Options
Corona-virus	Asymptomatic or mild respiratory illness that may progress to fatal respiratory failure (SARS)[40]	Fever > 100.4° F (38° C) Chills Headache Myalgia Cough Shortness of breath Dyspnea Hypoxia Lymphopenia Thrombocytopenia Mild ↑ in transaminases[40]	No definitive recommendations	Chest radiograph (evidence of pneumonia or adult respiratory distress syndrome) Detection of viral RNA by real-time reverse transcription PCR Detection of acute and convalescent antibodies to SARS by enzyme immunoassay[40]	Supportive care Empiric antimicrobial agents Intravenous administration of ribavirin* Corticosteroids* *Investigational[40]
Parvovirus B19	Severe, refractory anemia Pancytopenia Thrombotic microangiopathy Fibrosing cholestatic hepatitis Graft dysfunction[40]	Chronic anemia ↓ platelets ↓ white blood cell count Fever Malaise Pancytopenia[39]	No definitive recommendations	Detection of parvovirus B19 DNA in serum by PCR assay[40]	High-dose IVIG ↓ in immunosuppression Discontinuing tacrolimus (if possible)[40]
Human papilloma-virus	Cutaneous warts Anogenital warts Carcinoma of cervix and bladder Squamous cell carcinoma Anogenital carcinoma[40]	Warts Cutaneous Urogenital Anal Squamous cell carcinoma that arises in beds of flat warts[39]	Avoidance of excessive sun exposure and ultraviolet light Sun precautions Sunscreen with high sun protection factor (≥ 15)	Tissue biopsy	Topical keratolytic agents Caustic agents Topical retinoids Oral retinoids Podophyllin, 5-fluorouracil Bleomycin Ablation[40] Carcinoma (skin, cervix, urinary tract): Resection Reduction or withdrawal of immunosuppression Radiation Chemotherapy[39]

(Continued next page.)

Organism	May Cause	Clinical Manifestations	Prophylaxis/Preemptive Therapy	Diagnostic Tests	Treatment Options
Listeria monocytogenes	Bacteremia Meningitis Meningioencephalitis Myocarditis Cerebritis without meningitis[9,74] Less common manifestations: Pneumonia Arthritis Endophthalmitis Endocarditis Peritonitis Myocarditis Hepatitis[3]	Fever (1-5 days) Headache Decreased LOC Focal neurological deficits Meningismus Nuchal rigidity Spinal fluid: neutrophils, lymphocytes; glucose may be normal Abdominal cramps, diarrhea Seizures[3,9,10]	TMP-SMZ Dietary precautions regarding milk, cheeses, undercooked meats and uncooked vegetables[9,63,74]	Blood, sputum cultures CT scan MRI CSF cell count, Gram stain, culture, and protein and sugar determination Note: Organism may be confused with diphtheroids in Gram stain smears of pus or sputum Diagnosis confirmed by isolation of *Listeria monocytogenes* from culture of blood, CSF, or other sterile source[3]	Treatment of choice: ampicillin + aminoglycoside[3] Meningial doses of penicillin or ampicillin Gentamicin TMP-SMZ for penicillin-allergic patients[9,10]
Nocardia	Pulmonary and extrapulmonary infection (CNS, skin, and bone)[10,74]	Subacute onset is typical Subacute symptoms: Fever Cough Chest pain Pulmonary nodules, abscesses, cavitating lesions, infiltrates, effusions[10]	TMP-SMZ[63] Typical pneumocystis pneumonia prophylaxis with TMP-SMZ offers some protection[3]	Cultures: sputum, BAL fluid Gram stain Modified acid-fast stain[10] Diagnosis confirmed by presence of *Nocardia* species in culture[3]	Sulfonamides preferred[3] Sulfasoxazole TMP-SMZ Amikacin Imipenem Third generation cephalosporins Minocycline Linezolid Isolated pulmonary infection: 3-6 months of therapy Disseminated disease: 12 months of therapy[10]

Organism	May Cause	Clinical Manifestations	Prophylaxis/Preemptive Therapy	Diagnostic Tests	Treatment Options
Legionella	Pneumonia	Fever, chills Focal pulmonary infiltrate Headache Confusion Minimally productive cough Diarrhea Chest pain Malaise Dyspnea[3, 8]	Routine culture of hospital water supply Water treatment to control nosocomial infection	Cultures: sputum, BAL fluid Direct fluorescent antibody stain of respiratory secretions Urinary antigen detection: can only detect serogroup 1 of *Legionella pneumophila* species Fine needle aspiration of lung Open lung biopsy[10, 78] Chest radiograph: Dense infiltrates (unilateral or bilateral) that may → cavitation[3] Diagnosis confirmed by: *Legionella* antigen in urine Direct fluorescent antibody stain (respiratory secretions or tissue biopsy) Culture of lower respiratory tract secretions[3]	Quinolones (particularly levofloxacin or ciprofloxacin) Rifampin (may interact with other drugs via the hepatic cytochrome p450 system) Macrolides (azithromycin, erythromycin) interact with immunosuppressive medications and should generally be avoided) TMP-SMZ (but the side effects include bone marrow suppression, hepatitis, rash)[3, 8]

(*Continued next page.*)

Organism	May Cause	Clinical Manifestations	Prophylaxis/Preemptive Therapy	Diagnostic Tests	Treatment Options
Myco-bacteria	Pulmonary infection Extrapulmonary infection (intestinal, skeletal, bone, genitourinary, cutaneous, CNS) Disseminated disease[3,74]	Pulmonary: Nonproductive cough Mucopurulent secretions Hemoptysis Dyspnea Chest pain Fever Excessive sweating Weight loss Organ-specific manifestations[3,8]	Test and treat before transplantation Isoniazid (controversial)[9,10]	Tuberculin test: positive in 25%–33% of recipients infected with this disease[3] Chest radiograph Bronchoscopy with BAL Transbronchial biopsy Pleural needle biopsy Tuberculin test: often negative Smears for acid-fast bacilli and mycobacterial culture Organ-specific histology[8] Isolates require antimicrobial susceptibility testing[3]	Isoniazid *† (hepatotoxic) Rifampin*† (hepatotoxic) Pyrazinamide Ethambutol (may → optic neuritis) Streptomycin† (ototoxic; nephrotoxic) *Increases catabolism of steroids and cyclosporine and tacrolimus; monitor levels of cyclosporine and tacrolimus; monitor patient for rejection †Monitor renal and hepatic function Recipients with active disease: 9–12 months of therapy with two agents to which pathogen is susceptible[3,9]

Organism	May Cause	Clinical Manifestations	Prophylaxis/Preemptive Therapy	Diagnostic Tests	Treatment Options
Aspergillus	Pulmonary and extrapulmonary infection[3] Disseminates to: Brain Liver Spleen Kidneys Heart Blood vessels Bones Joints GI tract[3]	Depend on site(s) involved[3] Pulmonary involvement: Nonproductive cough Pleuritic chest pain Pulmonary infiltrates or nodules Dyspnea Low-grade fever[28] Invasive/disseminated infection: Refractory fever Sinusitis Epistaxis; nasal pain Periorbital pain or swelling Cutaneous embolic lesions Progressive erythema or induration along tunneled venous catheter[79] Focal neurologic findings Hemoptysis: sign of invasive disease[3]	No definitive recommendations[3] Heart, lung, heart-lung recipients: aerosolized amphotericin B[80] Lung recipients: oral itraconazole for patients with airway colonization[3] Epidemiologic: Minimize contact with fungal spores; shield patient from nosocomial environmental hazards: high-efficiency particulate air filters; high-performance masks Preemptive: Amphotericin B if respiratory tract is colonized[63]	Chest radiography Note: may be normal BAL Transbronchial biopsy Open lung biopsy CT scan (e.g., lung, sinuses) Tissue biopsy CT or MRI for brain abscesses[3] Sputum cultures Repeated positive cultures suggest invasive disease Positive sputum cultures plus cavitary lung disease suggest invasive disease[79]	Amphotericin B† Itraconazole (Oral* or IV) †† Voriconazole: recently shown to have greater efficacy than amphotericin B for invasive disease[3]; Use of voriconazole with sirolimus is contraindicated[18] Caspofungin: approved for refractory aspergillosis[3] *Absorption may be erratic, especially in patients with low gastric acidity; monitor plasma concentration of drug[9, 28, 79] † May → nephrotoxicity in patients on calcineurin inhibitors; monitor renal function (lipid formulations are less likely to be nephrotoxic; may be preferable for chronic treatment)[18] ††Associated with higher relapse rates than amphotericin B[18]

(Continued next page.)

Organism	May Cause	Clinical Manifestations	Prophylaxis/Preemptive Therapy	Diagnostic Tests	Treatment Options

Candida	Mucocutaneous candidiasis
	Oropharyngeal thrush
	Candidal esophagitis
	Vaginitis
	Intertrigo
	Paronychia
	Onychomycosis
	Sternal wound infection; mediastinitis
	Intra-abdominal abscesses
	UTI
	Endocarditis
	Disseminated infection[3,9,74]
		Thrush:
		  White patches or ulcers in mouth
		Vaginitis:
		  White or yellow vaginal discharge
		  Pruritus
		Intertrigo:
		  Erythematous, papular skin rash
		Paronychia:
		  Redness, swelling, suppuration around nail edge
		Onychomycosis:
		  Thickened, discolored nails
		Intravascular catheter infections
		Fever, sepsis
			Clotrimazole troches[18]
			Oral Nystatin[18]
			Liver transplant recipients:
			  Preoperative oral bowel decontamination with nystatin to ↓ gut colonization[3]
			Kidney and pancreas-kidney transplant recipients:
			  Preemptive therapy for asymptomatic candiduria[3]
			Pancreas transplant recipients:
			  Anecdotal reports of fluconazole prophylaxis for high-risk patients:
			    Enteric drainage
			    Pretransplant peritoneal dialysis
			    Pancreas after kidney transplant
			    Reperfusion pancreatitis
			    Retransplantation[3]
				Direct fluorescent antibody stain of respiratory secretions
				Localized infection:
				  Cultures with Gram stain
				Disseminated candidiasis:
				  Blood cultures
				  CT scan
				  Biopsy of skin lesions
				  Tissue biopsy[62,79]
				Diagnosis confirmed by isolating Candida species from culture specimens[3]
					Amphotericin B and lipid-based preparations[3,18]
					Lipid-based preparations: less nephrotoxic
					Clotrimazole
					Mycostatin
					Fluconazole for esophagitis and refractory candidiasis*†
					Candidemia in unstable or critically ill patients: Amphotericin B followed by fluconazole if organism is sensitive to fluconazole
					Candidemia in stable patients: Fluconazole, if organism is sensitive to fluconazole[63,74,81]
					Candida albicans:
					  Fluconazole*
					  Itraconazole*[3]
					Candida krusei:
					  Typically resistant to fluconazole
					  Requires maximal doses of amphotericin B[18]
					Newer agents: for Candida species
					  Caspofungin††
					  Voriconazole
					*Monitor renal function and cyclosporine levels; adjust dose accordingly
					†Effective for most Candida species except Candida krusei and Candida glabrata
					††When used with cyclosporine, may ↑ risk of hepatotoxicity; monitor liver function
					††When used with tacrolimus, may → ↓ tacrolimus levels; monitor tacrolimus levels

Organism	May Cause	Clinical Manifestations	Prophylaxis/Preemptive Therapy	Diagnostic Tests	Treatment Options
Crypto-coccus neoformans	Predilection for CNS	Pulmonary infection:	Primary prophylaxis: not recommended[3]	Lumbar puncture	Amphotericin B*
	Meningitis	Cough		CT scan	Amphotericin B* with 5-flucytosine†
	Brain abscesses[3]	Lung nodules		MRI	Fluconazole* with 5-flucytosine†
	Secondary seeding of skin, CNS, eye, urinary tract, and skeletal system	CNS involvement:		Blood culture	Fluconazole*
	Pulmonary infection[9]	Progressive headache		CSF analysis: cell count; protein and sugar; Gram stain; acid-fast and fungal stains and cultures (fungal, bacterial, and mycobacterial)	Course of treatment: minimum of 8-10 weeks [3]
		Memory or attention deficits			*Requires monitoring of renal function and cyclosporine levels
		Emotional disturbance			†Requires monitoring of 5 flucytosine levels to minimize hepatic and bone marrow toxicity[10, 29, 79]
		Disorders of balance		Cryptococcal antigen test on blood, CSF and pleural fluid[9, 79]	
		Cranial nerve dysfunction			
		Fever		CSF in meningitis:	
		Meningismus		Lymphocytic pleocytosis	
		Confusion		↑ protein	
		Dysphagia		↓ sugar	
		Muscle weakness, tremor		↑ opening pressure[3]	
		Urinary incontinence			
		Focal neurologic signs		Definitive diagnosis: detection of antigen in serum and CSF[3]	
		Seizures[10]			
		Subacute presentation:			
		Low-grade fever			
		Headache			
		Altered mental status[3]			
		Cutaneous involvement:			
		Ulcers			
		Papules or pustules			
		Subcutaneous swelling or tumors			
		Ecchymoses			
		Granulomata			
		Abscesses			
		Vesicles			
		Palpable purpura or papules			
		Necrotizing vasculitis			
		Cellulitis[10, 28]			

(Continued next page.)

Organism	May Cause	Clinical Manifestations	Prophylaxis/Preemptive Therapy	Diagnostic Tests	Treatment Options
Pneumo-cystis carinii	Pneumonitis[74]	Presentation typically subacute Fever Nonproductive cough Dyspnea Hypoxemia Tachypnea Diffuse pulmonary infiltrates[3, 63, 82]	TMP-SMZ (low-dose for 6 months) Dapsone* Aerosolized pentamidine Atovaquone[3, 18] *In patients with G6PD deficiency, evaluate risk of dose-dependent hemolytic anemia[18]	Transbronchial lung biopsy Needle biopsy of lung Bronchoalveolar lavage Chest radiograph (may be negative) Confirmatory diagnosis: direct staining of specimens: sputum, BAL lavage or lung tissue[3, 12]	TMP-SMZ (high-dose)* for 21 days Pentamidine Dapsone-trimethoprim Clindamycin-primaquine (if not G6PD deficient) *Dose may have to be adjusted for renal dysfunction [3]
Histo-plasma Capsulatum	Disseminated infection (most common presentation)[3]	Subacute respiratory illness with either focal or disseminated interstitial or miliary infiltrates Fever (not always present) Night sweats Chills Cough Headache Arthritis, myalgias CNS manifestations Hepatosplenomegaly Cutaneous, intestinal, oral mucosal lesions[3, 9, 28]	No firm recommendations; some centers use itraconazole for seropositive recipients[3, 28]	Methenamine-silver stain Peripheral blood stains Cultures: blood, respiratory secretions, tissue Serology Antigen detection (urine, serum, CSF, BAL fluid) Chest radiography (may be normal)[3, 28, 79]	Amphotericin B* Itraconazole† for maintenance therapy *Requires monitoring of renal function and cyclosporine levels †Absorption may be erratic, especially in patients with low gastric acidity; monitor plasma concentration of drug[3, 8]

Organism	May Cause	Clinical Manifestations	Prophylaxis/Preemptive Therapy	Diagnostic Tests	Treatment Options
Toxoplasma gondii	Myocarditis	Mononucleosis-like syndrome of fever, malaise, and lymphadenopathy	Particularly for seronegative recipient/seropositive donor:	Endomyocardial biopsy	Pyrimethamine with folinic acid and sulfadiazine
	Pericarditis			Antibody titers	
	Pneumonitis	Myocardial dysfunction that mimics rejection	Pyrimethamine (for sulfa allergy)	Lung lavage and/or biopsy	Sulfa allergy: dapsone used instead of sulfadiazine
	Encephalitis			CT scan of head	
	Hepatitis	Pulmonary: fever, dyspnea, cough, hemoptysis	Pyrimethamine + sulfonamide	Chest radiograph	Clindamycin and pyrimethamine with folinic acid
	Retinochoroiditis[74, 83, 84]	CNS involvement: multiple focal neurologic deficits, altered mental status; fever with headache[3, 83]	Pyrimethamine + folinic acid	Tissue and/or blood culture	Folinic acid given to prevent myelotoxity
			Co-trimoxazole	Serologic assays[63, 83]	Continue therapy for 2 to 3 weeks after acute infection has resolved[3, 18, 28]
			Atovaquone	Definitive diagnosis: histological detection of trophozoites + inflammation[3]	
			TMP-SMZ		
			Avoid changing cat litter boxes		
			Avoid raw or undercooked meat[3, 10, 18, 63, 84]		
Crypto-sporidium	Gastroenteritis	Profuse, watery diarrhea	Boil water for 5 minutes or use distilled or filtered water	Stool testing	Replace fluid and electrolytes
	Gallbladder infection[83]	Abdominal pain		Antibody detection assays	Maintain nutritional status
		Nausea and vomiting	Avoid ice cubes in restaurants	Small or large bowel biopsy[83]	Spiramycin effective for some patients; adverse effects reported (increased stool output and volume loss)[83]
		Fever	Avoid soda fountain drinks		
		Myalgias[83]			

(Continued next page.)

Organism	May Cause	Clinical Manifestations	Prophylaxis/Preemptive Therapy	Diagnostic Tests	Treatment Options
Strongyloides stercoralis	Ulcerating hemorrhagic enterocolitis Hemorrhagic pneumonia Disseminated disease: Pulmonary CNS (gram-negative meningitis)[9]	GI: Abdominal pain and distention Diarrhea Nausea and vomiting Adynamic ileus Small bowel obstruction Hemorrhage Pulmonary: Tachypnea Dyspnea Bronchospasm Cough Hemoptysis CNS: Headache Fever Eosinophilic meningitis Mental status changes Coma Focal neurologic deficits Gram-negative meningitis Skin manifestations: Migratory, raised, linear rash that may move at a rate of 10 cm/hour Crops of urticarial eruptions; immediate hypersensitive reactions to migrating worms, especially on the waist and buttocks)[3, 28]	Consider preemptive ivermectin for transplant candidates who have traveled to or lived in endemic areas Screen at-risk candidates for infection Treat established infection before transplantation[3]	Stool specimen for rhabditiform larvae (may be negative) Papanicolaou stain of duodenal aspirates, urine, ascitic fluid, sputum, and stool Jejunal biopsy Serologic testing Chest radiograph (frequently inconclusive) Definitive diagnosis: presence of larvae in stool[3]	Albendazole Ivermectin* Thiobendazole Taper immunosuppressive agents Systemic antibacterial therapy for bacteremia or meningitis *Periodic retreatments may be necessary[9, 28] Hyperinfection: 7 to 10 days of antimicrobial therapy[3]

BAL = bronchoalveolar lavage; CT = computed tomography; CMV = cytomegalovirus; CSF = cerebrospinal fluid; CBC = complete blood count; CNS = central nervous system; EBV = Epstein-Barr virus; ELISA = enzyme-linked immunosorbent assay; EEG = electroencephalogram; G6PD = glucose-6-phosphate dehydrogenase; GI = gastrointestinal; LFT = liver function tests; HBV = hepatitis B virus; HbsAg = hepatitis B surface antigen; HCV = hepatitis C virus; HCV-RNA = hepatitis C virus-ribonucleic acid; HHV = human herpes virus-6; HSV = herpes simplex virus; IV = intravenous; IVIG = intravenous immunoglobulin; LOC = level of consciousness; MRI = magnetic resonance imaging; PCR = polymerase chain reaction; PTLD = post-transplant lymphoproliferative disease; SARS = severe acute respiratory syndrome; TMP-SMZ = trimethoprim-sulfamethoxazole; VZV = varicella zoster virus; UTI = urinary tract infection.

Adapted from Cupples SA, Lucey DR. Infectious disease in transplant recipients. In Cupples, SA, Ohler L (Eds). *Solid Organ Transplantation: A Handbook for Primary Health Care Providers.* New York: Springer, 2002; pp. 16-63.

      c. Primary infections occur in approximately 70% to 80% of EBV-seronegative recipients.[8]

      d. EBV infection typically occurs during the first 6 months post-transplant.[18]

B. Effects of EBV infection: The sequelae of EBV infection range from a mononucleosis-like syndrome to post-transplant lymphoproliferative disease (PTLD).

    1. Risk factors for PTLD include:

      a. Pretransplant EBV-seronegativity

      b. High EBV viral load

      c. Primary EBV infection

      d. CMV mismatch (donor CMV-seropositive; recipient CMV-seronegative)

      e. CMV disease

      f. High-dose monoclonal or polyclonal antilymphocyte antibody therapy, high-dose cyclosporine or tacrolimus therapy, or high-dose pulse corticosteroid therapy, particularly if used in combination

      g. Type of allograft[3, 12, 27]

C. Incidence of EBV infection by type of allograft is shown in Table 5-10.[3]

D. See Table 5-9 for the clinical manifestations, prevention/prophylaxis, diagnosis and treatment of EBV.

IV. Herpes simplex virus (HSV)

A. Overview[3, 9, 28, 29]

    1. Approximately 80% of adult transplant recipients are HSV-seropositive.

    2. Incidence highest in kidney transplant recipients[-8]

    3. Most common strains associated with mucocutaneous infections: HSV-1 and HSV-2[18]

    4. After a primary HSV infection, the virus remains latent in the sensory nerve ganglia.

    5. Reactivation infection occurs in up to 40% of recipients, typically during the first post-transplant month.

TABLE 5-10

■ **Incidence of EBV[3]**

Type of Allograft	Incidence
Multi-organ	13%-33%
Intestine	7%-11%
Kidney-pancreas	11%
Lung	2%-8%
Heart	2%-4%
Liver	2%
Kidney	1%

6. Oral lesions may extend beyond the lip; the oral cavity and esophagus may be involved.[10]
7. Squamous cell carcinoma must be ruled out in verrucous lip lesions that do not respond to antiviral therapy.
8. Herpes labialis is the most common clinical manifestation of HSV-1.
    a. Lesions may bleed, interfere with nutritional intake, and require local analgesia to control pain.

B. Risk factor for reactivation: OKT3
C. See Table 5-9 for the clinical manifestations, prevention/prophylaxis, diagnosis, and treatment of HSV.

V. Varicella zoster virus (VZV)
A. Overview
1. In transplant recipients, VZV can cause herpes zoster in VZV-seropositive recipients (about 90% of adult recipients).[3]
    a. Recipients with a reactivated infection:[18]
        i. May have a complicated course that involves two or more dermatomes
        ii. May develop disseminated infection
2. VZV can cause primary infection in the remaining 10% of adult recipients.[3]
3. Although VZV infection can occur at any time, it typically occurs between 3 months and 3 years post-transplant.
4. Chickenpox in a transplant recipient is a medical emergency; hospitalization is required for intravenous antiviral therapy.
5. VZV-seronegative recipients are advised to report any exposure to VZV so that zoster immune globulin may be promptly administered.
6. Cutaneous manifestations may be muted, especially if immune globulin is given; patient should be observed for primarily visceral manifestations.
7. Dermatomal pain without typical skin eruptions has been observed.[3]

B. See Table 5-9 for the clinical manifestations, prevention/prophylaxis, diagnosis, and treatment of VZV.

VI. Human herpesvirus-6 (HHV-6)
A. Most post-transplant infections result from reactivation of endogenous latent virus.
B. Onset typically occurs between 2 and 4 weeks post-transplantation.
C. CMV coinfection is common.[9]
D. See Table 5-9 for the clinical manifestations, prevention/prophylaxis, diagnosis, and treatment of HHV-6.

VII. Hepatitis viruses
A. Overview
1. Post-transplant liver disease may be due to drug-induced hepatotoxicity or virus-induced disease.
    a. Hepatotoxic drugs include certain:
        i. Immunosuppressants—particularly azathioprine and cyclosporine
        ii. Antimicrobial agents—particularly medications used to treat tuberculosis (for example, isoniazid, pyrazinamide, rifampin)
        iii. Antihypertensive agents
        iv. Diuretics[9]

      b. Virus-induced disease: hepatitis virus B (HBV) and hepatitis virus C (HCV)

          i. HBV and HCV are common causes of post-transplant liver disease.[30]

          i. Risk of recurrence of either hepatitis B or C is greater than 80%.

          ii. Viral hepatitis may be transmitted via the allograft.[3]

B. Hepatitis B

    1. In the transplant recipient, HBV can cause hepatitis, cirrhosis, and hepatocellular carcinoma.

    2. Approximately 50% of recipients with HBV infection will have end-stage liver disease and/or hepatocellular carcinoma at 10 years post-transplant.[9, 12]

C. Hepatitis C

    1. Between 10% and 20% of recipients with HCV infection will have end-stage liver disease and/or hepatocellular carcinoma at 10 years post-transplant.

    2. Combination therapy with interferon and ribavirin is the most effective therapeutic regimen for post-transplant HCV infection; however, this combined therapy is problematic because:

      a. It is effective in less than 50% of patients who are infected with the most common HCV genotype found in the U.S.

      b. Many recipients find this regimen intolerable.[12, 29]

D. See Table 5-9 for the clinical manifestations, prevention/prophylaxis, diagnosis, and treatment of hepatitis infections.

VIII. Polyomaviruses

A. Overview

    1. BK and JC viruses: only two members of polyomavirus family known to naturally infect humans.[31]

    2. Approximately 80% of the general adult population is seropositive for the BK and JC viruses.[3]

      a. Transmission: respiratory route[32]

    3. BK and JC viruses have latency properties and often reactivate in the immunosuppressed recipient.

      a. Viruses tend to persist in kidneys, ureters, brain, and spleen.[33]

    4. First reported in 1971; named "BK" virus and "JC" virus after the initials of the recipients who were first diagnosed with these infections.

B. BK virus[3, 34]

    1. Transplant recipients may have primary and reactivation infections.[33]

    2. BK virus reactivation in kidney transplant recipients is common (prevalence: 45%-50%[33]), but reactivation progresses to nephropathy only occasionally (prevalence: 1%-10%[35]).

    3. Reactivation after kidney transplantation may cause significant morbidity:

      a. Tubulointerstitial nephritis

      b. Ureteral stenosis that leads to obstructive nephropathy

      c. Progressive graft dysfunction

      d. Graft loss: ranges from 10% to 80% in kidney transplant recipients with polyomavirus-associated nephropathy[35]

    4. Risk factors:[33, 36]

        a. Higher number of HLA mismatches

        b. Recurrent rejection episodes

        c. Intense immunosuppression

    5. See Table 5-9 for the clinical manifestations, prevention/prophylaxis, diagnosis, and treatment of BK virus.

  C. JC virus[33, 37]

    1. Causes progressive multifocal leukoencephalopathy (PML)

        a. Opportunistic JC virus infects and lyses oligodendrocytes; this causes multifocal demyelination in brain and progressive neurological deficits.

        b. Timing of onset: typically more than 6 months to several years post-transplant

        c. Noninflammatory CNS infection; not associated with fever or meningeal signs (nuchal rigidity)

        d. May occur concurrently in subset of kidney transplant recipients with documented BK virus-induced interstitial nephritis[33]

    2. Reported in renal, liver, heart, and lung transplant recipients[38]

    3. See Table 5-9 for the clinical manifestations, prevention/prophylaxis, diagnosis, and treatment of JC virus.

IX. Parvovirus B19

  A. Typically acquired during school-age period

    1. Results in "slapped cheek" rash that may be accompanied by lacy erythematous exanthem of extremities[39]

    2. Can cause pure red blood cell aplasia with low hematocrit

  B. See Table 5-9 for the clinical manifestations, prevention/prophylaxis, diagnosis, and treatment of parvovirus B19.

X. Human papillomavirus

  A. Associated with the development of warts (cutaneous and anogenital), cervical cancer, and squamous cell carcinoma[39]

  B. Cutaneous warts

    1. Incidence of warts: increases with duration of immunosuppression

    2. Tend to develop on areas of body exposed to sun

    3. More common in patients prone to sunburn

    4. May be refractory to treatment and tend to recur

  C. Squamous cell carcinoma

    1. Rate increases with duration of immunosuppression

    2. Risk factor: chronic sun exposure

  D. See Table 5-9 for the clinical manifestations, prevention/prophylaxis, diagnosis, and treatment of human papillomavirus.

XI. Community-acquired respiratory infections[40, 41]

  A. Community respiratory viruses[42]

    1. Respiratory syncytial virus (RSV)

    2. Influenza viruses

    3. Parainfluenza viruses

    4. Coronaviruses

  B. Epidemiology[41]

    1. RSV, influenza, parainfluenza infections: typically occur in winter months

    2. Parainfluenza virus 3 and adenovirus infections: occur throughout the year

    3. Viral respiratory infections can occur at any time post-transplant

        a.   Early post-transplant infection: may be associated with nosocomial infection or reactivation of latent virus

           i.   Transmission of adenovirus from donor organ has been reported.

        b.   Late post-transplant infection: typically community-acquired

    4.   Transplant patients may be the first individuals within a community to become infected with a community-acquired respiratory infection.

C. Mode of transmission[40]

    1.   Virus-laden respiratory droplets and aerosols

    2.   Direct contact (person-to-person)

    3.   Contact with fomites

    4.   Transmission can occur in community and hospital environment

D. Clinical presentation (general)

    1.   Upper respiratory tract symptoms

    2.   Elevated temperature

    3.   Myalgia, arthralgia

    4.   Anorexia

    5.   Inflammation of mucosa

E. Range of sequelae: mild, self-limiting upper respiratory infection to viral pneumonia, respiratory failure, and secondary infection with fungal or bacterial pathogens[42]

    1.   CMV may be reactivated secondary to immunomodulation

F. Respiratory syncytial virus (RSV)

    1.   Transmission[43]

        a.   Primarily through large droplets and fomites

        b.   Can survive on surfaces (nonporous), skin, and gloves for hours

        c.   Requires close person-to-person contact or contact with contaminated surfaces

    2.   See Table 5-9 for the clinical manifestations, prevention/prophylaxis, diagnosis, and treatment of RSV.

G. Influenza viruses

    1.   Infections with influenza viruses range from mild, self-limiting syndromes to serious secondary infections—typically bacterial.

    2.   See Table 5-9 for the clinical manifestations, prevention/prophylaxis, diagnosis, and treatment of influenza virus infections.

H. Parainfluenza viruses (PIV)

    1.   There are three types: PIV 1, 2, and 3; PIV types 1 and 3 infect transplant recipients most frequently.

    2.   In healthy individuals, viral shedding after PIV infection lasts for approximately 1 week; in transplant recipients, particularly those on long-term steroid therapy, shedding may be prolonged (greater than 4 weeks).[42]

    3.   See Table 5-9 for the clinical manifestations, prevention/prophylaxis, diagnosis, and treatment of parainfluenza virus infections.

I. Coronavirus

    1.   Associated with a range of infections from mild upper respiratory infections to severe acute respiratory syndrome (SARS).

    2.   See Table 5-9 for the clinical manifestations, prevention/prophylaxis, diagnosis, and treatment of coronavirus infections.

BACTERIAL INFECTIONS

I. Overview
   A. Bacteria are the most common causes of infection in transplant recipients.
      1. Bacterial infections are associated with increased morbidity and mortality in transplant recipients, particularly the rapidly emerging multi-drug resistant bacteria:
         a. Gram-negative: (for example, *Pseudomonas aeruginosa*; extended-spectrum B lactamase- [ESBL] producing *Enterobacteriaceae*)
         b. Gram-positive (for example, vancomycin-resistant enteroccocus [VRE] and methicillin-resistant *Staphylococcus aureus* [MRSA])
   B. Bacterial infections most commonly occur at the transplant site.
   C. Bacterial pneumonias are common among all types of solid organ transplant recipients.
II. Bacterial infections in specific transplant populations are shown in Table 5-11.
III. Listeriosis
   A. Typically occurs within first two post-transplant months, but can occur years later[3]
   B. One of the most frequent causes of CNS infection in transplant recipients
   C. Meningitis secondary to *Listeria monocytogenes* has a high mortality rate (approximately 25%)[9, 10]
   D. Mode of transmission: ingestion of contaminated food[3]
   E. See Table 5-9 for the clinical manifestations, prevention/prophylaxis, diagnosis, and treatment of listeriosis.
IV. Nocardiosis[3]
   A. Most common species: *Nocardia asteroides*
   B. Most common site: lung (pneumonitis, pulmonary nodules, pulmonary abscesses)
   C. Extrapulmonary sites: brain (abscesses, meningitis), skin, bone[10]
   D. Transmission: inhalation into lungs or inoculation into skin[10]
   E. All patients should have CNS imaging to rule out possibility of brain abscess.
   F. See Table 5-9 for the clinical manifestations, prevention/prophylaxis, diagnosis, and treatment options for nocardiosis.
V. Legionellosis[3, 8]
   A. May occur at any time post-transplant
      1. Nosocomial sources: contaminated hospital water supply, ventilators, nebulizers
      2. Community-acquired sources: drinking water, water heaters, room humidifiers, water aerosolization sources, shower heads
   B. Should be considered whenever a transplant recipient presents with pneumonia-like symptoms
   C. Simultaneous infection by other pulmonary pathogens may occur.
   D. Urine antigen test for *Legionella* only detects *Legionella pneumophilia* serotype 1.
   E. Mortality in transplant recipients is high (often over 50%).
   F. See Table 5-9 for the clinical manifestations, prevention/prophylaxis, diagnosis, and treatment of legionellosis.

TABLE 5-11

■ **Bacterial Infections in Specific Transplant Complications**

Allograft	General Considerations	Clinical Manifestations	Diagnosis	Treatment	Prevention

Lung	Pneumonia: common
	Overall prevalence: 60%
	Bacteria are the cause of the majority of infections in lung transplant recipients[44]
	The most frequent infection is bacterial pneumonia[45]
	Pneumonia: most common pathogens:
	  Gram-negative bacteria:
	    Enterobacteriaceas
	    Pseudomonas aeruginosa[3]
	  Other significant pathogens:
	    Staphylococcus aureus
	    Haemophilus influenzae
	    Streptococcus pneumoniae[3]
	Lung susceptible to infections due to:
	  Impaired cough reflex
	  Poor mucociliary clearance
	  Ischemia
	  Abnormal lymph drainage
	  Reperfusion injury
	  Airway inflammation secondary to rejection → bacterial colonization[3]
	Single lung transplantation:
	  Infection spreads from native lung to allograft[3]
	Pathogens with high morbidity and mortality in lung transplantation for cystic fibrosis:
	  Burkholderia cepacia
	  Pseudomonas pathogens[3,46]
		Pneumonia:
		  Persistent respiratory failure
		  Failure to wean from ventilator
		  Fever
		  Purulent respiratory secretions
		  Lung consolidations
		Mediastinitis:
		  Fever
		  Leukocytosis
		  Systemic toxicity
		Sternal wound infection:
		  Early:
		    Poor wound healing
		    Dehiscence
		  Late:
		    Sinus tract formation
		    Purulent discharge[3]
		NOTE: fever and leukocytosis may not be present
			Pneumonia:
			  Respiratory tract cultures
			Mediastinitis: CT scan
			Sternal wound infection:
			  CT scan
			  Nuclear imaging studies[3]
				Pneumonia:
				  Pathogen-specific antimicrobials
				  Dual antimicrobial regimen for:
				    Pseudomonas aeruginosa
				    Burkholderia cepacia
				    Enterobacteriaceae (multi-drug resistant)
				Mediastinitis:
				  Surgical wound debridement
				  Antimicrobial therapy
				Sternal wound infection:
				  Surgical wound debridement
				  Antimicrobial therapy[3]
					Antimicrobial prophylaxis guided by respiratory tract cultures from donor and recipient
					Patients colonized with *Burkholderia cepacia* or multiple drug-resistant gram-negative bacteria:
					  Double or triple antibiotic therapy
					  Inhaled aminoglycosides
					Perioperative prophylaxis for sternal wound infections:
					  Antimicrobials for gram-positive bacteria[3]

Allograft	General Considerations	Clinical Manifestations	Diagnosis	Treatment	Prevention
Liver	Most common bacterial infections: Intra-abdominal Surgical wound[3] Other bacterial infections: Wound Cholangitis Abscesses Device-related[3] Most common sites of infection: Liver Biliary tract Peritoneal cavity Surgical site Bloodstream[47] Risk factors for intra-abdominal infections: Long surgical time Blood transfusions Reoperation Early rejection CMV infection Retransplantation Roux-en-y choledocojejunostomy anastomosis (due to reflux of intestinal material and microbial flora into biliary system)[3]	Wound infections or intra-abdominal abscess: Fever Abdominal pain Dehiscence Purulent drainage Pain Guarding Rebound tenderness Cholangitis: Fever RUQ pain Rebound tenderness Hyperbilirubinemia ↑ transaminases[3] ↑ alkaline phosphatase[3]	Wound infections: Cultures CT scans Ultrasound MRI Cholangitis: Cholangiogram LFTs	Surgical or CT- or US-guided drainage of abscess Pathogen-specific antimicrobials Complicated infections: Cephalosporins Fluoroquinolones Carbapenems Beta-lactam and beta-lactamase inhibitor combinations Cholangitis: Obstruction: ERCP with dilation No obstruction: IV antibiotics[3]	Good surgical technique Gram-negative infections: Oral selective bowel decontamination (↓ gram-negative aerobic bacteria and fungi; spares gram-positive and anerobic microbes that exert antagonistic effect on gram-negative organisms) Wound infections: Perioperative administration of extended-spectrum cephalosporin Antibiotic therapy typically continued for 24 to 48 hours after surgery Antimicrobial prophylaxis before post-transplant cholangiograms, biopsies, or any other procedure that involves manipulation of the biliary tract[3]

(Continued next page.)

Allograft	General Considerations	Clinical Manifestations	Diagnosis	Treatment	Prevention
Kidney	80% of infections are bacterial[40] Urinary tract: Site of most bacterial infections[3] Most common primary site associated with secondary bacteremia[40] UTIs: common pathogens *Enterobacteriaceae* *Pseudomonas aeruginosa* *Enterococcus* sp.[40] Risk factors: DM Renal insufficiency Prolonged catheter use ↓ urine flow through urinary epithelium Neurogenic bladder Anatomic abnormalities[3, 40] Risk factors for recurrent UTIs: Serum creatinine > 2 mg/dL Prednisone dose > 20 mg/day Multiple treated rejection episodes Chronic viral infections[48] Etiology of surgical wound infections: gram-positive cocci; gram-negative bacilli[3] Lymphoceles can → abscess formation secondary to repeated percutaneous drainage[40]	UTI: Acute pylonephritis Fever Pain: graft site Leukocytosis Active urinary sediment Note: UTIs may be asymptomatic [3] Lymphoceles: Fever Graft tenderness Unilateral leg edema on side of kidney transplant may be a sign of a lymphocele (infected or not infected)	Surveillance urine cultures: Clean catch, midstream urine specimen[40] Culture of genitourinary stents[40] Febrile patients: Blood cultures Recurrent UTIs: Imaging studies to detect anatomic problems or obstruction[3]	UTIs: Pathogen-specific antimicrobial Fluoroquinolones Cephalosporins Vancomycin for infections due to coagulase-negative staphylococci or ampicillin-resistant enterococci Pyeloenephritis: typically requires 2 or more weeks of therapy Wound infections: Surgical debridement Antimicrobial therapy[3]	Incidence of asymptomatic UTIs is high; therefore surveillance cultures are frequently required[47] Early catheter removal UTIs: TMP/SMX Ciprofloxacin[40] TMP/SMX to ↓ incidence of septicemia For patients with sulfa allergy: Fluoroquinolones Surgical wound infections: Perioperative cephalosporin antibiotic[3]

Allograft	General Considerations	Clinical Manifestations	Diagnosis	Treatment	Prevention
Heart	Types of infection:[3] Main infection: ventilator-associated pneumonia due to gram-negative bacteria (*Pseudomonas aeruginosa, Klebsiella pneumoniae*, other *Enterobacteriaceae*) Sternotomy infection: *Staphylococcus aureus,* coagulase-negative staphylococci Mediastinitis Bacteremia[3] Pneumonia: most common bacterial infection[47] Mediastinitis typically caused by gram-positive bacteria (*Staphylococcus aureus,* coagulase-negative *staphylococcus aureus*); gram-negative organisms can also cause mediastinitis[11]	Pneumonia: Persistent respiratory failure Failure to wean from ventilator Fever Purulent respiratory secretions Lung consolidations Mediastinitis: Fever Leukocytosis Systemic toxicity Sternal wound infection: Early: Poor wound healing Dehiscence Late: Sinus tract formation Purulent discharge[3]	Pneumonia: Respiratory tract cultures Mediastinitis: CT scan Sternal wound infection: CT scan Nuclear imaging studies[3]	Pneumonia: Pathogen-specific antimicrobial Mediastinitis: Surgical wound debridement Antimicrobial therapy directed toward gram-positive organisms Sternal wound infection: Surgical wound debridement Antimicrobial therapy directed toward gram-positive organisms[3]	Pneumonia: Early weaning from ventilator Aggressive pulmonary hygiene Sternal wound infection: Perioperative antimicrobials Endocarditis: Standard dental prophylaxis[3]

(Continued next page.)

Allograft	General Considerations	Clinical Manifestations	Diagnosis	Treatment	Prevention
Pancreas	Most common: Wound infections Intra-abdominal abscesses[3, 47] Most common pathogen associated with wound and intra-abdominal infections: enteric bacteria[47] UTIs commonly associated with urinary drainage of exocrine secretions (due to bacterial overgrowth in bladder) Other infections: Cellulitis (abdominal wall) Peri-pancreatic abscesses Peritonitis Common pathogens: Gram-positive cocci Gram-negative bacteria Anaerobic bacteria[3] Pancreatic duct infection: Gram-negative bacteria appear to grow more readily in pancreatic secretions than gram-positive bacteria[49]	Wound infections or intra-abdominal abscess: Fever Abdominal pain Dehiscence Purulent drainage Pain Guarding Rebound tenderness[3]	Wound infections: CT scan Abdominal US MRI CBC count LFTs Fluid cultures[3] UTIs: Surveillance urine cultures: clean catch, midstream urine specimen[40] Febrile patients: Blood cultures Recurrent UTIs: Imaging studies to detect anatomic problems or obstruction[3]	Wound infections: Surgical or CT- or US-guided drainage of abscess Pathogen-specific antimicrobials[3] UTIs: Pathogen-specific antimicrobial Fluoroquinolones Cephalosporins	Early catheter removal UTIs: TMP/SMX Ciprofloxacin[40] TMP/SMX to ↓ incidence of septicemia For patients with sulfa allergy: Fluoroquinolones Surgical wound infections: Perioperative cephalosporin antibiotic[3]

CBC = complete blood cell; CT = computed tomography; DM = diabetes mellitus; ERCP = endoscopic retrograde cholangiopancreatography; LFTs = liver function tests; MRI = magnetic resonance imaging; RUQ = right upper quadrant; SPK = simultaneous pancreas kidney; TMP/SMX = trimethoprim/sulfamethoxazole; US = ultrasound; UTI = urinary tract infection.

VI. Myobacterium tuberculosis
   A. Worldwide incidence in transplant recipients: 0.35%–15%[3]
   B. Mortality in transplant recipients: approximately 30%[3]
   C. Transplant recipients are at risk for primary and reactivation infections
   D. The atypical and extra-pulmonary manifestations may prolong diagnosis and delay appropriate treatment.
   E. See Table 5-9 for the clinical manifestations, prevention/prophylaxis, diagnosis, and treatment of tuberculosis.
VII. Nosocomial infections
   A. *Clostridium difficile*[18, 40, 50]
      1. Pathogen produces protein endotoxins
      2. Risk factors
         a. Antimicrobial agents (but can occur without prior antibiotic therapy)
            i. Broad-spectrum antibiotics (for example, ampicillin, clindamycin, and the cephalosporins) disrupt the normal flora in the bowel; this in turn permits the overgrowth of *C. difficile*.
            ii. *C. difficile* produces a toxin that causes mucosal inflammation, secretion of fluids from the colon, and injury to the colon.
         b. Hospitalization
         c. Older age
         d. Immunosuppression
         e. Inflammatory bowel disease
      3. Potential clinical manifestations may include: (onset may be abrupt)
         a. Fever
         b. Abdominal cramps, pain
         c. Diarrhea
            i. May be profuse and watery
            ii. Stools may be bloody
         d. Ileus
         e. Toxic megacolon
         f. Perforation of colon
      4. Complications
         a. Fluid and electrolyte imbalances
         b. Inadequate absorption of medications
      5. Treatment options
         a. Metronidazole 250 to 500 mg by mouth, 3 to 4 times per day, for 10-14 days
            i. Intravenous metronidazole may be required for patients with severe dysmotility or ileus, as oral medication may not reach the colonic mucosa
         b. For patients who do not respond to metronidazole: vancomycin 125 mg by mouth 4 times per day for 10 to 14 days
         c. For patients with multiple relapses:
            i. Prolonged vancomycin tapering
            ii. Prolonged vancomycin tapering and cholestramine (to absorb *C. difficile* toxin)
            iii. Intravenous immunoglobulin (potential option)
      6. Prevention
         a. Prudent use of antibiotics
         b. Strict adherence to infection control guidelines

       c.   Proper and thorough environmental cleaning

B. Vancomycin-resistant enterococcus (VRE)[40, 50-52]

   1. Enterococci typically found in gastrointestinal tract and female genitourinary tract

   2. Two most common species

      a. *Enterococcus faecalis*

      b. *Enterococcus faecium*

   3. Enterococci first became resistant to gentamicin (reported in 1979) and then penicillin. In the 1990s, the emergence of VRE resulted from the acquisition of vancomycin resistance by multidrug-resistant enterococci, particularly *Enterococcus faecium*.

   4. VRE colonization

      a. Risk of colonization involves exposure to VRE and host susceptibility.

      b. Important risk factors

         i. Proximity to patients with VRE colonization, especially patients with diarrhea

         ii. Length of hospital stay

      c. Intestinal colonization has no symptoms, may persist for long periods of   time, and is a mechanism for transmission of VRE to other patients.

      d. Colonization rates after solid organ transplantation: 11%–63%[40]

      e. VRE-colonized transplant recipients are at risk of infection.

   5. VRE infection

      a. Develops in patients with VRE colonization

      b. Infection rate among solid organ transplant recipients: 1%–16%[40]

      c. Recipients of abdominal allografts are particularly susceptible to infection.

      d. Potential portals of entry

         i. Urinary tract

         ii. Intra-abdominal or pelvic sources

         iii. Wounds

         iv. Intravascular catheters

      e. Risk factors

         i. Immunosuppressive therapy

         ii. Lengthy intensive care unit stay

         iii. Prolonged hospitalization

         iv. Severity of illness

         v. Exposure to patients with VRE

         vi. Administration of broad-spectrum antibiotics

         vii. Renal insufficiency

         viii. Hemodialysis

         ix. CMV seropositive allograft

         x. Prolonged surgical time

         xi. Reoperation

         xii. Total parental nutrition

         xiii. Enteral tube feedings

         xiv. Indwelling bladder catheters

   6. Transmission

      a. Within institution: direct or indirect contact

         i. Staff hands

        ii. Organism has been isolated from virtually all objects in health care environment

        iii. Organism can survive on stethoscope diaphragm for 30 minutes; on telephone handset for 60 minutes; on bedrail for 24 hours; on tourniquet for 4 days, and on countertop for 1 week[50]

    b. Between institutions

        i. Via health care professionals who work at more than one hospital

        ii. Transfer of infected patients between institutions

  7. Potential treatment options

    a. Removal of nidus of infection (for example, by draining abscesses, surgical debridement of wounds)

    b. Antimicrobial agents[40]

        i. Test organism for susceptibility to ampicillin, linezolid, quinupristin/dalfopristin, daptomycin, chloramphenicol, doxycycline, gentamicin, streptomycin

        ii. Ampicillin, aminopenicillin or ureidopenicillin derivatives: for ampicillin-susceptible organisms

        iii. For severe infections: combination therapy with aminoglycosides; monitor kidney function

        iv. Linezolid or quinupristin/dalfopristin (for *Enterococcus faecium* only), or daptomycin: for organisms that are not susceptible to ampicillin or for patients allergic to penicillin and vancomycin

        v. Linezolid: oral or intravenous preparation; side effects: bone marrow suppression including anemia and thrombocytopenia (this may preclude long-term therapy with linezolid); serotonin syndrome (fever, hypertension, tachycardia, confusion) when used with some antidepressants; some resistance to linezolid has been noted

        vi. Quinupristin/dalfopristin: intravenous preparation; requires central catheter to prevent phlebitis; side effects: arthralgias, myalgias; most *Enterococcus faecalis* are intrinsically resistant to this agent.

  8. Prevention

    a. Strict adherence to infection control guidelines

        i. Gowns, gloves, hand washing

    b. Prudent use of antimicrobial agents

    c. Surveillance cultures (rectal or stool) for early identification and isolation of patients colonized with VRE

    d. Tracking of VRE colonization in high-risk units

    e. Continuation of isolation procedures per protocol (for example, until three weekly cultures have been negative)

    f. Proper and thorough environmental cleaning

  9. Epidemiological pattern is changing:

    a. In U.S.: community dissemination is developing.[53]

    b. In Europe: "very resistant enterococci" are emerging.

C. Methicillin-resistant *Staphylococcus aureus* (MRSA)

  1. Colonization occurs mainly in the nasopharynx and on the skin.[54]

  2. *S. aureus* infections can occur as:

    a. Wound infections

b. Bacteremia
c. Metastatic infections (for example, arthritis, osteomyelelitis, meningitis)

3. Transmission:[54]
    a. Colonized or infected patient
    b. Colonized healthcare worker
    c. Allograft

4. Reported clinical manifestations[54]
    a. Solid organ transplant recipients in general
        i. Pneumonia: *S. aureus* is the most common gram-positive organism that causes bacterial pneumonia in the first 3 months following solid organ transplantation.
        ii. Wound infections
        iii. Bacteremia
    b. Liver transplant recipients
        i. Wound infection
        ii. Bacteremia
        iii. Chest infection
    c. Heart, heart-lung, and lung transplant recipients
        i. Mediastinal abscess
        ii. Mediastinitis
        iii. Endocarditis
        iv. Pericarditis
    d. Kidney transplant recipients
        i. Urinary tract infection

5. Treatment options[54, 55]
    a. Vancomycin or teicoplanin
    b. Linezolid
    c. Quinupristin/dalfopristin
    d. For severe infections: rifampin (in combination with another agent) or gentamicin

6. Prevention[56]
    a. Surveillance cultures to detect nasal colonization on admission and periodically thereafter
    b. Intranasal mupirocin to eradicate MRSA in colonized patients
    c. Strict adherence to and monitoring of infection control measures
    d. Staff cohorting for MRSA-positive and MRSA-negative patients
    e. Use of vascular catheters impregnated with antibiotics
    f. Proper and thorough environmental cleaning

7. Note: *Community-acquired* (CA-MRSA) has also been observed.
    a. Transmission
        i. Person-to-person
        ii. Person-to inanimate objects-to person
    b. Rapidly spreading in many communities across the world
    c. Clinical manifestations
        i. Skin infection: boils
        ii. Soft tissue infection
        iii. Pneumonia
    d. Treatment
        i. Incision and drainage if possible

       ii. Often responds to TMP/SMZ, clindamycin, and doxycycline

D. Extended-spectrum beta-lactamase (ESBL) gram-negative bacilli[50, 57, 58]

   1. The use of broad-spectrum beta lactam antibiotics has resulted in the development of gram-negative bacilli that produce ESBL.

   2. These bacilli are resistant to many antibiotics, including the penicillins, first-generation and newer cephalosporins, cephamycins, carbapenems, and fluoroquinolones.

   3. Resistance to these antibiotics has been acquired primarily by *Klebsiella pneumoniae* and *Escherichia coli* as well as additional pathogens such as other *Klebsiella* strains, *Enterobacter* spp., *Proteus* spp., etc.

   4. Clinical sequelae: UTIs, septicemia, hospital-acquired pneumonia, intra-abdominal abscesses, brain abscesses, device-related infections

   5. Risk factors:

     a. Antibiotic therapy (especially with newer cephalosporins)

     b. Surgery

     c. Intensive care unit stay

     d. Prolonged hospitalization

   6. Treatment

     a. Removal of source of infection (for example, colonized intravascular line)

     b. Drainage of abscesses

     c. Antibiotic therapy, taking into consideration site and severity of the infection, liver and renal function, and patient's age

       i. Bacteremia: carbapenems (imipenem, meropenem)

       ii. Non-bacteremic UTIs: oral agents (for example, trimethoprim, nitrofurantoin, mecillinam) or intravenous agents (for example, piperacillin-tazobactam)

       iii. Aminoglycosides interact with cyclosporine and may result in nephrotoxicity

       iv. Colistin (polymyxin E): highly nephrotoxic

       v. Tigecycline

   7. Prevention

     a. Prudent use of antibiotics

     b. Prompt identification and separation of patients colonized or infected with ESBL bacilli

     c. Cohorting of nurses and patients

     d. Strict adherence to infection control guidelines

     e. Proper and thorough environmental cleaning

FUNGAL INFECTIONS

I. Overview

A. Fungal infections are a major cause of post-transplant morbidity and mortality.[3]

B. The incidence of fungal infection among transplant recipients is lower than that of bacterial or viral infections; however the mortality is typically higher.[8]

   1. Reported incidence: 5% (renal transplant recipients) to approximately 50% (liver transplant recipients)

C. Fungal infections typically occur in first 6 months post-transplant but can occur over the first several years.

D. Fungal infections may be categorized as opportunistic infections (aspergillosis, candidiasis, cryptococcosis, and pneumocystis) and infections with geographically-restricted mycoses (histoplasmosis, coccidioidomycosis, and blastomycosis).

E. Potential portals of entry:[59]
   1. Respiratory tract (most common)
   2. Gastrointestinal tract
   3. Skin (for example, via intravascular catheters)

F. Risk factors for fungal infections:[3]
   1. High-dose corticosteroid therapy
   2. Broad-spectrum antimicrobial agents
   3. Rejection requiring increased immunosuppression
   4. Allograft dysfunction
   5. Concurrent infection with immunomodulating virus (for example, CMV)

G. Fungal colonization: "the isolation of yeast or mold from a nonsterile body site without local or systemic evidence of infection"[40, p. 309]

H. Clinical manifestations are frequently nonspecific and often overlap with other infectious and noninfectious processes.[4]

I. When a fungal infection is diagnosed, it is important to look for metastatic infection, particularly to skin, skeleton, and CNS.[28]

II. *Candida* species

A. Found in human gastrointestinal tract (oropharynx to anus), gynecological tract, and skin[59]
   1. Pretransplant colonization of gastrointestinal tract is a risk factor for post-transplant candidal infection.

B. Most common sources: gastrointestinal tract and intravascular catheters[3]

C. Risk factors for invasive disease:
   1. Total parenteral nutrition
   2. Central venous catheters
   3. Acute renal failure
   4. Diabetes mellitus
   5. Corticosteroid therapy
   6. Neutropenia
   7. Abdominal surgery
   8. Use of broad-spectrum antibiotics
   9. Use of muromonab-CD3 monoclonal antibody (OKT$_3$)
   10. Immunomodulating viral infections (for example, CMV, human herpes virus 6)

D. See Table 5-9 for the clinical manifestations, prevention/prophylaxis, diagnosis, and treatment of candidal infections.

III. Aspergillus species

A. Epidemiological characteristics[60]
   1. Aspergillus infections occur in 1%–15% of solid organ transplant recipients.
   2. The mortality rate for transplant recipients with invasive aspergillosis ranges from 74%–92%.
   3. Between 9.3% and 16.9% of all deaths within the first post-transplant year are due to invasive aspergillosis.

B. *Aspergillus fumigatus* is the most common human pathogen.[59]
C. Portal of entry in majority of cases: respiratory tract via environmental exposure[3]
   1. Once the pathogen invades lung tissue, ulceration, necrosis ensues, as well as invasion of the tissues and blood vessels.
   2. If the pathogen invades blood vessels, widespread dissemination can occur.
D. The lung is the most common site of primary infection.[8]
E. Historically, aspergillosis typically occurred during the first 3 months post-transplant; newer data indicate that late-onset infections are becoming more frequent.[3]
F. Chronic obstructive pulmonary disease (COPD) predisposes patients to colonization of the airway with *Aspergillus*.[60]
G. Risk factors for invasive infections:[3]
   1. Neutropenia
   2. Potent immunosuppression (particularly high-dose steroid therapy and OKT3)
   3. Prolonged operative time
   4. Renal failure
   5. Neutropenia
   6. CMV infection
H. See Table 5-9 for the clinical manifestations, prevention/prophylaxis, diagnosis, and treatment of *aspergillus* infections.
I. A synopsis of candidal and aspergillus infections in specific transplant populations is shown in Table 5-12.

IV. *Cryptococcus neoformans*[3, 59]
   A. Pathogen is ubiquitous in the environment, especially in soil and bird excrement.
   B. Disease is acquired through inhalation.
   C. Infections can occur throughout the entire post-transplant course.
   D. *Cryptococcus neoformans* is the most common cause of fungal CNS infection.[8, 9]
   E. See Table 5-9 for the clinical manifestations, prevention/prophylaxis, diagnosis, and treatment of *Cryptococcus neoformans* infections.

V. *Pneumocystis carinii*
   A. Originally classified as a protozoan, but now classified as a fungal pathogen.[8]
   B. Infection typically occurs during first 6 months after transplantation in those recipients who do not receive prophylaxis.[3]
   C. A number of diseases may mimic pneumocystis: CMV, influenza, adenovirus infection, miliary tuberculosis, disseminated fungal infections, adult respiratory distress syndrome, and respiratory syncytial virus.[8, 10]
   D. See Table 5-9 for the clinical manifestations, prevention/prophylaxis, diagnosis, and treatment of *Pneumocystis carinii* infections.

VI. Endemic mycoses
   A. Overview
      1. Endemic mycoses include: *Coccidioides immitis, Histoplasma capsulatum, Blastomyces dermatitidis,* and *Paracoccidiodes brasiliensis.*[3]

TABLE 5-12

■ *Candida* and *Aspergillus* Infections in Specific Transplant Populations

Type of Allograft	Fungal Infections: General Considerations	*Candida* Infections	*Aspergillus* Infections
Lung	Abdominal cavity: frequent site of fungal infections; may be associated with fungemia[8]	Colonization may preclude optimal healing of bronchial anastomosis and thereby precipitate tracheobronchitis and leakage[8, 61]	Risk factors: 　Positive airway specimen cultures 　Obliterative bronchiolitis[3] COPD predisposes recipients to colonization with *aspergillus*[60] Cystic fibrosis patients: colonization with *aspergillus* common prior to transplantation[60] Most frequent infections during first 3 post-transplant months: 　Tracheobronchitis 　Anastomotic infections[60] Most frequent late-occurring infections: 　Invasive pulmonary infections 　Systemic infections[60] Overall mortality rate: 52%–55% Mortality rate: tracheobronchial infections: 23%–29%[60] Mortality rate: invasive pulmonary infections: 67%–82%[60] Fever may not be present; patients with tracheobronchitis or bronchial anastomotic infections are typically afebrile[60] Invasive aspergillosis:[60] 　Reported in 3%–15% of recipients 　Median time to first occurrence: 3.2 months post-transplant 　Majority of infections occur within 6 months after transplantation Single lung transplant recipients: 　More likely to develop infection later after transplantation 　Have ↑ incidence of invasive pulmonary (vs tracheo-bronchial) aspergillosis and ↑ mortality rate than other types of lung recipients 　Invasive aspergillosis often documented in native lung, thus suggesting that the infection originated from a preexisting focus Bilateral lung transplant recipients: 　May be at ↑ risk of colonization and infection at site of anastomosis due to: 　　Longer surgical procedure 　　↑ risk of ischemia 　　↑ impairment of cough reflex and mucociliary clearance

(Continued next page.)

Type of Allograft	Fungal Infections: General Considerations	Candida Infections	Aspergillus Infections
Liver	Of all SOT recipients, liver transplant recipients have highest incidence of invasive fungal infections[29] Risk factors for fungal infections: Roux-en-Y choledoco-jejunostomy CMV infection OKT3 Retransplantation[3] Opportunistic fungi cause up to 37% of post-transplant pneumonias – typically during the first 2–3 post-transplant months[59]	Risk factor for invasive infection: extensive abdominal surgery[61]	Invasive infections: Incidence: 1 – 8% of recipients[60] Mortality rate: approximately 60%[60] Infections typically occur early following transplantation[60] Infection frequently disseminates beyond the lungs[60] Risk factors for invasive infection: Renal dysfunction Retransplantation CMV infection HHV-6 infection Fulminant hepatic failure as reason for liver transplantation[3, 60]
Kidney	Opportunistic fungi cause 2%–14% of infectious complications[59] Recipients at risk for UTIs caused by fungal pathogens due to DM and indwelling urinary catheters Most common pathogens: *Candida* spp. *Aspergillus* spp. *Candida neoformans*[40]	*Candida albicans*: most commonly isolated species[40] Typically occur during first month; associated with technical complications, early rejection, ↑ immunosuppression[40] Typically associated with an endogenous source[40] Asymptomatic candiduria: poses serious threat due to formation of obstructing fungal balls, ascending pyelonephritis, and sepsis[9]	Invasive aspergillosis:[60] Reported incidence: 0.17%–4% Mortality rate – invasive aspergillosis: 75%–80% Risk factors for invasive aspergillosis: High-dose corticosteroid therapy Prolonged corticosteroid therapy Graft failure + hemodialysis Potent immunosuppression

Type of Allograft	Fungal Infections: General Considerations	Candida Infections	Aspergillus Infections
Heart	Fungal agents implicated in mediastinal infections include *Aspergillus fumigatus* and *Candida* spp.	May result in the development of mycotic aneurysm and subsequent rupture of aortic anastomosis[8]	Aspergillus is the most common fungal pathogen and accounts for approximately 70% of all invasive fungal infections[60] Invasive aspergillosis:[60] Invasive infections occur in about 6% of recipients (range: 3%–14%) Approximately 75% of invasive infections occur within first 3 months post-transplant Post-transplant risk factors for invasive aspergillosis: Reoperation CMV disease Hemodialysis Incidence of invasive infection at institution 2 months before or after transplant date Mortality rates: Invasive pulmonary aspergillosis: 53%–78% Disseminated infections: 90% Disseminated infections with CNS involvement: 100%
Pancreas-Kidney	At risk because urinary pH associated with drainage of exocrine secretions predisposes recipient to bladder colonization with *Candida*[3] Risk of fungal infection in SPK and PAK transplant recipients equals that of liver transplant recipients[40] Risk factors: Older donor or recipient age Enteric vs. bladder drainage in SPK recipients Retransplant vs primary transplant in PAK recipients Vascular graft thrombosis[40]	More than 45% of fungal infections are caused by *Candida* species[40] SPK recipients: bladder drainage may favor colonization of the urinary tract with *Candida* species[40] Other risk factors: DM Indwelling bladder catheters[29]	Similar to those in kidney transplant recipients[61]

COPD: chronic obstructive pulmonary disease; DM = diabetes mellitus; SPK = simultaneous pancreas-kidney; PAK = pancreas after kidney; SOT = solid organ transplant

2. The endemic mycoses should be considered in symptomatic patients who have traveled to or lived in Central or South America, Southeast Asia, or the midwestern or southwestern areas of the United States.
   a. Endemic areas for *Histoplasma capsulatum* and *Blastomyces dermatitidis* include the Mississippi and Ohio River valleys[18]
   b. Endemic areas for *Coccidioides immitis*: primarily southwestern United States
3. Theoretically, infection (primary or reactivation) can occur at any time during the post-transplant period[3]; however, these infections typically occur 6 or more months post-transplant.[18]
4. The pathogenesis of histoplasmosis, coccidioidomycosis, and blastomycosis is similar to that of tuberculosis. The following clinical presentations should prompt consideration of endemic disease in the differential diagnosis:
   a. Subacute respiratory illness with focal or disseminated infiltrates on chest radiograph
   b. Non-specific febrile illness
   c. Illness in which metastatic aspects predominate (for example, mucocutaneous manifestations in histoplasmosis or blastomycosis; CNS manifestations in coccidioidomycosis)[9, 62]

B. See Table 5-9 for the clinical manifestations, prevention/prophylaxis, diagnosis, and treatment of *Histoplasma capsulatum*.

PARASITIC INFECTIONS

I. Overview
   A. The major protozoal pathogens are *Toxoplasma gondii* and *Cryptosporidium parvum*.
II. *Toxoplasma gondii*[3, 8, 10, 29, 63]
   A. Toxoplasmosis typically results from reactivation of latent disease.
   B. Toxoplasmosis is more common in heart and heart-lung recipients than in any other transplant groups because the pathogen encysts in the heart muscle.
      1. The overall incidence of toxoplasmosis in heart transplant recipients ranges from 4% to 12%.
      2. Incidence increases to more than 50% for *toxoplasma*-seronegative recipients who receive allografts from *toxoplasma*-seropositive donors who do not receive prophylaxis.
   C. Infection typically occurs during first 2 months following transplantation.
   D. Toxoplasmosis can mimic rejection; endomyocardial biopsy is required for a definitive diagnosis.
   E. See Table 5-9 for the clinical manifestations, prevention/prophylaxis, diagnosis, and treatment of toxoplasmosis.
III. *Cryptosporidium parvum*
   A. Diarrhea caused by this pathogen is frequently fatal in immunocompromised patients; hospitalization may be required to reverse dehydration and wasting.
   B. Infection of the proximal small bowel is common; however, organisms can also be harbored in the hepatobiliary tree.

C. Organisms shed by patients are infectious; universal precautions are mandatory.

D. The disease is transmitted by fecal-oral contamination or water transmission.

E. Transplant recipients whose water supplies may be contaminated with *Cryptosporidium* may be advised to take special precautions such as:

1. Boiling water for 5 minutes prior to drinking or using in food preparation OR using bottled distilled water

2. Avoiding ice cubes that have been made with tap or well water

3. Adding a filter to faucet

4. Avoiding soda fountain drinks that have been reconstituted with tap water

F. See Table 5-9 for the clinical manifestations, prevention/prophylaxis, diagnosis, and treatment of cryptosporidiosis.

IV. *Strongyloides stercoralis*[3]

A. A helminthic (worm) parasite and intestinal nematode

B. Found in 36 states in the U.S.; endemic in Southeast Asia, the Caribbean, and West Africa.

C. Organism can live (asymptomatically) in the gastrointestinal tract for decades.

D. Organism causes diarrhea and peripheral eosinophilia (a typical marker for parasitic infection).

1. Autoinfection: process by which the larvae transform into an infectious form within the intestine

2. Larvae invade intestinal mucosa.

3. Constant reintroduction of infectious forms into the host sustains the infection.

4. In transplant recipients, autoinfection may precipitate a hyperinfection syndrome (disseminated strongyloidiasis).

5. Hyperinfection accelerates the organism's lifecycle and leads to excessive helminth burden.

   a. Disruption of normal intestinal barrier results in gram-negative bacteremia and shock.

   b. Mortality rate of hyperinfection: approximately 70%

E. See Table 5-9 for the clinical manifestations, prevention/prophylaxis, diagnosis, and treatment of strongyloidiasis.

INFECTIONS IN SPECIFIC TRANSPLANT POPULATIONS: KEY POINTS

I. Lung and heart-lung transplant recipients[3, 64]

A. Pneumonia is a common complication: overall prevalence approximately 60%[3]

1. Increased susceptibility is associated with the following factors:

   a. Decreased cough reflex

   b. Impaired mucociliary clearance

   c. Graft ischemia; reperfusion injury

   d. Altered lymphatic drainage

   e. Inflammation of airway secondary to rejection

2. Bacterial pathogens are the most common cause of pulmonary infections.

a. Most common early pathogens: gram-negative bacteria such as *Enterobacteriaceae* and *Pseudomonas aeruginosa*

3. Clinical presentation of nosocomial pneumonia:
    a. Respiratory failure that requires mechanical ventilation
    b. Consolidation on chest radiograph
    c. Fever and leukocytosis may be muted or absent.
4. Treatment
    a. Guided by antimicrobial susceptibilities of pathogens
    b. Therapy is aggressive and may involve multiple agents.
5. Prevention
    a. Tailored antimicrobial prophylaxis based on respiratory tract cultures of donor and recipient
        i. Patients colonized with *B. cepacia* or gram-negative bacteria that are resistant to several agents may require multiple antimicrobial medications and inhaled aminoglycosides.
    b. Wound infections: perioperative prophylaxis for gram-positive bacteria
    c. Cystic fibrosis patients may require post-transplant prophylactic therapy for 14 days or until purulent secretions subside.

B. CMV is the most lethal infection.
C. The donor lung is only type of allograft that is frequently infected or colonized with bacterial pathogens.
D. The native lung of single lung transplant recipients is also susceptible to infection.
    1. Radiographic changes in the native lung (for example, those caused by fibrosis) may make diagnosis of infection difficult.
E. *Pseudomonas* infections are particularly problematic among recipients who undergo lung transplantation for cystic fibrosis.
F. Other serious post-transplant infections include:
    1. Mediastinitis and sternal wound infections
        a. Wound infections: perioperative prophylaxis for gram-positive bacteria may be given
        b. May require debridement in addition to antimicrobial agents
    2. Infections that lead to leakage or dehiscence of the bronchial or tracheal anastomoses
        a. Nosocomial bacteria, *candida,* and *aspergillus* are commonly associated with anastomotic infections.
G. Toxoplasmosis
    1. More common in heart transplant recipients than in any other transplant group because *toxoplasma gondii* encysts in the heart muscle.
    2. Symptoms of toxoplasmosis may appear from 3 weeks to 6 months post-transplant.
    3. Toxoplasmosis can mimic rejection; therefore an endomyocardial biopsy is required for definitive diagnosis.

II. Liver transplant recipients[3, 8, 30, 52, 65-67]
A. Early after transplant, intra-abdominal and liver abscesses, peritonitis, wound infections, and cholangitis are common.
B. The abdomen is the most common site of bacterial infection.
    1. Abdomen is most common source of VRE bacteremia (particularly periotoneal space and biliary tract).
    2. Risk factors for abdominal infections:
        a. Long surgical time

      b.   Biliary leaks, obstruction, stenosis
      c.   Hepatic artery stenosis or thrombosis
      d.   Large number of blood transfusions
      e.   Reoperation
      f.   Early rejection
      g.   CMV infection
      h.   Retransplantation

3. The type of biliary anastamosis may affect the risk of infection.
   a. Choledochostomy (duct-to-duct): Risk of infection may be less because of maintenance of the native sphincter of Oddi.
   b. Roux-en-Y choledochojejunostomy anastomoses: Rate of abdominal infections may be higher due to potential for reflux of enteric organisms into the biliary system.

C. The incidence of invasive fungal infections is high.

D. Clinical presentation[3]
   1. Wound infections and intra-abdominal abscesses
      a. Abdominal pain
      b. Fever in some, but not all, patients
         i. Fever may not develop with some pathogens.
      c. Wound dehiscence
      d. Purulent drainage from wound
      e. Pain with palpation
      f. Guarding, rebound
      g. Laboratory findings: leukocytosis in some, but not all, patients
   2. Cholangitis
      a. Fever
      b. Pain in right upper quadrant
      c. Abdominal tenderness
      d. Rebound
      e. Laboratory findings: leukocytosis, elevated bilirubin, transaminases, alkaline phosphatase

E. Diagnosis requires imaging studies: computed tomography scans, ultrasound, magnetic resonance imaging.

F. Treatment[3]
   1. Intra-abdominal and surgical wound infections
      a. Antimicrobial therapy
         i. Based on cultures and sensitivities
         ii. Empiric therapy for known colonizing pathogens may be initiated until culture and sensitivity results are available.
      b. Intra-abdominal abscess: drainage
   2. Cholangitis
      a. Intravenous antibiotics in setting of adequate biliary flow
      b. In setting of biliary tree obstruction: ERCP with dilatation

G. Prevention[3]
   1. Pre- and post-transplant: selective bowel decontamination
   2. Perioperative antimicrobials to decrease risk of wound infections
   3. Post-transplant: antimicrobial prophylaxis prior to invasive procedures such as liver biopsies

H. Almost all liver transplant recipients who had pretransplant HCV infections remain viremic after transplantation.
   1. Recurrent HCV infection occurs in 30%–70% of these patients during the first post-transplant year.

I.   Without adequate immunoprophylaxis, HBV graft infection recurs in 80%–100% of hepatitis B surface antigen-positive liver transplant recipients.

    1.   With the appropriate use of hepatitis B immune globulin and new antiviral agents (for example, lamivudine, adefovir), this recurrence rate is significantly reduced.

III. Kidney transplant recipients[3, 8, 40]

A.   Approximately 80% of infections are caused by bacteria.

    1.   Risk factors for bacterial infections:

        a.   Decreased urine flow

        b.   Renal insufficiency

        c.   Prolonged catheterization of bladder

        d.   Comorbidities such as diabetes mellitus

B.   Common infectious syndromes include:[40]

    1.   Genitourinary tract infections (particularly UTIs associated with catheters)

    2.   Pneumonia

    3.   Primary bacteremia (often associated with use of vascular catheters)

    4.   Intra-abdominal infections

    5.   Surgical site infections (superficial or deep), often associated with fluid collections or devitalized tissues

C.   Bloodstream infections

    1.   The urinary tract is the most common site of primary infection that is associated with secondary bacteremia.

    2.   Poor outcomes are associated with the following causative agents:

        a.   Gram-negative bacteria

        b.   Organisms that are multidrug resistant

        c.   *Candida* species

D.   Genitourinary tract infections

    1.   Incidence of UTIs has decreased due to the routine use of trimethoprim-sulfamethoxazole (TMP-SMX) and early catheter removal.

    2.   Risk of genitourinary tract infections is related to surgical complications (for example, urine leaks, wound hematomas, lymphoceles).

    3.   Asymptomatic candiduria can be serious because of the potential for the development of obstructing candidal fungal balls, ascending candidal pyelonephritis, and sepsis, particularly in diabetic recipients with bladder dysfunction.

    4.   For patients with suspected UTIs, obtain a clean-catch midstream urine specimen for bacterial and fungal culture (quantitative).

    5.   Clinical presentation—UTIs:

        a.   Acute pyelonephritis

        b.   High fever

        c.   Pain at site of graft

        d.   Renal allograft dysfunction

        e.   Laboratory findings: leukocytosis, urinary sediment

        f.   May be asymptomatic (no urgency, frequency, dysuria); pyuria may be absent

E.   Treatment[3]

    1.   UTIs:

        a.   Antimicrobial therapy is based on culture and sensitivities.

        b.   Duration of therapy is based on severity of the infection.

        c.   Pyelonephritis typically requires at least 2 weeks of therapy.

        d.   Recurrent infections require imaging studies to detect any anatomic anomalies or obstruction.

     2. Surgical wound infections

        a.   May require debridement in addition to antimicrobial therapy

        b.   Empiric coverage may be initiated until results of culture and sensitivities are available.

F. Prevention[3]

     1. UTIs and bloodstream infections:

        a.   Routine surveillance urine cultures

        b.   Antimicrobial prophylaxis with trimethoprim/sulfamethoxazole (TMP-SMX) or fluoroquinolones

     2. Surgical wound infections: perioperative antibiotic such as a cephalosporin

G. Unilateral leg edema on the side of the kidney transplant may be a sign of a lymphocele, either infected or not infected, near the allograft

H. Fever

     1. Requires blood cultures

     2. Differential diagnosis includes:

        a.   Infection and/or rejection

        b.   Adverse effect of medications

        c.   Noninfectious systemic inflammatory response, for example:

           i.   Pancreatitis

          ii.   Cytokine-release syndromes associated with the administration of monoclonal or polyclonal antibodies

         iii.   Pulmonary embolism

     3. Fever of unknown origin may be associated with a deep wound infection; diagnosis requires needle aspiration of wound and ultrasound or CT scanning of both pelvic implantation and nephrectomy operative sites.

I. Female recipients are at increased risk of intraepithelial and invasive squamous cell tumors of the cervix associated with human papillomavirus.

IV. Heart transplant recipients[3, 8, 13]

A. The lung is a common site of infection.

     1. Major bacterial infection: ventilator-associated pneumonia caused by gram-negative bacteria

     2. Clinical presentation[3]

        a.   Respiratory failure and inability to wean from ventilator

        b.   Fever in some, but not all, patients

        c.   Purulent respiratory secretions

        d.   Consolidation on chest radiograph

     3. Treatment

        a.   Based on results of cultures and sensitivities

     4. Prevention

        a.   Early extubation

        b.   Aggressive pulmonary toilet

B. Mediastinitis

     1. Most common during first 2 to 4 weeks post-transplant

     2. Clinical presentation

        a.   Initial symptoms may be subtle: mild chest discomfort, slight edema and/or erythema along sternal incision

        b.   Some patients may present with fever and bacteremia.

      c. Laboratory findings: leukocytosis
   3. Treatment[3]
      a. Surgical debridement
      b. Antimicrobial therapy
 C. Sternal wound infections
   1. Clinical presentation[3]
      a. Early postoperative period
         i. Poor wound healing
        ii. Dehiscence
      b. Later postoperative period
         i. Formation of sinus tract
        ii. Purulent drainage
   2. Treatment[3]
      a. Surgical debridement
      b. Antimicrobial therapy directed at gram-positive pathogens
   3. Prevention: perioperative antimicrobial agents directed at gram-positive pathogens
 D. CMV
   1. Single most common and most important pathogen that affects heart transplant recipients
   2. The risk of developing symptomatic CMV disease is significantly greater when the virus that is activated is of donor origin rather than recipient origin.
   3. The GI tract is the most common site of CMV infection.
   4. CMV pneumonitis has the highest morbidity and mortality rate of any CMV infection.
 E. Toxoplasmosis
   1. More common in heart transplant recipients than in any other transplant group because *toxoplasma gondii* encysts in the heart muscle.
   2. Symptoms of toxoplasmosis may appear from 3 weeks to 6 months post-transplant.
   3. Toxoplasmosis can mimic rejection; therefore, an endomyocardial biopsy is required for definitive diagnosis.
V. Pancreas transplant recipients[8]
 A. Recipients are particularly susceptible to candidiasis due to:
   1. Underlying diabetes
   2. Indwelling bladder catheters
   3. Drainage of exocrine secretions into bladder
 B. Bacterial UTIs may also be associated with drainage of exocrine secretions into bladder (promotes bacterial overgrowth).
 C. The most common bacterial infections are wound and intra-abdominal infections.
 D. Treatment: similar to treatment of infections in liver and renal transplant recipients
 E. Prevention[3]
   1. TMP-SMX to prevent UTIs
   2. Standard perioperative antibiotics
VI. Kidney-pancreas transplant recipients[8, 40]
 A. Wound infections and UTIs are more common in kidney-pancreas transplant recipients than in isolated kidney transplant recipients.
 B. Factors associated with increased risk of UTI include:

1. Enzymatic digestion of the glycosaminoglycan layer that normally protects the urothelium
2. Change in the urinary pH secondary to pancreatic exocrine secretions
3. Underlying glycosuria

C. Pancreatic abscess associated with gram-negative organisms or fungi may necessitate surgical draining or removal of the graft.

PREVENTION OF INFECTION

I. Pharmacologic measures
   A. Antimicrobial therapy
      1. Therapeutic: to treat an established infection
      2. Prophylactic: administration of antimicrobials to an entire population of patients to prevent common infections
      3. Preemptive: administration of antimicrobials to a subgroup of patients who are at high risk for a particular infection (for example: CMV hyperimmune globulin for CMV-seronegative recipients of an allograft from a CMV-seropositive donor)
   B. Antibiotic prophylaxis against infective endocarditis per American Heart Association guidelines
   C. Periodic post-transplant vaccinations per Centers for Disease Control and Prevention guidelines for immunocompromised individuals.
      1. Post-transplant vaccination protocols vary among transplant centers; commonly recommended vaccines include:
         a. Annual influenza vaccine (for recipients and household contacts unless otherwise contraindicated)
         b. Pneumococcal vaccine approximately every 5–6 years
         c. Tetanus booster every 10 years; some transplant centers prefer to treat tetanus-related wounds with tetanus immunoglobulin alone
      2. It is important to note that vaccinations in transplant recipients may be less effective due to:[3]
         a. Loss of previous immunity due to declining antibody levels and decreased antibody responses to previous vaccine antigens
         b. Reduced vaccine efficacy: decreased responsiveness to vaccine immunization
      3. Live attenuated vaccines[3, 68]
         a. Typically contraindicated in adults due to the potential for viral replication in the immunocompromised host
            i. Oral polio vaccine
            ii. Measles-mumps-rubella vaccine
            iii. Bacilli Calmette-Guerin
            iv. Small pox vaccine
            v. TY21a typhoid vaccine
            vi. Yellow fever vaccine—if severely immunocompromised[68]
            vii. Varicella vaccine
         b. Household contacts of transplant recipients should not receive live attenuated vaccines due to the potential for secondary infections in the recipient

II. Nonpharmacologic measures
- A. Health care providers and institutions (**Box 5-1**)
- B. Patients and family members (**Box 5-2**)

BOX 5-1

■ Nonpharmacologic Measures for Health Care Providers and Institutions

Health Care Providers

Wash hands frequently and thoroughly with antimicrobial soap or alcohol gel products.

Use aseptic technique per post-transplant protocols (for example, central line dressing changes).

Follow reverse isolation procedures per post-transplant protocol.

Housekeeping per post-transplant hospital protocol

Use leukocyte-depleted and CMV-negative blood products for CMV- seronegative recipients.

Use high-efficiency leukocyte blood filters.

Discontinue indwelling lines and catheters as soon as possible.

Obtain post-transplant infection surveillance tests per protocols and in a timely manner.

Avoid cross-contamination by staff members caring for patients with contagious infections.

Use special masks to transport recipients through high-risk areas of hospital (e.g., construction sites that might contain *Aspergillus* spores).

Institutions

Monitor showers, toilet facilities, and air-conditioning systems for *Legionella.*

Use high-efficiency particulate air-filtered air-handling systems if air supply is potentially contaminated, especially from construction.

From Cupples, SA. Infectious disease. In SA Cupples & L Ohler (Eds). *Transplantation Nursing Secrets.* Philadelphia: Hanley & Belfus, 2003; pp. 247-270.

SUMMARY: KEY POINTS[1, 12, 13, 69]

I. Because immunosuppressed patients may have a suboptimal response to vaccinations, it is important to update transplant candidates' immunizations before transplantation. These immunizations should be given as early as possible in the disease course because vaccines are often less effective in patients with severe end-organ dysfunction.

II. Immunosuppressed patients are more vulnerable to infection with organisms that are relatively avirulent (in immunocompetent individuals) or at lower innoculum.

III. Diagnosis of infection in transplant recipients may be difficult due to the following:
- A. Muted inflammatory response
- B. Presence of dual infections
- C. Advanced infection at time of presentation
- D. Simultaneous toxic side effects of medications
- E. Anatomic alterations secondary to transplant surgery

BOX 5-2

■ **Nonpharmacologic Measures for Patients and Family Members**

Wash hands frequently and thoroughly with antimicrobial soap.

Avoid people with obvious signs of illness.

Avoid raw or partially cooked foods of animal origin.

Avoid cross-contamination between raw and cooked foods.

Avoid unpasteurized products.

Wash raw fruits and vegetables thoroughly before eating.

Avoid potential animal sources of infection (e.g., cleaning cat litter boxes, bird cages, fish aquaria; petting zoos).

Avoid close contact with infants and others who have recently received live virus vaccines (oral polio, varicella, or measles-mumps-rubella vaccines).

Avoid potential sources of fungal infections during first post-transplant year (e.g., live plants, fresh flowers).

Obtain yearly influenza vaccine (patients and household contacts) unless otherwise contraindicated.

Use boiled (for at least 1 full minute) water or distilled water if safety of drinking water is questionable.

Avoid intravenous drug use.

Follow safer sex guidelines.

Consult with transplant or infectious disease physician about travel to areas requiring malaria prophylaxis and/or vaccines.

From Cupples, SA. Infectious disease. In SA Cupples & L Ohler (Eds). *Transplantation Nursing Secrets.* Philadelphia: Hanley & Belfus, 2003; pp. 247-270.

IV. For patients whose source of infection is linked to an anatomical or technical abnormality, surgical correction of the abnormality is mandatory; otherwise, antimicrobial therapy will fail.

V. Antimicrobial therapy often is not prescribed for "fixed" courses, but rather is based on microbial burden. The greater the burden, the longer and more intense the therapy. Therapy is continued until clinical and laboratory evidence demonstrates that active infection has been eradicated.

VI. In general, pathogen-specific antimicrobial therapy is preferred over broad-spectrum, empiric antibiotics.

VII. Certain antimicrobial agents can significantly interact with cyclosporine and tacrolimus and/or cause additive nephrotoxicity (see Table 5-9). Macrolide antibiotics, in particular, should be avoided whenever possible, because they elevate levels of calcineurin inhibitors.

REFERENCES

1. Fishman JA. Curve Balls—New Diseases in Transplantation and Donation. NATCO 31st Annual Conference. August 27, 2006. Chicago, IL.
2. Avery RK. Recipient screening prior to solid organ transplantation. *Clin Infect Dis*, 2002; 35: 1513-1519.
3. Stosor V. Infections in transplant recipients. In: Stuart FP, Abecassis MM, Kaufman DB (Eds.). *Organ Transplantation*, 2nd ed., Georgetown, TX: Landes Bioscience, 2003; 399-425.
4. Cupples SA. Infectious disease. In: Cupples SA, Ohler L, (Eds.). *Transplantation Nursing Secrets*. Philadelphia: Hanley & Belfus, 2003; 247-270.
5. Fishman JA, Rubin RH. Infection in solid organ transplant recipients. *N Eng J Med*, 1998; 338: 1741-1751.
6. Tucker PC. Infectious complications. In: Baumgartner WA, Reitz B, Kasper E, et al. (Eds.). *Heart and Lung Transplantation*, 2nd ed. Philadelphia: Saunders, 2002; 355-371.
7. Kontoyiannis DP, Rubin RH. Infection in the organ transplant recipient. *Infect Dis Clin North Am*, 1995; 9: 811-822.
8. Cupples SA, Lucey DR. Infectious diseases in transplant recipients. In: Cupples SA, Ohler L (Eds.). *Solid Organ Transplantation: A Handbook for Primary Health Care Providers*. New York: Springer, 2002; 16-63.
9. Rubin RH. Infection in the organ transplant recipient. In: Rubin RH, Young LS (Eds.). *Clinical Approach to Infection in the Compromised Host*, 3rd ed. New York: Plenum Medical Books, 1994; 629-705.
10. Dummer S. Infections in transplantation. In: Makowa L, Sher L (Eds.). *Handbook of Solid Organ Transplantation*. Austin,TX: Landes Bioscience, 1995; 305-335.
11. Tucker PC. Infectious complications. In: Baumgartner WA, Reitz B, Kasper E, et al. (Eds.). *Heart and Lung Transplantation*, 2nd ed. Philadelphia: Saunders, 2002; 355-371.
12. Tolkoff-Rubin NE, Rubin RH. Recent advances in the diagnosis and management of infection in the organ transplant recipient. *Sem Nephrol*, 2000; 20: 148-163.
13. Rubin RH. Prevention and treatment of cytomegalovirus disease in heart transplant patients. *J Heart Lung Transplant*, 2000; 19: 731-735.
14. Rubin RH, Kemmerly SA, Conti D, et al. Prevention of primary cytomegalovirus disease in organ transplant recipients with oral ganciclovir or oral acyclovir prophylaxis. *Transpl Infect Dis*, 2000; 2: 112-117.
15. Ljungman P, Griffiths P, Paya C. Definitions of cytomegalovirus infection and disease in transplant recipients. *Clin Infect Dis*, 2002; 34: 1094-1097.
16. Rubin RH, Snydman DR. State-of-the-art management of cytomegalovirus infection and disease in recipients of thoracic organ transplants [Monograph]. *Clinician*, 2006; 24: 1-12.
17. Singh N. Infectious diseases in the liver transplant recipient. *Semin Gastrointest Dis*, 1998; 9: 136-146.
18. Chiu LM, Domagala BM, Park JM. Management of opportunistic infections in solid-organ transplantation. *Prog Transplant*, 2004; 14: 114-129.
19. Strippoli GF, Hodson EM, Jones CJ, et al. Pre-emptive treatment for cytomegalovirus viraemia to prevent cytomegalovirus disease in solid organ transplant recipients. *Cochrane Database Syst Rev*, 2006; 1:CD005133: 1-33.
20. Razonable RR, Paya CV. Herpesvirus infections in transplant recipients: Current challenges in the clinical management of cytomegalovirus and Epstein-Barr virus infections. *Herpes*, 2003; 10: 60-65.
21. Limaye AP, Raghu G, Koelle DM, et al. High incidence of ganciclovir-resistant cytomegalovirus infection among lung transplant recipients receiving pre-emptive therapy. *J Infect Dis*, 2002; 185: 20-27.
22. Limaye AP, Corey L, Koelle DM, et al. Emergence of ganciclovir-resistant cytomegalovirus disease among recipients of solid organ transplants. *Lancet*, 2000; 356: 645-649.
23. Emery VC, Griffiths PD. Prediction of cytomegalovirus load and resistance patterns after antiviral chemotherapy. *Proc Natl Acad Sci USA*, 2000; 97: 8039-8044.
24. Humar A, Humar D, Preiksaitis J, et al. A trial of valganciclovir prophylaxis

for cytomegalovirus prevention in lung transplant recipients. *Am J Transplant*, 2005; 5: 1462-1468.

25. Kruger RM, Shannon WD, Arens MQ, et al. The impact of ganciclovir-resistant cytomegalovirus infection after lung transplantation. *Transplantation*, 1999; 68: 1272-1279.

26. Limaye AP. Ganciclovir-resistant cytomegalovirus in organ transplant recipients. *Clin Infect Dis*, 2002; 35: 866-872.

27. Fishman JS, Rubin RH. Medical progress: Infection in organ transplant recipients. *N Eng J Med*, 1998; 338: 1741-1751.

28. Patel R, Paya CV. Infections in solid organ transplant recipients. *Clin Microbiol Rev*, 1997; 10: 86-124.

29. Singh N. Infections in solid organ transplant recipients. *Am J Infect Control*, 1997; 25: 409-417.

30. Bzowej NH, Wright TL. Viral hepatitis in the transplant patient. In: Bowden RA, Ljungman P, Paya CV (Eds.). *Transplant Infections*. Philadelphia: Lippincott-Raven, 1998; 309-324.

31. Dugan AS, Eash S, Atwood WJ. Update on BK virus entry and intracellular tracking. *Transpl Inf Dis*, 2006; 8: 62-67.

32. Barber CEH, Hewlett TJC, Geldenhuys L, et al. BK virus nephropathy in a heart transplant recipient: Case report and review of the literature. *Transpl Infect Dis*, 2006; 8: 113-121.

33. Kazory A, Ducloux D. Renal transplantation and polyomavirus infection: Recent clinical facts and controversies. *Transpl Infect Dis*, 2003; 5: 65-71.

34. Khaled AS. Polyomavirus (BK virus) nephropathy in kidney transplant patients: A pathologic perspective. *Yonsei Med J*, 2004; 45: 1065-1075.

35. Josephson MA, Williams JW, Chandraker A, et al. Polyomavirus-associated nephropathy: Update on antiviral strategies. *Transpl Infect Dis*, 2006; 8: 95-101.

36. Nickeleit V, Klimkait T, Binet IF, et al. Testing for polyomavirus Type BK DNA in plasma to identify renal-allograft recipients with viral nephropathy. *N Eng J Med*, 2000; 342: 1309-1315.

37. Aksamit AJ. Central nervous system. In: Bowden RA, Ljungman P, Paya CV (Eds.). *Transplant Infections*. Philadelphia: Lippincott-Raven, 1998; 133-151.

38. Ouwens JP, Haaxma-Reiche H, Verschuuren EAM, et al. Visual symptoms after lung transplantation: A case of progressive multifocal leukoencephalopathy. *Transpl Inf Dis*, 2000; 2: 29-32.

39. Green M, Michaels MG. Adenovirus, parvovirus B19, and papillomavirus. In: Bowden RA, Ljungman P, Paya CV (Eds.). *Transplant Infections*. Philadelphia: Lippincott-Raven, 1998; 287-294.

40. Kubak BM, Maree C, Pegues DA, et al. Infections in kidney transplantation. In: Danovitch GM (Ed.). *Handbook of Kidney Transplantation*, 4th ed., Philadelphia: Lippincott Williams & Wilkins, 2005; 279-333.

41. Palmer SM, Henshaw NG, Howell DN, et al. Community respiratory viral infection in adult lung transplant recipients. *Chest*, 1998; 113: 944-950.

42. Whimbey EE, Englund JA. Community respiratory virus infections in transplant recipients. In: Bowden RA, Ljungman P, Paya CV (Eds.). *Transplant Infections*. Philadelphia: Lippincott-Raven, 1998; 295-308.

43. Falsey AR, Walsh EE. Respiratory syncytial virus infection in adults. *Clin Microbiol Rev*, 2000; 13: 371-384.

44. Alexander BD, Tapson VF. Infectious complications of lung transplantation. *Transpl Inf Dis*, 2001; 3: 128-137.

45. Speich R, van der Bij W. Epidemiology and management of infections after lung transplantation. *Clin Infect Dis*, 2001; 33 (Suppl 1): S58-S65.

46. Frost AE. Role of infections, pathogenesis, and management in lung transplantation. *Transplant Proc*, 1999; 31: 175-177.

47. Soave R. Prophylaxis strategies for solid-organ transplantation. *Clin Infect Dis*, 2001; 33(Suppl 1): S26-S31.

48. Munoz P. Management of urinary tract infections and lymphocele in renal transplant recipients. *Clin Infect Dis*, 2001; 33(Suppl 1): S53-S57.

49. Walker RC. Gram-negative infections. In: Bowden RA, Ljungman P, Paya CV (Eds.). *Transplant Infections*. Philadelphia: Lippincott-Raven, 1998; 181-194.

50. Chou T. Emerging infectious diseases and pathogens. *Nurs Clin North Am*, 1999; 34: 429-442.

51. Kauffman CA. Therapeutic and preventive options for the management of vancomycin-resistant enterococcal

infections. *J Antimicrob Chemother*, 2003; 51(Suppl 53): iii23-iii30.

52. Patel R. Clinical impact of vancomycin-resistant enterococci. *J Antimicrob Chemother*, 2003; 51(Suppl S3): iii13-iii21.

53. D'Agata EMC, Jirjis J, Gouldin C, et al. Community dissemination of vancomycin-resistant *Enterococcus faecium*. *Am J Infect Control*, 2001; 29: 316-320.

54. Engelhard D, Geller N. Gram-positive bacterial infections. In: Bowden RA, Ljungman P, Paya CV (Eds.). *Transplant Infections*. Philadelphia: Lippincott-Raven, 1998; 167-179.

55. Haddadin AS, Fappiano SA, Lipsett PA. Methicillin-resistant *Staphylococcus aureus* (MRSA) in the intensive care unit. *Postgrad Med*, 2002; 78: 385-392.

56. Singh N, Patterson D, Chang FY, et al. Methicillin-resistant *Staphylococcus aureus:* The other emerging resistant gram-positive coccus among liver transplant recipients. *Clin Infect Dis*, 2000; 30: 322-327.

57. Bhattacharya S. ESBL: From petri dish to patient. *Indian J Med Microbiol*, 2006; 24: 20-24.

58. Thomson KS. Controversies about extended-spectrum and AmpC beta-lactamases. *Emerg Inf Dis*, 2001; 7: 333-336.

59. Nicod LP, Pache J-C, Howarth N. Fungal infections in transplant recipients. *Eur Respir J*, 2001; 17: 133-140.

60. Singh N, Paterson DL. *Aspergillus* infections in transplant recipients. *Clin Microbiol Rev*, 2005; 18: 44-69.

61. Tollemar JG. Fungal infections in solid organ transplant recipients. In: Bowden RA, Ljungman P, Paya CV (Eds.). *Transplant Infections*. Philadelphia: Lippincott-Raven, 1998; 339-350.

62. dePauw BE. Advances in the management of invasive fungal infections in organ transplant recipients: Step by step. *Transpl Inf Dis*, 2000; 2: 48-50.

63. Thaler SJ, Rubin RH. Opportunistic infections in the cardiac transplant patient. *Cur Opin Cardiol*, 1996; 11: 191-203.

64. Cupples SA, Boyce SW, Stamou SC. Heart transplantation. In: Cupples SA, Ohler L (Eds.) *Solid Organ Transplantation: A Handbook for Primary Health Care Providers*. New York: Springer, 2002; 146-188.

65. Fontana RJ, Hann HL, Wright T, et al. A multicenter study of lamivudine treatment in 33 patients with hepatitis B after liver transplantation. *Liver Transplant*, 2001; 7: 504-510.

66. Keefe KB. End-stage liver disease and liver transplantation: Role of lamivudine therapy in patients with chronic hepatitis B. *J Med Virol*, 2000; 61: 403-408.

67. Paya CV. Prevention of fungal and hepatitis infections in liver transplantation. *Clin Infect Dis*, 2001; 33(Suppl 1): S47-S52.

68. Centers for Disease Control and Prevention. Recommendations of the Advisory Committee on Immunization Practices (ACIP): Use of vaccines and immune globulins in persons with altered immunocompetence. *MMRW Morb Mortal Wkly Rep*, 1993; 43(RR-4): 1-18.

69. Avery RK, Ljungman P. Prophylactic measures in the solid organ recipient before transplantation. *Clin Infect Dis*, 2001; 33(Suppl 1): S15-S21.

70. Avery RK. Infectious disease and transplantation: Messages for the generalist. *Cleve Clin J Med*, 1998; 65: 305-314.

71. Avery RK. Prevention and treatment of cytomegalovirus infection and disease in heart transplant recipients. *Cur Opin Cardiol*, 1998; 13: 122-129.

72. Miller LW. Long-term complications of cardiac transplantation. *Prog Cardiovasc Dis*, 1991; 33: 229-282.

73. Sia IG, Paya CV. Infectious complications following renal transplantation. *Sur Clin N Am*, 1998; 78: 95-112.

74. Love K. Prevention and prophylaxis of infection in thoracic transplantation. In: Emery RW, Miller LW (Eds.). *Handbook of Cardiac Transplantation*. Philadelphia: Hanley & Belfus, 1996; 17-30.

75. Trofe J, Hirsch HH, Ramos E. Polyomavirus-associated nephropathy: Update of clinical management in kidney transplant patients. *Transpl Infect Dis*, 2006; 8: 76-85.

76. Major EO, Amemiya K, Tornatore CS, et al. Pathogenesis and molecular biology of progressive multifocal leukoencephalopathy in JC virus-induced demyelinating disease of the human brain. *Clin Microbiol Rev*, 1992; 5: 49-73.

77. Baas LS, Bell B, Giesting R, et al. Infections in the heart transplant recipient. *Crit Care Nurs Clin North Am*, 2003; 15: 97-108.

78. Ampel NM, Wing EJ. Legionellosis in the compromised host. In: Rubin RH, Young LS (Eds.). *Clinical Approach to Infection in the Compromised Host*, 3rd ed. New York: Plenum, 1994; 335-353.

79. Wheat J. Fungal infections in the immunocompromised host. In: Rubin RH, Young LS (Eds.). *Clinical Approach to Infection in the Compromised Host*, 3rd ed. New York: Plenum, 1994; 211-237.

80. Reichenspurner H, Gamberg M, Nitschke H, et al. Significant reduction in number of fungal infections after lung, heart-lung, and heart transplantation using aerosolized Amphotericin B prophylaxis. *Transplant Proc*, 1997; 29: 627-628.

81. Avery RK. Infections and immunizations in organ transplant recipients: A preventive approach. *Cleve Clin J Med*, 1994; 61: 386-392.

82. Rickenbacher PR, Hunt SA. Long-term complications of transplantation. In: Emery RW, Miller LW (Eds.). *Handbook of Cardiac Transplantation*. Philadelphia: Hanley & Belfus, 1996; 201-216.

83. Fishman JA. *Pneumocystis carinii* and parasitic infections in the immunocompromised host. In: Rubin RH, Young LS (Eds.). *Clinical Approach to Infection in the Compromised Host*, 3rd ed. New York: Plenum, 1994; 275-334.

84. Parameshwar J. Follow-up after cardiac transplantation. *Br J Hosp Med*, 1996; 56: 350-354.

REVIEW QUESTIONS

1. The indirect effects of cytomegalovirus infection include:
   a. Opportunistic infections
   b. Allograft injury
   c. Rejection
   d. All of the above

2. Which statement is *most* accurate?
   a. The allograft is more likely to be affected by cytomegalovirus than a native organ.
   b. Native organs are more likely to be affected by cytomegalovirus than the allograft.
   c. Native organs and the allograft are equally affected by cytomegalovirus.
   d. Cytomegalovirus rarely affects either the allograft or native organs.

3. You are caring for a liver transplant recipient on the intermediate (step-down) care unit on postoperative day 10. Your patient has had a complicated postoperative course. Your patient was colonized with vancomycin-resistant enterococcus (VRE) prior to transplant. There are two other patients on the unit who are colonized with VRE. Which of the following statements is *least* accurate?
   a. You should not be assigned to take care of one of the other VRE-colonized patients.
   b. You should observe the abdominal incision for signs of infection.
   c. Your patient may not develop a fever in response to an infection.
   d. Because he was colonized with VRE prior to transplantation, your patient is less likely to develop a VRE infection.

4. Which transplant recipients are most likely to develop CMV?
   a. Recipient CMV seropositive, donor CMV seropositive
   b. Recipient CMV seropositive, donor CMV seronegative
   c. Recipient CMV seronegative, donor CMV seropositive
   d. Recipient CMV seronegative, donor CMV seronegative

5. You are caring for a 66-year-old male heart transplant recipient with insulin-dependent diabetes mellitus. His postoperative course was complicated; his first biopsy (on postoperative day 5) indicated severe cellular rejection. The patient was given a 3-day course of intravenous corticosteroids. Your patient is about to be discharged on postoperative day 13 when he complains of mild chest discomfort. His temperature is 100.4° F (38° C). His sternal incision is intact but appears slightly edematous. You notice that his white blood cell count is elevated. Your patient most likely is developing:
   a. Recurrent rejection
   b. Mediastinitis
   c. Pneumonia
   d. Pericarditis

6. Which of the following statements are true regarding lung transplant recipients?
   1. The donor lung is the only type of allograft that is frequently colonized or infected with bacterial pathogens.
   2. Radiographic changes in the native lung (for example, fibrosis) may make diagnosis of infection difficult.
   3. *Toxoplasma gondii* is commonly associated with anastomotic infections.
   4. Nosocomial bacteria are commonly associated with anastomotic infections.

   a. 1, 2, and 3
   b. 1, 2, and 4
   c. 2, 3, and 4
   d. 1, 3, and 4

7. A 37-year-old female transplant recipient is readmitted to your unit. She is 5 weeks status post kidney transplant. On admission, her temperature is 102.6° F (39.2° C). Her white blood cell count is 13,000/μL (SI units:13 x 10⁹ L) ; urinary sediment is present. She complains of pain at the graft site. She has no frequency, urgency, or dysuria. You suspect that this patient might have:
   1. Acute cellular rejection
   2. Acute pyelonephritis
   3. Urinary tract infection
   4. Humoral rejection

   a. 1 and 2 only
   b. 2 and 3 only
   c. 1 and 3 only
   d. 2 and 4 only

8. Pancreas transplant recipients are particularly susceptible to candidiasis due to:
   1. Underlying diabetes
   2. Indwelling bladder catheters
   3. Poor nutritional status
   4. Drainage of exocrine secretions into bladder

   a. 1, 2, and 3
   b. 1, 2, and 4
   c. 2, 3, and 4
   d. 1, 3, and 4

9. The most important pathogen that affects solid organ transplant recipients is:
   a. *Toxoplasma gondii*
   b. Cryptosporidium
   c. Cytomegalovirus
   d. Epstein-Barr virus

10. Which of the following statements about post-transplant infections are true?
   1. Immunosuppressive agents may decrease the inflammatory response.
   2. Fever may be associated with other phenomenon such as rejection.
   3. Most infections are treated with standard courses of antimicrobial agents.
   4. Certain infections may not be associated with fever.

   a. 1, 2, and 3 only
   b. 1, 2, and 4 only
   c. 1, 3, and 4 only
   d. 2, 3, and 4 only

11. In transplant recipients, risk factors for invasive fungal infections include which of the following?
   1. High-dose corticosteroid therapy
   2. Use of broad-spectrum antibiotics
   3. Diabetes mellitus
   4. Concurrent infection with an immunomodulating virus

   a. 1, 2, and 3 only
   b. 2, 3, and 4 only
   c. 1, 2, and 4 only
   d. 1, 3, and 4 only

12. The clinical manifestations associated with intra-abdominal abscesses and abdominal wound infections may include:
   a. Abdominal pain, wound dehiscence, purulent wound drainage
   b. Nausea, vomiting, diarrhea
   c. Ascites, abdominal bloating, constipation
   d. Hematemesis, reflux, diarrhea

Correct answers:

1. d	4. c	7. b	10. b
2. a	5. b	8. b	11. c
3. d	6. b	9. c	12. a

6 Transplant Complications: Noninfectious Diseases

NANCY STITT, MARIA ANGELA BARONE, MARCELLO CASTELLESE,
SANDRA GIAMMONA, GIOVANNI SCIANNA, MARIELLA ZIINO,
SANDRA A. CUPPLES

INTRODUCTION

I. Several factors have increased short- and long-term transplant survival rates:
   A. The development of potent immunosuppression regimens that have reduced graft loss and death from acute rejection
   B. Individualized immunosuppressive therapies
   C. Earlier detection and treatment of infection
II. Survival rates are also influenced by the emergence of long-term medical complications post-transplant.
III. This chapter will provide an overview of the following major (non-infectious, non-rejection) long-term complications following transplantation:
   A. Cardiovascular disease
   B. Renal insufficiency
   C. Hyperlipidemia
   D. Metabolic syndrome
   E. Diabetes mellitus
   F. Obesity
   G. Malignancy
   H. Bone disease
   I. Gastrointestinal dysfunction
   J. Gout
   K. Gingival hyperplasia
   L. Sexual dysfunction
   M. Neurocognitive impairment
IV. Monitoring of recipients for post-transplant complications
   A. While each transplant organ group may have unique post-transplant complications, the amount of evidence for post-transplant complications is highest in the renal transplantation population.
   B. The American Society for Transplantation (AST) has developed guidelines for routine surveillance of kidney transplant recipients in the outpatient setting.[1]
      1. These detection and prevention guidelines, which include specific recommendations, strength of evidence, and pertinent reviews of the

scientific literature, are designed to be used as a reference by health care professionals.

2. Given the similarities across organ transplant groups, many of the AST renal transplant guidelines are applicable to other types of solid organ transplant recipients.

CARDIOVASCULAR DISEASE (CVD)

I. For the purposes of this discussion, CVD refers to a wide range of vascular and heart-related diseases, disorders and events that include:
   A. Hypertension
   B. Arteriosclerosis
   C. Atherosclerosis
   D. Coronary artery disease (CAD)
   E. Myocardial infarction (MI)
   F. Congestive heart failure (CHF)
   G. Peripheral vascular disease
   H. Cerebral vascular disease
   I. Stroke
II. A discussion of each of these CVDs is beyond the scope of this chapter. Given, however, that hypertension is the most common disorder across all organ types, it will be discussed in detail below.
III. Cardiovascular complications are emerging as the major cause of late morbidity and mortality in all solid organ transplants groups.[2, 3]
   A. For example, CVD is the leading cause of death in renal transplant recipients and accounts for 40%-55% of all deaths.[4]
IV. There is some evidence that mortality rates due to CVD in transplant recipients are greater than in the general population;[5] for example:
   A. Renal transplant recipients have almost a two-fold risk of cardiovascular mortality compared to the general population.[6]
   B. Renal transplant recipients with graft failure have a seven- to eight-fold risk of cardiovascular mortality compared to the general population.[7]
V. Risk factors for CVD
   A. Transplant recipients may have CVD risk factors that are common to the general population as well as risk factors that are unique to transplantation.
   B. Risk factors common to the general population:[8]
      1. Male gender
      2. Older age
      3. Family history of premature CVD
      4. Elevated serum lipid concentrations
      5. Obesity
      6. Diet high in fat and cholesterol content
      7. Sedentary lifestyle
      8. Cigarette smoking
      9. Excessive alcohol consumption
      10. Prothrombic factors
      11. Left ventricular hypertrophy
   C. Transplant-specific risk factors:

1. Maintenance immunosuppressive therapy—particularly calcineurin inhibitors, mammalian target of rapamycin (mTOR) inhibitors, and corticosteroids[9]
2. Treatment of acute rejection episodes requiring increased dosing of immunosuppression
3. Chronic rejection

VI. Given the prevalence of CVD in the transplant population, pre- and post-transplant screening for CVD is imperative. Examples of screening tools include the following:

   A. Framingham Heart Study Risk Assessment Tool: estimates 10-year risk of myocardial infarction or coronary death in adults who do not have heart disease or diabetes[10] (available at http://hp2010.nhlbihin.net/atpiii/calculator.asp?usertype=prof)

   B. German Prospective Cardiovascular Munster (PROCAM) study score: considers sex, age, low-density lipoprotein (LDL) cholesterol, high-density lipoprotein (HDL) cholesterol, triglycerides, systolic blood pressure, smoking, diabetes mellitus (DM), and family history[11] (available at http://chdrisk.uni-muenster.de/calculator.php)

   C. Systematic Coronary Risk Evaluation Project (SCORE) risk chart: estimates 10-year risk of fatal CVD; considers age, gender, smoking status, systolic blood pressure, and total cholesterol[12, 13]

VII. Markers for coronary heart disease (CHD)[14]

   A. Non-modifiable risk factors
      1. Age
         a. Males: ≥ 45 years
         b. Females: ≥ 55 years
      2. Male gender
      3. Family history of premature CHD
         a. Myocardial infarction (MI) or sudden death before age 55 in father or other male first-degree relative
         b. MI or sudden death before age 65 in mother or other female first-degree relative

   B. Modifiable risk factors
      1. Hypertension
      2. Elevated LDL cholesterol
      3. Cigarette smoking
      4. Thrombogenic/hemostatic state
      5. Diabetes
      6. Obesity
      7. Physical inactivity
      8. Atherogenic diet

   C. Negative (protective) risk factor: HDL cholesterol >60 mg/dL (>1.5 mmol/L)

   D. Emerging risk factors
      1. Lipid risk factors
         a. Triglycerides
         b. Lipoprotein remnants
         c. Elevated lipoprotein(a)
         d. Small LDL particles
         e. HDL subspecies
         f. Apoliproteins
         g. Total cholesterol/HDL cholesterol ratio

   2. Non-lipid risk factors
       a. Elevated homocysteine level
       b. Thrombogenic/hemostatic factors
       c. Inflammatory markers (e.g., elevated high-sensitivity C-reactive protein)
       d. Impaired fasting glucose (110-125 mg/dL) (2.85-3.24 mmol/L)
       e. Subclinical atherosclerotic disease
VIII. Guidelines for primary and secondary prevention of cardiovascular disease and stroke are shown in Table 6-1.

HYPERTENSION

   I. Overview
       A. Common complication of all types of solid organ transplantation
       B. May develop as early as the first few days and weeks after transplantation and increase over time or may develop later in the post-transplant course.
  II. Etiology: general[17]
       A. Pretransplant hypertension
       B. Pretransplant renal disease
       C. Calcineurin inhibitors[18]
           1. Produce afferent arteriolar vasoconstriction through stimulation of sympathetic nervous system and upregulation of renin-angiotensin-aldosterone system
           2. Reduce nitric oxide (a vasodilating prostaglandin)
           3. Mediate elaboration of vasoconstrictor cytokines (for example, adenosine, platelet-derived growth factor, endothelin-1)
           4. Note: Tacrolimus typically does not cause as much hypertension as cyclosporine
       D. Corticosteroid therapy: increases sodium and water retention
       E. High body mass index
       F. Smoking
 III. Etiology: organ-specific
       A. Renal transplant recipients[3]
           1. Hypertension in donor
           2. Uncontrolled renin secretion from remaining kidney
           3. Renal artery stenosis
           4. Chronic allograft nephropathy
           5. Recurrence of intrinsic renal disease
       B. Heart transplant recipients
           1. Abnormal regulation of sodium balance associated with cardiac denervation and renal impairment
           2. Structural changes in resistance arteries[19]
  IV. Definition of hypertension—general population
       A. American Heart Association/National Heart Lung Blood Institute (Table 6-2)[20]
   V. Definition of hypertension—transplant population
       A. To date, there is no standard definition of hypertension for transplant recipients.
       B. Current target blood pressure goals include those shown in Table 6-3.

TABLE 6-1

■ **Guidelines for Primary and Secondary Prevention of Cardiovascular Disease and Stroke**

PARAMETER	GOALS	
	Primary Prevention[15]	Secondary Prevention[16]
Smoking	Cessation of smoking; No exposure to environmental smoke	Cessation of smoking; No exposure to environmental smoke
Blood pressure control	< 140/90 mm Hg RI or HF: < 130/85 mm Hg DM: < 130/80 mm Hg	< 140/90 mm Hg RI or DM: < 130/80 mm Hg
Diet	Heart healthy diet Optimize weight Saturated fat < 10% of total calories Cholesterol < 300 mg/day Salt intake < 6 grams/day Limit *trans*-fatty acids Limit alcohol intake	Heart healthy diet Optimize weight Saturated fat: < 7% of total calories Cholesterol: < 200 mg/day Limit *trans*-fatty acids
Lipid Management Primary goals	≤ 1 risk factor: LDL < 160 mg/dL (< 4.14 mmol/L) ≥ 2 risk factors + 10 yr risk < 20%: LDL < 130 mg/dL (< 3.36 mmol/L) ≥ 2 risk factors + 10 yr risk ≥ 20% or in setting of DM LDL < 100 mg/dL (< 2.59 mmol/L)	LDL < 100 mg/dL or < 70 mg/dL (< 2.59 mmol/L or < 1.81 mmol/L)
Lipid Management Secondary goals if LDL is at target goal and triglycerides are > 200 mg/dL (2.26 mmol/L)	≤ 1 risk factor Non-HDL < 190 mg/dL (< 4.92 mmol/L) ≥ 2 risk factors + 10 yr risk ≤ 20% Non-HDL < 160 mg/dL (< 4.14 mmol/L) ≥ 2 risk factors + 10 yr risk ≥ 20% Non-HDL < 130 mg/dL (< 3.36 mmol/L)	

(Continued next page.)

GOALS

PARAMETER	Primary Prevention[15]	Secondary Prevention[16]
Triglycerides	< 150 mg/dL (< 1.69 mmol/L)	For triglycerides ≥ 200 mg/dL (≥ 2.26 mmol/L) non-HDL should be < 130 mg/dL (< 3.36 mmol/L) Non HDL = total cholesterol minus HDL For triglycerides 200-499 mg/dL (2.26-5.63 mmol/L); non-HDL goal = < 130 mg/dL (< 3.36 mmol/L) or < 100 mg/dL (< 2.59 mmol/L)
HDL	Men: > 40 mg/dL (> 1.03 mmol/L) Women: > 50 mg/dL (> 1.29 mmol/L)	Men: > 40 mg/dL (> 1.03 mmol/L) Women: > 50 mg/dL (> 1.29 mmol/L)
Physical activity	30 minutes of moderately intense exercise on most, if not all, days of the week	30 minutes 7 days/week Minimum: 5 days/week
Weight	Optimize weight BMI: 18.5-24.9 kg/m² Waist circumference: Men: < 40 inches Women: < 35 inches Overweight/obese patients: 10% ↓ in weight during first year of therapy	BMI: 18.5-24.9 kg/m² Waist circumference: Men: < 40 inches Women: < 35 inches Initial goal: 10% ↓ in weight from baseline
Management of DM	Normal fasting blood glucose: < 110 mg/dL HgbA1c < 7%	HgbA1c < 7%
Anticoagulation/Antiplatelet therapy	In setting of chronic AF: anticoagulation to maintain INR between 2.0 and 3.0 (target: 2.5)	INR 2.0 to 3.0 for patients with AF or flutter and as indicated in MI patients Aspirin and/or clopidogrel as indicated

GOALS

PARAMETER	Primary Prevention[15]	Secondary Prevention[16]
RAA system blockers (Unless otherwise contraindicated)		ACEI — Indefinitely in setting of: EF ≤ 40%, Hypertension, DM, Chronic kidney disease, Consider in other settings
		ARBs — In setting of ACEI intolerance and HF or MI with EF ≤ 40%
		Aldosterone blockade — In combination with therapeutic ACEI and β-blocker doses for status post MI patients with potassium level < 5.0 mEq/L and creatinine < 2.5 mg/dL (men) or < 2.0 mg/dL (women) and with EF ≤ 40% and DM or HF
β-blocker therapy (Unless otherwise contraindicated)		Indefinitely in patients with MI, ACS, or LV dysfunction with or without HF symptoms. Consider for other patients in setting of CHD, DM, or vascular disease
Influenza vaccine		Recommended for all patients with CVD unless otherwise contraindicated

ACEI = angiotensin-converting enzyme inhibitors; ACS = acute coronary syndrome; AF = atrial fibrillation; ARB = angiotensin receptor blocker; BMI = body mass index; CHD = coronary heart disease; CVD = cardiovascular disease; DM = diabetes mellitus; HDL = high-density lipoprotein; HF = heart failure; HgbA$_{1c}$ = hemoglobin A$_{1c}$; INR = international normalized ratio; LDL = low-density lipoprotein; LV = left ventricular; MI = myocardial infarction; NSR = normal sinus rhythm; RAA = renin-angiotensin-aldosterone; RI = renal insufficiency

TABLE 6-2

■ Hypertension in the General Population[20]

Category	Systolic	Diastolic
Normal	Less than 120 mm Hg	Less than 80 mm Hg
Pre-hypertension	120-139 mm Hg	80-90 mm Hg
High blood pressure		
Stage 1	140-159 mm Hg	90-99 mm Hg
Stage 2	160 mm Hg or higher	100 mm Hg or higher

TABLE 6-3

■ Current Target Blood Pressure Goals for Transplant Recipients

Organization	Target Blood Pressure Goal
National Kidney Foundation Kidney Disease Outcomes Quality Initiative[21]	Recipients without proteinuria: ≤ 135/85 mm Hg
	Recipients with proteinuria: ≤ 125/75 mm Hg
American Society of Transplantation: Follow Joint National Commission VI Recommendations[8]	< 140 mm Hg systolic
	< 90 mm Hg diastolic
European Best Practice Guidelines Expert Group on Renal Transplantation[21]	Recipients without proteinuria: < 130/85 mm Hg
	Recipients with proteinuria: < 125/75 mm Hg

VI. Treatment options[3, 18]
   A. Goals
      1. Prevent damage to kidneys and heart
      2. Prevent cerebral vascular events
   B. Nonpharmacologic therapy
      1. Used alone, may be successful only if systolic blood pressure (SBP) is within 10 mm Hg of target SBP
      2. Strategies
         a. Smoking cessation
         b. Weight reduction
         c. Salt restriction
         d. Fluid restriction (as indicated)
         e. Regular exercise
   C. Pharmacologic therapy
      1. Antihypertensive agents are shown in Table 6-4.[18]
      2. Substitution of another immunosuppressive agent for cyclosporine
   D. Renal artery stenosis: stenting, angioplasty, bypass

TABLE 6-4

■ Antihypertensive Agents[18]

Medication	Advantages	Disadvantages
Specific β1 blockers (e.g., atenolol, metoprolol)	Agents of choice in patients with coronary artery disease (CAD) and good left ventricular function	↓ Cardiac output May ↓ renal blood flow
Alpha 1 blockers (e.g., terazosin)	May help in patients with benign prostatic hyperplasia; May ↑ renal blood flow	Orthostatic hypotension
Alpha 1 blocker + nonspecific β-blocker (e.g., labetolol)	May be effective for patients who need both vasodilatation and heart rate control	Bronchospasm Avoid with peripheral vascular disease Possible ↑ risk of cerebrovascular events May exacerbate cyclosporine-induced hyperkalemia ↓ Cardiac output
Calcium channel blockers: Dihydropyridines (e.g., nifedipine)	Best agents to prevent cyclosporine A-induced vasoconstriction	Edema (non-sodium retentive) Reflex tachycardia Avoid with active CAD May exacerbate cyclosporine-induced gingival hyperplasia
Calcium channel blocker: Diltiazem	Can prevent cyclosporine A-induced vasoconstriction	↑ Cyclosporine levels ↑ Tacrolimus levels
Calcium channel blocker: Verapamil	Can prevent cyclosporine A-induced vasoconstriction	↑ Cyclosporine levels ↑ Tacrolimus levels ↓ Cardiac output Bradycardia Constipation

(Continued next page.)

Medication	Advantages	Disadvantages
Angiotensin-converting enzyme inhibitors (ACEI) (e.g., enalapril)	May be best agents for patient with ↓ left ventricular function or left ventricular dilatation.	Hyperkalemia
Angiotensin II blockers (e.g., losartan)	May be best agents to ↓ proteinuria experimentally. May ↓ cyclosporine-mediated renal fibrosis	Deterioration in renal function (particularly in patients with renal artery stenosis)
Alpha 2 agonists (e.g., clonidine)	Effective in many people ↓ Central sympathetic discharge	Drowsiness Dry mouth
Direct vasodilators (e.g., hydralazine, minoxidil)	Hydralazine often used with patients intolerant to ACEI or alpha II blockers with congestive heart failure Minoxidil effective in refractory patients	Reflex tachycardia Sodium retention
Diuretics (e.g., furosemide)	Often necessary in volume extended patients	Electrolyte disorders Volume depletion may activate renin-angiotensin II system May exacerbate cyclosporine-induced fibrosis

Data from Kaplan B, Meier-Kriesche H-U. Late complications of transplantation. In Stuart FP, Abecassis MM, Kaufman DB (Eds.). *Organ Transplantation*, 2nd edition. Austin: Landes Bioscience, 2003: 437-447.

RENAL INSUFFICIENCY (RI)

    I. Overview
        A. Scope of problem (Table 6-5)
    II. Etiology:[26]
        A. Nonrenal transplant recipients: pretransplant RI associated with end-stage heart or liver disease
        B. Nephrotoxicity associated with:
            1. Calcineurin inhibitors (cyclosporine, tacrolimus)
            2. Antibiotics
            3. Certain non-maintenance immunosuppressants used to treat acute rejection
    III. Risk factors for post-transplant RI[26]
        A. Pretransplant RI
        B. Perioperative events
            1. Hypotension
            2. Use of pressor agents
            3. Sepsis
            4. Cytomegalovirus (CMV) infection
        C. Hypertension
        D. Hyperlipidemia
        E. Proteinuria
    IV. Types of cyclosporine-induced injury
        A. Acute[27]
            1. Severe vasoconstriction of afferent arterioles leads to decrease in renal blood flow and glomerular filtration rate (GFR)
            2. Effects are dose-related; effects are often reversed with withdrawal of cyclosporine
        B. Chronic[27]
            1. Characterized by structural changes in renal architecture
                a. Tubular atrophy
                b. Tubulointerstitial fibrosis
                c. Glomerulosclerosis
            2. Injury worsens over time and results in permanent renal dysfunction

---

TABLE 6-5

■ **Scope of the Problem of Renal Insufficiency**

Kidney	Heart	Lung	Heart-lung	Liver
The majority of survivors eventually develop acute and/or chronic graft dysfunction[1]	Cumulative prevalence: 32%, 33%, and 36% at 1, 5, and 8 years post-transplant, respectively[22]	Cumulative prevalence: 26%, 39%, and 43% within 1, 5, and 10 years post-transplant, respectively[23]	Cumulative prevalence: 18% and 28% within 1 and 5 years post-transplant, respectively[23]	At 10 years post-transplant, up to 20% of recipients have developed end-stage renal disease and require hemodialysis or renal transplantation[24,25]

V. Assessment
   A. Potential clinical manifestations:
      1. Decreased creatinine clearance
      2. Proteinuria
      3. Increased serum potassium level
      4. Increased serum uric acid level
      5. Decreased sodium excretion
      6. Hypertension
      7. Fluid retention
      8. Anemia
   B. Monitor trough levels of cyclosporine or tacrolimus.
      1. Nephrotoxicity typically occurs with high trough levels but may occur at low trough levels.[17]
   C. Assess patient's volume status to determine if dehydration is contributing to RI.
   D. Review patient's medication profile to identify other medications that may be contributing to nephrotoxicity, such as:
      1. Antibiotics
      2. Antihypertensive medications
      3. Diuretics
      4. Nonsteroidal anti-inflammatory drugs (NSAIDs)
VI. Interventions
   A. Target patients who have a significant increase in serum creatinine during first 6 months post-transplant.[27]
   B. Immunosuppression management
      1. If possible, reduce dose of cyclosporine or tacrolimus.
      2. Consider changing patient from cyclosporine to tacrolimus.
   C. Aggressive blood pressure control
      1. Diastolic hypertension has been linked to severe RI
      2. Antihypertensive agents[26] (see Table 6-4)
   D. Aggressive treatment of hyperlipidemia
   E. Screen for and treat renal artery stenosis

HYPERLIPIDEMIA

I. Overview
   A. Hyperlipidemia is a significant post-transplant problem. (Table 6-6)
II. Etiology: factors associated with hypercholesterolemia
   A. History of pretransplant hyperlipidemia and/or obesity
   B. Genetic factors
   C. Male gender
   D. Older age
   E. Post-transplant medications
      1. Immunosuppressive agents
         a. Cyclosporine
         b. Corticosteroids
         c. Rapamycin
      2. Antihypertensive agents
      3. Effect of post-transplant medications on lipoproteins (Table 6-7)
         [18, 29, 30]

TABLE 6-6

■ Hyperlipidemia

Type of Transplant	Scope of Problem
Kidney	50%-60% of kidney transplant recipients have hypercholesterolemia[3]
	Approximately 60% of recipients have total cholesterol levels > 240 mg/dL[1]
Heart	Cumulative prevalence in survivors at 1, 5, and 8 years post-transplant: 68.6%, 86.3%, and 91.4%, respectively[22]
	Total cholesterol, LDL, apolipoprotein B, and triglyceride levels may increase during the first 3 months post-transplant[28]
Lung	Cumulative prevalence in survivors during first post-transplant year: 24%
	Cumulative prevalence in survivors within 5 and 10 years post-transplant: 49% and 67%, respectively[23]
Heart-Lung	Cumulative prevalence in survivors within 1 and 5 years: 19.5% and 64.7%, respectively[23]
Liver	May affect up to half of recipients[25]

TABLE 6-7

■ Effect of Post-transplant Medications on Lipoproteins[18, 29, 30]

Medication	Effect
Cyclosporine	↑ 20-30% total and LDL cholesterol; ↑ triglycerides
Glucocorticoids	↑ 5-25% total, VLDL, and LDL cholesterol
Sirolimus	↑ triglycerides, ↑ VLDL cholesterol
Beta-blockers	↑ 15-50% triglycerides; ↓ 5-15% HDL cholesterol
Thiazide diuretics	↑ 0-10% total and LDL cholesterol; ↑ triglycerides 30-50%

LDL = low density lipoprotein; VLDL = very low density lipoprotein; HDL = high density lipoprotein

Data from Lake KL. Management of post-transplant obesity and hyperlipidemia. In Emery RW, Miller LW. (Eds). *Handbook of Cardiac Transplantation*. Philadelphia: Hanley & Belfus. 1996. pp. 147-164.

F. Comorbid conditions
1. Diabetes mellitus: associated with hypertriglyceridemia, hypercholesterolemia
2. Proteinuria: associated with elevated low-density lipoprotein (LDL) and lipoprotein A
3. Renal dysfunction
4. Obesity[30-32]
   a. Causes excessive production of very-low-density lipoprotein (VLDL) particles
   b. Increases triglyceride levels

        c. Increases LDL levels

        d. Decreases high-density lipoprotein (HDL) levels

   G. Diet high in saturated fat and/or cholesterol

III. Major consequences of post-transplant hyperlipidemia[1]

   A. Cardiovascular disease

   B. Chronic allograft vasculopathy

IV. Screening for post-transplant hyperlipidemia[1]

   A. Fasting (12-hour) total cholesterol, LDL, HDL, and triglyceride levels at least twice during the first post-transplant year

      1. More frequent screening for recipients with history of pretransplant hyperlipidemia and those at high risk for hyperlipidemia (e.g., patients on rapamycin)

   B. Regular screening throughout the post-transplant course, particularly for recipients with risk factors for cardiovascular disease

V. Treatment: given the multifactorial etiology of hyperlipidemia, a multifaceted and individualized treatment strategy is imperative

   A. Similar to treatment of hyperlipidemia in general population

   B. Nonpharmacologic interventions

      1. Optimization of weight

      2. Exercise

      3. Smoking cessation

      4. Diet low in saturated fat and cholesterol

   C. Pharmacologic interventions

      1. Indications for drug therapy vary among transplant populations and transplant centers.

         a. Some heart transplant centers prescribe 3-hydroxy-3-methylglu-taryl coenzyme A (HMG-CoA) reductase inhibitors, also known as statins, for all recipients, even those with normal cholesterol profiles.[33]

            i. There is evidence that pravastatin, in addition to lowering cholesterol levels in heart transplant recipients, may have additional beneficial effects.

            ii. For example, Kobashigawa and colleagues demonstrated that pravastatin also decreased the incidence of rejection associated with hemodynamic compromise, increased one-year survival, and decreased the development of coronary vasculopathy[34]

         b. Heart transplant recipients: drug therapy is typically initiated if:[19]

            i. Total or LDL cholesterol levels are elevated

            ii. Nonpharmacologic interventions have failed after a 3- to 6-month trial

            iii. Immuosuppressive medications have been reduced to a maintenance level and cholesterol levels remain elevated

      2. LDL is the primary target of therapy[14, 35]

      3. LDL goals are established on the basis of risk for coronary heart disease (CHD); however, goals may be lower in transplant recipients than in the general population.

      4. Risk assessment considers:

         a. LDL-cholesterol levels

         b. Presence or absence of CHD or other forms of atherosclerotic disease

    c. Risk factors other than LDL
  5. Once risks have been assessed, patient's risk category is determined and therapy is individualized (Table 6-8)[36]
    a. Ten-year risk calculator is available at: http://hp2010.nhlbihin. net/atpiii/calculator.asp?usertype=prof
D. Drugs that affect lipid metabolism (Table 6-9)[14]
E. Drug interactions
  1. Interactions may occur between calcineurin inhibitors (cyclosporine, tacrolimus) and statins[18] such that the serum concentration of statins is increased.
  2. Increased serum levels of statins can lead to the development of rhabdomyolysis.
    a. Rhabdomyolysis is a potentially fatal disease that is characterized by the destruction of striated muscle.
      i. As the muscle breaks down and becomes necrotic, intracellular muscle contents leak into the circulation and extracellular fluid.
    b. Rhabdomyolysis may be asymptomatic; however, symptoms typically include the classic triad of muscle pain, weakness, and dark urine.
      i. Muscle pain may be generalized or may involve specific muscle groups such as the thighs, calves, and lower back.[37]
      ii. Symptoms may develop acutely upon initiation of statin therapy or many months or years later.
    c. Additional risk factors associated with rhabdomyolysis include:[38]
      i. Older age
      ii. Female gender
      iii. Diabetes mellitus
      iv. Concurrent renal or liver disease
      v. Concurrent use of fibrate-type agents[18]
    d. Instruct patients to promptly report muscle pain, weakness, or any other untoward symptoms.
    e. If rhabdomyolysis is suspected, obtain hepatic function tests and a serum creatine kinase (CK).
      i. CK may be within normal range, but it typically begins to rise within 12 hours of development of rhabdomyolysis, peaks after 1 to 3 days, and then declines over a period of 3 to 5 days after the muscle injury ceases.
  3. Monitor lipid profile and hepatic function tests:
    a. When a statin is started.
    b. Anytime a statin dose is increased.
    c. Anytime a different statin is started.
  4. Some patients may not tolerate any statins; others may tolerate one statin, but not another.
F. Specific types of dyslipidemia (Table 6-10)[14]

TABLE 6-8

■ **Risk Category and Therapy[36]**

Risk Category	Explanation of Risk Category	LDL Cholesterol Goal	LDL Level at Which to Initiate TLC	LDL Level at Which to Consider Drug Therapy(c)
High	CHD includes: Evidence of clinically significant myocardial ischemia or History of: MI Angina Coronary artery procedures CHD risk equivalents include: Clinical manifestations of noncoronary forms of atherosclerotic disease, diabetes, and 2+ risk factors with 10-year risk for hard CHD >20%	<100 mg/dL (<2.59 mmol/L) Optional goal: <70 mg/dL (a) (<1.81 mmol/L)	>100 mg/dL(b) (>2.59 mmol/L) TLC = therapeutic lifestyle changes including reduced intake of saturated fats and cholesterol, weight reduction, and increased physical activity	>100 mg/dL (d) (>2.59 mmol/L) <100 mg/dL: (<2.59 mmol/L) consider drug options (c)
Moderately High	2+ risk factors: Cigarette smoking Hypertension (BP >140/90 mm Hg or on antihypertensive medications) Low HDL-C (<40 mg/dL[<1.03 mmol/L]) Family history of premature CHD (e) Age (men >45 years; women >55 years)	<130 mg/dL (<3.67 mmol/L) Optional goal: <70 mg/dL (<1.81 mmol/L)	>130 mg/dL (b) (>3.67 mmol/L)	>130 mg/dL (>3.67 mmol/L) (100–129 mg/dL: (2.59–3.34 mmol/L) consider drug options) (f)
Moderate Risk	2+ risk factors (see above) 10-year risk <10%	<130 mg/dL (<3.67 mmol/L)	>130 mg/dL (>3.67 mmol/L)	>160 mg/dL (>4.14 mmol/L)

Risk Category	Explanation of Risk Category	LDL Cholesterol Goal	LDL Level at Which to Initiate TLC	LDL Level at Which to Consider Drug Therapy(c)
Lower Risk	0-1 risk factors	< 160 mg/dL (< 4.14 mmol/L)	> 160 mg/dL (> 4.14 mmol/L)	> 190 mg/dL (> 4.92 mmol/L) 160-189 mg/dL: (4.14–4.89 mmol/L) LDL-lowering drug optional

BP = blood pressure; CHD: coronary heart disease; HDL–C = high-density lipoprotein cholesterol; LDL–C = low-Density lipoprotein cholesterol; MI = myocardial infarction; TLC = therapeutic lifestyle changes

(a) Very high risk favors the optional LDL-C goal of < 70 mg/dL (1.81 mmol/L), and in patients with high triglycerides, non-HDL-C < 100 mg/dL (< 2.59 mmol/L).

(b) Any person at high risk or moderately high risk who has lifestyle-related risk factors (e.g., obesity, physical inactivity, elevated triglyceride, low HDL-C, or metabolic syndrome) is a candidate for therapeutic lifestyle changes to modify these risk factors regardless of LDL-C level.

(c) When LDL-lowering drug therapy is used, it is advised that intensity of therapy be sufficient to achieve at least a 30% - 40% reduction in LDL-C levels.

(d) If baseline LDL–C is < 100 mg/dL (2.59 mmol/L), institution of a LDL-lowering drug is a therapeutic option on the basis of available clinical trial results. If a high-risk person has high triglycerides or low HDL-C, combining a fibrate or nicotinic acid with an LDL-lowering drug can be considered.

(e) Family history of CHD: CHD in male first-degree relative < 55 years of age; CHD in female first-degree relative <65 years of age.

(f) For moderately high-risk persons, when LDL-C level is 100-129 mg/dL (2.59-3.34 mmol/L) at baseline or on lifestyle therapy, initiation of a LDL-lowering drug to achieve an LDL-C level <100 mg/dL (< 2.59 mmol/L) is a therapeutic option on the basis of clinical trial results.

TABLE 6-9

■ **Drugs that Affect Lipid Metabolism[14]**

Drug Class	Dose Range	Effect	Potential Side Effects	Contraindications	Follow-up Monitoring
HMG CoA reductase inhibitors		↓ LDL	Myopathy	Absolute:	Monitor patient for:
Lovastatin	20-80 mg	↓ triglycerides	Rhabdomyolysis	Liver disease (acute or chronic)	Muscle pain, tenderness, soreness
Pravastatin	20-40 mg	↑ HDL	↑ liver enzymes	Relative:	Onset of therapy: Evaluate patient for muscle symptoms; check CK
Simvastatin	20-80 mg			Certain medications that are metabolized through the cytochrome p450 system:	Subsequent visit:
Fluvastatin	20-80 mg			Cyclosporine, Macrolide antibiotics	Evaluate patient for muscle symptoms
Atorvastatin	10-80 mg			Some antifungal agents	If patient develops muscle pain, tenderness or soreness: check CK
					Onset of therapy: monitor ALT and AST
					Monitor ALT and AST immediately after onset of therapy, 12 weeks after onset of therapy, and annually thereafter or as indicated
Bile acid sequestrants		↓ LDL	Mainly GI:	Absolute:	Monitor patient for side effects at onset of therapy and at each follow-up visit
Cholestyramine	4-24 grams	↑ HDL	Indigestion	Dysbeta-lipoproteinemia	May interfere with absorption of cyclosporine; check cyclosporine levels
Colestipol	5-30 grams	Triglycerides: ↑ or no change	Bloating	Triglycerides > 400 mg/dL (4.52 mmol/L)	
Colesevelam	2.6-4.4 grams		Constipation	Relative:	Cyclosporine and other medications should not be taken 1 hour before or 4 to 6 hours after bile acid sequestrant is taken
			Abdominal pain	Triglycerides > 200 mg/dL (2.26 mmol/L)	
			Flatulence		
			Nausea		
			↓ absorption of other medications		
			Side effects may preclude long-term compliance		

Drug Class	Dose Range	Effect	Potential Side Effects	Contraindications	Follow-up Monitoring
Nicotinic acid		↓ LDL	Flushing	Absolute:	Monitor patient for side effects at onset of therapy and at each follow-up visit
Immediate-release	1.5-3 grams	↓ triglycerides	Itching	Chronic liver disease	FBS and uric acid:
		↑ HDL	Tingling	Severe gout	At onset of therapy,
Extended-release	1-2 grams		Headache	Relative:	6-8 weeks later;
Sustained-release	1-2 grams		Nausea	Diabetes	Annually or as indicated thereafter
			Flatulence	Hyperuricemia	AST and ALT:
			Heartburn	Peptic ulcer disease	At onset of therapy;
			Fatigue		6-8 weeks later;
			Rash		At dose of 1500 mg;
			Hyperglycemia		6-8 weeks after reaching maximum dose;
			Hyperuricemia		Annually or as indicated thereafter
			Gout		For patients on cyclosporine: may ↑ LFTs and uric acid
			Hepatotoxicity		
Fibric acid derivatives		↓ LDL	Abdominal pain	Absolute:	Monitor patient for side effects at onset of therapy and at each follow-up visit
Gemfibrozil	600 mg BID	↓ triglycerides	Dyspepsia	Severe renal disease	Monitor PT/ INR:
		↑ HDL	Headache	Severe liver disease	May potentiate effects of warfarin
Fenofibrrate	200 mg daily		Drowsiness		Use with caution in diabetic patients: interacts with insulin and sulfonylureas
Clofibrate	1000 mg BID		Cholelithiasis		
			Myopathy		

ALT = alanine aminotransferase; AST = aspartate aminotransferase; CK = creatine kinase; GI = gastrointestinal; HDL = high density lipoprotein; FBS = fasting blood glucose; HMG CoA = 3-hydroxy-3methylglutaryl coenzyme A; LDL = low-density lipoprotein; LFT = liver function test; PT = prothrombin time; INR = international normalized ratio

TABLE 6-10

■ **National Cholesterol Education Program Adult Treatment Panel III Criteria for Metabolic Syndrome**[40, 41]

Type of Dyslipidemia	Treatment	Comment
Very high LDL cholesterol: ≥ 190 mg/dL (≥ 4.92 mmol/L)	Combined drug therapy: statin and bile acid sequestrant	Patient may have genetic hypercholesterolemia
Elevated serum triglycerides: Normal: < 150 mg/dL Borderline-high: 150-199 mg/dL High: 200-499 mg/dL Very high: ≥ 500 mg/dL SI Units: Normal: < 1.69 mmol/L Borderline-high: 1.69–2.24 mmol/L High: 2.26–5.63 mmol/L Very high: ≥ 5.65 mmol/L	Achieve target LDL goal Borderline high: • Weight reduction • ↑ physical activity High: • Intensify therapy to lower LDL or • Add nicotinic acid or fibrate Very high: • Prevent acute pancreatitis with very low fat diet (≤ 15% of total intake), weight reduction, ↑ physical activity, and fibrate or nicotinic acid	Contributing factors: Overweight Obesity Physical inactivity Smoking Excess alcohol intake High carbohydrate diet Certain disease states (e.g., type 2 diabetes mellitus) Certain drugs (e.g., corticosteroids), Genetic disorders
Low HDL cholesterol: < 40 mg/dL (< 1.03 mmol/L)	Achieve target LDL goal When LDL goal is reached: Weight reduction Physical activity Isolated low HDL: fibrates or nicotinic acid	Strong predictor of coronary heart disease Potential etiology: Insulin resistance Physical inactivity Type 2 diabetes mellitus Smoking High carbohydrate intake Certain drugs (e.g., beta-blockers)

METABOLIC SYNDROME[14]

I. Refers to a cluster or group of lipid and nonlipid risk factors for CHD that are of metabolic origin
II. Closely related to "insulin resistance"—a condition in which the normal function of insulin is hampered. Factors associated with insulin resistance include:
   A. Excess body fat, particularly in the abdominal area
   B. Physical inactivity
   C. Genetic predisposition (in certain individuals)
III. Definitions of metabolic syndrome
   A. World Health Organization clinical definition (Table 6-11)[39]

B. National Cholesterol Education Program Adult Treatment Panel III clinical definition of metabolic syndrome: Three or more of the five criteria in Table 6-12[40, 41]

IV. Management of metabolic syndrome[14]
A. Control LDL cholesterol
B. Weight reduction
C. Increase physical activity to:
1. Lower very low-density lipoprotein (VLDL) levels
2. Lower LDL levels (in certain patients)
3. Increase HDL cholesterol
4. Lower blood pressure
5. Decrease insulin resistance

TABLE 6-11
■ World Health Organization Clinical Definition of Metabolic Syndrome[39]

Clinical Measure	Description
Required criteria: Hyperglycemia/insulin resistance criteria and two or more of the following:	Insulin resistance: impaired glucose tolerance; impaired fasting glucose, type 2 diabetes mellitus or lowered insulin sensitivity (Insulin sensitivity measured under hyperinsulinemic euglycemic conditions; glucose uptake in lowest 25 percent of population of interest)
Central obesity	Waist/hip ratio: Males: > 0.9 Females: > 0.85 and/or body mass index > 30 kg/m²
Hyperglycemia	Impaired glucose tolerance Impaired fasting glucose Type 2 diabetes mellitus
Dyslipidemia	Elevated plasma triglyceride levels: ≥ 150 mg/dL (1.7 mmol/L) and/or High density lipoprotein cholesterol: Males: < 35 mg/dL (<0.9 mmol/L) Females: < 39 mg/dL (< 1.0 mmol/L)
Elevated blood pressure	Arterial blood pressure ≥ 140/90 mm Hg
Other	Microalbuminuria

TABLE 6-12

■ **Criteria for Metabolic Syndrome**[40, 41]

Clinical Measure	Description	
Central Obesity	Waist circumference: Caucasians Males: ≥ 40 inches (≥ 102 cm) Females: ≥ 35 inches (≥ 88 cm)	Waist circumference: Asians Males: ≥ 35.4 inches (≥ 90 cm) Females: ≥ 31.5 inches (≥ 80 cm)
	Note: Consider lower cut-offs for some non-Asian adults with strong genetic predisposition to insulin resistance (Males: ≥ 94 cm; females: ≥ 80 cm)	
Hyperglycemia	Fasting plasma glucose level ≥ 100 mg/dL (5.6 mmol/L) or current drug therapy for hyperglycemia	
Reduced high density lipoprotein (HDL) cholesterol levels	Males: < 40 mg/dL (< 1.0 mmol/L) Females: < 50 mg/dL (< 1.3 mmol/L) or current drug therapy for low HDL cholesterol level	
Elevated triglyceride levels	Triglyceride level ≥ 150 mg/dL (≥ 1.7 mmol/L) or current drug therapy for hypertriglyceridemia	
Elevated blood pressure	Systolic blood pressure ≥ 130 mm Hg Diastolic blood pressure ≥ 85 mm Hg or current drug therapy for hypertension	

DIABETES MELLITUS (DM)

I. Overview
  A. DM that develops *de novo* after transplantation is also referred to as new onset DM (NODM)[42]
  B. Incidence of DM is as follows:
    1. Kidney: 2.5% to 58%[42]
    2. Heart: 31%, 34%, and 37% at 1, 5, and 8 years post-transplant, respectively[22]
    3. Lung: 22% and 31% within 1 and 5 years post-transplant, respectively[23]
    4. Heart-lung: 14% and 22% within 1 and 5 years post-transplant, respectively[23]
  C. Onset[43]
    1. Can range from 3 weeks to 20 years post-transplant
    2. Typically occurs within first 3 post-transplant months or when corticosteroid therapy is augmented to treat rejection
  D. Approximately 40% of transplant recipients who develop DM will require insulin therapy[43]
II. Etiology[18]
  A. Primary cause: Immunosuppressive agents (Table 6-13)[1, 44]

B. Overweight/obesity
III. Screening: post-transplant DM[8]
    A. Tests
        1. Fasting blood glucose (FBG) (Table 6-14)[45]
        2. Oral glucose tolerance test: 2-hour plasma glucose (Table 6-15)
        3. HgbA$_{1c}$[45]
           a. Measures average glycemic levels over a period of weeks
           b. Elevated HgbA$_{1c}$ reflects chronic state of hyperglycemia
           c. May be more appropriately used to monitor the effectiveness of glycemic therapy rather than diagnose DM

TABLE 6-13
■ Immunosuppressive Agents[1, 44]

Immunosuppressive Agent	Inhibits insulin secretion	Causes insulin resistance	Directly affects release of insulin from islets	Causes temporary or permanent structural damage to islets
Cyclosporine*	X			X (at high doses)
Tacrolimus*†	X			X (at high doses)
Mycophenolate mofetil	X			
Sirolimus	X			
Corticosteroids	X	X	X	

* Has additive effect when given in combination with corticosteroids
† Tacrolimus appears to be more diabetogenic than cyclosporine

TABLE 6-14
■ Fasting Blood Glucose[45]

Diagnosis	FBG Test Results
Normal	< 100 mg/dL (< 5.6 mmol/L)
Impaired fasting glucose	100–125 mg/dL (5.5–6.9 mmol/L)
Diabetes (must be confirmed on a separate day)	≥ 126 mg/dL (≥ 7.0 mmol/L)

TABLE 6-15
■ Oral Glucose Tolerance Test

Diagnosis	2-hour Plasma Glucose Test Results
Normal	< 149 mg/dL (< 7.8 mmol/L)
Impaired glucose tolerance	140–199 mg/dL (7.8–11.0 mmol/L)
Diabetes (must be confirmed on a separate day)	≥ 200 mg/dL (≥ 11.1 mmol/L)

    B. Recommended frequency for testing
        1. Post-transplant months 1 to 3: FBG weekly
        2. Post-transplant months 2 to 6: FBG every other week
        3. Post-transplant months 6 to 12: FBG monthly
        4. After first year: FBG and/or glycosylated hemoglobin: at least yearly

IV. Transplant recipients at increased risk for post-transplant DM[1, 18, 43]
    A. Older recipients (> 45 years)
    B. Recipients with positive family history of DM
    C. African-American, Afro-Caribbean, or Hispanic ethnicity[42]

V. Treatment of post-transplant DM
    A. Similar to treatment of DM in general population
        1. Dietary therapy
            a. Very few transplant recipients can be managed by dietary therapy alone
        2. Oral hypoglycemic agents
            a. May be sufficient for some patients with moderate hyperglycemia (FBG < 250 mg/dL [<13.9 mmol/L]) or patients with normal FBG but with postprandial hyperglycemia[43]
        3. Insulin therapy
            a. Required for 40%–50% of transplant recipients with DM[43]
        4. Weight loss
        5. Exercise
    B. Components of Diabetes Control and Complications Trial (DCCT) recommendations[46]
        1. Strict control of blood glucose levels is essential[17]
        2. In the DCCT, a 2% decrease in average $HgbA_{1c}$ was associated with a 60% reduction in the risk of several complications of DM including retinopathy, nephropathy, and neuropathy.
    C. Surveillance for complications of DM
        1. Cardiovascular disease
            a. Post-transplant DM imposes a greater relative risk for cardiovascular morbidity and mortality than hyperlipidemia and hypertension.[42]
        2. Infections
        3. Retinopathy
        4. Nephropathy
        5. Neuropathy

VI. Transplant-specific treatment strategies
    A. Decrease dose of steroids and/or calcineurin inhibitors when possible
    B. Withdraw steroids when possible
    C. Change immunosuppression regimens (e.g., from tacrolimus to cyclosporine)

VII. Patient monitoring
    A. Oral hypoglycemic agents
        1. Most agents are excreted, at least partially, through kidneys
        2. Use with caution in patients with renal impairment
        3. Monitor renal function
    B. Monitor recipient for rejection in setting of:
        1. Immunosuppression dose reduction
        2. Steroid withdrawal
        3. Changes in immunosuppressive agents

VIII. Diabetes in specific transplant populations
  A. Lung transplant recipients: Additional contributing factor: pancreatic insufficiency associated with cystic fibrosis[47]
  B. Kidney transplant recipients: possible contributing factors: adult polycystic kidney disease[1], hepatitis C infection[48]
  C. Pancreas transplant recipients[44]
    1. HgbA$_{1c}$ is typically normal by 1 month post-transplant.
    2. Once euglycemia has been achieved, recurrent hyperglycemia that requires insulin therapy typically is associated with one or more of the following:
      a. Graft failure secondary to acute or chronic rejection
      b. Insulin resistance with new-onset type 2 DM
      c. Islet cell toxicity secondary to immunosuppression
      d. Immune-related islet cell destruction
    3. Follow-up screening for glucose intolerance includes a fasting glucose and HgbA$_{1c}$ at every clinic visit.
      a. An oral glucose tolerance test (with insulin concentrations) is done if there have been no recent rejection episodes and:
        i. The fasting blood glucose level > 100 mg/dL (5.55 mmol/L)
        ii. HgbA$_{1c}$ is elevated
    4. New-onset type 2 diabetes mellitus
      a. Typically represents a genetic predisposition to insulin resistance that is exacerbated by immunosuppressive agents and/or considerable weight gain
      b. Treatment options:
        i. Insulin therapy to protect function of islet cells until other treatment strategies become effective (e.g., treatment of rejection, weight loss, oral hypoglycemic agents, or manipulation of immunosuppression regimen)
        ii. Because post-transplant resumption of insulin therapy constitutes graft failure, some centers may be reluctant to reinitiate insulin—preferring, instead, to use oral hypoglycemic agents

OBESITY

I. Overview
  A. Obesity is a common problem among solid organ transplant recipients.
  B. Assessment of obesity
    1. Estimation of body fat
      a. Waist circumference: high-risk waistline
        i. Females: ≥ 35 inches
        ii. Males: ≥ 40 inches
    2. Body mass index (BMI)
      a. Assesses weight relative to height
      b. Two formulas:
        i. Weight (in kilograms) divided by height in meters squared
        ii. Multiply weight in pounds by 703, divide by height in inches, divide by height in inches again
      c. BMI calculator online: http://www.nhlbisupport.com/bmi/

d.   Body mass index values (Table 6-16)[49, 50]
II.   Determinants of obesity[51]
   A.   Age
   B.   Gender
   C.   Genetic factors
   D.   Environmental factors
III.   Obesity is a major risk factor for coronary heart disease[1, 52] and is associated with:
   A.   Dyslipidemia
      1.   Elevated blood cholesterols and triglyceride levels
      2.   Decreased HDL levels
   B.   Hypertension
   C.   DM
IV.   Obesity in the pretransplant period
   A.   Goal: optimize transplant candidate's weight prior to transplantation
   B.   Weight loss guideline: deficit of 500 to 1000 calories/day depending on patient's current intake, anticipated time on transplant waiting list, and ability to exercise[53]
   C.   Weight loss medications or bariatric surgery may be appropriate for certain patients
V.   Obesity in the post-transplant period
   A.   Associated with increased post-transplant morbidity[53-56] such as:
      1.   Delayed kidney graft function
      2.   Decreased kidney graft survival
      3.   Increased incidence of wound infection
      4.   Increased incidence of surgical complications (for example, thrombosis)
      5.   Decreased respiratory function and endurance
   B.   Contributing factors[53]
      1.   Excess caloric intake due to
         a.   Enhanced appetite secondary to corticosteroid use
         b.   Poor eating behaviors
         c.   Resolution of pretransplant malabsorption
      2.   Caloric intake that exceeds expenditure due to sedentary habits, lack of exercise
      3.   Genetic predisposition
      4.   Age, gender, race

TABLE 6-16
■ Body Mass Index Values[49, 50]

BMI	Interpretation
< 18.5	Underweight
1.5–24.7	Normal
25 – < 30	Overweight
≥ 30	Obesity
≥ 40	Extreme obesity

VI. Components of healthy post-transplant weight loss program[53]
   A. Reduction in calories
   B. Behavior modification
   C. Exercise
   D. Immunosuppressant modifications to consider
      1. Decrease or wean corticosteroids
      2. Substitute tacrolimus for cyclosporine
VII. Psychological aspects of weight loss[53]
   A. Assessment of patient's readiness and motivation
      1. If patient is not willing to embark on weight loss program, identify and remove barriers to weight loss.
   B. Establishment of reasonable goals with respect to desired:
      1. Amount of weight loss[50]
         a. Initial goal: reduce body weight by approximately 10% from baseline (typically over 6 months)
         b. When this goal is reached, further weight loss, if indicated, can be considered.
         c. When target weight is reached, weight maintenance program is initiated.
            i. Sustained physical activity is useful in preventing weight regain.
      2. Cholesterol level
      3. Glucose level
      4. Blood pressure
   C. Incorporation of behavioral strategies such as:[50]
      1. Self-monitoring of eating patterns and physical activity
      2. Stress management
      3. Stimulus control
      4. Problem-solving
      5. Contingency management
      6. Cognitive restructuring
      7. Incorporation of social support
VIII. Weight loss medications[53]
   A. To date, not tested for safety and efficacy in transplant population
   B. Certain medications are contraindicated in setting of congestive heart failure, coronary artery disease, severe liver or renal impairment, and poorly controlled hypertension.
   C. Orlistat can alter cyclosporine levels.
IX. Bariatric surgery
   A. Gastric stapling and other types of weight loss surgery carry inherent surgical risks and must first be discussed with the transplant team.
   B. Bariatric surgery may affect the absorption of medications; decreased absorpotion of immunosuppressive agents may put the patient at increased risk for rejection.

MALIGNANCY

I. Overview[57]
   A. Several factors have contributed to the increase in post-transplant malignancies and recipient mortality due to *de novo* malignancies:
      1. Improved graft survival and longer exposure to immunosuppression

   2. Use of more potent immunosuppressive agents
 B. Data regarding post-transplant malignancies comes from the following sources:
   1. Large tumor registries, for example:
      a. Israel Penn International Transplant Tumor Registry
      b. Australia and New Zealand Dialysis and Transplant Registry (ANZ)
      c. United States Renal Data System (USRDS)
      d. Scientific Registry of Transplant Recipients
      e. International Society for Heart and Lung Transplantation Registry
   2. Single center data
 C. Magnitude of the problem
   1. ANZ data over the past 25 years indicate a progressive increase in the incidence of cancer in kidney transplant recipients.
   2. ANZ, USRDS, and European registry data indicate a significantly higher incidence of cancer in kidney transplant recipients than in the general population.
   3. Compared to the general population, USRDS data indicate:
      a. A two-fold increase in common cancers in kidney transplant recipients (colon, lung, prostate, and breast cancer)
      b. A 15-fold higher incidence of kidney cancer in kidney transplant recipients
      c. A 20-fold higher incidence of Kaposi's sarcoma, non-Hodgkin's lymphoma, and non-melanoma skin cancer in kidney transplant recipients
   4. Single-center data (U.S.) indicate a 40% incidence of all types of cancers at 25 years following renal transplantation.
   5. Transplant recipients are at increased risk of specific types of carcinoma compared to the general population (Table 6-17)[58]
   6. Many transplant patients succumb to malignancy with a fully functioning allograft.
II. Etiologic factors associated with transplant recipients' increased risk of malignancy include:[58]

TABLE 6-17

■ **Increased Risk of Specific Types of Carcinoma[58]**

Type of Carcinoma	Increased Risk
Skin	4-fold to 21-fold
Kaposi's sarcoma	400-fold to 500-fold (compared to controls of same ethnic origin)
Lip	29-fold
Vulvular and anal	100-fold
Hepatocellular	20-fold to 38-fold
In situ uterine cervical	14-fold to 16-fold
Post-transplant lymphoproliferative disease	28-fold to 49-fold

A. Impaired immune surveillance caused by chronic immunosuppression therapy (decreased ability to eliminate malignant cells)

B. Mutagenic properties of immunosuppressive agents
  1. Azathioprine, cyclophosphamide, and cyclosporine can directly damage DNA.
  2. Immunosuppressants may augment the effects other carcinogens such as sunlight.

C. Chronic antigenic stimulation caused by foreign allograft antigens, repeated infections, or transfusions
  1. May overstimulate immune system and cause post-transplant lymphoproliferative disease (PTLD)
  2. Faulty feedback mechanisms may lead to impaired control of immune reactions and uninhibited lymphoid proliferation.

D. Environmental factors (for example, ultraviolet radiation, particularly in Australia)

E. Genetic factors that alter susceptibility to malignancy by modifying carcinogenic metabolism, interferon secretion, response to viral infections, or major histocompatibility regulation of the immune response

F. Chronic viral infections, particularly those shown in Table 6-18.[4, 59]

III. Pathogenesis of post-transplant malignancy:[59]
  A. *De novo* occurrence
  B. Recurrent malignancy
  C. Transmission of malignancy from donor[60]
    1. The United Network for Organ Sharing Tumor Registry lists 21 incidences of donor transmission in 125,092 organ transplants from 1994 to 2001.

IV. Characteristics of malignancies in transplant recipients
  A. Malignancies occur in a relatively short time period following transplantation. (Table 6-19)[58]
  B. The incidence of malignancies increases with time post-transplant.

V. Types of malignancies that occur in transplant recipients
  A. Most common *de novo* malignancies in order of decreasing frequency: (Cincinnati Transplant Tumor Registry data)[58]
    1. Skin and lips
    2. PTLD
    3. Lung
    4. Kaposi's sarcoma

TABLE 6-18
■ Chronic Viral Infections[4, 59]

Virus	Associated Malignancy
Human papilloma virus (HPV):	Carcinoma of lip, cervix, penis vulva, perineum, anus
HPV 8, 19:	Nonmelanoma skin cancer
HPV 16, 20:	Skin and tonsillar cancer
Epstein-Barr Virus (EBV):	Lymphomas; PTLD
Human herpes virus 8:	Kaposi's sarcoma; lymphoma
Hepatitis C virus (HCV):	Hepatocellular carcinoma
Hepatitis B virus (HBV):	Hepatocellular carcinoma

TABLE 6-19

■ **Occurrence of Malignancy after Transplantation**[58]

Type of Malignancy	Mean Time to Appearance	Median Time to Appearance
Kaposi's sarcoma	21 months	13 months
PTLD	34 months	13 months
Skin	66 months	51 months
Anogenital	115 months	114 months

Data from Cincinnati Transplant Tumor Registry.

     5. Uterus
     6. Kidney
     7. Colon and rectum
     8. Breast
     9. Head and neck
    10. Vulva, perineum, penis, scrotum
    11. Urinary bladder
    12. Prostate gland
    13. Metastatic carcinoma (unknown primary site)
    14. Leukemias
    15. Hepatobiliary carcinoma
    16. Sarcomas (excluding Kaposi's sarcoma)

  B. Carcinomas that are common in the general population (lung, breast, prostate, colon, and invasive uterine cervical cancer) do not occur more frequently in transplant recipients.[18, 58]

  C. Common types of malignancy noted in specific transplant populations are shown in Table 6-20.

VI. Skin cancer[58, 65]

  A. Overview

     1. The most commonly occurring type of cancer among transplant recipients; comprises 38% of all malignancies

     2. Tends to occur more often in light-skinned individuals with blue eyes and blond or red hair

     3. Post-transplant interval to appearance is shorter in:

       a. Older individuals

       b. Individuals who live in lower latitudes

  B. Basal cell versus squamous cell carcinoma

     1. Squamous cell carcinoma seen more frequently than basal cell carcinoma

       a. In the general population, the opposite is true: basal cell carcinomas are more frequently seen than squamous cell carcinomas.

  C. Evolution of cutaneous carcinomas in transplant recipients;[1] compared to the general population, in transplant recipients:

     1. Skin lesions are more aggressive.

     2, The incidence of multiple skin lesions is higher.

     3. The onset of basal and squamous cell carcinomas occurs at a younger age.

4. Relapses and metastasis are more common.
D. Characteristics of skin lesions (Table 6-21)[58, 66]

VII. PTLD
   A. Overview
1. Involves wide spectrum of disorders that range from benign polymorphic B-cell hyperplasia to malignant lymphomas[67]
2. Incidence ranges from 2% in kidney transplant recipients to 10% in combined heart-lung transplant recipients[67]
3. Often extranodal; may initially involve the gastrointestinal (GI) tract, lung, or kidney[18, 58]
   a. Can involve the GI tract in up to 10% of transplant recipients[68]
4. May involve single or multiple organs[58]
5. More common in nonrenal allograft recipients[58]
   a. Most likely due to the fact that intense anti-rejection therapy may be required in nonrenal allograft recipients as a life-saving mechanism
   B. Risk factors[58, 67]
1. Intense immunosuppression (for example, with anti-CD3 monoclonal antibody therapy)
2. Primary Epstein-Barr virus (EBV) infection (recipient EBV-seronegative; donor EBV-seropositive)
3. CMV infection
4. CMV mismatch (recipient CMV-seronegative; donor CMV-seropositive)
5. Type of transplant (lung; heart-lung)
   C. Clinical presentation: May be asymptomatic[58]
1. Symptoms that resemble infectious mononucleosis
2. Fever

TABLE 6-20

■ **Common Types of Malignancy Noted in Specific Transplant Populations**

Kidney[61]	Heart[62]	Heart-Lung[47, 63]	Lung[27]	Liver[64]	Pancreas[44]
Skin: KS	Skin: Squamous cell Basal cell	Skin: KS Squamous cell Basal cell Melanoma	Skin: Nonmelanoma	Skin: Squamous cell KS	Skin
PTLD	Respiratory tract (larynx, bronchi, lung)	PTLD	Lymphoma	PTLD	PTLD
	Gastrointestinal tract	Anogenital	Lung: particularly in setting of pretransplant COPD or pulmonary fibrosis		

COPD = chronic obstructive pulmonary disease; KS = Kaposi's sarcoma; PTLD = post-transplant lymphoproliferative disease

TABLE 6-21
■ Characteristics of Skin Lesions[58, 66]

Lesion	Tend to occur in	Treatment Options	Other
Premalignant cutaneous lesions: Warts	Sun-exposed areas of skin	Liquid nitrogen, Electrocoagulation, CO_2 laser Note: surgery typically avoided so as to prevent dissemination of HPV	Lesions tend to be multiple; HPV typically found in warts; High frequency of recurrence; Sign that lesion is transforming into squamous cell carcinoma: appearance of vegetation lesions on warts
Premalignant cutaneous lesions: Actinic keratosis	Uncovered areas	Electrocoagulation; Cryotherapy Retinoids for diffusely spreading forms	May be associated with warts; Sign that lesion is transforming into squamous cell carcinoma: infiltrate in lesion; rapid recurrence of lesion
Squamous cell	Sun-exposed areas of skin; Often develops on warts and lesions of keratosis	Surgical excision; Lymph node resection with radiotherapy in setting of lymph node metastasis Systemic retinoids in patients with large number of lesions	Location is age-dependent:[58] Patients transplanted before age 40: lesions typically on dorsum of hands, forearms, and trunk Patients transplanted after age 40: lesions typically on head
Basal cell	Sun-exposed areas of skin; Trunk		
Melanoma	Areas exposed to acute, intense exposure to ultraviolet radiation (via sunburn)[66]	Surgical excision Lymph node dissection for intermediate depth tumors Adjuvant therapy	Risk: 3 to 4 times higher than in general population Characteristics of lesion: Asymmetry Borders: notched, irregular Color: varies from light to dark; may be dark black or blue-black Diameter > 0.6 cm CTTR data: Melanomas represent 5% of skin cancers in adult transplant recipients; 32% of recipients who developed melanoma after transplantation died Median post-transplant time to development of melanoma: 46 months Transmission from donor with metastatic melanoma has been noted
Kaposi's sarcoma	Trunk and extremities Occurs rarely on face Mucocutaneous lesions: palate	Reduction in immunosuppression Mucocutaneous lesions: Cryotherapy Laser therapy Chemotherapy Radiotherapy	More common in blacks and patients of Mediterranean, African, or Caribbean origin Mean time to onset: 20 months post-transplant Onset shorter in liver transplant recipients

CTTR = Cincinnati Transplant Tumor Registry; HPV = human papilloma virus

3. Night sweats
4. Upper respiratory infection
5. Weight loss
6. Diarrhea
7. Abdominal pain
8. Lymphadenopathy
9. Tonsillitis
10. GI tract involvement: intestinal perforation, peritonitis
11. Lung lesion or visceral mass

D. Treatment options[67]
1. Reduction in or withdrawal of immunosuppression
2. Surgery for localized disease
3. Cytotoxic chemotherapy
4. Radiotherapy
5. Interferon-α
6. Antiviral therapy
7. Intravenous immunoglobulin

E. Prevention of PTLD[67]
1. EBV replication inhibitors (antiviral drugs such as ganciclovir)
2. Immunoglobulin

VIII. Prevention of cancer[17, 58]
1. Smoking cessation
2. Routine self-examination of skin
3. Hepatitis B vaccination in non-immune recipients (may help to prevent hepatitis B virus-related hepatocellular carcinoma)
4. Sun precautions
    a. Avoiding undue exposure to sunlight
    b. Avoiding tanning beds
    c. Wearing protective clothing
        i.   Broad-brimmed hats
        ii. Long-sleeve shirts and pants
    d. Wearing sunglasses and sun visors
    e. Using sunscreen lotion that provides protection against ultraviolet-B rays (minimum sun protection factor [SPF] = 15)
5. Routine cancer screening per American Cancer Society guidelines (Table 6-22)[69]
    a. These are minimum guidelines. Depending on the patient's family history, personal history, post-transplant course, and current medical status, more aggressive screening tests and/or more frequent screening intervals may be required.
    b. Post-transplant cancer-screening guidelines have been developed for renal transplant recipients and are applicable to most transplant recipients (Table 6-23).[1]

BONE DISEASE

I. Osteoporosis
    A. Definition: condition characterized by loss of bone mass and deterioration of bone tissue such that patients are at risk for bone fragility and fractures[17]

TABLE 6-22

■ **American Cancer Society Routine Cancer Screening Guidelines for General Population[69]**

Males and Females	Males	Females
Over 50 years: routine sigmoidoscopy, colonoscopy, fecal occult blood test, or fecal immunohistochemical test	Annual prostate specific antigen test	Age 20 and over: Monthly self- breast examination
	Annual digital rectal examination	Age 40 and over: Annual mammogram
		Clinical breast examination:
Note: colonoscopy is typically preferred for transplant recipients		Age 20-39: every 3 years
		Age 40 and over: yearly
		Annual pelvic examination with Papanicolaou test
Annual skin examination by dermatologist		
Semi-annual examination for oral cancer by dentist		

B. World Health Organization (WHO) diagnostic criteria for postmeno-pausal women:
   1. Osteopenia: Bone mineral density (BMD) between 1 standard devia-tion (SD) and 2.5 SD below the mean BMD of young adult women
   2. Osteoporosis: BMD greater than 2.5 SD below the mean BMD of adult women
C. Bone mass has been shown to be consistently lower in transplant recipi-ents than in age- and sex-matched controls.
D. Vertebral bone loss is typically highest in first 6 to 12 months post-transplant.
E. Etiology[17, 70, 71]
   1. General pretransplant factors that predispose patient to low bone density:
      a. Chronic renal failure
      b. Prolonged use of loop diuretics
      c. Prerenal azotemia
      d. Uncontrolled DM
      e. Abnormal thyroid function
      f. Liver congestion
      g. Smoking history
      h. Hypogonadism
      i. Insufficient intake of dietary calcium and/or vitamin D
      j. Decreased mobility; lack of weight-bearing exercise
   2. Organ-specific pretransplant factors:
      a. Lung transplant candidates[47]
         i. Hypoxemia
         ii. Prior glucocorticoid therapy
         iii. Cystic fibrosis patients: calcium malabsorption, delayed puberty, pancreatic insufficiency with vitamin D deficiency
      b. Pancreas transplant candidates[44]

TABLE 6-23
■ Post-transplant Cancer-Screening Guidelines for Renal Transplant Recipients[1]

Type of Carcinoma	Minimum Screening Recommendations
Anogenital	Yearly examination of anogenital area; pelvic examinations for women with cytologic studies
	Follow-up biopsy of suspicious lesions
	Prompt treatment of warts
Kaposi's sarcoma	Yearly examination of skin, conjunctiva, oropharyngeal mucosa; biopsy of suspicious lesions
	More frequent examination for high-risk patients (those of Arab, Italian, Greek or Jewish ethnicity; those living in Africa or Middle East; those with HHV-8 infection)
PTLD	History and physical examination with particular attention to any symptoms suggestive of disseminated or localized PTLD every 3 months during first post-transplant year and yearly thereafter
Hepatobiliary	Patients with liver disease: α-fetoprotein levels every 6-12 months may assist in early detection
	High-risk patients (e.g., those with chronic hepatitis): liver sonography every 6-12 months
Uterine cervix	Annual Pap tests for all women $\geq$ 18 years of age and for women < 18 years of age who are sexually active
Breast	Women age 50-69: screening mammography every 1-2 years, with or without clinical breast examinations
	Women age 40-49: may opt for screening mammography every 1-2 years, with or without clinical breast examinations
	Women $\geq$ age 70 with reasonable life expectancies: may opt for screening mammography every 1-2 years with or without clinical breast examinations
	High-risk women < age 50: screening mammography every 1-2 years with or without clinical breast examinations
Colorectal	Patients $\geq$ 50 years of age: annual fecal occult blood testing
	Flexible sigmoidoscopy or colonoscopy every 5 years
	More frequent screening for patients at higher risk
Prostate	Men $\geq$ 50 years with at least 10-year life expectancy: annual digital rectal examination and prostate-specific antigen test
	Men at higher risk (e.g., family history of prostate screening): start screening at younger age

HHV = human herpes virus; PTLD = post-transplant lymphoproliferative disease

       i.   Uncontrolled diabetes
   3. Post-transplant factors
       a.   Corticosteroid therapy—particularly high corticosteroid doses in early transplant period or following episodes of acute rejection; corticosteroid therapy is associated with:
           i.   Increased urinary calcium secretion
          ii.   Decreased intestinal absorption of calcium
        iii.   Increased parathyroid hormone level
        iv.   Decreased skeletal growth factors, including synthesis of androgen and estrogen

            v.   Increased bone resorption
            vi. Decreased formation of bone by osteoblasts
        b.   Cyclosporine: may be associated with high rates of bone turn-
             over
        c.   Hyperparathyroidism
        d.   Hypogonadism in males and postmenopausal females
        e.   Progressive aging
        f.   Kidney transplant recipients
            i.   Persistent metabolic acidosis associated with chronic
                 allograft dysfunction
    F.   Assessment:
        1.   Dual-energy x-ray absorptiometry (DEXA) of lumbar spine and hip
            a.   Pretransplant baseline assessment
            b.   Six months post-transplant
            c.   Periodically thereafter to monitor bone density and effectiveness
                 of therapy
        2.   Laboratory tests
            a.   Calcium
            b.   25-OH vitamin D
            c.   Osteocalcin
            d.   Intact parathyroid hormone
            e.   Alkaline phosphatase
            f.   Chemistry levels
            g.   Urinary calcium
            h.   Markers of resorption
                i.   Urinary pyridmoline cross-links
                ii. N-telopeptides
    G.   Therapeutic options
        1.   Inhibitor of bone resorption (bisphosphonates); for example, alen-
             dronate, etidronate
            a.   May be administered on daily, weekly, or monthly basis
            b.   To optimize absorption: medication must be taken with 8 ounces
                 of plain water 30 minutes prior to ingesting any food or liquid
                i.   Medication cannot be taken with mineral water, coffee, tea,
                     juice, or any other liquids
            c.   To prevent esophageal irritation: patient must remain fully
                 upright for 30 minutes after taking this medication (standing,
                 sitting, or walking)
            d.   Instructions to patients:
                i.   Promptly report any chest pain, new or worsening heart-
                     burn, or difficult or painful swallowing
                ii. Stop taking medication if above symptoms occur; notify
                     physician
        2.   Calcitonin: subcutaneous injections or nasal spray
        3.   Calcium supplements: 1500 mg per day
        4.   Vitamin D supplements: 800–1000 mg per day
        5.   Minimizing steroid dose
        6.   Withdrawing steroids in patients at high risk for osteoporosis
        7.   Parathyroidectomy for selected patients if calcium and vitamin D
             therapy do not effectively suppress parathyroid hormone secretion
    H.   Prevention of osteopenia/osteoporosis (Figure 6-1).[8]

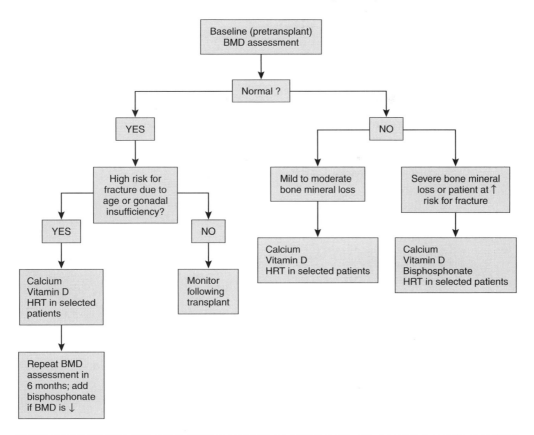

Figure 6-1. Prevention of osteopenia/osteoporosis.[8] HRT = hormone replacement therapy.

II. Avascular necrosis (AVN)[71, 72]
   A. Often associated with corticosteroid therapy
   B. Typical site in 90% of cases: femoral head
   C. Clinical presentation
      1. Hip or groin pain that worsens with weight bearing
      2. Pain may be referred to knee
   D. Diagnosis: magnetic resonance imaging
   E. Treatment options
      1. Core decompression (prior to collapse of femoral head)
      2. Total hip arthroplasty

GASTROINTESTINAL COMPLICATIONS

I. Overview
   A. Most immunosuppressive agents are associated with some type of GI complication.
   B. Corticosteroids may mask certain clinical manifestations of GI complications such as leukocytosis, abdominal guarding, and rebound.
   C. The most common post-transplant GI disorders include:[17, 68]
      1. Infections

    2. Mucosal injury and perforation

    3. Biliary tract diseases

    4. Diverticular disease

    5. Pancreatitis

    6. Malignancy

II. Infections[68] (See Chapter 5 for additional information)

  A. Chronic immunosuppression can lead to localized GI infections.

  B. Infections may occur in one or more portions of the gut between the mouth and the anus.

  C. Types of infections:

    1. Viral

    2 Bacterial

    3. Fungal

    4. Parasitic

  D. Viral infections

    1. CMV

      a. Enteric and/or gastric infections are common, especially in the first 6 to 12 post-transplant months.

      b. Any portion of the GI tract can be affected by CMV infection; clinical manifestations depend on the segment of the GI tract that is affected.

      c. Common symptoms associated with CMV infections of the GI tract include:

        i. Dysphagia (inability to swallow or difficulty swallowing)

        ii. Odynophagia (pain with swallowing)

        iii. Nausea, vomiting, diarrhea

        iv. Abdominal pain

        v. GI bleeding

        vi. GI perforation

      d. Diagnosis of CMV infection

        i. Endoscopy and biopsy to rule out CMV gastritis

        ii. Direct detection of CMV in blood by antigenemia or PCR

      e. Prompt investigation of symptoms such as vomiting, diarrhea, leukopenia, and/or elevated liver function tests is imperative, particularly for patients who are:

        i. In the early post-transplant phase

        ii. Undergoing intense immunosuppression to treat rejection

        iii. CMV seronegative and received an allograft from a CMV seropositive donor

      f. Undetected CMV infection in the GI tract can lead to:

        i. Spread of the infection to other organs

        ii. Perforation of the affected viscus

    2. Herpes simplex virus (HSV)

      a. Typically presents as reactivation of a latent HSV infection

      b. More common during the first 6 weeks post-transplant

      c. Common sites

        i. Mild, ulcer-like lesions in oral cavity and pharynx

        ii. Esophagus

      d. Common symptoms

        i. Dysphagia

        ii. Odynophagia

        iii. Orocutaneous lesions

      e. Prompt investigation of symptoms, particularly in patients who are undergoing intense immunosuppression therapy for rejection, is imperative.
         i. Untreated ulcers may lead to hemorrhage and esophageal perforation.

E. Bacterial infections
  1. Common pathogens
    a. *Clostridium difficile*
    b. *Yersenia enterocolitica*
  2. Bacterial infections may occur more often in recipients who have a concurrent CMV infection.
  3. Common presenting symptoms
    a. Diarrhea
    b. Abdominal tenderness
  4. *Helicobacter pylori*
    a. May cause gastritis and peptic ulcer disease
    b. Diagnosis: endoscopy and biopsy

F. Fungal infections
  1. Recipients are at greater risk during the first few months post-transplant.
  2. Risk factors for fungal infections include:
    a. Antibiotic therapy
    b. Corticosteroid therapy
    c. Hyperglycemia
    d. Indwelling catheters
    e. Recent treatment of rejection
  3. Candidal infection is the most common post-transplant GI infection.
    a. Risk factors for candidal infection in GI tract:
      i. Use of broad-spectrum antibiotics
      ii. Recent rejection therapy, particularly with high-dose steroids or antibodies
      iii. Liver transplant recipients: Roux-en-Y choledochojejunostomy
    b. Symptoms:
      i. Oral thrush
      ii. Esophagitis: odynophagia, dysphyagia (with or without oral thrush), fever, heartburn, epigastric pain, perforation
    c. Common pathogens
      i. *Candida albicans*
      ii. *Candida tropicalis*
  4. Diagnosis of fungal infections
    a. Histopathologic examination
    b. Cultures
  5. Fungal infections may occur concurrently with CMV infection.

G. Parasitic infections (protozoal or metazoal)
  1. Types of parasites
    a. Protozoa (e.g., microsporidia)
    b. Metazoa
    c. Nematodes (e.g., *Strongyloides stercoralis*)
      i. Endemic areas for *S. stercoralis*: West Indies, Far East

        ii.   Living donors with history of *S. stercoralis* infection should have stool and urine tested for larvae.

III. Mucosal injury and perforation[68]

    A. Diarrhea

        1. Potential etiology:

            a. Infection

            b. Immunosuppressive agents (e.g., tacrolimus, mycophenolate mofetil [MMF])

        2. Management strategies if etiology is due to immunosuppressive agents:

            a. Reduction in total daily dose (as indicated)

            b. Dose splitting (e.g., giving medication 4 times daily instead of 2 times daily)

            c. Changing immunosuppressive agents

    B. Ulceration

        1. Potential etiology

            a. Stress associated with surgery

            b. Corticosteroid therapy

                i. Ironically, corticosteroid therapy may also mask symptoms of ulceration.

            c. Medication-induced (e.g., azathioprine, MMF) slowing of intestinal cell turnover which may lead to impairment of normal gastroduodenal cytoprotection

            d. Sequelae associated with post-transplant dialysis

                i. Increased secretion of gastric acid

                ii. Heparin-induced ulcers

                iii. Increased levels of histamine and gastrin

            e. Use of NSAIDs

        2. Symptoms (may also be asymptomatic)

            a. Abdominal pain

            b. GI bleeding

        3. Prophylaxis

            a. Purpose

                i. Decrease acid secretion

                ii. Protect GI mucosa from effects of excessive acid secretion

            b. Types of preventive medications

                i. H_2-receptor antagonists

                ii. Proton-pump inhibitors

                iii. Coating agents

                iv. Prostaglandins

                v. Note: transplant recipients typically are advised to avoid NSAIDs

        4. Potential problems with prophylactic medications:

            a. H_2-receptor antagonists and coating agents may alter cyclosporine levels; monitor cyclosporine levels carefully.

            b. H_2-receptor antagonists and proton-pump inhibitors may:

                i. Decrease acid secretion and thus alter flora in the upper gut

                ii. As a result, the patient may be at increased risk for colonization with pathogens; monitor patient for infections such as fungal esophagitis.

            c. Coating agents may block the absorption of cyclosporine; monitor cyclosporine levels carefully.

     5.   Diagnosis: endoscopy

     6.   Treatment options for bleeding ulcers

        a.   Injection of epinephrine or alcohol

        b.   Heater probes

        c.   Vicaps electrodes

        d.   Surgical intervention

IV. Perforations[68]

   A. Can occur in any segment of the GI tract

   B. Etiology is typically multifactorial; perforations in lower GI tract have been associated with:

     1.   Diverticular disease

     2.   Medications that compromise the integrity of the GI tract (e.g., corticosteroids and other immunosuppressants, NSAIDs)

     3.   Infections such as CMV and mycormycosis

   C. Prevention

     1.   Steroid-sparing immunosuppression regimen

     2.   Prompt treatment of infections

     3.   Early diagnosis of GI complications

   D. Management: aggressive surgery

V. Biliary tract disease[68]

   A. Types reported in literature

     1.   Biliary calculi

        a.   Transplant recipients are at high risk for biliary calculi.

        b.   Post-transplant cholecystectomy is often required; mortality rate associated with this procedure is high, particularly in heart and lung transplant recipients.[73]

     2.   Dilated bile ducts

     3.   Cholelithiasis

     4.   Gallbladder hydrops

   B. Etiology

     1.   Multifactorial

     2.   May be due to cyclosporine-induced cholestasis and decreased bile flow

VI. Acute pancreatitis[68]

   A. A rare but serious complication with published mortality rates that range from 64% to 100% in liver and kidney transplant recipients, respectively[68]

   B. Precipitating factors in liver and kidney transplant recipients include:

     1.   Liver transplantation:

        a.   Biliary manipulation

        b.   Alcohol use

        c.   Hepatitis B infection

        d.   Malignancy in area around pancreas

     2.   Renal transplantation

        a.   CMV infection

        b.   Hypercalcemia

        c.   Alcohol use

        d.   Cholelithiasis

   C. A possible association between azathioprine and acute pancreatitis has been reported.[74, 75]

   D. Diagnosis

     1.   Computed tomography

E. Treatment options
   1. If drug-induced, discontinuation of drug
   2. Fasting
   3. Administration of intravenous fluids
   4. Parenteral nutrition
   5. Surgery if indicated

VII. Malignancy[68] (also see section on malignancy above)
   A. Post-transplant lymphoproliferative disease (PTLD)
      1. Can involve the GI tract in up to 10% of transplant recipients[68]
      2. Diagnosis: endoscopy
      3. Late sequelae
         a. Perforation
         b. Obstruction
         c. Bleeding
   B. Low-grade gastric mucosa-associated lymphoid tissue-type lymphomas
      1. Occurrence is rare
      2. May be associated with *H. pylori*

VIII. GI complications in specific transplant populations (Table 6-24)

TABLE 6-24
■ GI Complications in Specific Transplant Population

Type of transplant	Gastrointestinal Complication

Pancreas[76]	Pancreatitis: Bladder drained procedure:
	• Reflux pancreatitis may cause acute inflammation of graft
	• May mimic rejection
	• Clinical manifestations: Pain; ↑ serum amylase levels
	• Potential etiology
	  o Reflux of urine through ampula and into pancreatic ducts
	  o In older males: hypertrophy of prostate gland
	• Management:
	  o Foley catheter
	  o Resolution of bladder dysfunction
	Pancreatitis: Enteric-drained procedure:
	• GI bleeding
	• Potential etiology:
	  o Preoperative anticoagulation
	  o Bleeding from duodenoenteric anastomosis

Liver	Types of GI complications:[77] • Bile leakage • Biliary tract stricture • Cholangitis • Obstruction of ampullae • Biliary obstruction due to sludge or calculi Most common complications:[77] • Biliary tract stricture • Bile leakage

Type of transplant	Gastrointestinal (GI) Complication

Liver *(continued)*	Clinical manifestations:[77]
	• Vary with type of complication
	• Fever and jaundice are common
	• Biliary obstruction:
	  o ↑ bilirubin
	  o ↑ alkaline phosphatase
	  o ↑ gamma glutamyl transpeptidase (γ-GTP)
	Diagnosis:[77]
	• Cholangiography (gold standard)
	• Endoscopic retrograde cholangiography (ERCP)
	• Magnetic resonance cholangiopancreatography (MRCP)
	Anastomotic leaks:[78]
	• May occur in early postoperative period
	• May result in localized or general peritonitis
	• Monitor biliary output from drains and serum bilirubin
	Etiology of leaks:[78]
	• Technical problems with surgery
	• Ischemic bile duct secondary to hepatic artery thrombosis
	Treatment:[78]
	• Surgical revision
	• ERCP and sphincterotomy with stenting of the leak
	Biliary casts and stones:[78]
	• Long-standing T- tubes may lead to the formation of biliary casts and stones and subsequent biliary obstruction that may necessitate ERCP intervention
	
	Recurrence of Hepatitis B—Prevention and treatment[79]
	• Human hepatitis B immunoglobulin (HBIG) during anhepatic phase then daily for a period of time (e.g., 1 week)
	• Subsequent HBIG dosing as needed to maintain adequate Hepatitis B antibody titer
	• Lamuvidine
	Recurrence of Hepatitis C—Treatment[79]
	• Interferon and ribavirin

Intestine	Most common GI complication: bleeding
	• May be due to rejection or infection
	• Requires prompt assessment via endoscopy and biopsy[80] and initiation of appropriate treatment
	Leaks from anastomoses: more common
	• May occur during first postoperative week
	• Etiology: surgical technique, poor wound healing secondary to immunosuppression and/or malnutrition
	• Clinical presentation: peritonitis, abdominal distention, fever
	• Treatment: surgical revision and removal of peritoneal contaminants
	Hypermotility
	• Potential etiology
	  o Alteration in baseline motility of denervated graft
	  o Infection
	  o Rejection (particularly in setting of fever and/or abdominal distention)
	• Management
	  o Antidiarrheal agents, fiber
	  o Treatment of rejection or infection

Kidney	Diverticular disease and colonic perforation[68] • Increased incidence reported in kidney transplant recipients with polycystic kidney disease

GOUT

I. Pathogenesis of hyperuricemia[81-83]
   A. Adverse effects of calcineurin inhibitors, particularly cyclosporine, on renal excretion of uric acid secondary to vasoconstriction in the renal vasculature; results in decreased secretion of uric acid into urine
   B. RI
   C. Volume contraction secondary to diuretic use
II. Diagnosis
   A. Aspiration of affected joint is required for definitive diagnosis.
      1. Polymorphonuclear leukocytes contain uric acid crystals.
III. Treatment options[83]
   A. Colchicine
      1. May cause gastrointestinal toxicity
      2. May be administered on an alternate day schedule
   B. Glucocorticoids
      1. Prednisone: oral bolus followed by gradual taper
      2. Adrenocorticotrophic hormone (ACTH)
   C. Allopurinol
      1. Given only after acute gout attack has subsided
      2. Allergic reactions may occur with chronic use
      3. Rarely given in conjunction with azathioprine
         a. Allopurinol potentiates myelosuppression associated with azathioprine by inhibiting the metabolism of the active metabolite of azathioprine (mercaptopurine); this can result in mercaptopurine toxicity.
         b. Concurrent administration of allopurinol and azathioprine requires:
            i. Reduction in azathioprine dose by 75%
            ii. Decrease in the initial allopurinol dose to 50 mg daily
            iii. Careful monitoring of white blood cell count
      4. If allopurinol is to be used, mycophenolate mofetil is often substituted for azathioprine to decrease the risk of leukopenia.
   D. NSAIDs should be avoided as they may precipitate RI

GINGIVAL HYPERPLASIA

I. Overview
   A. Definition: excessive proliferation of gingival tissue
   B. Clinical presentation
      1. Can affect labial, buccal, palatal, and lingual tissues in all areas of mouth[84]
      2. Hyperplasia typically more severe in the maxillary and mandibular anterior regions of the mouth
      3. Overgrowth of soft tissue begins between the teeth and spreads in all directions[85]
         a. Tissue becomes thick and lobulated
         b. Overgrowth may encroach upon the tooth surface, including the chewing surface
   C. Incidence: average incidence is solid organ transplant recipients is approximately 25%; incidence varies with:[86]

   1. Genetic factors
   2. Duration of drug therapy (incidence increases with length of therapy)
   3. Drug dose (higher incidence with higher drug doses)
   4. Serum drug levels
   5. Salivary concentrations
   6. Oral hygiene
   7. Age (incidence tends to be higher in older patients)
   8. Gender (higher incidence in males)
II. Etiology: known side effect of certain mediations:
   A. Major causative agents:[87]
      1. Cyclosporine
      2. Calcium channel blockers (e.g., amlodipine, diltiazem, felodipine, nicardipine, nifedipine, verapamil)
      3. Anticonvulsants (e.g., phenytoin)
III. Pathophysiology[86]
   A. The mechanism by which hyperplasia is localized in the gingiva, as opposed to other tissues, is unknown.
      1. Proposed mechanisms include higher concentration of drugs (e.g., cyclosporine, calcium channel blockers, phenytoin) in gingival tissues directly through gingival blood supply or from the oral cavity itself.
   B. Drug-mediated expression of cytokines and growth factors may affect the growth and function of gingival fibroblasts and epithelial cells.
IV. Potential sequelae of gingival hyperplasia[88]
   A. Interference with normal oral function
      1. In certain patients, may lead to alveolar bone loss and tooth loss[84]
   B. Difficulty in maintaining oral hygiene with subsequent bacterial overgrowth and secondary inflammatory response
   C. Altered appearance; poor self-image
   D. Noncompliance with medical therapy
V. Treatment options[85]
   A. Plaque control
   B. Removal of local irritants
   C. Periodontal surgery
      1. As with any dental cleaning or procedure, heart transplant recipients with cardiac valvulopathy require preprocedure dental prophylaxis per American Heart Association guidelines. (Table 6-25)[89]

TABLE 6-25
■ Preprocedure Dental Prophylaxis[89]

Standard adult prophylaxis	Amoxicillin 2 grams orally one hour before procedure
If allergic to amoxicillin, ampicillin, or penicillin	Clindamycin 600 mg orally one hour before procedure OR
	Cephalexin or cefadroxil 2 grams orally one hour before procedure OR
	Azithromycin or clarithromycin 500 mg orally one hour before procedure

2. Depending upon the extent of the surgery, postprocedure antibiotics may also be indicated.
- D. Laser therapy[90]
- E. Changing immunosuppression regimen (e.g., from cyclosporine to tacrolimus)

VI. Prevention
- A. Pretransplant
  1. Optimization of oral hygiene
  2. Regular dental examinations
  3. Periodontal prophylaxis as indicated
  4. Treatment of dental disease
- B. Post-transplant
  1. Meticulous oral hygiene
  2. Regular dental examinations
  3. Removal of plaque and calculus deposits

SEXUAL DYSFUNCTION

I. Overview
- A. Definition of sexual health
  1. World Health Organization definition of sexual health: "the integration of somatic, emotional, intellectual and social aspects of sexual being in ways that are positive, enriching, and that enhance personality, communication, and love"[91]

II. Etiologic factors associated with sexual dysfunction[7, 92-94]
- A. Pretransplant factors: sexual dysfunction associated with:
  1. Medical conditions
     - a. Chronic debilitating illness such as:
       - i. Renal failure and dialysis
       - ii. Hepatic failure
       - iii. Alcohol abuse
     - b. Endocrine disorders
       - i. DM
       - ii. Hyperthyroidism or hypothyroidism
       - iii. Hypogonadism
     - c. Cardiovascular disease
       - i. Arteriosclerosis
       - ii. Peripheral vascular disease
     - d. Neurologic disorders
       - i. Peripheral neuropathy
       - ii. Nerve injury secondary to prostate surgery
       - iii. Stroke
  2. Chronic fatigue
  3. Loss of libido
  4. Medications
     - a. Types of pharmacologically induced sexual dysfunction
       - i. Erectile dysfunction
       - ii. Ejaculatory disorder
       - iii. Loss of libido
       - iv. Orgasmic disorder
       - v. Priapism

        b.   Medications associated with sexual dysfunction (Table 6-26)[92, 94]

   B. Post-transplant factors

      1. Residual pretransplant fears about sexual activity, particularly in heart transplant recipients

      2. Side effects of medications

         a. Immunosuppressive agents

         b. Medications associated with erectile dysfunction (see list above)

      3. Loss of libido

      4. Irregular menstrual cycles

      5. Onset of menopause

      6. Vaginal dryness secondary to medications, low estrogen levels, or vascular damage due to poorly controlled DM

      7. Vaginal yeast infections due to elevated blood glucose levels

      8. Fear of infection, pregnancy

      9. Loss of intimacy

     10. Poor body image secondary to:

         a. Weight gain

         b. Acne

         c. Hirsutism

         d. Hair loss

         e. Surgical scars

     11. Altered roles and relationships

     12. Depression

     13. Partner's fears about safety of resuming sexual activity

III. Treatment options following thorough history and physical examination

   A. Manipulation of medication regimen as indicated and tolerated

   B. Referral to a urologist, gynecologist, or mental health provider as indicated

   C. Medications to treat erectile dysfunction (for example, phosphodiesterase-5 [PPD-5] inhibitors such as sildenafil) have been used in selected transplant recipients.[95]

      1. Approximately 60% of transplant recipients responded to sildenafil treatment.

      2. Metabolism of sildenafil

         a. Metabolized via the same pathway as cyclosporine (the cytochrome P450 isozyme 3A4 enzymatic pathway)

         b. Studies in the kidney transplant population indicate that although cyclosporine and sildenafil are metabolized via the same pathway, no changes in cyclosporine dose were required.

      3. PDE-5 inhibitors in setting of cardiovascular disease

         a. Many transplant recipients have cardiovascular disease

         b. For general population: cardiovascular risk stratification and recommendations for treatment with PDE-5 inhibitors (Table 6-27)[96]

IV. Patient education[93]

   A. Clinicians may be reluctant to discuss sexual issues with patients and their partners. It is important to identify and resolve potential barriers such as:

      1. Viewing topic as irrelevant to nursing practice

      2. Embarrassment

      3. Lack of knowledge

TABLE 6-26

■ **Medications Associated with Sexual Dysfunction**[92, 94]

Category	Medication
Antihypertensive agents	β-blockers
	Thiazide diuretics
	Clonidine
	Methyldopa
	Spironolactone
	Calcium channel blockers
	α-adrenoceptor antagonists
	ACE inhibitors
Psychotherapeutic agents	Antidepressants
	Heterocyclic agents
	MAOIs
	SSRIs
	Tricyclic antidepressants
	Lithium carbonate
	Neuroleptics
	Thioridazine
	Anxiolytics
	Clonazepam
H_2-antagonists	Cimetidine
Anticonvulsants	Phenytoin
	Carbamazepine
	Phenobarbital
	Primidone
Lipid-lowering agents	Fibrates
	Statins
5-α-reductase inhibitor	Finasteride
Drugs of abuse	Nicotine
	Alcohol
	Anabolic steroids
	Heroin
	Marijuana

ACE = angiotensin converting enzyme; MAOI = monoamine oxidase inhibitors; SSRI = selective serotonin re-uptake inhibitors

TABLE 6-27

■ **Cardiovascular Risk Stratification and Recommendations for Treatment with PDE-5 Inhibitors for General Population[96]**

Level of Risk	Description	Recommendation
Low	Asymptomatic CVD with < 3 major risk factors for CAD	Can be treated with PDE-5 inhibitor without further CV diagnostic evaluation
	Controlled hypertension with ≥ 1 antihypertensive medications	
	Successful coronary revascularization	Exception: Patients taking nitrates in any form
	Uncomplicated post-MI (> 6–8 weeks)	
	Mild valvular disease	
	LV dysfunction/CHF (NYHA Class I)	
	Mild, stable angina	Require noninvasive evaluation before treatment with PDE-5 inhibitor
Intermediate	Asymptomatic, ≥ 3 major risk factors for CAD, excluding gender	Require further cardiac evaluation before restratification into low- or high-risk category
	Moderate, stable angina	
	Recent MI (> 2 weeks and < 6 weeks)	
	LV dysfunction/CHF (NYHA Class II)	
	Noncardiac sequelae of atherosclerotic disease (peripheral arterial disease, history of stroke or TIAs)	
High	Unstable or refractory angina	Require cardiac assessment and treatment before considering use of PDE-5 inhibitors
	Uncontrolled hypertension	
	LV disease/CHF (NYHA Class III/IV)	
	Recent MI (< 2 weeks)	
	High-risk arrhythmias	
	Obstructive hypertrophic cardiomyopathy	
	Moderate/severe valvular disease, particularly AS	

AS = aortic stenosis; CAD = coronary artery disease; CHF = congestive heart failure; CV = cardiovascular; CVD = cardiovascular disease; LV = left ventricular; MI = myocardial infarction; NYHA = New York Heart Association; PVD = peripheral vascular disease; TIA = transient ischemic attack

Adapted from DeBusk RF, Drory Y, Goldstein I, et al. Management of sexual dysfunction in patients with cardiovascular disease: Recommendations of the Princeton Consensus Panel. *Am J Cardiol* 2000, 86: 175-181.

    4.   Lack of time

    5.   Lack of privacy

    6.   Fear of offending patient and/or partner

  B. Create an environment in which patients and their partners feel comfortable in discussing sexual concerns.

  C. Convey to patients and their partners that post-transplant sexual dysfunction is common.

D. Extended PLISSIT Model[93, 97-99]
   1. Four levels of nursing interventions (Table 6-28)
   2. Permission-giving is a core aspect of each level.
      a. At each level, nurses should begin with reflection and review.
      b. Seek the patient's perspective by asking questions such as:[99, p.40]
         i. "What do you think about that?"
         ii. "Are there any other things that you might have thought of?"
         iii. "What have we not covered fully?"
      c. This review process further validates permission-giving which in turn encourages patients/partners to further discuss problems and concerns.
      d. At each level, review interactions with patients/partners.

NEUROCOGNITIVE IMPAIRMENT

I. Overview
   A. Neurocognitive function is a dynamic process that involves the ability to perceive, retain, reason, and flexibly respond to information in the environment.
   B. Four major classes of neurocognitive function[100]
      1. Receptive functions: ability to select, acquire, integrate and classify information

TABLE 6-28

■ **Extended PLISSIT Model: Levels of Nursing Interventions**[93, 97-99]

Level		Description	Example
P	Permission	Inform patient and partner that sexual concerns are an important component of the nursing assessment.	"Transplant recipients often experience sexual problems such as a loss of desire. What has been your experience?"
		Introduce topic and give patient permission to think about the impact of his or her illness/transplant on his or her sexuality.	"Tell me about any sexual changes you have experienced since your transplant."
LI	Limited information	Provide information about the impact of transplant on sexuality and the effects of medications on sexual function.	Discuss the sexual side effects of patient's medications. Provide limited educational materials.
SS	Specific suggestions	Employ problem-solving approach; suggest specific solutions to patient's particular problem.	Use of lubricants for discomfort or pain associated with intercourse
		Address all aspects of sexuality rather than just sexual behavior.	If a female transplant recipient is concerned about her femininity and body image, discuss what femininity means to her and identify specific strategies to enhance femininity.
IT	Intensive therapy	Refer patients to additional resources as indicated.	Individuals who require psychosexual counseling should be referred to a mental health provider.

  2. Memory and learning: ability to store and retrieve information

  3. Thinking: ability to mentally organize and reorganize information

  4. Expressive functions: ability to communicate or act upon information

 C. Each class is distinct but the functions are interdependent.

 D. Neurocognitive impairment is a deficit or dysfunction in one or more of these functions.

 E. Biological, psychological, and social factors affect both the pattern and severity of neurocognitive impairment.

II. Pretransplant neurocognitive impairment[17]

 A. Occurs in a significant number of patients with end-stage organ disease

 B. Examples of organ-specific etiologic factors:

  1. End-stage renal disease: uremia, hyperphosphatemia; metabolic abnormalities

  2. End-stage heart disease: decreased cardiac output

  3. End-stage lung disease: hypoxia

  4. End-stage liver disease: encephalopathy; metabolic abnormalities; nutritional deficits

III. Post-transplant neurocognitive impairment

 A. The precise prevalence of neurocognitive impairment among transplant recipients is unknown; however, subsets of patients in each transplant population have significant post-transplant neurocognitive dysfunction.

 B. Etiologic factors

  1. Medications

   a. Immunosuppressive agents

   b. Antimicrobial agents

    i. Antivirals

    ii. Antifungal agents

    iii. Antibiotics

  2. Iatrogenic factors: for example, effects of cardiopulmonary bypass

  3. Comorbidities such as:

   a. Infections

   b. Cerebrovascular events

   c. Psychiatric illness

  4. Substance abuse

  5. Acute rejection

IV. Medications

 A. Immunosuppressants

  1. Can cause neurocognitive impairment through:

   a. Direct effects on central nervous system (CNS)

   b. Indirect effects through

    i. Infections that involve CNS

    ii. Neoplasms that cause neurological impairment

  2. Neurotoxicity can occur in setting of immunosuppressant blood levels within the therapeutic range.

  3. Neuropsychiatric side effects of common immunosuppressive agents (Table 6-29)[101]

 B. Side effects of antimicrobial agents[101]

  1. Antiviral agents (Table 6-30)

  2. Antifungal agents (Table 6-31)

  3. Antibacterial agents (Table 6-32)

TABLE 6-29

■ **Neuropsychiatric Side Effects of Common Immunosuppressive Agents**[101]

Medication	Reported Neuropsychiatric Side Effects	Comments
Cyclosporine	Fine tremors Confusion Paresthesias Headache Insomnia Anxiety/agitation Blurred vision Apathy Delirium Seizures Stupor/coma Psychosis Encephalopathy Sensorimotor disturbances Cerebrovascular events	Symptoms are typically mild in most patients but may be more pronounced in liver transplant recipients due to advanced liver insufficiency and subsequent blood-brain barrier abnormalities Predisposing factors: Hypomagnesemia Hypocholesterolemia <120 mg/dL) High-dose corticosteroids Aluminum overload Fever Infection Intravenous administration of cyclosporine Advanced liver failure Malignant hypertension Renal insufficiency Drug interactions that ↑ cyclosporine levels
Tacrolimus	Tremulousness Sleep disturbance Headache Dysesthesia Mood changes Visual symptoms Vivid dreams/nightmares	Predisposing factors: Intravenous administration of tacrolimus Drug interactions that ↑ tacrolimus levels
Corticosteroids	Anxiety Irritability Mania Depression Emotional lability Obsessional thoughts Delirium Encephalopathy	Females may be at higher risk for side effects. Side effects may be dose-related (side effects more severe with dose > 40 mg/day). Alternate day dosing may ↓ risk and severity of side effects. Dose must be gradually tapered in order to avoid rebound psychiatric symptoms or relapse in medical condition. Side effects may occur months after continuous treatment; however, most side effects occur within first three weeks.
Mycophenolate Mofetil	Tremor Insomnia Anxiety Depression Hypertonia Parathesia Somnolence	Adverse effects are higher with dose of 3 grams/day.
Muromonab-CD3	Delirium Tremors Impaired cognition Hallucinations Acute psychosis Aseptic meningitis (fever, headache, delirium)	Possible etiology: release of lymphokines and lymphotoxins from T cells Aseptic meningitis: Occurs in 5%–14% of patients Symptoms typically resolve within 72 hours (without treatment or discontinuation of drug)
Azathioprine	None reported	

TABLE 6-30

■ **Antiviral Agents**[101]

Medication	Reported Neuropsychiatric Side Effects	Comments
Acyclovir	Tremor/myoclonus Confusion Agitation Lethargy Hallucinations Clouding of consciousness Extrapyramidal symptoms Unilateral focal symptoms Seizures Psychotic depression	Symptoms typically develop within first 24 to 72 hours of treatment. Symptoms are typically reversible. Renal failure is associated with ↑ risk of neurotoxicity.
Ganciclovir	Nightmares Visual hallucinations Agitation Delirium Headache	Renal insufficiency is a risk factor for side effects. Reduce dose in setting of renal insufficiency. Side effects may occur immediately or two weeks after administration has been started. Side effects typically resolve after dose reduction or stopping medication. For amelioration of side effects: temporarily stop medication and then reintroduce at a lower dose.
Alpha-Interferon	Delirium Anxiety Irritability Depression with affective lability Initial dose associated with: Headache Lethargy ↓ concentration Insomnia Fatigue-induced psychomotor retardation and dulled cognition	Used in liver transplant population in setting of chronic hepatitis C infection Side effects are dose-related

TABLE 6-31

■ **Antifungal Agents**[101]

Medication	Reported Neuropsychiatric Side Effects	Comments
Amphotericin	Delirium	Does not cross blood-brain barrier; therefore, central nervous system (CNS) toxicity is low
	Confusion	
	Restlessness	CNS toxicity associated with intrathecal administration
	Headache	
	Tremor	
Metronidazole	Sensory peripheral neuropathy	Peripheral neuropathy reversed by discontinuing medication
	Ataxia	
	Seizures	
	Hallucinations	
	Depression	
	Agitation	

TABLE 6-32

■ **Antibacterial Agents**[101]

Medication	Reported Neuropsychiatric Side Effects	Comments
Penicillins	Seizures	Side effects ↑ in setting of renal insufficiency
Cephalosporins	Delirium	
Quinolones	Ciprofloxacin: visual hallucinations, disorientation, impaired thinking	Side effects typically uncommon but ↑ when nonsteroidal anti-inflammatory agents are administered
Aminoglycocides	Delirium	Side effects ↑ in setting of renal insufficiency
	Neuromuscular blockade: hypoactive deep tendon reflexes, flaccid paralysis, mydriasis	
	Gentamicin: delirium, particularly with intrathecal administration	

    V. Infections
        A. Polymicrobial and multi-organ infections are common in transplant recipients.
        B. CNS infections are particularly serious.
            1. CNS infections are difficult to treat due to reduced penetration of antimicrobial agents.
            2. The CNS dose not tolerate inflammation or pressure effects.
            3. The CNS has minimal capacity for regeneration.

   VI. Stroke—etiology
    A. Angioinvasive infections
        1. Invade intracranial vessels directly
        2. Produce *in situ* thrombosis or hemorrhage
    B. Vasculitis
        1. Example: intracranial extension of varicella zoster along trigemino-vascular network
    C. Endocarditis with subsequent cerebral embolization
        1. Example: virulent organisms (*Aspergillus;* pseudomonas) associated with friable vegetation
    D. Accelerated atherosclerotic disease associated with diabetes mellitus, hypertension, or hypercholesterolemia
   VII. Acute rejection
    A. Can precipitate encephalopathy
    B. Immunosuppressant levels must be carefully monitored.
        1. Rejection can lead to decreased drug clearance.
        2. Decreased drug clearance can lead to toxic immunosuppression levels even with standard doses.
   VIII. Potential indications of neurocognitive impairment:
    A. Impairment in attention/memory/processing speed
        1. Inability to focus and resist distractions
        2. Slowness in learning new information
        3. Difficulty in remembering critical information
        4. Failure to comprehend multi-step directions
        5. Inability to carry out instructions
    B. Frontal/executive deficits
        1. Failure to generalize information to new situations
        2. Mental inflexibility
        3. Deficient self-awareness about cognitive problems
        4. Lack of initiation when a problem is recognized
   IX. Potential consequences of unrecognized neurocognitive impairment:
    A. Noncompliance with medical regimen
    B. Graft rejection
    C. Infections
    D. Failure to inform health care clinicians about important symptoms and side effects
    E. Depression/anxiety
    F. Feelings of loss of control
    G. Conflict between patient and staff
   X. Assessment and treatment of neurocognitive impairment
    A. Formal neurocognitive assessment to:
        1. Identify presence of cognitive impairment and potential etiology
        2. Establish differential diagnosis
        3. Determine impact of neurocognitive impairment on patient's ability to cope with demands of transplant process
        4. Prevent negative outcomes by:
            a. Teaching patient compensatory strategies
            b. Modifying demands placed on patient
        5. Intervene as indicated to:
            a. Ameliorate negative effects of previously unrecognized neurocognitive impairment
            b. Address newly developed neurocognitive problems

      c.   Refer patient to formal rehabilitation program

XI. Strategies to manage neurocognitive impairment

    A. Optimize organization, structure and ease of use of all educational materials.

    B. Begin transplant teaching early in transplant process.

       1. Break information up into small, manageable units.

       2. Provide short educational sessions.

       3. Use multimodal cues (words, colors, symbols) as indicated.

       4. Individualize teaching according to patient's needs.

    C. Strategies for specific disorders

       1. Memory disorders

          a. Provide patient with log book for medication list and other important medical information.

          b. Provide pill dispensers to minimize demands on memory.

          c. Develop alarm system to cue patient to perform daily tasks.

          d. Provide deliberate reminders for non-routine tasks (via postcards, email, phone calls).

          e. Involve patient's family and friends.

       2. Executive disorders

          a. Don't expect patient to spontaneously report critical information; deliberately check for important symptoms.

          b. Enlist the assistance of another person to provide cues and directions for the patient.

    D. For all intervention and prevention strategies

       1. Verify the effectiveness of these strategies with the patient/family member.

       2. Ask patient/family members what works best for them.

       3. Each transplant team member must implement and reinforce strategies.

SUMMARY: STRATEGIES TO PREVENT LONG-TERM COMPLICATIONS[71]

I. Tailor immunosuppression therapy to decrease the risk of CVD, cancer, and infection.

    A. Maintain patient on minimum amount of immunosuppression that is needed to prevent acute rejection.

       1. Consider individual recipient's risk factors.

          a. Recipients who *may* require more immunosuppression:

             i   Recipients of prior transplants

             ii   Younger recipients

             iii. African-American recipients

             iv. Female recipients, particularly those who have had one or more pregnancies

             v. Recipients with history of severe vascular rejection

             vi. Recipients with history of more than one acute rejection episode

             vii. Kidney transplant recipients with greater than 1 major histocompatibility mismatches

          b. Recipients who *may* require less immunosuppression

             i. *De novo* transplant recipients

      ii. Older recipients

     iii. White recipients

     iv. Male recipients

      v. Recipients with history of no or mild cellular rejection

     vi. Recipients with no or only one acute rejection episodes

    vii. Kidney transplant recipients with zero major histocompatibility mismatches

B. Select the most effective and least toxic immunosuppressants.

C. Adapt immunosuppression regimen to patient's risk profile and/or most bothersome adverse side effects; for example:

   1. For patients with severe hyperlipidemia: avoid use of or minimize dose of cyclosporine, prednisone, or sirolimus.

   2. For patients with hypertension: reduce dose of cyclosporine or prednisone as indicated and tolerated.

   3. For patients with diabetes: wean or minimize prednisone dose; switch patient from tacrolimus to cyclosporine.

II. Adopt strategies to prevent medication noncompliance.

A. Use medications that can be dosed once daily whenever possible.

B. Educate patients and family members.

C. Help patient to develop a system that reminds them to take their medications.

D. Maintain regular contact with patient.

E. Develop solutions for financial problems associated with cost of medications.

F. Identify patients who are at high risk for noncompliance .

G. Develop targeted risk factor interventions for patients who are at high risk for noncompliance.

III. Monitor renal function at regular intervals.

A. Identify potential etiology of renal insufficiency.

B. Develop targeted interventions.

IV. Monitor graft function closely for acute and chronic rejection.

A. Biopsies and labwork per protocol

B. Monitor patient for signs and symptoms of rejection.

V. Treat hyperlipidemia aggressively.

A. Assess lipid profile.

   1. Elevated total cholesterol levels are typically associated with elevated low-density lipoprotein (LDL) cholesterol and triglycerides.

   2. In the general population, treatment of elevated LDL levels has been shown to decrease the risk for ischemic events and reduce mortality.

B. Treat specific dyslipidemia(s).

C. Monitor patient's response with regard to:

   1. Improvement in lipid profile

   2. Side effects of medications

VI. Treat hypertension aggressively.

A. Assess patient's risk factors.

B. Monitor response to antihypertensive therapy with regard to:

   1. Blood pressure

   2. Side effects of antihypertensive agents

VII. Encourage a healthy lifestyle.

A. Regular aerobic exercise to

   1. Optimize weight

        2.   Counteract effects of corticosteroid therapy

        3.   Improve mood state

    B. Smoking cessation

    C. Heart-healthy diet

        1.   Therapeutic lifestyle changes (TLC): nutrient composition of TLC diet (Table 6-33)[14]

VIII. Screen for cancer routinely. (Table 6-34)

  IX. Prevent infection.

    A. Infection prophylaxis during periods of anti-rejection therapy

    B. Annual influenza vaccination unless otherwise contraindicated

    C. Strict control of blood glucose levels in patients with DM

   X. Preserve bone health.

    A. Screen for decreased bone mineral density with dual-energy x-ray absorptiometry of the lumbar spine and hip.

        1.   Baseline (pretransplantation)

        2.   6-months post-transplant

        3.   Every 12 months thereafter if abnormal at 6 months post-transplant

    B. Prevent or treat osteopenia/osteoporosis.

        1.   Calcium and vitamin D supplements

        2.   Bisphosphonates to reverse bone loss and increase bone mass

        3.   Calcitonin

        4.   Hormone replacement therapy in carefully selected patients

TABLE 6-33

■ **Therapeutic Lifestyle Changes—Diet[14]**

Nutrient	Recommended Intake
Saturated fat	< 7% of total calories
Polyunsaturated fat	Up to 10% of total calories
Monounsaturated fat	Up to 20% of total calories
Total fat	25%–35% of total calories
Carbohydrate	50%–60% of total calories
Fiber	20–30 grams per day
Protein	Approximately 15% of total calories
Cholesterol	< 200 mg/day
Total calories	Balance energy intake and expenditure to maintain desirable body weight or prevent weight gain

TABLE 6-34

■ **Cancer Screening**

Males	Females
Skin cancer: Self-examination and annual examination by dermatologist; biopsy of suspicious lesions	Skin cancer: Self-examination and annual examination by dermatologist; biopsy of suspicious lesions
Colorectal cancer: Colonoscopy; stool for occult blood	Colorectal cancer: Colonoscopy; stool for occult blood
Prostate cancer: Annual digital rectal examination of prostate; annual prostate specific antigen (PSA) testing	Breast cancer: Monthly self-examination; annual mammography
	Cervical cancer: Annual pelvic examination and Papanicolaou smear

REFERENCES

1. Kasiske BL, Vazquez MA, Harmon WE, et al. Recommendations for the outpatient surveillance of renal transplant patients. American Society of Transplantation. *J Am Soc Nephrol*, 2000, 11: S1-S86.
2. Guckelberger O, Byram A, Klupp J, et al. Coronary event rates in liver transplant recipients reflect the increased prevalence of cardiovascular risk-factors. *Transpl Int*, 2005, 18: 967-974.
3. Ojo AO. Cardiovascular complications after renal transplantation and their prevention. *Transplantation*, 2006, 82: 603-611.
4. Briggs D. Causes of death after renal transplantation. *Nephrol Dial Transplant*, 2001, 16: 1545-1549.
5. Fellstrom B. Risk factors for and management of post-transplantation cardiovascular disease. *BioDrugs*, 2001, 15: 261-278.
6. Kaplan B. Relationship of renal function and cardiovascular mortality in renal transplant recipients. www.medscape.com/viewarticle/504271. Accessed January 28, 2007.
7. Kaplan B, Meier-Kriesche H-U. Mortality risk assessment after renal transplantation. *Clin Transpl*, 2002, 13: 131-136.
8. Kasiske BL. Long-term health risks after transplantation. http://www.medscape.com/viewprogram/314_pnt. Accessed May 4, 2005.
9. Jardine AG. Assessing the relative risk of cardiovascular disease among renal transplant patients receiving tacrolimus or cyclosporine. *Transpl Int*, 2005; 18: 379-84.
10. National Cholesterol Education Program Risk Assessment Tool for Estimating 10-year Risk of Developing Hard CHD (Myocardial Infarction and Coronary Death). http://hp2010.nhlbihin.net/atpiii/calculator.asp?usertype=prof. Accessed January 25, 2007.
11. Von Birgelen C, Hartmann M, Mintz GS, et al. Relationship between cardiovascular risk as predicted by established risk scores versus plaque progression as measured by serial intravascular ultrasound in left main coronary artery. *Circulation*, 2004, 110: 1579-1585.
12. Conroy RM, Pyorala K, Fitzgerald AP, et al. Estimation of ten-year risk of fatal cardiovascular disease in Europe: The SCORE project. *Eur Heart J*, 2003, 24: 987-1003.
13. SCORE (Systematic Coronary Risk Evaluation) Risk Charts http://www.escardio.org/initiatives/prevention/prevention-tools/SCORE-Risk-Charts.htm. Accessed January 25, 2007.
14. National Cholesterol Education Program. National Cholesterol Education Program (NECP) Expert Panel on Detection, Evaluation, and Treatment of High Blood Cholesterol in Adults (Adult Treatment Panel III). Final

Report. *Circulation*, 2002, 106: 3143-3421.

15. Pearson TA, Blair SN, Daniels SR, et al. AHA guidelines for primary prevention of cardiovascular disease and stroke: 2002 update. *Circulation*, 2002, 106: 388-391.

16. Smith SC, Allen J, Blair SN, et al. AHA/ACC guidelines for secondary prevention for patients with coronary and other atherosclerotic vascular disease: 2006 update. Endorsed by the National Heart, Lung, and Blood Institute. *Circulation*, 2006, 113: 2363-2372.

17. Augustine SM, Flattery MP. Long-term complications of solid organ transplantation. In: Cupples SA, Ohler L, (Eds.). *Transplantation Nursing Secrets*. Philadelphia: Hanley & Belfus, 2003, pp. 271-278.

18. Kaplan B, Meier-Kriesche H-U. Late complications of transplantation. In: Stuart FP, Abecassis MM, Kaufman DB, (Eds.). *Organ Transplantation*, 2nd ed. Georgetown, TX: Landes Bioscience, 2003, pp. 437-447.

19. Cupples SA, Boyce SW, Stamou SC. Heart transplantation. In: Cupples SA, Ohler L (Eds.). In: *Solid Organ Transplantation: A Handbook for Primary Health Care Providers*. New York. Springer: 2002, pp. 146-188.

20. American Heart Association. American Heart Association Recommended Blood Pressure Levels. www.americanheart.org. Accessed February 19, 2007.

21. Prasad SA, Kasiske BL, Curtis JJ, et al. Impact and measurement of cardiovascular risks after kidney transplantation. www.medscape.com/viewprogram/4237. Accessed February 19, 2007.

22. Taylor DO, Edwards LB, Boucek MM, et al. Registry of the International Society for Heart and Lung Transplantation: Twenty-second official adult heart transplant report—2006. *J Heart Lung Transplant*, 2006, 25: 869-879.

23. Trulock EP, Edwards LB, Taylor DO, et al. Registry of the International Society for Heart and Lung Transplantation: Twenty-third official adult lung and heart-lung transplantation report—2006. *J Heart Lung Transplant*, 2006, 25: 880-892.

24. Gonwa TA. Hypertension and renal dysfunction in long-term liver transplant recipients. *Liver Transpl*, 2001, 7(Suppl 1): S22-S26.

25. Levitsky J, Martin S. The liver transplant recipient: What you need to know for long-term care. *J Fam Pract*, 2006, 55: 136-144.

26. Wilkinson AH, Cohen DJ. Renal failure in the recipients of nonrenal solid organ transplants. *J Am Soc Nephrol*, 1999, 10: 1136-1144.

27. Kotloff RM, Ahya VN. Medical complications of lung transplantation. *Eur Respir J*, 2004, 23: 334-342.

28. Lindenfeld J. Drug therapy in the heart transplant recipient Part III: Common medical problems. *Circulation*, 2005, 111: 113-117.

29. Spinelli GA, Felipe CR, Machado PG, et al. Relationship of cyclosporine and sirolimus blood concentrations regarding the incidence and severity of hyperlipidemia after kidney transplantation. *Braz J Med Biol Res*, 2006, 39: 19-30.

30. Lake KL. Management of post-transplant obesity and hyperlipidemia. In: Emery RW, Miller LW, (Eds). *Handbook of Cardiac Transplantation*. Philadelphia: Hanley & Belfus, 1996. pp. 147-164.

31. Carr MC, Brunzell JD. Abdominal obesity and dyslipidemia in the metabolic syndrome: Importance of Type 2 diabetes and familial combined hyperlipidemia in coronary artery disease risk. *J Clin Endocrinol Metab*, 2004, 89.

32. Orzano AJ, Scott JG. Diagnosis and treatment of obesity in adults: An applied evidence-based review. *J Am Board Fam Pract*, 2004, 17: 359-369.

33. Yamani MH, Starling RC. Long-term medical complications of heart transplantation: Information for the primary care physician. *Cleve Clin J Med*, 2000, 67: 673-680.

34. Kobashigawa JA, Katznelson S, Laks H, et al. Effect of pravastatin on outcomes after cardiac transplantation. *N Eng J Med*, 1995, 333: 621-627.

35. Grundy SM, Cleeman JI, Merz NB, et al. Implications of recent clinical trials for the National Cholesterol Education Program Adult Treatment Panel III Guidelines. *Circulation*, 2004, 110: 227-239.

36. National Cholesterol Education Program (1) Third report of the National Cholesterol Education Program (NCEP) Expert Panel on Detection, Evaluation, and Treatment of High Blood Cholesterol in Adults (Adult Treatment Panel III), (2) Implications of recent clinical trials for the National Cholesterol Education Program Adult Treatment Panel III Guidelines. www.guideline.gov/summary/summary.aspx?doc_id=5503&nbr=003746&string=cholesterol. Accessed March 15, 2007.

37. Huerta-Alardin AL. Bench-to-bedside review: Rhabdomyolysis—an overview for clinicians. *Crit Care*, 2005, 9: 158-169.

38. Bellosta S, Paoletti R, Corsini A. Safety of statins: Focus on clinical pharmacokinetics and drug interactions. *Circulation*, 2004, 109 (Suppl III): S50-S57.

39. World Health Organization. Definition, Diagnosis, and Classification of Diabetes Mellitus and Its Complications: Part 1: Diagnosis and Classification of Diabetes Mellitus. Geneva. World Health Organization, 1999. pp. 1-65.

40. Chew GT, Gan SK, Watts GF. Revisiting the metabolic syndrome. *Med J Aust*, 2006, 185: 445-449.

41. Grundy SM, Cleeman JI, Daniels SR, et al. Diagnosis and management of the metabolic syndrome: An American Heart Association/National Heart, Lung, and Blood Institute Scientific Statement. *Circulation*, 2005, 112: 2735-2752.

42. Ravindran V, Baboolal K, Moore R. Post-transplant diabetes mellitus after renal transplantation: The emerging clinical challenge. *Yonsei Med J*, 2004, 45: 1059-1064.

43. Shihab FS. Metabolic complications. In: Norman DJ, Turka LA, (Eds.). *Primer on Transplantation*, 2nd ed. Mt. Laurel, NJ: American Society of Transplantation, 2001. pp. 247-256.

44. Larsen JL. Pancreas transplantation: Indications and consequences. *Endocrine Rev*, 2004, 25: 919-946.

45. The Expert Committee on the Diagnosis and Classification of Diabetes Mellitus. Follow-up report on the diagnosis of diabetes mellitus. *Diabetes Care*, 2003, 26: 3160-3167.

46. The Diabetes Control and Complications Trial Research Group. The effect of treatment of diabetes on the development and progression of long-term complications in insulin-dependent diabetes mellitus. *N Eng J Med*, 1993, 329: 977-986.

47. Singer LG, Weinacker AB, Theodore J. Long-term management and outcome of heart-lung and lung transplant recipients. In: Baumgartner WA, Reitz B, Kasper E, et al., (Eds). *Heart and Lung Transplantation*. Philadelphia: Saunders, 2002. pp. 434-455.

48. Bloom RD, Rao V, Weng F, et al. Association of hepatitis C with post-transplant diabetes in renal transplant patients on tacrolimus. *J Am Soc Nephrol*, 2002, 13: 1374-1380.

49. American Heart Association. Body Composition Tests. www.americanheart.org/presenter.jhtml?identifier=4489. Accessed February 28, 2007.

50. National Heart, Lung, and Blood Institute. Clinical Guidelines on the Identification, Evaluation, and Treatment of Overweight and Obesity in Adults (Report No. 228) Bethesda, MD: National Institutes of Health, 1998.

51. American Heart Association. Obesity: Impact on cardiovascular disease. www.americanheart.org/presenter.hjtml?identifier=1818. Accessed February 28, 2007.

52. Kobashigawa J, Starling RC, Mehra MR, et al. Multicenter retrospective analysis of cardiovascular risk factors affecting long-term outcome of de novo cardiac transplant recipients. *J Heart Lung Transplant*, 2006, 25: 1063-1069.

53. Hasse J. Nutritional issues in adult organ transplantation. In: Cupples SA, Ohler L, (Eds). *Solid Organ Transplantation: A Handbook for Primary Health Care Providers*. New York: Springer, 2002. pp. 64-87.

54. Humar A, Kandaswamy R, Granger D, et al. Decreased surgical risks of pancreas transplantation in the modern era. *Ann Surg*, 2000, 231: 269-275.

55. Kanasky WF, Anton SD, Rodrigue JR, et al. Impact of body weight on long-term survival after lung transplantation. *Chest*, 2002, 121: 401-406.

56. Pischon T, Sharma AM. Obesity as a risk factor in renal transplant patients. *Nephrol Dial Transplant*, 2001, 16: 14-17.

57. Prasad SA, Kasiske BL, Curtis JJ, et al. Awareness and management of post-transplant malignancies. 2006, Califon, NJ: SynerMed Communications.

58. Penn I. Neoplasia following transplantation. In: Norman DJ, Turka LA, (Eds.). *Primer on Transplantation*, 2nd ed. Mt. Laurel, NJ: American Society of Transplantation, 2001. pp. 268-275.

59. Morath C, Mueller M, Goldschmidt H, et al. Malignancy in renal transplantation. *J Am Soc Nephrol*, 2004, 15: 1582-1588.

60. Feng S, Buell JF, Chari RS, et al. Tumors and transplantation. *Am J Transplant*, 2003, 3: 1481-1487.

61. Desai U. Management of malignancy after kidney transplantation. *The Immunology Report*, 2007, 3 (Winter 2007): 30-36.

62. Barr ML, Kobashigawa JA. Improving long-term outcomes of heart transplantation: cardiac allograft vasculopathy, malignancy, and treatment options. *Transplantation Updates*, 2006, 1: 1-12.

63. Opelz G, Ohler B. Lymphomas after solid organ transplantation: A collaborative transplant study report. *Am J Transplant*, 2004, 4: 222-230.

64. Fung JJ, Jain A, Kwan EJ, et al. *De novo* malignancies after liver transplantation: A major cause of late death. *Liver Transplant*, 2001, 7: S109-S18.

65. Dreno B. Skin cancers after transplantation. *Nephrol Dial Transplant*, 2003, 18: 1052-1058.

66. Stasko T, Russell MA. Diseases of the skin following transplantation. In: Norman DJ, Turka LA, (Eds.). *Primer on Transplantation*, 2nd ed. Mt. Laurel, NJ: American Society of Transplantation, 2001. pp. 287-295.

67. Razonable RR, Paya CV. Herpesvirus infections in transplant recipients: Current challenges in the clinical management of cytomegalovirus and Epstein-Barr virus infections. *Herpes*, 2003, 10: 60-65.

68. Helderman JH, Goral S. Gastrointestinal complications of transplant immunosuppression. *J Am Soc Nephrol*, 2002, 13: 277-287.

69. Smith RA, Cokkinides V, Eyre HJ. American Cancer Society guidelines for the early detection of cancer. *CA Cancer J Clin*, 2006, 56: 11-25.

70. Rodino MA, Shane E. Osteoporosis after organ transplantation. *Am J Med Sci*, 1998, 104: 459-469.

71. Sahadevan M, Kasiske BL. Long-term post-transplant management and complications. In: Danovitch GM, (Eds.). *Handbook of Kidney Transplantation*, 4th ed. Philadelphia: Lippincott, Williams & Wilkins, 2005. pp. 234-278.

72. Silkensen JR. Long-term complications in renal transplantation. *J Am Soc Nephrol*, 2000, 11: 582-588.

73. Gupta D, Sakorafas GH, McGregor CG, et al. Management of biliary tract disease in heart and lung transplant patients. *Surgery*, 2000, 128: 641-649.

74. Eland IA, van Puijenbroek EP, Sturkenboom MJ, et al. Drug-associated acute pancreatitis: Twenty-one years of spontaneous reporting in the Netherlands. *Am J Gastroenterol*, 1999, 94: 2417-2422.

75. Soderdahl G, Tyden G, Groth CG. Incidence of gastrointestinal complications following renal transplantation in the cyclosporin era. *Transplant Proc*, 1994, 26: 1771-1772.

76. Kaufman DB. Pancreas transplantation. In: Stuart FP, Abecassis MM, Kaufman DB, (Eds.). *Organ Transplantation*, 2nd ed. Georgetown, TX: Landes Bioscience, 2003. pp. 155-182.

77. Liang T-B. Biliary tract complications after liver transplantation. *Hepatobiliary Pancreat Dis Int*, 2005, 4: 10-11.

78. Abecassis MM, Blei A, Koffron A, et al. Liver transplantation. In: Stuart FP, Abecassis MM, Kaufman DB, (Eds.). *Organ Transplantation*, 2nd ed. Georgetown, TX: Landes Bioscience, 2003. pp. 205-243.

79. Flynn BM. Liver transplantation. In: Cupples SA, Ohler L, (Eds.). *Transplantation Nursing Secrets*. Philadelphia: Hanley & Belfus, 2003. pp. 151-171.

80. Kosmach B. Intestinal transplantation. In: Cupples SA, Ohler L, (Eds.). *Transplantation Nursing Secrets*. Philadelphia: Hanley & Belfus, 2003. pp. 173-190.

81. Chanard J, Toupance O, Lavaud S, et al. Amlodipine reduces cyclosporine-induced hyperuricemia in hypertensive renal transplant recipients. *Nephrol Dial Transplant*, 2003, 18: 2147-2153.

82. Clive DM. Renal transplant-associated hyperuricemia and gout. *J Am Soc Nephrol*, 2000, 11: 974-979.

83. Leventhal JP, Schlueter WA. Early medical problems common to many recipients. In: Stuart FP, Abecassis MM, Kaufman DB, (Eds.). *Organ Transplantation*, 2nd ed. Georgetown, TX: Landes Bioscience, 2003. pp. 426-436.

84. Gomez E, Sanchez-Nunez M, Sanchez JE, et al. Treatment of cyclosporine-induced gingival hyperplasia with azithromycin. *Nephrol Dial Transplant*, 1997, 12: 2904-2997.

85. Taylor BA. Management of drug-induced gingival enlargement. *Aust Prescr*, 2003, 26: 11-13.

86. Das SJ, Newman NH, Olson I. Keratinocyte growth factor receptor is up-regulated in cyclosporin A-induced gingival hyperplasia. *J Dent Res*, 2002, 81: 683-687.

87. Abdollahi M, Radfar M. A review of drug-induced oral reactions. *J Contemp Dent Pract*, 2003, 4: 10-31.

88. Argani H, Pourabbas R, Hassanzadeh D, et al. Treatment of cyclosporine-induced gingival overgrowth with azithromycin-containing toothpaste. *Exp Clin Transplant*, 2006, 4: 420-424.

89. American Heart Association. Endocarditis prophylaxis information. www.americanheart.org/presenter.jhtml?identifier=11086. Accessed March 3, 2007.

90. Mattson JS, Blankenau R, Keene JJ. Use of an argon laser to treat drug-induced gingival overgrowth. *J Am Dent Assoc*, 1998, 129: 78-83.

91. World Health Organization. Education and treatment in human sexuality: The training of health professionals. Geneva: World Health Organization, 1975.

92. Thomas JA. Pharmacological aspects of erectile dysfunction. *Jpn J Pharmacol*, 2002, 89: 101-112.

93. Schroeder B. Renewing intimacy and sexuality after organ transplantation. American Society of Transplantation 10th Annual Winter Symposium. February 16, 2006. Cancun, Mexico.

94. Viera AJ, Clenney TL, Shenenberger DW, et al. Newer pharmacologic alternatives for erectile dysfunction. *Am Fam Physician*, 1999, 60: 1159-1172.

95. Hatzichristou DG. Sildenafil citrate: Lessons learned from 3 years of clinical experience. *Int J Impot Res*, 2002, 14(Suppl 1): S43-S52.

96. Kostis JB, Jackson G, Rosen R, et al. Sexual dysfunction and cardiac risk (The Second Princeton Consensus Conference). *Am J Cardiol*, 2005, 96: 313-321.

97. Annon J. The PLISSIT model: A proposed conceptual scheme for the behavioral treatment of sexual problems. *J Sex Educ*, 1976, 2: 1-15.

98. Davis S, Taylor B. From PLISSIT to Ex-PLISSIT. In: Davis S, (Eds.). *Rehabilitation: The use of theories and models in practice*. Edinburgh: Elsevier, 2006. pp. 101-129.

99. Taylor B, Davis S. Using the Extended PLISSIT model to address sexual healthcare needs. *Nurs Stand*, 2006, 21: 35-40.

100. Lezak MD. *Neuropsychological Assessment*, 3rd ed. 1995, New York: Oxford University Press.

101. Trzepacz PT, Gupta B, DiMartini AF. Pharmacologic issues in organ transplantation: Psychopharmacology and neuropsychiatric medication side effects. In: Trzepacz PT, DiMartini AF, (Eds.). *The Transplant Patient: Biological, Psychiatric, and Ethical Issues in Organ Transplantation*. Cambridge: University Press, 2000. pp. 187-213.

REVIEW QUESTIONS

1. You are caring for a 68-year-old gentleman who is 13 years post-heart transplantation. He has been readmitted to your unit for renal insufficiency. His current immuno-suppressants are cyclosporine 125 mg every 12 hours and CellCept 1500 mg every 12 hours. As you are taking the patient's medical history, he reports recent onset of pain in his thighs. He mentions that his primary care physician increased his dose of simvastatin three weeks ago. In particular, you would antici-pate orders for which of the follow-ing lab tests?
   a. CBC
   b. Hepatic function panel
   c. Total iron binding capacity
   d. Creatine kinase
   e. A and D
   f. B and D

2. Your patient reports that his pri-mary care physician has given him a prescription for sildenafil for erectile dysfunction. Your patient wants to know if he may take sildenafil. His current medications include cyclosporine, mycophe-nolate mofetil, pravastatin, isosor-bide mononitrate, furosemide, and potassium chloride. His provider will most likely respond:
   a. "Yes, you may take sildenafil."
   b. "No, you may not take sildena-fil because it increases serum cyclosporine levels."
   c. "No, you may not take silde-nafil because, in combination with nitrates, it may precipitate severe hypotension."
   d. "No, you may not take sildena-fil because, in combination with furosemide, it may precipitate severe renal insufficiency."

3. Which of the following statements are true with regard to allopurinol?
   1. It is given only after an acute gout attack has subsided.
   2. It is given immediately upon the onset of an acute gout attack.
   3. It is rarely given with cyclospo-rine.
   4. It is rarely given with azathio-prine.

   a. 1 and 4
   b. 1 and 3
   c. 2 and 3
   d. 2 and 4

4. Mrs. K. is a 45-year-old woman who underwent kidney transplan-tation 5 years ago. She has been readmitted to your unit for intra-venous antibiotics for community-acquired pneumonia. In caring for Mrs. K., you note that she is very depressed about her 75 pound weight gain since transplantation. Nutrition and psychology consults have been requested. In reviewing the dietitian's note, you learn that the following weight-loss goal has been recommended:
   a. 25% reduction in weight from Mrs. K.'s baseline weight over 12 months
   b. 10% reduction in weight from Mrs. K.'s baseline weight over 6 months
   c. 5% reduction in weight from Mrs. K.'s baseline weight over 9 months
   d. 10% reduction in weight from Mrs. K.'s baseline over 3 months

5. The most common cardiovascular complication across all types of solid organ transplantation is:
   a. Coronary artery disease
   b. Peripheral vascular disease
   c. Myocardial infarction
   d. Hypertension

6. Clinical manifestations of renal insufficiency include:
   1. Increased serum potassium level
   2. Decreased serum potassium level
   3. Increased serum creatinine
   4. Decreased serum creatinine
   5. Increased sodium excretion
   6. Decreased sodium excretion

   a. 2, 4, and 5
   b. 1, 3, and 6
   c. 1, 3, and 5
   d. 1, 4, and 5

7. Which of the following statements are true?
   1. Neurotoxicity can occur in the setting of normal cyclosporine levels.
   2. Neurocognitive functions are independent of one another.
   3. Pretransplant neurocognitive impairment rarely influences post-transplant neurocognitive function.
   4. Immunosuppressants and antimicrobials may have neurocognitive side effects.

   a. 2 and 4
   b. 1 and 4
   c. 2, 3, and 4
   d. All of the above

8. Patients at risk for post-transplant diabetes mellitus include:
   1. Patients with steroid-treated rejection
   2. Recipients < 45 years of age
   3. Recipients > 45 years of age
   4. Recipients of Caucasian and Asian ethnicity
   5. Recipients of African-American and Hispanic ethnicity

   a. 1, 2, and 5
   b. 1, 2, and 4
   c. 1, 3, and 5
   d. 2, 4, and 5

9. The most common malignancy in solid organ transplant recipients is:
   a. Lung
   b. Skin
   c. Colon
   d. Bladder

10. Of the following types of antihypertensive medications, which type is most likely to affect cyclosporine or tacrolimus levels:
    a. β-blockers
    b. Calcium channel blockers
    c. Angiotensin-converting enzyme inhibitors
    d. Alpha-adrenergic receptor blockers

11. Which of the following statements about post-transplant malignancy are true?
    1. Squamous cell carcinoma is seen more frequently than basal cell carcinoma.
    2. Basal cell carcinoma is seen more frequently than squamous cell carcinoma.
    3. Carcinomas that are common in the general population (e.g., breast and prostate cancer) also occur more frequently in transplant recipients.
    4. The incidence of post-transplant malignancy and recipient mortality due to *de novo* malignancy are increasing.

    a. 1 and 2
    b. 2 and 3
    c. 3 and 4
    d. 1 and 4

12. You are caring for a 19-year-old woman who had a heart and lung transplant 6 months ago. She has received antibody therapy for several rejection episodes. In reviewing her medical record, you note that at the time of transplant she was both Epstein-Barr virus (EBV) seronegative and cytomegalovirus (CMV) seronegative. The donor was both EBV and CMV seropositive. Your patient has had one post-transplant readmission for CMV gastritis which was treated with ganciclovir. Her symptoms on this readmission include fever, night sweats, lymphadenopathy, diarrhea, abdominal pain, and weight loss. Her CMV-PCR is negative. You suspect that she may have:
    a. Tuberculosis
    b. Post-transplant lymphoproliferative disease
    c. A recurrence of CMV gastritis
    d. Cholecystitis

13. Which of the following statements about post-transplant bone disease are true?
    1. Vertebral bone loss typically is highest during the first 6 to 12 months post-transplant.
    2. Corticosteroids can cause increased bone resorption.
    3. Hypogonadism contributes to bone loss.
    4. Pain associated with avascular necrosis may be referred to the knee.

    a. 1, 3, and 4
    b. 2, 3, and 4
    c. 1, 2, and 3
    d. All of the above

14. Which of the following medications are typically associated with the development of gingival hyperplasia?
    1. Cyclosporine
    2. Diuretics
    3. Anticonvulsants
    4. Antihyperlipidemic agents
    5. Calcium channel blockers

    a. 1, 3, and 5
    b. 1, 4, and 5
    c. 2, 3, and 4
    d. 1, 2, and 5

15. In order to prevent gastric ulceration, transplant recipients may take all of the following medications *except*:
    a. H$_2$-receptor blockers
    b. Proton-pump inhibitors
    c. Nonsteroidal anti-inflammatory drugs
    d. Prostaglandins
    e. Coating agents

16. The hallmarks of metabolic syndrome include:
    1. Central obesity
    2. Hyperglycemia
    3. Renal insufficiency
    4. Hypertension
    5. Metabolic acidosis
    6. Dyslipidemia

    a. 1, 2, 3, and 6
    b. 1, 2, 5, and 6
    c. 2, 3, 4, and 6
    d. 1, 2, 4, and 6

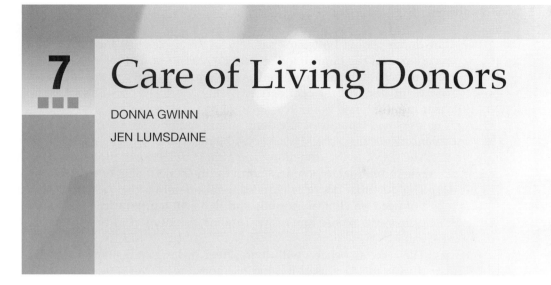

7 Care of Living Donors

DONNA GWINN

JEN LUMSDAINE

INTRODUCTION

I. The evolution of living organ donation
   A. The first successful human living donor transplant was performed in 1954 in Boston, MA, U.S., between identical twin brothers.
   B. The advent of immunosuppressant drugs in the 1970s facilitated transplantation from non-identical family members and a subsequent increase in organ transplantation from cadaveric donors.
   C. This permitted a reduction in the number of living donor transplants and thus relieved the operating surgeon from the responsibility of removing an organ from a healthy person.
   D. However, the steady decrease in cadaveric donors worldwide has demanded more focus on living donation.
      1. The benefits for the recipient of a living donor transplant are clear—the organ is from a fit and healthy person who has undergone an intense medical evaluation.
      2. The time the organ is without a blood supply (ischemic time) is very short compared to the time involved in cadaveric transplantation.
      3. The negative side for the recipient is in having a family member or close friend undergo major surgery, which they themselves do not medically require, on behalf of the recipient.
II. Selection and education of the living donor
   A. Each living donor is carefully evaluated to ensure there is maximum benefit to the recipient and minimum risk to the donor.[1]
   B. This evaluation encompasses both the physical and psychosocial health of the donor.
   C. The idea of living donation may be broached at the transplant assessment clinic or by health professionals involved in the early treatment of organ failure.
   D. Families may have heard about other living donor transplants within the hospital/community setting or via the media.
   E. In some countries, the recipient team will contact family members directly and ask if they wish to be considered as donors.
   F. Care must be taken that potential donors are not pressured or coerced by the recipient or other family members.

G. The donor should be seen separately, in the absence of the prospective recipient and the family, and should be reassured that his or her views with respect to donation, as well as his or her medical and social history, will be treated in strict confidence.

III. Ethical issues for living donor transplantation

A. The risks and benefits of live donor transplantation need to be carefully balanced as many ethical issues may be raised.

1. The act of living donation is an almost unique situation—exposing one individual to potential harm for the benefit of another.[2]

2. The potential donor is requesting an operation that he or she does not need on clinical grounds and that will temporarily disable him or her and expose him or her to some risk of morbidity and mortality.

3. The risks associated with living liver or lung transplant are higher due to the increased morbidity/mortality of the donor procedure along with the absence of alternative replacement therapies for the recipient.

4. The Hippocratic Oath states "Primum non nocere"—firstly, do no harm.[3] Is the removal of a healthy organ from an otherwise fit person "harm" or would the donor be "harmed" by not being allowed to donate an organ to improve the life quality (or in some cases save the life) of a closely linked individual?

5. A broader ethical view may be argued that an increase in living donation reduces the number of individuals waiting on the transplant list.[4]

B. The ethical principles of autonomy, beneficence, non-maleficence, and justice may be applied to the living donor.

1. Autonomy is the right of self-government, personal freedom, and freedom of will.

2. Beneficence is doing good, active kindness.

3. Non-maleficence is doing no harm.

4. Justice is the moral obligation to act on the basis of fair adjudication between competing claims.

5. These four principles are "prima facie"—binding unless it conflicts with another moral principle—if it does, then we have to choose between them.[5]

C. Informed consent. Respect for an individual's autonomy is the central reason that each person has the right to consent to or refuse treatment.

1. Individuals should have the necessary information about the choices available and the potential consequences of each course of action. Hence the term "informed consent."

2. While potential donors may be given an appropriate, detailed description of the risks of donation, it is much less clear that all donors will listen.

3. There is a well-described tendency for some people to decide at an early stage that they wish to donate and then to be impervious to any suggestion that they should make a more informed decision in the light of further counseling.[6] The consent may be real but whether it is truly informed may be questionable.[7]

D. It is also important to recognize that the clinical team involved also has rights as well as responsibilities.

       1. If a fully informed donor wishes to proceed with a course of action that involves risks of mortality or morbidity more severe than the team finds acceptable, they are under no obligation to proceed. Referral for a second opinion would be appropriate in such circumstances.[7]

  E. Key issues of consent

       1. Donors should be approached "neutrally."

       2. Potential donors should be fully informed about risks, benefits, and alternatives as early as possible.

       3. Coercive, inherent, and external pressures should be probed for and detected wherever possible.

       4. Independent clinicians and other health care professionals should be involved where possible.

       5. An opportunity to withdraw discreetly should be offered.[8]

  F. Payment for organs

       1. Most international bodies, such as the World Health Organization and the Transplantation Society, oppose payment for human organs.

       2. In 2000, the World Medical Association issued the following statement: "Payment for organs and tissues for donation and transplantation should be prohibited. A financial incentive compromises the voluntariness of the choice and the altruistic basis for organ and tissue donation. Furthermore, access to needed medical treatment based on ability to pay is inconsistent with the principles of justice. Organs suspected to have been obtained through commercial transaction should not be accepted for transplantation."[2]

  G. Provision of information should include:

       1. A wide range of literature, including the risks and benefits of living donation with both national and local perspectives. This may be in the form of booklets, leaflets, and videos.

       2. The opportunity to talk to a person who has been a living donor.

       3. A flow-chart or algorithm that summarizes the donor evaluation process.[7]

  H. Good communication throughout the donor assessment period is essential. A clinical nurse specialist or transplant coordinator usually acts as the key contact during the process.

IV. The medical evaluation

  A. The medical evaluation encompasses three main areas:

       1. Immunological compatibility—although incompatibility no longer excludes transplantation of some organs, appropriate treatment of the recipient may be required to overcome potential incompatibility and acute rejection.

       2. General health—to exclude comorbidities that may increase the risk to the donor of major complications peri-operatively and postoperatively and to reduce the risk of disease transmission to the recipient (e.g., viral or malignancy).

       3. Organ function—to ensure the donor has adequate organ reserve for both the short- and long term, and that the recipient receives a well-functioning transplant

       4. See Tables 7-1 to 7-4.

  B. Both recipient and donor criteria must be considered when assessing the risk/benefit balance.

TABLE 7-1

■ **Basic Investigations for Living Donor Assessment—General**

History	General health
	Psychiatric history
	Potential contraindications: obesity, hypertension, diabetes, smoking
Examination	General
	Cardiovascular
	Respiratory
	Abdominal
Immunology screen	Blood group
	Human leucocyte antigen (HLA type)
	Lymphocytotoxic crossmatch
Hematology screen	Full blood count
	Coagulation studies
Biochemistry screen	Urea and electrolytes
	Creatinine clearance
	Liver function tests
	Blood glucose
Urinalysis	Protein
	Blood
	Sugar
	Culture
	Sensitivity and microscopy
Cardiovascular	Serial blood pressure measurements
	ECG
Microbiological screen	Hepatitis B and C
	HIV
	CMV
	Epstein-Barr virus
	Syphilis
	Toxoplasma
Radiology	Chest x-ray
	Organ-specific imaging

TABLE 7-2
■ **Specific Additional Investigations for Living Donor Assessment—Renal**

History	Risk of renal disease: family history, particularly if disease in recipient is familial
	Past history of renal infections, hematuria, renal calculi
Urinalysis	Protein
	Blood
	Sugar
	Creatinine clearance
	Culture
	Sensitivity and microscopy
Radiology	Isotope GFR
	Renal ultrasound
	Angiogram/spiral CT/MRA

TABLE 7-3
■ **Specific Additional Investigations for Living Donor Assessment—Liver**

History	History of liver disease
	Alcohol intake
Radiology	Liver ultrasound
	MRCP
	Angiogram/spiral CT/MRA

TABLE 7-4
■ **Specific Additional Investigations for Living Donor Assessment—Lung**

History	History of respiratory disease
	Smoking
Cardiovascular	Echocardiogram
Radiology	Chest x-ray
	Spiral CT/MRA
	Ventilation-perfusion scan
Other	Spirometry
	Pulmonary function tests

1. Specific recipient issues include any comorbidities, the primary disease with risk of recurrence, and psychosocial concerns, such as compliance with drug regimen post-transplantation.
2. The donor evaluation is usually performed over a period of 3 months to ensure that all results are satisfactory and to allow the donor time to consider the risks and benefits of the procedure.
3. In some cases, such as the situation where a liver or lung patient is acutely ill, the assessment may be performed in a much shorter time frame.
4. See Figure 7-1.

V. The surgical procedure
  A. It is considered best practice that the donor and recipient operations are undertaken synchronously in parallel operating theatres staffed by two full teams of theatre personnel.
    1. This minimizes cold ischemic time.
    2. It also ensures that the donor organ is removed from the donor only after it has been confirmed that there are no unforeseen problems with the recipient that prevent implantation.[7]
  B. Living kidney donor
    1. Living kidney donation is increasing significantly.[9]
    2. The most common method, until recently, has been to remove a kidney for transplantation by open nephrectomy.
      a. This involves an incision on the side of the upper abdomen (flank incision) using a retro-peritoneal approach.
      b. It is sometimes necessary to remove part of a rib for better exposure.
      c. This technique has been shown to be safe and effective with a low peri-operative mortality rate, acceptable risk of peri-operative complications, and excellent preservation of graft function.
      d. However, the extensive flank incision may result in significant wound discomfort and a prolonged convalescence.[7]
      e. The left kidney is frequently the preferred kidney for donation, unless there is anatomically some reason to use the right, such as blood supply or position.[10]
    3. Laparoscopic (keyhole surgery) donor nephrectomy has been used increasingly in the past decade.
      a. It has been shown that donors have a reduced requirement of analgesia, a shorter hospital stay, and an earlier return to normal activity.[11]
      b. The surgeon makes two or three small incisions close to the umbilicus, and the kidney is removed through a central incision.
      c. Various techniques can be used, including hand-assisted laparoscopic nephrectomy.
  C. The living lung donor
    1. The lower lobe of one lung is the most ideal for living donor transplantation.[9] Living lung donation requires two donors—one donating a right lower lobe and the other donating a left lower lobe.
    2. The donor lobectomy is performed through a postero-lateral thoracotomy through the fourth or fifth intercostal space.[12]
    3. Living lung donation is usually reserved for children or young adults with cystic fibrosis.

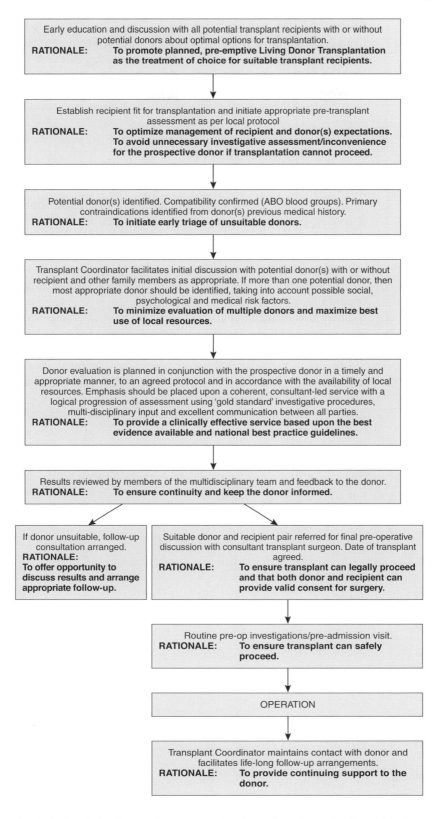

Figure 7-1. Donor evaluation: Summary and organizational chart

D. The living liver donor
   1. Living donor liver transplantation was initially performed only in the pediatric setting, usually a parent donating the left lateral segment of the liver to his or her child.
   2. In adult transplantation this segment is too small, thus the right liver has to be donated to provide enough liver mass in adult recipients.[13]
   3. The liver has the ability to regenerate itself in both the donor and recipient after transplantation.

VI. Complications of living organ donation
   A. Kidney donor
      1. Kidney donation has a very low morbidity rate as compared to liver and lung donation, but risk is still there, just from the surgery and anesthesia.
      2. Common short-term complications are pulmonary problems such as atelectasis and pneumonia.
      3. Deep vein thrombosis and pulmonary emboli are a risk from the immobility of surgery and anesthesia.
      4. Urinary tract infections and bowel ileus have been reported.
      5. The spleen can sometimes be damaged during the removal of the left kidney, requiring removal to prevent bleeding.
      6. Siddins et al.[14] report that some donors have complained of persistent shoulder discomfort and neurologic symptoms, probably due to phrenic nerve irritation.
      7. Table 7-5 compares complication rates following different kinds of nephrectomy.

TABLE 7-5

■ **Complications Following Donor Nephrectomy[24]**

Complication	Open nephrectomy (5660) %	Laparoscopic hand assisted (2239) %	Full laparoscopic nephrectomy (2929) %
Re-operation	0.4	1.0	0.9
Complications not needing re-operation	0.3	1	0.8
Bleeding	0.15	0.18	0.45
Bowel obstruction	0.05	0.27	0.1
Bowel injury	-	0.1	0.14
Hernia	0.18	0.5	0.03
DVT/pulmonary embolus	0.02	0.09	0.1
Pneumothorax	0.09	0.05	-
Prolonged ileus	-	0.05	0.06
Rhabdomyolysis	-	0.09	0.13

Readmission rate: open 0.6%, laparoscopic 1.6%

B. Living lung donor
1. Although mortality is low, morbidity is high in lung lobectomy donation.[15] Battafarano and colleagues[15] reported that only 38.7% of lung lobe donors did not experience any complications in their study of 62 donors.
2. Major complications included pleural effusions and air leaks, hemorrhage requiring a transfusion, permanent phrenic nerve injury, arrhythmias, airway complications, pneumonia and atelectasis, and infections.
    a. Hemorrhage risk after thoracic surgery is high due the vascular nature of the lungs.
    b. The lungs must move with each breath; therefore, air leaks are also a risk. Resolving such leaks may require chest tubes, bronchoscopy, or exploratory surgery.
    c. Pneumonia and atelectasis are often complications of any surgery and anesthesia, but the risk is increased greatly when the lungs are operated on. Pulmonary toilet and aggressive respiratory therapy are imperative to prevent pneumonia.
    d. Pain must be addressed because it can interfere with inspiratory effort and contribute to the development of atelectasis and pneumonia.
    e. Bronchial stump fistulas, strictures, and air leaks are other problems that the donor may face if healing is interrupted at the site of surgery. The sutures that closed the bronchus can open from the tension of inspiration. Scarring can cause strictures to form.
    f. Atrial arrhythmias are also a common complication because the surgery requires dissection of the inferior pulmonary vein and the suture line is over the left atrium.
    g. This suture line also increases the risk of pericarditis.
3. Due to the high risk of complications, lung lobectomy donation continues to be reserved for only selected recipients who cannot wait for cadaveric allografts.[15]
C. Living liver donor
1. Living donation for liver transplant has been discouraged because of the increased pre-operative mortality and risk; several deaths have been reported.[9]
2. The removal of enough liver tissue for the adult recipient is often dangerous for the donor; therefore, living liver donation is usually confined to pediatric recipients.[9]
3. The incidence of major and minor complications of liver donation is estimated at 15%-20%, a risk that some transplant centers consider to be too high.[10]
4. The organ-specific complications are the result of the hepatic resection. These include bile leaks, bleeding, strictures and adhesions from scarring and infection, hepatic artery or portal vein thrombosis, and an extended recovery time.
    a. Severe pain of the abdomen or referred pain to the shoulder can signify a bile leak from the cut surface of the liver. These leaks usually resolve on their own without additional surgery,[10] but can be quite discouraging to the donor because recovery can be slow.

          b.   Intestinal obstruction from adhesions is another possible complication, especially if there has been delayed healing.

          c.   Abdominal pain, bloating, nausea, and vomiting can signify an ileus which can be treated conservatively with suction decompression and mobilizing the patient to facilitate peristalsis.

    5.   Severe complications have occurred, including liver failure (resulting in the need for the donor to receive a transplant) and pulmonary emboli.

    6.   There have been at least five liver donor deaths reported in 2500 cases.[10] Rao and colleagues in Hong Kong believe the key to low morbidity in liver donation is a thorough pre-operative workup.[16]

VII.   General post-operative nursing care

  A. The immediate post-operative care of living organ donors should be the same as any routine surgical patient in the recovery room.[17]

  B. These patients tend to be very healthy and recover quickly because they have been pre-screened extensively for possible problems and potential complications, but post-operative complications can occur even in healthy individuals due to immobility, anesthesia, and the removal of a whole, or portion of a, vital organ.

  C. The donor's airway must be maintained at all times to ensure adequate oxygenation.

  D. Continuous monitoring of oxygen saturation is imperative as well as monitoring vital signs.

  E. Hypotension or hypertension may be present after surgery and the cause must be determined.

    1.   Because arteries are cut to remove the organ, hemorrhage risk is high. An increase in pulse rate and a small drop in blood pressure could be the first sign of hemorrhage.

    2.   Fluid intake and loss should be documented and deficits or excess corrected with fluid resuscitation or diuresis.

    3.   Pain and nausea should be liberally treated with medication.

    4.   Upon arrival in the postanesthesia care unit, the surgical incision(s) should be inspected for drainage and/or bleeding.

    5.   If the patient has a wound drain, the color, consistency, and odor of drainage should be observed, measured, and documented.

    6.   Prophylactic antibiotics are routinely administered for the first 24 hours after surgery.

    7.   Transfer to the post-operative floor can occur when the donor is sufficiently recovered from anesthesia and vital signs are stable.

  F. The nursing care after transfer to the ward is, again, routine for the post-surgical patient, but with a special emphasis on the organ-specific surgery.[18]

    1.   Good respiratory toilet is essential in preventing post-operative pulmonary problems.[18]

          a.   Encouragement of deep-breathing exercises and/or incentive spirometer exercises is important to prevent atelectesis.

          b.   The chest is auscultated to detect rales, rhonchi, or any other abnormality.

    2.   Deep vein thrombosis (DVT) prevention protocol should be followed.

    3.   Early ambulation and activity are essential to prevent DVT, pneumonia, and ileus; therefore, adequate pain control is essential.

      a.   Assess for pain and document response to medications.

      b.   Pain medication can be administered either intravenously or by epidural catheter initially or then orally as soon as the patient is able to tolerate intake.

      c.   Patient-controlled analgesia (PCA) is very effective in the pain management of the post-surgical patient.[19] Instructions should be given to the patient and family regarding proper usage to prevent overdose. Only the patient him- or herself should administer the medication via the PCA to prevent overdosage.

      d.   It is not uncommon for the donor to experience more pain than the organ recipient. This may be due to the fact that the recipient is receiving steroids and pain perception is diminished. (The kidney recipient may not have as extensive surgery as the donor due to placement of the kidney in the abdominal cavity.)

      e.   The application of cold/heat therapy may be beneficial in helping with pain control.

      f.   Splinting the incision or applying an abdominal binder may decrease pain.

   4.   Vital signs should be monitored as per hospital policy and as needed.

      a.   Heart rate and pulse can indicate fluid volume deficits or overload.

   5.   Temperature elevations should be evaluated for etiology. If infection is suspected, the source should be determined and treatment instituted.

   6.   Monitor intake and output.

      a.   Changes in heart sounds, such a new murmur, may be the first indication of a fluid imbalance.

      b.   Fluids are important to provide hydration and flush the effects of anesthesia out of the body.

      c.   Urinary output should be monitored; an output less than 30 ml/hour should be reported to the physician.

   7.   Diet is advanced as tolerated.

   8.   The operative site should be monitored for signs of infection or bleeding.

  G.   The nurse must also address the emotional well-being of the donor and family.

   1.   Because there is often a significant amount of pain post-operatively, the donor may exhibit remorse and anxiety.

   2.   Exploring the donor's feelings and keeping the lines of communication open is very important as he or she recovers.

   3.   Donors are concerned about the recipient, but may also have feelings of jealousy if the family does not recognize the contribution and sacrifice the donor has made.

   4.   Post-donation depression is not uncommon.[20]

      a.   This can result from changes in body image or fatigue.

      b.   Referrals to appropriate support such as counseling may be indicated.

VIII. Organ-specific post-operative nursing care of the living donor

  A.   Kidney

1. New surgical techniques such as laparoscopic nephrectomy have made it easier to consider living donation because it is perceived as less invasive and risky.[14]
   a. It often surprises donors when they still experience significant post-operative pain.[14]
   b. Nephrotoxic medications such as ketorolac for pain should be avoided.
   c. Often the patients have received diuretics and mannitol intra-operatively and they may be dehydrated.
      i. Meticulous attention to recording of intake and output is mandatory.
      ii. Because there has been a 50% reduction in kidney function, intravenous fluids are given to hydrate and flush the remaining kidney and maintain urine output of at least at 50 ml/hour.[17]
   d. Post-operatively, a chest x-ray and laboratory studies such as serum electrolytes, BUN, and creatinine will be ordered to monitor the donor's recovery from the surgical procedure.
   e. Discharge from the hospital will vary depending on the center and the condition of the donor.
      i. Some centers have discharged the donor the evening after a laparoscopic nephrectomy if vital signs are stable,[18] but this is uncommon.
      ii. Most donors will spend the night in the hospital following a laparoscopic nephrectomy.
      iii. An open nephrectomy requires a longer hospitalization, up to 5 days or longer.
B. Lung
   1. Routine thoracotomy post-operative care is instituted.
      a. The donor will return from surgery with an incision on the chest wall and a chest tube.
      b. The patient should be assessed first, then the chest tube drainage system.[23]
   2. Respiratory status should be monitored closely and any distress addressed quickly.
      a. Lungs should be auscultated frequently to assure that breath sounds are clear and are heard throughout.
      b. A chest x-ray will provide the status of the lung expansion and presence of pleural effusion.
      c. Oxygen saturation should be monitored with oxygen supplied via nasal cannula or mask as needed.
      d. A sudden drop in oxygen saturation and respiratory distress could be indicative of a pneumothorax, pulmonary emboli, or bleeding.
      e. The trachea should be assessed to determine if there is a midline shift. If this occurs, emergency measures should be instituted.
      f. Incentive spirometry with coughing and deep-breathing exercises will promote lung expansion and healing.
   3. Pain should be addressed because inadequate pain management will prevent the donor from breathing deeply and expanding the lungs.
   4. Inspect the chest of the donor.

      a. The dressing on the chest tube or tubes should be occlusive to prevent any air leaks. If an air leak is detected, the dressing should be reinforced with occlusive tape.

      b. The skin around the dressing should be examined for subcutaneous emphysema.

  5. Drainage from the chest tube should be monitored for amount, color, consistency, and odor and collected in a closed water-sealed system connected to suction.

      a. The chest tube should be checked for flow and position.

      b. Drainage should be measured and charted.

      c. The surgeon should be notified immediately if profuse, bright red, and copious drainage is noted.

         i. Transfusion of packed cells may be ordered and protamine may be indicated for heparin reversal.

      d. The chest tubes are removed when the lung has completely expanded into the pleural space and the drainage has slowed.

      e. An occlusive dressing should be applied to the site when the tubes are removed.

C. Liver

  1. Daily laboratory testing will be ordered to monitor hepatic and renal function.

      a. These tests will include the liver profile studies: aspartate aminotransferase (AST), alanine aminotransferase (ALT), total bilirubin, complete blood count (to monitor hemoglobin and white counts), electrolytes, blood urea nitrogen (BUN), creatinine, and prothrombin time (PT) and international normalized ratio (INR).

      b. The indicators of liver function, the values of AST, ALT, total bilirubin, and PT/INR, will peak abnormally high 1-2 days postoperatively.

      c. These values should fall quite rapidly and approach normal levels by days 7-14 if the liver is recovering and growing.

  2. These patients require frequent mental status evaluations, since liver failure is often heralded by a change in mental status.

      a. Because the liver metabolizes opioids and liver function may be decreased, it is very important to assess the mental status of the donor patient receiving these medications for pain.

      b. The physician should be notified immediately if there is a change in mental status. Laboratory tests will be ordered.

      c. A Doppler ultrasound may be ordered to evaluate healing and blood flow.

  3. A drain may be placed in the operative site to drain any bile that leaks from the cut surface of the liver.

      a. Drainage should be assessed for color, consistency, and amount.

      b. A biliary tube may also be placed to prevent a stricture of the bile ducts and to assess the function of the liver.

      c. Bile resembles the color and consistency of motor oil.

  4. Living liver donors require expert medical and nursing management to ensure favorable outcomes.

  5. An uncomplicated hospital course typically lasts 5-7 days.

  6. The remaining portion of the liver will regenerate rapidly to about 70% of its original size in 2 weeks.[22]

IX. Discharge teaching for living donors
    A. The donor should be given verbal and written discharge instructions regarding post-operative care.
    B. Wound or incision care will vary depending on the transplant team's policy.
        1. Usually, a sterile dressing will be applied in the operating room and will be removed the morning after the surgery.
        2. The site should be cleaned with saline, and at some centers, the incision may be "painted" with betadine.
        3. It is important that the incision is kept clean and dry.
        4. If the incision has staples or sutures, they will be removed in 7-10 days.
        5. If the surgery was laparoscopic, there may not be visible sutures, but adhesive strips of tape or "steristrips."
        6. The donor should be instructed to allow the tapes to "fall off by themselves."
    C. Tub bathing and swimming should be avoided until the incision is completely healed.
    D. Showering is usually allowed when the patient is discharged home.
    E. Drains may be connected to collection devices or suction after surgery. It is important to protect the skin from the moisture or drainage.
        1. The drains should be emptied and the amount, color, consistency, and odor noted.
        2. The surgeon will remove the drains when the drainage has decreased.
        3. The area around the drains should be cleansed with saline; dry sterile dressings should be applied to collect any additional drainage.
        4. Ostomy bags have been used to collect drainage around a tube if the amount is copious.
    F. Follow-up care
        1. Follow-up care is very important to insure that the donor recovers without complications.
            a. At discharge from the hospital, the donor should have written instructions on what to expect in recovery.
            b. Some donors may live a distance from the transplant hospital.
                i. Decisions about discharge may be related to the distance the donor must travel to go home.
                ii. Communication with the donor's family physician is very important for follow-up care.
        2. There should be a contact number to call if the donor or donor family has questions or problems.
        3. Instructions should include which symptoms need immediate attention and which can wait until office hours.
            a. Symptoms such as chest pain, light-headiness, excessive bleeding, or shortness of breath should be considered a medical emergency.
            b. If the donor complains of severe pain or temperature is elevated above 38.5° C, the transplant team should be notified.
        4. The donor should also be told what to expect in the healing process and that fatigue is common after surgery. The donor should be encouraged to rest as needed.
        5. Lifting more than 10 pounds should be avoided for 4 weeks.

6. Light activity such as walking should be encouraged as soon a possible to help improve healing and return of strength. The donor can return to normal activities in approximately 4-6 weeks after the surgery.
7. Diet should be nutritious with ample fluids.
8. While the donor is taking opioid medications for pain control postoperatively, a stool softener should be prescribed.
9. The donor will usually return to see the surgeon or transplant team for follow-up visits at least once in the 6-week period after surgery.
10. If the recipient was a relative and the outcome was poor, some centers have found that grieving donors may be reluctant to return to the transplant center where their loved one died.[15]
11. Lab tests will be ordered to ascertain whether the remaining organ is functioning properly.

X. Long-term outcomes
  A. The long-term outcomes of organ donation can range from an uncomplicated, short-term recovery to sequelae that include disability, chronic organ failure, or even death.
  B. The key to positive outcomes is directly related to the donor selection process.
  C. There can be long-term psychological effects of live organ donation.
    1. Psychological evaluations are very important to rule out subclinical mental illness or depression prior to donation.
    2. There have been several reported suicides in living donors.
      a. The donor may experience grief in adjusting to a new body image and may actually mourn the loss of an organ.
      b. When the transplant outcome is poor, dissatisfaction with the donation process is higher in non-related donation than when the donor is biologically related.[18]
      c. If the donor experiences any severe complications, this too may impact the quality of life and there may be resentment and regret.
      d. It is important that the donor have psychological counseling available to help heal emotionally after donation.
  D. Some other long-term issues the donor may face are related to financial and/or social issues.
    1. There is concern that health or life insurance may be difficult or expensive to obtain after organ donation.
    2. Time lost during the recovery period may affect income.
    3. Future employment or promotions may be hampered for fear of the donor's health.
    4. The donor's family may experience stress and may not support the donation. This conflict could lead to marital discord.
    5. The donor may also express anger if the recipient "doesn't take care" of the donated organ, as evidenced by lifestyle choices.
  E. Organ-specific long-term outcomes
    1. Kidney
      a. It has been reported that a very small number of donors have developed end-stage renal failure in their remaining kidney, but the uninephrectomy has not been substantiated in clinical studies as the cause.[9]

  b. Women donors have successfully carried pregnancies without the risk of renal failure.

  c. In the United States, if a kidney donor needs a transplant due to failure of the remaining organ, they receive additional points to move up on the transplant list.

2. Lung
  a. Lung capacity is reduced in relation to the amount of lung tissue removed.

  b. There have been reports of pulmonary hypertension in the remaining lung when a pneumonectomy was performed.[23]

  c. Pulmonary function is decreased, but most patients are able to resume normal activity and lifestyle.[9]

3. Liver
  a. Liver donors tend to do very well in the long term, once they recover from the initial surgery and/or complications.

  b. The liver will regenerate to the pre-surgical size.

  c. Because the gallbladder is often removed, there may be some fat absorption delays in the gut.

  d. Other long-term effects may include adhesions or biliary strictures that formed from bile leaks or the surgery itself.

  e. The scar can be disturbing cosmetically for some patients and might require a revision.

F. Living organ donors are truly the heroes of organ donation; they save lives with sacrifice and live by the golden rule, do unto others as you would have done to you. It is very important that these generous people receive support from the transplant team.

REFERENCES

1. *United Kingdom guidelines for living donor kidney transplantation*. British Transplantation Society and Renal Association; 2000.

2. Wigmore S, Plant W. *The ethics of transplantation*. UK: Elsevier Saunders; 2005: 11.

3. Bakker D. Living related and living unrelated organ donation: A clinician's view of the ethical aspects. *Living Organ Donation in the Nineties: European Medico-Legal Perspectives*. Leicester: Eurotold; 1995: 26.

4. Kasiske BL, Bia MJ. The evaluation and selection of living kidney donors. *Am J Kidney Dis*, Aug 1995; 26(2): 387-398.

5. Gillon R. Medical ethics: Four principles plus attention to scope. *Br Med J*, July 16, 1994; 309(6948): 184-188.

6. Russell S. Living related organ donation: The donor's dilemma. *Patient Education and Counselling*, 1993; 21: 89-99.

7. *United Kingdom guidelines for living donor kidney transplantation*. British Transplantation Society and Renal Association; 2005: Section 3.0, p. 1.

8. Rice D. Legal and ethical dilemmas in living donor kidney transplantation. *Living Donor Kidney Transplantation, Current Practices, Emerging Trends and Evolving Challenges*. UK: Taylor & Francis Group; 2005: 163.

9. O'Connor K, Delmonico F. Donor selection and management. In: Ginns L, Cosimi A, Morris P (Eds.). *Transplantation*. Malden, MA: Blackwell Science, Inc; 1999: 942.

10. O'Rouke M. Care of living donors. In: Cupples S, Ohler L (Eds.). *Transplantation Nursing Secrets*. Philadelphia: Hanley & Belfus, Inc; 2003: 213-226.

11. Wolf JS, Jr., Merion RM, Leichtman AB, et al. Randomized controlled trial of hand-assisted laparoscopic versus open surgical live donor nephrectomy. *Transplantation*, July 27, 2001; 72(2): 284-290.

12. Bowdish ME, Barr ML. Living lobar lung transplantation. *Respir Care Clin N Am*, Dec 2004; 10(4): 563-579.

13. Farge O. *Liver transplantation in the third millennium*. UK: Elsevier Saunders; 2005: 180.

14. Siddins M, Hart G, He B, Kanchanabat B, et al. Laparoscopic donor nephrectomy: Meeting the challenge of consumerism? *ANZ J Surg,* Nov 2003; 73(11): 912-915.

15. Battafarano RJ, Anderson RC, Meyers BF, et al. Peri-operative complications after living donor lobectomy. *J Thorac Cardiovasc Surg,* Nov 2000; 120(5): 909-915.

16. Rao AR, Chui AK, Chan HL, Hui AY, et al. Complications of liver donation for living related liver transplantation. *Transplant Proc,* Oct 2004; 36(8): 2224-2225.

17. Barone CP, Lightfoot ML, Barone GW. The post-anesthesia care of an adult renal transplant recipient. *J Perianesth Nurs,* Feb 2003; 18(1): 32-41.

18. Ford EA, Leshko ME, Corsini JM. Nursing care of the living renal donor. In: Cupples S, Ohler L (Eds.). *Transplantation Nursing Secrets*. Philadelphia: Hanley & Belfus, Inc; 2003: 201-211.

19. O'Rourke M, Arnott L, Goldman JS. Living liver donors: A coordinator's perspective. *Prog Transplant,* June 2003; 13(2): 82-87; quiz 88-89.

20. Wright L, McQuarrie M, Haines J. Psychosocial issues of living donors. In: Cupples S, Ohler L (Eds.). *Transplantation Nursing Secrets*. Philadelphia: Hanley & Belfus, Inc; 2003: 227-234.

21. St. John R, Reichert P. Nursing interventions common to respiratory disorders. In: Beare P, Myers J (Eds.). *Adult Health Nursing,* 3rd ed. St. Louis: Mosby; 1998: 270-317.

22. Yokoi H, Isaji S, Yamagiwa K, et al. Donor outcome and liver regeneration after right-lobe graft donation. *Transpl Int,* Aug 2005; 18(8): 915-922.

23. Kramer MR, Sprung CL. Living related donation in lung transplantation: Ethical considerations. *Arch Intern Med,* Sep 11, 1995; 155(16): 1734-1738.

24. Matas AJ, Bartlett ST, Leichtman AB, Delmonico FL. Morbidity and mortality after living kidney donation, 1999-2001: Survey of United States transplant centers. *Am J Transplant,* July 2003; 3(7): 830-834.

REVIEW QUESTIONS

1. An open nephrectomy for living kidney donors using a retroperitoneal approach often includes removal of which of the following?
   a. Appendix
   b. Gallbladder
   c. Portion of a rib
   d. a and b

2. Nurses should assess living lung donors for which of the following major complications?
   a. Ruptured spleen
   b. Pleural effusions
   c. Atelectasis
   d. Phrenic nerve damage
   e. All of the above
   f. b, c, and d

3. Atrial arrhythmias are a common complication of lung donation because of which of the following factors?
   a. Surgery requires removal of ¼ inch of the left atrium.
   b. Surgery requires dissection of the inferior pulmonary vein.
   c. The development of atelectasis post-donation.
   d. a and c
   e. All of the above

4. Which of the following symptoms may indicate a bile leak in a living liver donor?
   a. Severe abdominal pain
   b. Diarrhea
   c. Referred pain to the shoulder
   d. a and b
   e. a and c

5. Which of the following severe complications have been reported in living liver donors?
   a. Liver failure resulting in a donor needing a liver transplant
   b. Death of the donor
   c. Pulmonary emboli
   d. All of the above
   e. a and b

6. The indicators of liver function values of the AST, ALT, total bilirubin, and PT/INR will peak abnormally high 1-2 days post-operatively. As the liver recovers, these levels will decrease within which of the following time periods?
   a. 3-4 weeks
   b. 3-4 days
   c. 3-4 hours
   d. 7-14 days

7. The donor and recipient operations are undertaken synchronously in parallel operating rooms staffed by two full teams of OR personnel. This is done for which of the following reason(s)?
   a. Convenience of the families and staff
   b. Ensure there are no unforeseen problems with the recipient that prevent transplantation
   c. Minimize warm ischemic time
   d. Minimize cold ischemic time
   e. b and c
   f. b and d

8. Living kidney donors have a shorter hospital stay and decreased pain with which of the following procedures?
   a. Laparoscopic donor nephrectomy
   b. Right kidney nephrectomy
   c. Flank incision
   d. Open nephrectomy

9. Living lung donation requires two live donors. The most ideal lobes for living lung donation are which of the following?
   a. Left lower lobe and right middle lobe
   b. Apices on both left and right side due to the high oxygen content
   c. Right and left lower lobes
   d. Middle lobes of both lungs provide the greatest expansion in the recipient

10. For living liver donation in pediatric transplantation, which of the following lobes is used?
    a. Right lateral segment
    b. Right frontal segment
    c. Left lateral segment
    d. Left posterior segment

Correct answers:

1. c	5. d	9. c	
2. f	6. d	10. c	
3. b	7. f		
4. e	8. a		

8 Professional Issues in Transplantation

REBECCA WINSETT

JANELLE YORKE

SANDRA A. CUPPLES

INTRODUCTION

I. A professional is one who:
   A. Is engaged in a practice that requires training or education
   B. Is characterized by or conforms to the technical and ethical standards of a vocation
II. Professional attributes
   A. Individual attributes include characteristics that professionals emulate so that they will be recognized as members of a profession (e.g., honesty, integrity)
   B. Group attributes consist of professional activities associated with:
      1. Evidence-based practice
      2. The development, evaluation, and updating of practice and certification standards
      3. Research-based expansion of the body of knowledge relative to the profession
      4. Dissemination of new knowledge through professional publication
      5. Membership and participation in a professional organization
III. Organizations that advance the individual and group attributions of transplant professionals include, but are not limited to, those shown in Table 8-1.
IV. Major professional issues in transplantation nursing include the following:
   A. Legal issues
   B. Ethical issues
   C. Evidence-based practice
   D. Transplant research
   E. Transplant education

LEGAL ISSUES

I. State Nurse Practice Acts (NPAs)[1]
   A. The purpose of NPAs is to protect the public health, safety, and welfare by ensuring that competent and quality nursing care is provided by qualified nurses.

TABLE 8-1

■ **Organizations Advancing Individual and Group Attributions of Transplant Professionals**

Professional Organizations in Transplantation	Local Chapters	Web address
Association of Nurses Endorsing Transplantation	Yes	none
Australasian Transplant Co-ordinators Association		none
Transplant Nurses Association	No	http://www.tna.asn.au
Canadian Association of Transplantation	No	http://www.transplant.ca/index.htm
European Transplant Coordinators Organization	No	http://www.etco.org/index.htm
International Transplant Coordinators Society	No	http://med.kuleuven.be/itcs/about/about_ITCS.html
International Transplant Nurses Society	Yes	http://www.itns.org/
Japan Transplant Coordinators Organization	No	none
NATCO—The Organization for Transplant Professionals	No	http://www.natco1.org
Society for Transplant Social Workers	No	http://www.transplantsocialworker.org/index.cfm
United Kingdom Transplant Coordinators' Association	No	http://www.uktca.co.uk

    B. Statutory laws direct entry into nursing practice, define the scope of nursing practice within that state, and establish disciplinary procedures; state boards of nursing oversee statutory law.

  II. Scope of practice

    A. State-specific guidelines that define the roles and practices for nurses

  III. Standards of care[1]

    A. The terms "standards of care," "standards of practice," "clinical practice guidelines," "policies," and "procedures" are often used interchangeably. However, all of these terms describe aspects of patient care that have undergone a review process and are based on an agreed-upon and established level of performance or excellence of care.

    B. The purpose of standards of care is to improve patient outcomes.

    C. Standards of care may be established by usual and customary practice, legal precedent, or guidelines promulgated by institutions or professional associations.

    D. Standards of care may be specific to a nation (e.g., Joint Commission on Accreditation of Healthcare Organizations [JCAHO] standards); a state; a community or region (e.g., regional United Network for Organ Sharing organ allocation policies); a health care facility; or a unit within a health care facility (e.g., isolation procedures for an intensive care unit).

IV. Certification[1]

    A. Certification is a process that uses preestablished standards to validate a nurse's ability to practice within a given functional or clinical area.

    B. Within the transplant community, certification acknowledges that an individual has met a standard of competency and possesses the requisite knowledge and skills to provide quality care for transplant donors and recipients.[2]

    C. Transplant certifications awarded by the American Board for Transplant Certification include the following:

        1. Certified Clinical Transplant Coordinator (CCTC)

        2. Certified Clinical Transplant Nurse (CCTN)

        3. Certified Procurement Transplant Coordinator (CPTC)

V. Documentation

    A. Documentation requirements may be mandated by federal or state agencies, local or facility standards, or voluntary oversight organizations (for example, JCAHO).[1]

    B. Accurate documentation:[1]

        1. Enhances communication among health care providers

        2. Promotes continuity of care

        3. Protects the patient from harm

        4. Reduces the risk of litigation

        5. Promotes performance evaluation and improvement

    C. Documentation in the organ donation phase

        1. For each patient who dies, documentation is required regarding the patient's organ and tissue donation eligibility status, whether donation was requested, and the outcome of the donation request.[3]

            a. A recent study indicated that this documentation is often missing, inaccurate, or contradictory and that completion rates of hospital-specific forms range between 12% and 82.6%.[3]

    D. Documentation in the transplant candidate evaluation phase

        1. Documentation during this phase focuses on:

            a. Physiological test results and psychosocial data that will determine the patient's eligibility for transplantation

            b. Patient and family education

                i. Purpose: to provide patients/families with information to make an informed decision regarding the option for transplantation

    E. Documentation during the transplant hospitalization phase focuses on:

        1. Findings from patient assessments and reassessments

        2. Reports of all test results

        3. Goals of treatment and the treatment plan; modifications to the treatment plan

        4. Patient's response to care

        5. Medications administered; drug allergies; adverse drug reactions

        6. Referrals for consultants or community agencies (for example, home health visits)

        7. Patient education

            a. Barriers to learning; willingness to learn; learning needs

            b. Education about diagnostic and therapeutic procedures

  c. Discharge teaching: detailed instructions about every aspect of post-transplantation care (for example, medications, side effects of medications, home monitoring, return visits, biopsies, signs/symptoms of rejection, how to contact the transplant center, etc.)

 F. Documentation during the outpatient follow-up phase (clinic visits) includes, but is not limited to, the following:

  1. Findings from patient assessment

  2. Reports of all test results

  3. Goals of treatment and the treatment plan; modifications to the treatment plan

  4. Patient's response to care

  5. Current medication regimen; drug allergies; adverse drug reactions

  6. Ongoing patient/family education

  7. Date of next follow-up visit

VI. Declaration of brain death

 A. World Medical Association Declaration on Death statement: "It is essential to determine the irreversible cessation of all functions of the entire brain, including the brain stem. This determination will be based on clinical judgment supplemented if necessary by a number of diagnostic aids. However, no single technological criterion is entirely satisfactory in the present state of medicine nor can any one technological procedure be substituted for the overall judgment of the physician. If transplantation of an organ is involved, the decision that death exists should be made by two or more physicians and the physicians determining the moment of death should in no way be immediately concerned with performance of transplantation"[4]

 B. Uniform Determination of Death Act[5]

  1. Was developed by the Uniform Law Commissioners in cooperation with American Medical Association, the American Bar Association, and the President's Commission on Medical Ethics

  2. States that "An individual who has sustained either (1) irreversible cessation of circulatory and respiratory functions, or (2) irreversible cessation of all functions of the entire brain, including the brain stem, is dead. A determination of death must be made in accordance with accepted medical standards."

  3. Has been adopted by most states, the District of Columbia, Puerto Rico, and the U.S. Virgin Islands

 C. Declaration of death: procedure[1]

  1. Once the responsible physician suspects that there has been an irreversible loss of all brain functions, the patient's neurologic status is determined by the appropriate tests.

   a. Family members or others may obtain a second opinion regarding the declaration of brain death.

  2. Declaration of death: cardiopulmonary criteria[1]

   a. Responsible physician determines that there has been an irreversible cessation of cardiopulmonary function.

   b. Patient is declared dead.

   c. Consent of family members or others is not required.

   d. In the setting of organ donation, the declaration of death should not be made by health care clinicians who:

    i. Are members of the transplant team

   ii. Are members of the patient's family

   iii. Have pending malpractice charges related to the case

   iv. Have any special interest in the declaration of the patient's death

  3. Cessation of treatment: Once death has been declared, treatment ordinarily stops unless:[1]

   a. The body or parts of the body will be used for the purposes stated in the Uniform Anatomical Gift Act[6]

    i. Organ transplantation

    ii. Therapy

    iii. Medical or dental education or research

    iv. Advancement of medical or dental science

   b. The patient is pregnant and treatment is given to save the life of the fetus

VII. Organ donation

 A. Required request laws

  1. All U.S. hospitals must have policies and procedures that identify potential organ and tissue donors. Hospitals with Medicare and Medicaid programs must also notify an organ procurement organization of potential donors.

 B. Types of organ donors[1]

  1. Deceased donors

   a. Heart-beating donors:

    i. Donor is brain dead.

    ii. Respiration is supported by mechanical ventilation.

    iii. Cardiac function is spontaneous.

   b. Non–heart-beating donors

    i. Donor is brain dead.

    ii. Organ procurement occurs immediately after cardiac and respiratory function stops.

  2. Living donors

   a. Living-related: donation is made to a relative, spouse, or friend of the donor

   b. Living-unrelated or "Good Samaritan": donation is made, often anonymously, to an unrelated recipient

VIII. Privacy of individually identifiable health information: the "Privacy Rule"[7]

 A. The *Standards for Privacy of Individually Identifiable Health Information* (the "Privacy Rule") established national standards regarding the protection of health information.

  1. These standards are reflected in the Health Insurance Portability and Accountability Act (HIPAA) of 1996 (Public Law 104-91).

  2. The Office of Civil Rights is responsible for implementing and enforcing the Privacy Rule.

 B. The goal of the Privacy Rule is to assure that health information is protected while at the same time permitting the flow of health information required for quality health care and protection of the public's health.

 C. The Privacy Rule protects all individually identifiable health information that is held or transmitted in any form or media: electronic, paper, or oral. This information is known as "protected health information."

 D. Protected health information includes the following:

  1. Demographic data

2. Information regarding an individual's past, present, or future physical or mental health
3. Any health care that has been provided to an individual
4. The past, present, or future payment for an individual's health care

E. Transplant nurses must be aware of and adhere to the standards regarding the privacy of protected health information, particularly with respect to donor and recipient identities

ETHICAL ISSUES

I. Professional ethics
   A. Many professions espouse a code of ethics that articulates the ethical obligations, duties, and standards of that profession—for example, the American Nurses Association Code of Ethics[8]
   B. The American Nurses Association Code of Ethics contains provisions regarding:[1, 8]
      1. Respect for persons regardless of their socioeconomic status, personal attributes, or health problems
      2. Commitment to the patient
      3. Patient advocacy
      4. Responsibility and accountability for individual nursing practice
      5. Professional competency; personal and professional growth
      6. Establishing, maintaining, and improving the health care environment
      7. Advancement of the nursing profession
      8. Collaboration with other health care professionals and the public
      9. Responsibility of the profession to articulate nursing values, maintain the integrity of the profession, and shape social policy

II. Clinical ethics
   A. Clinical ethics is "the systematic identification, analysis, and resolution of ethical problems associated with the care of particular patients."[1, 9]
   B. The goals of clinical ethics are to:[1]
      1. Facilitate clinical decision-making that focuses on the patient and respects the patient's rights and interests
      2. Promote the participation of all relevant professionals (for example, transplant physicians, surgeons, coordinators, staff nurses, advanced practice nurses, social workers, chaplains, ethicists, and so forth)
      3. Enhance organizational commitment and cooperation such that all involved parties develop and implement plans in support of the patient
   C. Clinical ethics extend across the entire life-span continuum.[1] Examples in the field of transplantation include the following:
      1. Pre-pregnancy (the pros and cons of pregnancy in transplant recipients)
      2. During pregnancy (the pros and cons of terminating a pregnancy that is endangering the life of the transplant recipient)
      3. Infancy (the pros and cons of transplantation in an infant with multiple congenital anomalies)
      4. Childhood and adolescence (the extent to which children and adolescents should be involved in making decisions about transplantation)

       5.   Adulthood (the pros and cons of retransplantation)

       6.   Old age (the pros and cons of transplantation in the elderly)

   D.   Transplant nurses must transcend their own values and emotional responses towards potential ethical conflicts associated with, for example, transplantation of patients who are HIV-positive, substance abusers, or noncompliant; post-transplant pregnancy, etc.

III. Major ethical principles[10, 11]

   A.   Autonomy: a competent individual's independence, self-reliance, and ability to decide

       1.   The principle of autonomy and self-determination supports the informed consent process with respect to decision-making regarding therapeutic options and participation in research.

       2.   Informed consent means that the patient has:

          a.   The legal capacity to provide consent

          b.   The ability to exercise free power of choice without any form of constraint or coercion

          c.   Sufficient knowledge and comprehension to make an enlightened decision

   B.   Nonmaleficence: the principle that one must "do no harm"

       1.   Prohibits intentional harm

       2.   Requires the justification of risks by probable benefits

       3.   Requires that agents exercise due care and meet the legal and moral standards regarding knowledge, skills, and diligence

   C.   Beneficence: the principle to provide benefits and balance benefits and harms

       1.   More altruistic and far-reaching than the principle of nonmaleficence

       2.   Requires positive acts to prevent harm, remove harmful conditions, confer benefits, and balance benefits and harms

   D.   Justice: principle that one has been treated justly when one has been given what one is due or owed—that is, what one deserves and can legitimately claim

       1.   Comparative vs. noncomparative justice

          a.   Comparative justice: the desert (that which one person deserves) is determined by balancing the competing claims of others (for example, transplant eligibility criteria)

          b.   Noncomparative justice: the desert is judged by a standard that is independent of others' claims (for example, innocent individuals do not deserve punishment)

       2.   Distributive justice: refers to the distribution of benefits under conditions of scarcity (for example, scarcity of donor organs)

          a.   Macroallocation issues involve decisions regarding social justice and public health policy (for example, equality and rights in health care; the ability to pay and access to organ transplantation[12])

          b.   Microallocation issues involve decisions regarding who shall live when not all can live[13] (for example, the allocation of scarce life-saving medical resources such as donor organs)

IV. Ethics consultations

   A.   Many situations in the field of transplantation present ethical dilemmas and can benefit from ethics consultations.

B. Key elements of ethics consultations include the following:[1]
1. Identification of individuals who can initiate ethics consultations (for example, health care providers, clinicians, patients, family members)
2. Identification of individuals who should be notified that the ethics consultation has been initiated
3. Complete and accurate documentation in the patient's record
4. Promotion of accountability through case review or quality improvement process

EVIDENCE-BASED PRACTICE

I. Evidence-based practice is "the conscientious, explicit, and judicious use of current best evidence in making decisions about the care of individual patients."[14]
II. The current best evidence can inform transplant nursing care.
III. Web-based resources for evidence-based practices include the Cochrane Collaboration and the National Institute for Health and Clinical Evidence.
   A. Cochrane Collaboration
      1. International non-profit, independent organization dedicated to making up-to-date, accurate information about the effects of health care readily available worldwide
      2. Cochrane Database of Systematic Reviews
         a. Provides systematic reviews of health care interventions
         b. URL: www.cochrane.org/reviews/index.htm
   B. National Institute for Health and Clinical Evidence (NICE)—United Kingdom
      1. Independent organization that provides national evidence-based guidance regarding the promotion of good health and the prevention and treatment of ill health
      2. URL: www.nice.org.uk
IV. Taxonomies
   A. Several taxonomies are available to evaluate the evidence associated with a particular practice.
      1. An example of a hierarchical taxonomy used to evaluate the evidence regarding practice guidelines in liver transplantation is shown in Table 8-2.[15]

TRANSPLANT RESEARCH

I. Research is the systematic collection of information in order to increase generalizable knowledge.[16, 17]
II. Protection of human subjects
   A. Many research studies involve human subjects. A human subject is defined as a living person.
   B. Research investigators must:

TABLE 8-2

■ **Hierarchical Taxonomy Used to Evaluate the Evidence Regarding Practice Guidelines in Liver Transplantation[15]**

Grade	Explanation
I	Evidence from multiple, well-designed, randomized controlled trials, each involving a number of participants to be of sufficient statistical power
II	Evidence from at least one large, well-designed clinical trial with or without randomization from cohort or case-controlled analytic studies or well-designed meta-analysis
III	Evidence based on clinical experience, descriptive studies, or reports of expert committees

1. Prevent undo risk to human subjects who choose to participate in research studies
2. Have sufficient study guidelines and procedures in place that will minimize or handle risks to research participants
3. Obtain a scientific review of the study protocol to ensure that the study guidelines and procedures meet or exceed federal standards for the protection of human subjects
    a. In the U.S., this review process is called "institutional review;" in Europe and Australia, it is referred to as "ethics review"
C. In the U.S., the institutional review must be completed prior to implementing a research study.
    1. The research protocol must meet the regulatory guidelines set forth by the federal government and the local institutional review board (IRB). These guidelines include requirements for reporting untoward or adverse events and an annual review of study outcomes.
        a. Sufficient data must be submitted annually (or as stated by the IRB) to demonstrate that the benefit and risk ratio has been maintained and the data provide sufficient evidence to warrant continuation of the study.
        b. If the annual data are not reported or indicate that the risk outweighs the benefit, the IRB has the authority to stop the research study.
    2. IRB or ethics review board requirements are summarized in Table 8-3.
III. Informed consent: overview
    A. Definition: Informed consent is "the knowing consent of an individual or his/her legally authorized representative, under circumstances that provide the prospective subject or representative sufficient opportunity to consider whether or not to participate without undue inducement or any element of force, fraud, deceit, duress, or other forms of constraint or coercion"[18]
        1. Informed consent is a continuing process that involves providing information to patients and their families so that they understand the research study and have enough information to make an informed decision regarding whether or not they want to participate in the research study.

TABLE 8-3

■ **IRB or Ethics Review Board Requirements**

Requirement	Explanation
Investigator and research team qualifications	Is there sufficient evidence that the investigators have the knowledge and background to carry forth the intended study? Is there departmental support for the investigator and the project?
Study purpose and aims	Are the research aims and questions clearly stated and are they in line with the mission of the institution?
Study design and procedure	Will the study methodology answer the question outlined and is there a clear procedure of what the subjects will need to do and what the investigator will be doing?
Risk and benefits to the study subject	What are the risks—psychological, physical, and financial—to the subject? Are there procedures in place to minimize risks? What will happen if there is an untoward event and what is in place to identify and treat a subject in the event of a serious adverse event? How will the subject know his/her rights and responsibilities?
Benefits to society	In conducting this study what benefits will society see? In other words, what is the "so what?" of this study.
Procedures in place to minimize risk and maximize benefits	The investigator outlines the procedures to minimize risks, both actual and potential, and what procedures are in place to identify and minimize risks.
Conflict of interest	Is there a monetary or other benefit to the investigators for doing this study? Is there a family member who works for a company that the investigators are using? Is there a financial arrangement between the investigators and a company involved in the study? Is there a reason that the investigator may be biased for positive or negative outcomes?
Copy of informed consent or conditions outlined where no written informed consent is needed.	A research consent document typically has specific guidelines that must be followed. The IRB or the ethics committee will review the consent to insure that the consent complies with the federal guidelines.

  B. Informed consent is based on the principles of respect for persons, beneficence, and justice as defined in the 1979 Belmont Report.
    1. This report arose from the National Commission for the Protection of Human Subjects of Biomedical and Behavioral Research in 1974.[16]
    2. These principles contributed to the "Common Rule" which was described and accepted by 17 different areas in the Department of Health and Human Services in 1991.
  C. Knowledge of these principles enables transplant nurses to better protect the rights of patients who are invited to participate in research studies.
 IV. Principles of informed consent in research
  A. Respect for persons

1. This principle is grounded in the belief that individuals can and will provide informed consent if given sufficient information.
2. Transplant nurses have the responsibility to provide accurate, clear and comprehensive information about the research study and to maintain confidentiality about the data collected during the course of the study.
3. Transplant nurses are often perceived by patients/families to hold positions of power and authority. Therefore, it is essential that transplant nurses refrain from any actions or statements that might in any way influence a patient's decision regarding participation in a research study.

B. Beneficence
1. With regard to research studies, the principle of beneficence requires a balancing of benefits and harms.
2. Researchers make every effort to maximize the benefits and minimize the risks that may be associated with a research study.
3. Transplant nurses have a responsibility to inform patients/families when risk/benefit considerations change so that they can decide whether to continue their participation in the research study.

C. Justice
1. In the research setting, justice requires that all persons have an equal opportunity to participate so that no one specific gender, ethnic, or cultural group bears the burden of research participation.
2. For example, this principle requires that researchers refrain from using a particular group of potential research subjects solely because that group is easily accessible.

V. Factors that influence a patient's ability to provide informed consent appear in Table 8-4.[19]

VI. Transplant nurses may be more familiar with the informed consent process prior to surgical or other invasive procedures. Table 8-5 outlines the differences in informed consent for invasive procedures and research studies.

VII. Research studies: Transplant nurses' responsibilities
A. Create an environment, conducive to listening, in which the consenter can explain the research study by making certain that:
1. The room is quiet and that interruptions are minimized
2. The patient is free from pain, fatigue, anxiety, etc.

B. Assess the patient's understanding of the procedure so that the nurse and the patient are confident that an *informed* decision was made.
1. If the patient/family has questions, notify the consenter.

C. Verify that informed consent was obtained *before* initiating a research protocol.

D. Place copies of the research study and IRB approval in the designated location.
1. If multiple studies are being conducted simultaneously, it may be useful to create a chart that lists each study, the investigators and/or study coordinators, and their contact information.

E. Place the signed informed consent document in the designated area of the medical record.

F. Obtain research data per protocol (e.g. drawing laboratory samples, documenting vital signs, administering medications).

G. Notify the principal investigator or study coordinator of any patient-related factors that may impact the study protocol.

TABLE 8-4

■ **Factors That Influence a Patient's Ability to Provide Informed Consent**[19]

Factor	Example
Development-related	Cognitive status; external factors that may inhibit patients' ability to make decisions in concordance with their developmental stage (e.g., pain, stress, mental acuity, disease process)
Illness-related	Past and current illness history; past experiences with health care system
Psychological issues; cultural and religious values	Desire to "please" health care providers
External pressures	Lack of insurance coverage; threat of catastrophic health events; family pressure

TABLE 8-5

■ **Differences in Informed Consent for Invasive Procedures and Research Studies**

Invasive procedure requiring written informed consent	Research study requiring written informed consent
The decision to undergo a procedure is based on a perceived health need.	Participation is not based on a health need.
Risks and benefits are presented and patient may choose to undergo procedure even if there are great risks.	Risks and benefits are weighed against current and future risks and benefits. These risks include psychological, physical, and financial risks to participating. The patient does not have to participate in research study to have ongoing health care.
Patient expects to have improved health based on procedure.	Patient expects not to have health compromised by participating in the study.
Patient is provided enough information to be able to make an informed decision. If patient is not able to make an informed decision due to health status, next of kin is provided with information and gives consent according to local or state laws.	Patient is provided with enough information to make an informed decision. In the case where an experimental procedure is planned, there is additional oversight with a medical ethics committee or institutional review board (IRB).
The consent process is a hospital-based procedure and is considered a legal document. The patient has the right to cancel participation at any time; however, if the consent is for a procedure that will improve his or her health, revoking the consent may be difficult for the patient and difficult for the health care provider to accept the patient canceling the procedure.	The IRB or ethics committee oversees the consent process; approval from this body must be obtained before approaching a potential subject about participation. The informed consent document itself must be approved by this body. The consent is a legal document; the participant has the right to withdraw participation at any time.

TRANSPLANT EDUCATION

I. Education of self
 A. In order to educate others, transplant nurses themselves must continuously update their knowledge and skills—particularly in this era of accelerated changes and unprecedented challenges.
 B. Educational opportunities for transplant nurses include formal coursework, affiliations with professional organizations, professional conferences, peer-reviewed journals, and dialogue with other health care providers.
 C. Continued education, coupled with clinical practice, enables the transplant nurse to progress from "novice" to "expert" practitioner, and engage in complex decision-making processes.[20]
  1. Critical thinking is the ability to deconstruct events and to determine the origins of situations.[21] It involves the ability to:
   a. Consider the relationship among events and to anticipate what might happen next
   b. Ask probing questions and relate this information to the history and current status of the patient
II. Education of other health care providers
 A. Transplant nurses have a responsibility to educate other health care providers, particularly new staff nurses and nursing students, about organ donation and transplantation.
 B. Education about organ donation
  1. In the U.S. and many other Western countries, hospitals have been mandated to implement specific protocols to assist in the identification and evaluation of potential donors and ensure that every potential donor family is informed of the option to donate.
  2. However, health care providers' lack of knowledge about organ donation may contribute to the limited availability of donor organs.[22]
  3. Health care professionals are the most critical link in the organ procurement process, because they are the first individuals who establish rapport with a potential donor's family and consequently have the opportunity to discuss the option of organ donation.[22, 23]
  4. Therefore, the education of all health care workers, particularly those who work in emergency departments and intensive care units, is an essential component of any transplant program.
 C. Education about transplantation
  1. Transplant nurses must continually educate new transplant staff members and students about the complex and ever-changing field of transplantation.
  2. Given the growing number of transplant recipients in the general population and their increasing longevity, transplant nurses must also educate non-transplant staff members who may care for recipients upon readmission to the hospital or in an outpatient setting.
   a. Transplant standards of care are a valuable resource and should be readily available to non-transplant health care providers.
III. Education of the general public
 A. The importance of public education cannot be underestimated. Family refusals to donate constitute a major source of lost donations.[24]

B. It has been demonstrated that the majority of people would be willing to donate a family member's organs if the family member had expressed the wish before death.[25]

C. Misconceptions about brain death remain a barrier to organ donation.
   1. In one study, over 98% of participants had heard of the term "brain death," but only 34% believed that someone who was brain dead was legally dead[26]. The majority of participants were unaware, misinformed, or held beliefs that were not congruent with current definitions of brain death.

D. Transplant nurses may facilitate organ donation by educating the public about:
   1. The benefits and procedures of organ donation
   2. The importance of the fact that individuals who wish to be organ donors must communicate this intention to their families
   3. The concept of brain death

E. Education of the public may be formal or informal. Transplant staff may have opportunities to provide this education in academic and community settings or via the media.

F. Despite education and public policy efforts, increasing organ donation rates has proven to be a considerable challenge.[27]
   1. A number of research efforts have been made to identify factors that can be targeted for change in education interventions designed to improve organ donation rates.[28-30]
   2. These studies highlight the importance of incorporating belief and attitude change strategies into educational programs.
   3. Therefore, it is essential that transplant nurses involved in public education not only deliver factual information but also allow individuals to discuss their beliefs and attitudes in a safe and supportive environment.

REFERENCES

1. Molter NC. Professional caring and ethical practice. In: Alspach JG, (Ed.). *Core Curriculum for Critical Care Nursing*. St. Louis: Saunders Elsevier, 2006. pp. 1-44.
2. American Board for Transplant Certification. www.abtc.net/certification.html. Accessed June 18, 2006.
3. Siminoff LA, Nelson KA. The accuracy of hospital reports of organ donation eligibility, requests, and consent: A cross-validation study. *Joint Commission Journal on Quality Improvement*, 1999; 25: 129-136.
4. World Medical Association. World Medical Association Declaration on Death. www.wma.net/e/policy/d2.htm. Accessed June 24, 2006.
5. Uniform Law Commissioners. Uniform Determination of Death Act. http://www.law.upenn.edu/bll/ulc/fnact99/uaga87.htm. Accessed June 24, 2006.
6. Uniform Law Commissioners. Uniform Anatomical Gift Act. http://www.nccusl.org/nccusl/uniformact_factsheets/uniformacts-fs-aga87.asp. Accessed June 24, 2006.
7. Department of Health and Human Services. Summary of the HIPAA Privacy Rule. www.hhs.gov/ocr/privacysummary.pdf. Accessed June 25, 2006.
8. American Nurses Association. Code of Ethics for Nurses with Interpretive Statements. 2001, Washington, DC.
9. Ahronheim JC, Moreno JD, Zuckerman C. Ethics in clinical practice. Gaithersburg, MD: Aspen, 2001, p. 2.
10. Beauchamp TL, Childress JF. *Principles of Biomedical Ethics*, 5th ed. Oxford: Oxford University Press, 2001.
11. Beauchamp TL, Childress JF. *Principles of Biomedical Ethics*. New York: Oxford University Press, 1979.

12. Daniels N. Ability to pay and access to transplantation. In: Coelho DH, (Ed.). *The Ethics of Organ Transplants*. Amherst, NY: Prometheus, 1998, pp. 243-245.

13. Childress JF. Who shall live when not all can live? In: Waters L, (Ed.). *Contemporary Issues in Bioethics*. Belmont, CA: Wadsworth, 1978, pp. 389-398.

14. Sackett DL, Rosenberg WMC, Gray JAM, et al. Evidence-based medicine: What it is and what it isn't? *Br Med J*, 1996; 312: 71-72.

15. Carithers RL Jr. Liver Transplantation. American Association for the Study of Liver Diseases. *Liver Transplant*, 2000; 6: 122-135.

16. National Commission for the Protection of Human Subjects of Biomedical and Behavioral Research. The Belmont Report: Ethical principles and guidelines for the protection of human subjects of research. Washington, DC: U.S. Department of Health, Education, and Welfare. April 18, 1979. GPO 887-809.

17. Department of Health and Human Services Common Rule. 56 Federal Register (45 CFR part 46 Subpart A), Washington, DC, 1991: 28002-28032.

18. Code of Federal Regulations, Title 45, Part 46, Washington, DC. January 26, 1981, 9-10.

19. Roberts LW. Informed consent and the capacity for voluntarism. *Am J Psychiatry*, 2002; 159: 705-712.

20. Benner P. From novice to expert. *Am J Nurs*, 1982; 82: 407-17.

21. Brookfield S. *Developing Critical Thinkers: Challenging Adults to Explore Alternative Ways of Thinking Critically*. United Kingdom: Open University Press, 1987.

22. Schaeffner ES, Windisch W, Freidel K, et al. Knowledge and attitudes regarding organ donation among medical students and physicians. *Transplantation*, 2004; 77: 1714-1718.

23. Prottas J, Batten HL. Health professionals and hospital administrators in organ procurement: Attitudes, reservations and their resolutions. *Am J Public Health*, 1988; 78: 642-645.

24. Reeves RR, Agin WS, Rose E, et al. When is an organ donor not an organ donor? *S Med J*, 2004; 97: 1259-1261.

25. Evans R, Orians C, Ascher N. The potential supply of organ donors: An assessment of the efficiency of organ procurement efforts in the United States. *J Am Med Assoc*, 1992; 267: 239-246.

26. Siminoff LA, Burant C, Youngner SJ. Death and organ procurement: Public beliefs and attitudes. *Soc Sci Med*, 2004; 59: 2325-2334.

27. Rodrigue J, Cornell DL, Jackson SI, et al. Are organ donation attitudes and beliefs, empathy, and life orientation related to donor registration status? *Prog Transplant*, 2004; 17: 56-60.

28. Akgun S, Tokalak I, Erdal R. Attitudes and behavior related to organ donation and transplantation: A survey of university students. *Transplant Proc*, 2002; 34.

29. Danielson BL, LaPree AJ, Odland MD, et al. Attitudes and beliefs concerning organ donation among Native Americans in the upper midwest. *J Transpl Coord*, 1998; 8: 153-156.

30. Radecki CM, Jaccard J. Psychological aspects of organ donation: A critical review and synthesis of individual and next-of-kin donation decisions. *Health Psychol*, 1997; 16: 183-185.

REVIEW QUESTIONS

1. The transplant nurse's responsibilities regarding research studies include which of the following?
   1. Creating a quiet environment in which the study can be explained to the patient
   2. Explaining the research study to the patient
   3. Verifying that informed consent was obtained before initiating the research study
   4. Placing the signed consent document in a designated area of the chart

   a. 1, 2, and 3 only
   b. 1, 2, and 4 only
   c. 1, 3, and 4 only
   d. 2, 3, and 4 only

2. Standards of care are established by:
   a. Usual and customary practice
   b. Legal precedent
   c. Guidelines promulgated by institutions or professional organizations
   d. All of the above

3. The term "beneficence" refers to:
   a. The principle to "do no harm"
   b. The competent individual's independence, self-reliance, and ability to decide
   c. The principle to provide benefits and balance benefits and harms
   d. None of the above

4. The implementation of the Privacy Rule is the responsibility of the:
   a. Office of Civil Rights
   b. Department of Health and Human Services
   c. Food and Drug Administration
   d. Health Care Finance Administration

5. Protected health information includes information about:
   a. An individual's past, present, or future physical or mental health
   b. Any health care that has been provided to an individual
   c. The past, present, or future payment for an individual's health care
   d. All of the above

6. In the U.S., institutional review of a research study must be completed before the:
   a. Study is published
   b. Study is implemented
   c. Data are analyzed
   d. Study is presented at a professional conference

7. If a patient has questions about a research study in which he/she is participating, the transplant nurse should first:
   a. Notify the Institutional Review Board
   b. Contact the patient's physician
   c. Contact the consenter
   d. Notify the primary investigator

8. The goals of clinical ethics are to:
   1. Facilitate decision-making that focuses on the patient
   2. Promote the participation of all relevant professionals
   3. Enhance organizational commitment and cooperation such that all involved parties develop and implement plans in support of the patient
   4. Resolve clinical dilemmas

   a. 1, 2, and 4 only
   b. 2, 3, and 4 only
   c. 1, 2, and 3 only
   d. 1, 3, and 4 only

9. The Uniform Declaration of Death Act states that an individual is dead if he/she has sustained irreversible cessation of:
   1. Circulatory and respiratory functions
   2. Neurologic functions
   3. All functions of the entire brain, including the brain stem
   4. Function of the brain stem

   a. 1 and 2 only
   b. 1 and 3 only
   c. 1 and 4 only
   d. 1 or 3 only

10. The Privacy Rule protects individually identifiable health information that is transmitted in:
    a. Electronic and paper format
    b. Paper format and orally
    c. Electronic format and orally
    d. Electronic and paper format and orally

11. With respect to informed consent for patients participating in a research study, which of the following statements are true?
    1. The patient's participation is based on a health need.
    2. The patient's participation is not based on a health need.
    3. The IRB or ethics committee oversees the consent process.
    4. Risk and benefits are weighed against current and future risks and benefits.
    5. The patient may withdraw from the study at any time.

    a. 1, 3, and 4 only
    b. 2, 3, 4, and 5 only
    c. 1, 3, 4, and 5 only
    d. 1, 3, and 5 only

12. Aspects of patient care that have undergone a review process and are based on an agreed-upon and established level of performance are known as:
    a. Standards of care
    b. Clinical practice guidelines
    c. Policies and procedures
    D. All of the above

Correct answers:

1. c	4. a	7. c	10. d
2. d	5. d	8. c	11. b
3. c	6. b	9. d	12. d

9 Heart Transplantation

CHRISTINE HARTLEY

GRANT FISHER

SANDRA A. CUPPLES

INTRODUCTION

The topics in this chapter are discussed generally in the order presented in the American Board for Transplant Certification candidate handbook for the Certified Clinical Transplant Nurse examination (available at www.abtc.net).

OVERVIEW OF HEART FAILURE (HF)

I. Definition: "Heart failure is a complex clinical syndrome that can result from any structural or functional cardiac disorder that impairs the ability of the ventricle to fill with or eject blood."[1, p. 5]
II. HF is an important cause of morbidity and mortality worldwide.
III. End-stage heart disease (ESHD) is a common endpoint for which heart transplantation is the only remaining therapeutic option.

PATHOPHYSIOLOGY OF HEART FAILURE

I. The heart cannot pump blood at a rate commensurate with the body's metabolic needs and/or can pump effectively only if the diastolic volume is abnormally elevated.[2]
II. Left ventricular (LV) versus right ventricular (RV) failure[2, 3]
   A. Overview
      1. HF may be described in terms of the ventricle that is initially impaired.
         a. Fluid accumulates behind (upstream to) the affected chamber.
         b. LV failure: fluid accumulates in the pulmonary capillary bed.
         c. RV failure: fluid accumulates in the systemic venous circulation.
   B. LV failure[2-4]
      1. The LV can no longer adequately pump oxygen-rich blood from the lungs into systemic circulation. This results in decreased cardiac output (CO) and increased LV pressure and volume.

2. Because the left atrium (LA) cannot completely empty its contents into the LV, left atrial pressure increases.

3. In turn, elevated pressures in the LA lead to elevated pulmonary capillary pressures and the signs and symptoms of pulmonary congestion.

C. RV failure[2, 3, 5]

1. Increased pressure in the pulmonary vasculature leads to elevated right heart pressure.

2. The RV is not able to pump blood into the pulmonary system.

3. As the RV fails, there is systemic venous congestion.

4. LV failure typically precedes RV failure except in the setting of:

   a. RV infarct

   b. Arrhythmogenic right ventricular dysplasia

   c. Certain primary pulmonary disease processes

III. Systolic versus diastolic failure

A. Overview

1. HF can also be characterized by abnormalities in systolic and/or diastolic function—based on whether the dysfunction stems from an inability of the ventricle to contract normally and pump sufficient blood (systolic HF) or an inability of the heart to relax and fill normally (diastolic HF).[2]

2. Isolated systolic and diastolic failure occurs in approximately two-thirds and one-third of HF patients, respectively.[3, 6]

3. Some patients may have concurrent systolic and diastolic dysfunction—for example, patients with ventricular hypertrophy and dilatation.[2]

B. Systolic failure

1. Impaired myocardial contractility leads to weakened systolic contraction.

2. Hemodynamically, systolic failure is associated with:

   a. Decreased CO

   b. Reduced stroke volume (SV)

   c. Increased ventricular diastolic pressure

   d. Decreased ejection fraction (EF): the amount of blood ejected in a single heartbeat relative to the total LV volume; normal EF is approximately 60%

   e. Eventual cardiac dilatation

C. Diastolic failure[6]

1. Defined as pulmonary or systemic venous congestion in the setting of near normal systolic function

2. Principal abnormality is the inability of the ventricles to relax and fill adequately. This leads to elevated ventricular end diastolic pressure.

3. May result from altered ventricular relaxation (Table 9-1)

EVALUATION OF OBJECTIVE MEASURES OF END-STAGE HEART DISEASE: POTENTIAL FINDINGS[1, 10-12]

I. Vital signs

A. Heart rate (HR)

1. May be increased due to decreased CO

TABLE 9-1
■ Etiology of Heart Failure[7-9]

Cardiomyopathy	Infection	Metabolic Disorders	Electrolyte Deficiency	Nutritional Disorders	Systemic Diseases	Toxins
Dilated (idiopathic)	Chagas' disease	**Endocrine:**	Hypokalemia	Kwashiorkor	**Connective tissue disorders**	Alcohol
Hypertrophic		Diabetes mellitus	Hypomagnesemia	Anemia	Systemic lupus erythematosus	Cocaine
Restrictive	Infection	Thyroid disease		Thiamine deficiency (Beriberi)	Scleroderma	Radiation therapy
Ischemic	Viral	Adrenal insufficiency		Selenium deficiency	Sarcoidosis	Chemotherapeutic agents (e.g., anthracyclines)
Valvular:	Bacterial	Pheochromocytoma		Carnitine deficiency	Rheumatoid arthritis	Chemicals (e.g., hydrocarbons, lead)
Obstruction	Fungal	Acromegaly			Polyarteritis nodosa	
Insufficiency		**Familial storage disease:**			Polymyositis	
Hypertensive		Hemachomatosis			**Neuromuscular disorders**	
Peripartum		Glycogen storage disease			Duchenne's dystrophy	
Inflammatory:					Becker's dystrophy	
Infective					Myotonic dystrophy	
Noninfective					**Amyloidosis**	

       a.   With systolic and diastolic dysfunction, contractility and EF decrease; this may precipitate a compensatory increase in HR.

    2.   May be decreased due effects of β-blockers

  B. Heart rhythm

    1.   May be irregular due to atrial fibrillation, atrial flutter, or supraventricular tachycardia with variable atrioventricular block

    2.   Pulsus alternans: Pulse regular but strong beats alternate with weak beats. Typically indicative of impaired LV systolic function.

  C. Blood pressure

    1.   Typically maintained as low as tolerable without causing symptoms such as lightheadedness or dizziness, so as to decrease myocardial workload

    2.   May be low in right-sided heart failure

II. Hemodynamic parameters: see "Clinical Findings in Left-Sided and Right-Sided Heart Failure"

III. Radiologic tests

  A. Chest radiograph may be normal in some patients

  B. Abnormal chest radiograph findings may include:

    1.   Pulmonary vasculature: Pulmonary edema or congestion associated with left-sided HF

    2.   Cardiac silhouette: Heart may be enlarged

    3.   Enlarged RA or RV: Indicative of right-sided heart failure

    4.   Pleural effusions: May be associated with left-sided failure

    5.   Valve calcifications: May be associated with valvular disease

IV. Electrocardiogram

  A. May indicate nonspecific changes

  B. Atrial dysrhythmias and bundle branch blocks common

    1.   High incidence (70%–80%) of atrial fibrillation[12]

    2.   Atrial fibrillation often is secondary to left atrial enlargement

  C. Dysrhythmias may be associated with ischemic heart disease, conduction abnormalities, electrolyte imbalances, and other factors

  D. Increased QRS voltage may indicate LA and/or LV enlargement

V. Echocardiogram: Used to assess:

  A. Chamber size:

    1.   Dilated cardiomyopathy: as myocardial fibers degenerate and become fibrotic, atria and ventricles dilate

  B. Wall thickness

    1.   LV hypertrophy is common in hypertrophic cardiomyopathy

  C. Ejection fraction:

    1.   Dilated cardiomyopathy: EF typically <20% in patients referred for heart transplantation

  D. Thrombus formation

    1.   Atrial fibrillation: Potential for thrombi formation in atria (requires anticoagulation therapy)

    2.   Left ventricular hypokinesis and systolic dysfunction: Potential for thrombi formation in left ventricle

  E. Valve function: Dilatation of mitral annulus may occur secondary to LV dilatation

  F. Systolic and diastolic function

VI. Cardiac catheterization: purposes

  A. Right-sided catheterization: Used to assess:

1. Right heart pressures: see "Clinical Findings in Left-Sided and Right-Sided Heart Failure"
2. Pulmonary vascular resistance
   B. Left-sided catheterization: Used to assess coronary anatomy and determine potential for coronary revascularization
   C. Determine ventricular contractility (EF)
   D. Evaluate valve function
   E. Detect structural defects
VII. Electrophysiology study: Purpose
   A. To determine patient's risk of ventricular tachycardia or ventricular fibrillation
   B. To guide therapy (for example, cardiac resynchronization therapy; anti-arrhythmic medications; automatic implantable cardiac defibrillator)
VIII. Laboratory tests (Table 9-2)
   IX. Physical assessment: potential abnormal findings (Table 9-3)
   X. Clinical findings in left-sided and right-sided heart failure (Table 9-4)[12]
   XI. New York Heart Association Classification of Heart Failure (Table 9-5)[13]
   XII. Heart failure progression: American College of Cardiology/American Heart Association Stages of Heart Failure (Table 9-6)[14]

TREATMENT OF HEART FAILURE

I. Patients with end-stage HF may be on a medical regimen that includes:[15]
   A. Routine exercise to increase exercise tolerance
   B. Sodium restriction (for example, ≤ 2 g/day) to prevent fluid accumulation or facilitate diuresis
   C. Fluid restriction (for example, ≤ 2 L/day) to help prevent fluid accumulation
   D. Smoking cessation
   E. Pharmacologic therapy with one or more of the medications shown in Table 9-7[11, 12, 16-18]
II. Patients with refractory HF who fail to respond to inotropic therapy may require mechanical circulatory support to maintain cardiac output and prevent irreversible failure of other organs.
III. Monitoring of subjective and objective signs of worsening heart failure (Box 9-1)[1, 11, 15, 19]

HEART TRANSPLANTATION

I. Historical perspective
   A. First heart transplant: December 3, 1967, Capetown, South Africa by Dr. Christiaan Barnard[20]
      1. Confirmed that heart transplantation was technically possible and that a transplanted heart could indeed sustain life
   B. This early success gave rise to the worldwide development of heart transplant centers in the late 1960s and early 1970s. However, without effective immunosuppression, heart transplantation was not a viable therapeutic option.
   C. In the 1970s, two important advances revolutionized the field of heart transplantation: The development of the endomyocardial biopsy procedure[21] and the discovery of cyclosporine[22]

TABLE 9-2

■ Laboratory Tests

Liver function tests	Total bilirubin and liver enzymes: May be ↑ due to ↓ CO and ↑ liver congestion
Renal function tests:	Serum creatinine and BUN may be ↑ due to:
	↓ CO and subsequent ↓ perfusion to kidneys
	Nephrotoxic side effects of medications such as calcineurin inhibitors and certain diuretics
BNP	↑ may reflect myocyte stretch and ↑ ventricular pressures
	Note: falsely low levels may occur in obese patients because adipose tissue removes BNP from circulation; falsely elevated levels may occur in elderly and female patients and in the setting of hypertension and treatment with niseritide
C-reactive protein	↑ indicates inflammation
Cardiac troponin I and troponin T	Sensitive markers of myocyte injury
	↑ in acute MI
Creatine kinase	MB isoenzyme sensitive for cardiac tissue; ↑ creatine kinase MB may be associated with myocardial muscle damage (cardiomyopathy, congestive heart failure, myocardial infarction)
ABG	To assess patient for hypoxemia: O_2 pressure and/or O_2 saturation in arterial blood is lower than normal; Generally defined as $PaO_2 < 55$ mm Hg or SaO_2 below 88% on room air (at sea level)
	Cardiogenic shock: Metabolic acidosis on ABGs (↓ pH; ↓ HCO_3)

Serum electrolytes (See Appendix A for additional information on electrolyte imbalances)	Electrolyte Imbalance	Potential Etiology	CV signs and symptoms
	Hyponatremia	Inadequate Na intake	Concurrent hypovolemia: weak, rapid pulse; ↓ CVP; ↓ PAWP; ↓ PA pressures
		Excessive Na loss	Concurrent hypervolemia: Rapid, bounding pulse; ↑ CVP; ↑ PA pressure; ↑ jugular venous pressure
		Certain loop or thiazide diuretics	
	Hypernatremia	Retention of Na	↑ ECF: weak, thready pulse; hypertension
		Impaired renal function	↓ ECF: tachycardia often → bradycardia;
		Osmotic diuretics	Hypotension (may or may not be associated with postural changes)
		Osmotic diuresis associated with DM	
	Hypokalemia	Excessive K loss via GI fluid loss	Weak, irregular pulses;
		Certain diuretics	Palpitations;
			Orthostatic hypotension;
			Dysrhythmias (PACs; PVCs; sinus bradycardia; PAT; AV blocks; AV or ventricular tachycardia;
			EKG changes (flat or inverted T wave; ST segment depression; U wave)
			Digoxin toxicity
	Hyperkalemia	Renal failure (↓ K excretion)	Irregular pulse; ↓ CO; hypotension;
		ACE inhibitors	EKG changes (tall peaked T waves; flat P wave; prolonged PR interval; wide QRS interval; depressed ST segment)
			Dysrhythmias (bradycardia, heart block, ventricular dysrhythmias, asystole)
	Hypomagnesemia	Poor absorption of Mg	Irregular pulse
		Excessive loss of Mg via GI fluid loss	Hypotension in some patients
		Loop or thiazide diuretics	Dysrhythmias (tachycardia, atrial fibrillation, heart block, torsades de pointes, PAT, PVCs, SVT, VT, VF)
		Osmotic diuresis associated with DM	EKG changes (prolonged PR interval, wide QRS, prolonged QT interval; depressed ST segment, U wave; flat T wave)
	Hypermagnesemia	Overuse of Mg supplements	Dysrhythmias (bradycardia; heart block)
		Overuse of antacids or laxatives that contain Mg	EKG changes (prolonged PR interval, wide QRS complex, tall T wave)
		Impaired Mg excretion due to renal failure	Hypotension due to ↓ myocardial contractility may → cardiac arrest
	Hypophosphatemia	Hyperglycemia	Hypotension
		Thiazide or loop diuretics	Tachycardia
		↓ absorption of PO$_4$ due to diarrhea, prolonged use of PO$_4$-binding antacids or laxatives	↓ CO
	Hyperphosphatemia	Impaired renal excretion of PO$_4$	Irregular HR
		Excessive use of PO$_4$-containing laxatives	

ABG = arterial blood gas; ACE = angiotensin converting enzyme; AV = atrioventricular; BNP = brain natriuretic peptide; BUN = blood urea nitrogen; CO = cardiac output; CVP = central venous pressure; DM = diabetes mellitus; ECF = extracellular fluid; EKG = electrocardiogram; GI = gastrointestinal; HCO$_3$ = bicarbonate; HR = heart rate; K = potassium; Mg = magnesium; MI = myocardial infarction; Na = sodium; O$_2$ = oxygen; PA = pulmonary artery; PACs = premature atrial contractions; PaO$_2$ = arterial partial pressure of oxygen; PAT = paroxysmal atrial tachycardia; PO$_4$ = phosphorous; PAWP = pulmonary artery wedge pressure; PVCs = premature ventricular contractions; SaO$_2$ = arterial oxygen saturation; SVT = supraventricular tachycardia; VF = ventricular fibrillation; VT = ventricular tachycardia.

TABLE 9-3
■ Potential Abnormal Findings

Finding	Comment
Jugular venous distention	When patient is reclining at 45 degree angle, jugular veins are distended
	Indicative of ↑ right atrial and right ventricular filling pressures (right-sided heart failure)
S_3 (Ventricular gallop)	Related to early diastolic filling; Can be normal in young adults;
	Typically indicative of severely ↑ left ventricular end-diastolic pressure; common in patients with restrictive or constrictive disease; may be associated with left- or right-sided HF, ischemia, and fluid overload
S_4 (Atrial gallop)	Related to late diastolic filling; Associated with ischemia or infarction, systemic and pulmonary hypertension, ventricular failure
S_3 and S_4 (Summation gallop)	Associated with tachycardia (due to shortened diastole) and HF
Splenomegaly	May be associated with right-sided heart failure
Hepatomegaly	Common in right-sided heart failure
Hepatojugular reflux	Upper right abdomen is compressed for approximately 10 seconds; this results in ↑ venous return to the heart from the liver; Hepatojugular reflux: jugular pulses are prominent; level of filling of neck veins ↑; this ↑ is associated with the inability of the right side of the heart to manage added volume
Peripheral cyanosis	Bluish discoloration of lips, nose, earlobes, extremities: indicative of poor peripheral perfusion associated with ↓ cardiac output or pronounced vasoconstriction
Dependent edema	Ambulatory patients: typically localized in lower extremities
	Bedridden patients: typically localized in sacral and presacral areas
Cachexia	State of malnutrition, wasting, and loss of skeletal muscle mass; associated with severe heart failure
Ascites	Accumulation of fluid in peritoneal cavity; associated with right-sided heart failure
Cough or wheeze	Wheeze may be associated with intolerance of β-blocker therapy
	Cough may be associated with pulmonary venous congestion or intolerance of ACE inhibitor therapy
Crackles	May present initially in dependent lung fields; as pulmonary congestion ↑, crackles become more diffuse
Altered mental status	Cognitive dysfunction (e.g., confusion, memory impairment, inability to focus) may be associated with ↓ cardiac output and ↓ blood flow to the brain

TABLE 9-4

■ **Clinical Findings in Heart Failure**[12]

Left-Sided Heart Failure		Right-Sided Heart Failure
Systolic	*Diastolic*	
Anxiety	Exercise intolerance	• Dependent pitting edema
Sudden light-headedness	Orthopnea	• Fatigue, weakness
Fatigue, weakness, lethargy	Dyspnea, dyspnea on exertion	• ↓ exercise tolerance
Orthopnea		• Weight gain or loss
Dyspnea, dyspnea on exertion	Paroxysmal nocturnal dyspnea	• Anorexia
Paroxysmal nocturnal dyspnea	Cough with frothy white or pink sputum (in pulmonary edema)	• Ascites
		• Cachexia
Tachypnea (on exertion)	Tachypnea (on exertion)	• Nausea, vomiting
Cheyne-Stokes respirations (if severe)	Basilar crackles, rhonchi, wheezes	• Abdominal pain (from liver congestion)
Diaphoresis	CXR: Pulmonary edema	• Hepatomegaly
Palpitations	Hypoxia	• Hepatojugular reflux
Sacral edema, pitting of extremities	Respiratory acidosis: ↑ pH and ↑ $PaCO_2$	• Venous distention
Basilar rales, rhonchi, crackles, wheezes	↑ pulmonary artery diastolic pressure	• Splenomegaly
		• Hypotension
Cool, moist, cyanotic skin	↑ Pulmonary capillary wedge pressure	• Bounding pulses
Hypoxia	S_3, S_4 heart sounds	• S_3, S_4 heart sounds
Respiratory acidosis: ↑ pH and ↑ $PaCO_2$	Holosystolic murmur (if tricuspid, mitral regurgitation)	• Murmur of tricuspid insufficiency
↑ Pulmonary artery diastolic pressure	Symptoms of right-sided heart failure	• ↑ CVP, RA, RV pressures
↑ Pulmonary capillary wedge pressure		• CXR: Enlarged RA, RV
		• Dysrhythmias
Nocturia		• Oliguria
Mental confusion		• Nocturia (secondary to ↑ renal perfusion when patient is lying in bed)
↓ Pulse pressure		
Pulsus alternans		• Kussmaul's sign (constrictive cardiomyopathy): Paradoxical ↑ in venous distention and pressure during inspiration
Lateral displacement of point of maximal impulse		
S_3, S_4 heart sounds		
Murmur of mitral insufficiency		

CXR = chest x-ray; CVP = central venous pressure; $PaCO_2$ = arterial partial pressure of carbon dioxide; RA = right atrium; RV = right ventricle.

Adapted from Lessig ML. The cardiovascular system. In Alspach JG (Ed.). *Core Curriculum for Critical Care Nursing*, 6th ed. Philadelphia: Elsevier, pp. 185-380.

TABLE 9-5

■ **New York Heart Association Classification of Heart Failure**[13]

Functional Capacity	Objective Assessment
Class I. Patients with cardiac disease but without resulting limitation of physical activity. Ordinary physical activity does not cause undue fatigue, palpitation, dyspnea, or anginal pain.	**A.** No objective evidence of cardiovascular disease
Class II. Patients with cardiac disease resulting in slight limitation of physical activity. They are comfortable at rest. Ordinary physical activity results in fatigue, palpitations, dyspnea, or anginal pain.	**B.** Objective evidence of minimal cardiovascular disease
Class III. Patients with cardiac disease resulting in marked limitation of physical activity. They are comfortable at rest. Less than ordinary activity causes fatigue, palpitations, dyspnea, or anginal pain.	**C.** Objective evidence of moderately severe cardiovascular disease
Class IV. Patients with cardiac disease resulting in inability to carry on any physical activity without discomfort. Symptoms of heart failure or the anginal syndrome may be present even at rest. If any physical activity is undertaken, discomfort is increased.	**D.** Objective evidence of severe cardiovascular disease

TABLE 9-6

■ **Heart Failure Progression**[14]

Stage	Description	Example
A	Patients are at high risk of developing heart failure (HF) Patients have conditions that are strongly associated with development of heart failure (HF) Patients have no identified structural or functional abnormalities of pericardium, myocardium or valves Patients have never shown signs or symptoms of HF	Systemic hypertension Coronary artery disease Diabetes mellitus
B	Patients have developed structural heart disease that is strongly associated with the development of HF Patients have never shown signs or symptoms of HF	Left ventricular (LV) hypertrophy LV dilatation or hypocontractility Valvular heart disease Previous myocardial infarction
C	Patients have current or prior symptoms of HF associated with underlying structural heart disease	Dyspnea or fatigue secondary to LV systolic dysfunction Asymptomatic patients who are undergoing treatment for prior HF symptoms
D	Patients with advanced structural heart disease and marked HF symptoms at rest and who are on maximal medical therapy and require specialized interventions	Patients who are frequently hospitalized for HF and cannot be safely discharged Hospitalized patients awaiting heart transplantation Patients at home who are receiving continuous intravenous support for symptom relief Patients on mechanical circulatory assist device Patients in hospice setting for HF management

TABLE 9-7
■ Pharmacologic Therapy for Heart Failure[11, 12, 16-18]

Medication	Action(s)
Diuretics	↓ intravascular and extravascular fluid volume, thereby ↓ preload
Angiotensin converting enzyme (ACE) inhibitors	↓ afterload by blocking the formation of angiotensin II and inhibiting the release of aldosterone, thereby ↓ sodium retention ↓ preload via vasodilatation
Angiotensin II receptor blockers (ARBs)	↓ blood pressure by blocking the vasoconstrictor and aldosterone-secreting effects of angiotensin II
β-adrenergic receptor antagonists (β-blockers)	↓ preload
Aldosterone antagonists (spironolactone)	↓ preload by ↑ excretion of sodium and water
Direct acting vasodilators (hydralazine/nitrates)	↓ preload
Nitrates	↓ preload via dilatation of systemic veins and by ↓ venous return, thereby ↓ LV filling pressure ↓ afterload by vasodilatation of systemic arteries
Anticoagulants	↓ risk of thromboembolism associated with atrial fibrillation, LV hypokinesis, or systolic dysfunction
Digitalis glycosides	↓ preload May be used for rate control in setting of atrial fibrillation or atrial flutter
Inotropic agents: Milrinone	↑ myocardial contractility without ↑ heart rate ↓ afterload and preload via arterial and venous smooth muscle relaxation and by ↑ peripheral vasodilatation
Inotropic agents: Dobutamine	↑ myocardial contractility ↑ stroke volume and cardiac output ↓ systemic vascular resistance
Neseritide (human B-type natriuretic peptide)	↑ vasodilatation; ↓ pulmonary capillary wedge pressure; ↑ renal blood flow; ↑ urinary output
Vasopressors: Dopamine	Dose: 2-10 micrograms/kilogram/minute (β-adrenergic effects): ↑ vasoconstriction; ↑ blood pressure; ↑ renal and cerebral perfusion Dose: > 10 micrograms/kilogram/minute: α-adrenergic effects: Peripheral vasoconstriction; ↑ systemic vascular resistance, ↑ afterload and blood pressure; may possibly ↓ cardiac output
Vasopressors: Phenylephrine hydrochloride	↑ blood pressure via arteriolar vasoconstriction; ↑ stroke volume May ↓ heart rate

BOX 9-1

■ **Subjective and Objective Signs of Worsening Heart Failure**[1, 11, 15, 19]

Subjective:

- ↑ dyspnea at rest or with exertion
- ↑ orthopnea
- ↑ paroxysmal nocturnal dyspnea
- ↑ weakness, fatigue
- ↓ appetite and/or early satiety
- ↑ abdominal fullness
- Difficulty sleeping
- Development of or ↑ in angina

Objective:

- ↑ edema (abdominal, peripheral)
- New onset or worsening dysrhythmias
- Weight gain > 3 pounds for more than 2 consecutive days
- Vomiting
- Development of cardiac cachexia
- New onset or increasing frequency of syncope
- ↑ serum creatinine > 2.0 mg/dL (may be secondary to use of diuretics and ACE inhibitors)
- ↑ blood urea nitrogen > 50 mg/dL (unless patient has intrinsic renal disease)
- Serum sodium < 134 mEq/L
- ↑ liver enzymes and bilirubin over baseline
- Diuretic unresponsiveness
- ↑ brain natriuretic peptide level over baseline level *in certain patients*

Note: Brain natriuretic peptide (BNP) increases with age and is higher in women than men. Research has shown that BNP may be related to a number of other factors such as weight, kidney function, and indicators of cardiovascular damage such as hypertension, previous myocardial infarction or stroke, angina, and diabetes mellitus. Serum BNP levels may parallel the severity of heart failure (HF); however, at this time there is insufficient clinical evidence to warrant the use of BNP levels as targets for the adjustment of therapy in individual patients. Patients on optimal HF medications may have markedly increased BNP levels and patients with advanced HF may have normal BNP levels. Further clinical trials are needed to determine the role of BNP measurement in diagnosing and managing HF.

  D. Since 2000, approximately 3000 heart transplant procedures per year have been reported to the International Society for Heart and Lung Transplantation.
 II. The goals of heart transplantation: To extend survival and improve quality of life
III. Indications: Heart transplantation is considered when:[23]

A. The patient's symptoms can no longer be managed by optimal medical therapy.

B. There are no other surgical options that would offer better long-term survival.

C. The patient's short-term prognosis (without transplantation) is poor.

IV. International Society for Heart and Lung Transplantation (ISHLT) Recommendations: Listing criteria and contraindications are shown in Table 9-8.[24]

V. Selection process. Patients undergo a comprehensive, multidisciplinary pretransplant evaluation to identify the following[25] (see also Table 9-9):

A. Severity of the patient's functional impairment

B. Prognosis

C. Physiologic or psychologic cormorbidities

D. Likelihood that the patient will be able to resume an active and relatively normal lifestyle following transplantation

E. Potential to comply with the post-transplant regimen

F. Level of psychosocial support

VI. Reassessment of patients while on the waiting list

A. While on the waiting list, patients undergo periodic reassessment. The ISHLT Recommended Schedule for Heart Transplant Evaluation is shown in Table 9-9.[24]

VII. Survival rates: Current ISHLT Registry survival rates are:[26]

A. Adult one- and five-year survival rates for patients (N = 16, 227) undergoing heart transplantation between 1999 and June 2004 are approximately 88% and 73%, respectively (Figure 9-1).[26]

VIII. Diagnoses: ISHLT diagnoses for patients who underwent heart transplantation between January 2001 and June 2005 are shown in Figure 9-2.[26]

EDUCATION FOR PATIENTS/FAMILIES AWAITING HEART TRANSPLANTATION

I. Education should include an explanation of the following:

A. Description of and rationale for preoperative tests and procedures

B Postoperative course (for example, length of stay in ICU and step-down unit, progressive ambulation, use of incentive spirometer)

C. Lines that will be inserted (for example, IV lines, arterial line, urinary catheter, chest tubes, drains, pacing wires, endotracheal tube, naso- or orogastric tube)

D. Incisional care

E. Pain management plan

F. Activity limitations, lifestyle, and body image changes

G. Medications and side effects

H. Importance of compliance with post-transplant medical regimen (for example, endomyocardial biopsies, follow-up lab work, vital sign monitoring, prompt reporting of symptoms of illness)

TABLE 9-8

■ **International Society for Heart and Lung Transplantation (ISHLT) Recommendations: Listing Criteria and Contraindications[24]**

Parameter	Recommendation
Maximal Cardiopulmonary Exercise Test (CPX) (on optimal medical therapy) with respiratory exchange ratio (RER) > 1.05 and achievement of anaerobic threshold	Patients intolerant of β-blocker: use cutoff for peak VO_2 of ≤ 14 ml/kg/min to guide listing decision
	In presence of β-blocker: use cutoff for peak VO_2 of ≤ 12 ml/kg/min to guide listing decision
	Patients < 50 years and women: consider use of alternate standards in addition to peak VO_2 to guide listing decision, including percent of predicted peak VO_2 (≤ 50%)
	If CPX is submaximal (RER < 1.05), consider use of ventilation equivalent of carbon dioxide (V_E/V_{CO_2}) slope of > 35 to guide listing decision
	In obese patients (Body Mass Index [BMI] > 30 kg/m²), consider adjusting VO_2 to lean body mass. Lean body mass-adjusted peak VO_2 of < 19 ml/kg/min can serve as an optimal threshold to guide prognosis
Heart Failure Survival Score (HFSS)	When CPX VO_2 is ambiguous (e.g., peak VO_2 > 12 and < 14 ml/kg/min), consider HFSS as adjunct to guide listing decision for ambulatory patients. (The HFSS is a multivariable predictive index that includes 7 measurements: resting heart rate, mean blood pressure, ejection fraction, serum sodium level; peak VO_2; intraventricular conduction delay, and presence of ischemic cardiomyopathy).
Right heart catheterization	Right heart catheterization (RHC) should be performed on all candidates in preparation for listing for cardiac transplantation and annually until transplantation.
	RHC should be performed at 3- to 6-month intervals in listed patients, especially in the presence of reversible pulmonary hypertension or worsening heart failure symptoms.
	A vasodilator challenge should be administered when the pulmonary artery systolic pressure is ≥ 50 mm Hg and either the transpulmonary gradient (TPG) is ≥ 15 or the pulmonary vascular resistance is > 3 Wood units while maintaining a systolic arterial blood pressure > 85 mm Hg.
	When an acute vasodilator challenge is unsuccessful, hospitalization with continuous hemodynamic monitoring should be performed, as often the PVR will decline after 24 to 48 hours of treatment consisting of diuretics, inotropes, and vasoactive agents.
	If medical therapy fails to achieve acceptable hemodynamics and if the left ventricle cannot be effectively unloaded with mechanical adjuncts including an intra-aortic balloon pump (IABP) and/or left ventricular assist device (LVAD), it is reasonable to conclude that pulmonary hypertension is irreversible.

(Continued next page.)

Parameter	Recommendation
Pulmonary artery hypertension and elevated PVR	Should be considered as a relative contraindication to cardiac transplantation when the PVR is > 5 Wood units or the PVR index is > 6 or the TPG exceeds 16 to 20 mm Hg.
	If the pulmonary artery systolic pressure exceeds 60 mm Hg in conjunction with any of the preceding three variables, the risk of right heart failure and early death is increased.
	If the PVR can be reduced to ≤ 2.5 with a vasodilator but the systolic pressure falls < 85 mm Hg, the patient remains at high risk of right heart failure and mortality after heart transplantation.
Age	Patients should be considered for cardiac transplantation if they are ≤ 70 years of age.
	Carefully selected patients > 70 years of age may be considered for cardiac transplantation. For centers considering these patients, the use of an alternate-type program (e.g., use of older donors) may be pursued.
Cancer	Patients with preexisting neoplasms: Collaboration with oncologists is recommended to stratify each patient with regard to risk of tumor recurrence. Cardiac transplantation should be considered when tumor recurrence is low based on tumor type, response to therapy, and negative metastatic work-up. The specific amount of time to wait to transplant after neoplasm remission will depend on the aforementioned factors and no arbitrary time period for observation should be used.
Obesity	Pretransplant BMI > 30 kg/m^2 or percent ideal body weight (PIBW) > 140% are associated with poor outcome after cardiac transplantation. For obese patients, weight loss is recommended to achieve a BMI of < 30 kg/m^2 or PIBW of < 140% before listing for cardiac transplantation.
Diabetes	Diabetes with end-organ damage other than non-proliferative retinopathy or poor glycemic control (Glycosylated hemoglobin [HbA$_{1c}$] > 7.5) despite optimal effort is a relative contraindication for transplant.
Renal dysfunction	Renal function should be assessed using estimated glomerular filtration rate (eGFR) or creatinine clearance under optimal medical therapy. Evidence of abnormal renal function requires further investigation, including renal ultrasonography, estimation for proteinuria, and evaluation for renal artery disease, to exclude intrinsic renal disease. It is reasonable to consider the presence of irreversible renal dysfunction (eGFR < 40 ml/min) as a relative contraindication for heart transplantation alone.
Cerebrovascular disease	Clinically severe cerebrovascular disease, which is not amenable to revascularization, may be considered a contraindication to transplantation.
Peripheral vascular disease (PVD)	PVD may be considered as a relative contraindication to transplantation when its presence limits rehabilitation and revascularization is not a viable option.

Parameter	Recommendation
Tobacco use	Education on the importance of tobacco-cessation and reduction in environmental or second-hand exposure should be performed before the transplant and continue throughout the pre- and post-transplant periods.
	It is reasonable to consider active tobacco smoking as a relative contraindication to transplantation. Active tobacco smoking during the previous 6 months is a risk factor for poor outcomes after transplantation.
Substance abuse	A structured rehabilitation program may be considered for patients with recent (24 months) history of alcohol abuse if transplantation is being considered.
	Patients who remain active substance abusers (including alcohol) should not receive heart transplantation.
Psychosocial assessment	Psychosocial assessment should be performed before listing for transplantation. Evaluation should include an assessment of the patient's ability to give informed consent and comply with instruction including drug therapy, as well as assessment of the support systems in place at home or in the community.
	Mental retardation or dementia may be regarded as a relative contraindication to transplantation.
	Poor compliance with drug regimens is a risk factor for graft rejection and mortality. Patients who have demonstrated an inability to comply with drug therapy on multiple occasions should not receive transplantation.

Adapted from Mehra MR, Kobashigawa J, Starling R, et al. Listing criteria for heart transplantation: International Society for Heart and Lung Transplantation Guidelines for the Care of Cardiac Transplant Candidates – 2006. *Journal of Heart and Lung Transplantation,* 2006: 25(9): 1024-1042.

TABLE 9-9

■ ISHLT Recommended Schedule for Heart Transplant Evaluation[24]

TEST	BASELINE	REPEAT			
		3 MONTHS	6 MONTHS	9 MONTHS	12 MONTHS (AND YEARLY)
Complete H & P	X				
• Follow-up assessment		X	X	X	X
• Weight/BMI	X	X	X	X	X
Immunocompatibility					
• ABO	X				
• Repeat ABO	X				
HLA tissue typing	Only at transplant				
PRA and flow cytometry:	X				
• > 10%	Every 1-2 months				
• VAD	Every 1-2 months				
• Transfusion	2 weeks after transfusion then per protocol				
Assessment of heart failure severity					
• CPX with RER	X				X
• Echocardiogram	X				X
• RHC (vasodilator challenge as indicated)	X		X		X
• ECG	X				X
Evaluation of multi-organ function					
Routine lab work (BMP, CBC, LFT)	X	X	X	X	X
PT/INR More frequently per protocol if on VAD or Coumadin	X	X	X	X	X
Urinalysis	X	X	X	X	X
GFR (MDRD quadratic equation)	X	X	X	X	X
Urine sample for protein excretion	X	X	X	X	X
PFT with arterial blood gases	X				
CXR (PA and lateral)	X				X
Abdominal ultrasound	X				
Carotid Doppler (if indicated or > 50 years)	X				
ABI (if indicated or > 50 years)	X				
DEXA scan (if indicated or > 50 years)	X				
Dental examination	X				X
Ophthalmologic examination (if diabetic)	X				X
Infectious serology and vaccination					
Hep B surface Ag	X				
Hep B surface Ab	X				
Hep B core Ab	X				
Hep C Ab	X				

| | | REPEAT | | | |
TEST	BASELINE	3 MONTHS	6 MONTHS	9 MONTHS	12 MONTHS (AND YEARLY)
HIV	X				
RPR	X				
HSV IgG	X				
CMV IgG	X				
Toxoplasmosis IgG	X				
EBV IgG	X				
Varicella IgG	X				
PPD	X				
Flu shot (yearly)	X				
Pneumovax (every 5 years)	X				
Hep B immunizations 1, 2, & 3	X				
Hep B surface Ab (immunity)	6 weeks after third immunization				
Preventive and malignancy					
Stool for occult blood x 3	X				X
Colonoscopy (if indicated or > 50 years)	X				
Mammography (if indicated or > 40 years)	X				X
Gyn/PAP (if indicated ≥ 18 years sexually active)	X				X
PSA and digital rectal exam (men > 50 years)	X				X
General consultations					
Social work	X				
Psychiatry	X				
Financial	X				
Neurologic/psychiatric (if applicable)	X				

ABI = ankle brachial index; BMI = body mass index; BMP = basic metabolic panel; CBC = complete blood count; CMV = cytomegalovirus; CXR = chest x-ray; DEXA = dual-energy X-ray absorptiometry; EBV = Epstein Barr virus; ECG = electrocardiogram; GFR = glomerular filtration rate; GYN = gynecology; H & P = history and physical; Hep B core Ab = hepatitis B core antibody; Hep B surface Ab = hepatitis B surface antibody; Hep B surface Ag = hepatitis B surface antigen; Hep C Ab = hepatitis C antibody; HIV = human immunodeficiency virus; HLA = human leukocyte antigen; HSV = herpes simplex virus; INR = international normalized ratio; LFT = liver function test; MDRD = modification of diet in renal disease; PA = posterior-anterior; PAP = Papanicolaou; PFT = pulmonary function test; PPD = purified protein derivative; PRA = panel reactive antibody; PSA = prostate specific antigen; PT = prothrombin time; RER = respiratory exchange ratio; RPR = rapid plasma reagin; VAD = ventricular assist device

Adapted from Mehra MR, Kobashigawa J, Starling R, et al. Listing criteria for heart transplantation: International Society for Heart and Lung Transplantation Guidelines for the Care of Cardiac Transplant Candidates – 2006. *Journal of Heart and Lung Transplantation*, 2006; 25(9): 1024-1042.

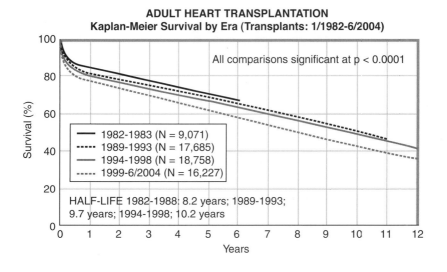

Figure 9-1. Adult heart transplantation survival by era. Taylor DO, Edwards LB, Boucek MM, et al. Registry of the International Society for Heart and Lung Transplantation: Twenty-third Official Adult Heart Transplant Report–2006. *J Heart Lung Transplant*, 2006; 25: 869-879.

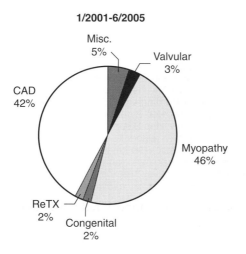

Figure 9-2. ISHLT diagnoses for patients who underwent heart transplantation between January 2001 and June 2005. Taylor DO, Edwards LB, Boucek MM, et al. Registry of the International Society for Heart and Lung Transplantation: Twenty-third Official Adult Heart Transplant Report–2006. *J Heart Lung Transplant,* 2006; 25: 869-879. CAD = coronary artery disease; ReTX = retransplantation.

PREPARATION OF PATIENT FOR SURGERY

(Preoperative protocols differ among transplant centers. Typical preoperative procedures follow.)

I. Obtain preoperative tests and results in timely manner
   A. Chest radiograph
   B. Lab tests: Complete blood cell count, complete metabolic profile (renal and hepatic function tests; electrolyte panel), coagulation tests, urinalysis
   C. Recipient/donor prospective crossmatch (if required)
   D. Obtain blood type and crossmatch per protocol
      1. Blood products: (for example, packed red blood cells, fresh frozen plasma, platelets) before, during, and after surgery are often required to correct coagulation abnormalities and replace blood volume lost during the surgery
      2. Leukocyte-depleted blood is ordered in some centers[27]
      3. CMV-negative blood is ordered for CMV-negative patients
   E. Electrocardiogram (particularly in patients who will have a re-do sternotomy; abnormal findings alert the anesthesiologist and surgeon to potential cardiac problems that may arise before cardiopulmonary bypass is initiated).
II. Ensure that patient has nothing by mouth
   A. Oral preoperative medications may be administered with a small sip of water
III. Initiate telemetry monitoring, especially if patient's implantable cardioverter/defibrillator (ICD) has been deactivated
   A. ICD is deactivated at some point prior to surgery because the electrocautery used during the procedure can cause the device to discharge unexpectedly
IV. Measure and record patient weight
V. Measure and record vital signs per protocol
VI. Ensure that surgical informed consent document has been signed
VII. Start intravenous line
VIII. Administer preoperative medications as directed or per protocol
   A. Phytonadione (vitamin K) if patient has been on anticoagulant therapy
   B. Immunosuppressant(s)
   C. Anti-anxiety agent(s)
   D. Induction therapy: intense perioperative immunosuppression, typically involves use of poly- or monoclonal antibodies or relatively high doses of conventional immunosuppressants[28, 29]
   E. Prophylactic antimicrobial therapy
IX. Provide emotional support to patient and family
   A. Give patient/family opportunity to ask questions or verbalize their concerns
X. Review immediate preoperative, intraoperative, and postoperative procedures with patient and family, such as:
   A. Approximate time surgery will begin, duration of surgery (typically 4–8 hours)
      1. Duration of surgery is typically longer if the recipient has had prior cardiac surgery, including implantation of a ventricular assist device

      B. Location of family waiting room
      C. Provision of periodic updates by surgical team member
      D. Location of recovery room and/or intensive care unit (ICU)
  XI. Address cultural, religious, or psychosocial concerns such as:
      A. Administration of blood products
      B. Spiritual care for patient, family
 XII. Other
      A. Have patient take antimicrobial shower per protocol
XIII. If surgical procedure is canceled:
      A. Make certain that ICD is turned back on
      B. Make certain that patient is adequately anticoagulated if anticoagulation had been reversed
      C. Provide emotional support to patient and family
          1. Explain reason for cancellation of surgery
          2. Given the long waiting times for donor hearts, patient and family are typically very distraught over this "missed opportunity" and often wonder if another donor heart will be found in time
          3. Allow patient and family opportunity to express their emotions and disappointment
          4. If needed, arrange consultation with mental health and/or spiritual care provider

SURGICAL PROCEDURE

    I. Placement of lines and catheters
      A. Hemodynamic monitoring lines (for example, pulmonary artery catheter, arterial line) that will facilitate intra- and postoperative monitoring of:
          1. Blood pressure
          2. Pulmonary artery pressure
          3. Pulmonary capillary wedge pressure
          4. Central venous pressure
          5. Arterial blood gases
          6. Cardiac output/cardiac index
      B. Foley catheter to monitor urine output
      C. Large-bore peripheral lines
      D. Naso- or orogastric tube to decompress the stomach and remove secretions
   II. Initiation of cardiopulmonary bypass
  III. Surgical techniques[30]
      A. Median sternotomy
      B. Biatrial (standard) technique[31, 32]
          1. Cuffs of the recipient's native right and left atria are sutured to the donor right and left atria; donor aorta is sutured to recipient's aorta; donor pulmonary artery is sutured to recipient's pulmonary artery.
          2. The donor heart is denervated.
             a. With explantation of the donor heart, the sympathetic and parasympathetic nervous system fibers are severed (See "Denervation of the Cardiac Allograft").

      b.   The recipient's remaining *native* atrial tissue may still have electrical activity; however, these impulses do not cross the suture line.

    3.   Disadvantages of biatrial technique are related to the large and anatomically abnormal atria created during the surgery and include the risk of mitral and tricuspid valve regurgitation, thrombus formation within the atria, and tachydysrythmias; permanent pacemaker may be required for persistent sinus node dysfunction.[30]

    4.   Biatrial technique is shown in Figure 9-3. Anastomoses include left atrium, right atrium, pulmonary artery, and aorta.

C. Bicaval technique[33, 34]

    1.   More commonly used

    2.   Leaves recipient with more anatomically normal atria

    3.   Intact donor right atrium is preserved; anastomoses are at recipient's superior and inferior vena cavae; left atrial cuff is reduced in size to a small area around the pulmonary veins.[30]

    4.   Advantages: Preserved sinoatrial node function, decreased sinus node dysfunction, decreased incidence of atrial dysrhythmias and mitral and tricuspid regurgitation[30, 35, 36]

    5.   Disadvantages: Longer surgical procedure prolongs ischemic time

    6.   Bicaval technique for orthotopic heart transplantation is shown in Figure 9-4.

D. Heterotopic transplantation is a procedure in which the donor heart is "piggy-backed" onto the recipient's native heart.

    1.   This procedure was first successfully performed in 1974;[37] During the 1970s, it was the primary method of heart transplantation due to the ability of the recipient's native heart to maintain cardiac function during acute rejection episodes.

    2.   With the advent of cyclosporine and improved outcomes with orthotopic heart transplantation, use of the heterotopic technique subsequently waned.[38]

    3.   More recently, heterotopic heart transplantation has increased in some centers owing to a number of factors, including:

        a.   Increased number of large (>80 kg) candidates with refractory pulmonary hypertension

        b.   Under-use of small donor hearts and marginal allografts

        c.   Small donor pool in some areas of the world

    4.   Advantages of heterotopic transplantation include[39]:

        a.   More lenient size matching between recipient and potential donor

        b.   Ability of recipient's native heart to maintain hemodynamic stability during acute rejection episodes

        c.   Prevention of RV failure in recipients with severe pulmonary hypertension

    5.   Disadvantages of heterotopic transplantation include:[39]

        a.   Continued pathology of native heart (for example, ischemic disease, HF)

        b.   Difficulty in performing endomyocardial biopsy

        c.   Persistent angina in recipients with ischemic cardiomyopathy

        d.   Need for anticoagulation in the setting of hypokinesis, clot formation

e. Pulmonary complications associated with compression and subsequent atelectasis of the right lung by the heterotopically placed donor heart

6. Example of a heterotopic heart transplant technique is shown in Figure 9-5.

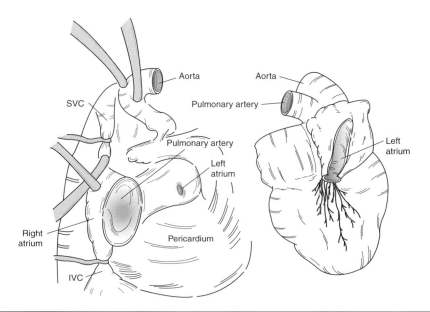

Figure 9-3. Biatrial technique. Augustine SM, Baumgartner WA, Stuart RS, et al. Heart and lung transplantation and cardiomyoplasty for end-stage cardiopulmonary disease. In Baumgartner WA, Owens SG, Cameron DE, et al. (Eds.). *The Johns Hopkins Manual of Cardiac Surgical Care*. St. Louis: Mosby, 1994; pp. 461-484. SVC = superior vena cava; IVC = inferior vena cava

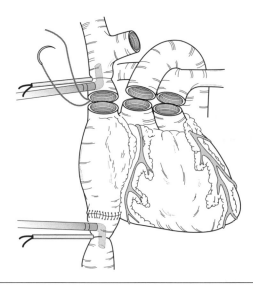

Figure 9-4. Bi-caval technique for orthotopic heart transplantation. Blanche C, Lawrence SC, Czer C, et al. Alternative technique for orthotopic heart transplantation. *Ann Thorac Surg*, 1994; 57: 765-767.

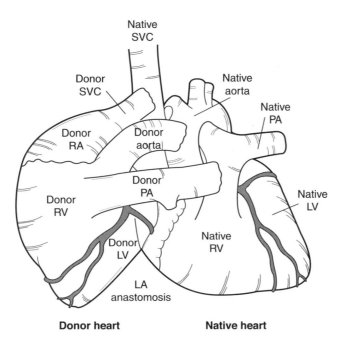

Figure 9-5. Heterotopic heart transplant technique. LA = left atrium; LV = left ventricle; PA = pulmonary artery; RA = right atrium; RV = right ventricle; SVC = superior vena cava. From Allen MD, Naasz CD, Popp RL, et al. Noninvasive assessment of donor and native heart function after heterotopic heart transplantation. *J Thorac Cardiovasc Surg*, 1988; 95: 75-81.

DENERVATION OF CARDIAC ALLOGRAFT[30, 40, 41]

I. In the normal heart, sympathetic and parasympathetic (vagal) chains affect the speed of electrical conduction, heart rate, and contractility.

II. Donor cardiectomy severs both sympathetic and parasympathetic nervous system connections. These connections are not restored when the donor heart is implanted. As a result, the transplanted heart is denervated; that is, it lacks sympathetic or parasympathetic innervation. This unique physiology has several effects:

A. Bradydysrhythmias may be observed in the immediate postoperative period; chronotropic support with isoproterenol or pacing may be temporarily required.

B. Unique response to activity, exercise, and stressors such as hypovolemia, hypoxia, hemorrhage, ischemia

C. See Table 9-10 for a comparison of normal (innervated) and denervated heart.

III. Major implications of cardiac denervation are as follows:[30, 40, 42, 43]

A. Response to vigorous physical activity and exercise

1. Recipients require a longer warm-up period before exercise so that circulating catecholamines and increased venous return can increase HR.

a. Because the denervated heart's response to activity is slow, it is essential to have the patient do appropriate warm-up exercises (for example, 5 to 10 minutes of leg pumping, ankle rotations) prior to engaging in activity (getting out of bed, ambulating). Failure to do so can result in orthostatic hypotension.

    2.   Similarly, recipients require a longer cool-down after exercise so that HR can gradually decrease as circulating catecholamines dissipate.

        a.   Patients should not abruptly stop vigorous physical activity. Instead, they should gradually decrease their level of activity.

  B. The denervated heart does not respond well to stress that requires an abrupt increase in HR (for example, hypoxia, hemorrhage, hypovolemia) in order to maintain or increase CO.

  C. The denervated heart will have an altered response to certain cardiac drugs. In particular, atropine is not useful in the setting of bradycardia, because atropine's mechanism of action is to block input from the parasympathetic nerves. (See "Response of Denervated Cardiac Allograft to Medications.")

    1.   Isoproterenol is typically used to treat bradycardia because it directly stimulates cardiac adrenergic receptors. (See "Hemodynamic Monitoring and Support.")

  D. The normal diurnal variation in blood pressure is eliminated.

  E. The transplanted heart lacks afferent innervation.[1] Although there is some evidence that partial reinnervation may develop over time,[44-46] most recipients with myocardial ischemia or infarction typically do not have angina, as there is no direct afferent sensory input.

    1.   Clinical manifestations of ischemia in heart transplant recipients include the *sequelae* of ischemia or infarction such as shortness of breath, increased fatigue, decreased ability to perform usual activities, etc.

    2.   However, it is important to teach recipients not to disregard angina, as angina can be a symptom of ischemia in some patients.

TABLE 9-10

■ **Comparison of Normal and Denervated Heart**

Factor	Normal Heart	Denervated Heart
Parasympathetic innervation	Resting HR 60–100 bpm due to inhibitory effect of parasympathetic stimulation	No parasympathetic stimulation; resting HR = 90 to 110 BPM[30]
Sympathetic innervation	Direct sympathetic stimulation that automatically increases CO with exercise	No direct sympathetic stimulation; other mechanisms increase CO with exercise:[40] (1) Early in exercise: ↑ venous return augments preload and ↑ CO (2) Later in exercise: inotropic and chronotropic effects of catecholamines released from noncardiac sites results in ↑ CO

BPM = beats per minute; CO = cardiac output; HR = heart rate.

ROUTINE POSTOPERATIVE MONITORING AND MAINTENANCE: EVALUATE OBJECTIVE CRITERIA

I. Arrival in ICU
   A. Patient arrives in ICU sedated and intubated with:
      1. Dressings in place over sternal incision, pacemaker/ICD removal site
         a. The surgical dressing is typically left in place for approximately 24–48 hours, unless bleeding from the surgical wound necessitates removal of the dressing.
      2. Mediastinal, pericardial, and if necessary, pleural drains
         a. Mediastinal and pleural drains are typically placed to 20 cm of underwater seal suction[27]
      3. Epicardial pacing wires (see "Telemetry and Epicardial Pacemaker")
   B. Goals of nursing care:
      1. Maintenance of graft function and hemodynamic stability
      2. Ensuring proper ventilation and oxygenation
      3. Maintenance (or recovery) of all organ system functions
      4. Prevention or early recognition of complications
   C. Patients are placed in protective isolation status per center protocol (see "Prevention of Infection")
II. Vital signs:
   A. Systolic blood pressure is typically maintained at 90–110 mm Hg.
   B. HR is typically maintained at 100–120 bpm.[27]
III. Hemodynamic monitoring and support
   A. Hemodynamic monitoring includes:
      1. Blood pressure via an arterial line
      2. Pulmonary artery pressure
      3. Central venous pressure
      4. Cardiac output and cardiac index
      5. SvO_2 (mixed venous oxygen saturation)
      6. Pulse oximetry
   B. Obtain specific guidelines from the physician regarding acceptable hemodynamic parameters; monitor hemodynamic profile and notify physician if patient deviates from acceptable parameters.
      1. Acceptable hemodynamic parameters differ from patient to patient and depend on a number of factors including preoperative conditions such as pulmonary hypertension and renal insufficiency, the intraoperative course, and ischemic time of the donor heart.
      2. Decreased diastolic compliance requires higher than normal filling pressures; typically, an adequate cardiac output is achieved by maintaining preload with:[23]
         a. Right atrial pressures between 10 and 15 mm Hg
         b. Left atrial pressures between 10 and 20 mm Hg
   C. It is important to monitor, document, and report *trends.*
   D. Normal hemodynamic parameters are shown in Table 9-11.[12, 47, 48]
   E. The function of the allograft is influenced by denervation and the preceding cold ischemic time[49] (see "Denervation of the Cardiac Allograft").
   F. Contractility, systolic function, and heart rate may be impaired and may necessitate inotropic or chronotropic support. Certain IV medications

may be required, depending upon the patient's hemodynamic state;[27] however, the response to many of these medications may be altered due to the fact that the heart is denervated.

    G. Response of denervated cardiac allograft to medications is shown in Table 9-12.

  IV. Ventilator settings

    A. Maintain ventilator settings per protocol.

    B. Monitor blood gases[50]

      1. Normal adult blood gases (at sea level) are shown in Table 9-13.

      2. Blood gases are used to guide weaning from ventilator.

    C. Weaning from mechanical ventilation typically begins 6–8 hours postoperatively when the patient:

      1. Has recovered from anesthesia and is alert and awake

      2. Is hemodynamically stable and has no dysrhythmias or excessive bleeding

      3. Is able to maintain adequate ventilation and oxygenation; can maintain airway and clear secretions

      4. Meets weaning criteria per protocol

    D. Weaning may be delayed due to:[51]

      1. Pretransplant ventilation

      2. Preexisting pretransplant pulmonary complications

      3. Post-transplant complications such as:

        a. Decreased metabolism of anesthetic agents and muscle relaxants secondary to hepatic dysfunction

        b. Elevated pulmonary vascular resistance

        c. Pleural effusions

    E. Following extubation, maintain aggressive pulmonary toilet to decrease atelectasis and prevent risk of pneumonia through chest physiotherapy, turning, coughing, deep breathing, and early ambulation.

  V. Neurologic status

    A. Assess neurologic status upon admission to ICU and monitor closely throughout postoperative period. Depending on the patient's condition, elements of the neurologic assessment may include an evaluation of:

      1. Level of consciousness: Spontaneous activity and responsiveness (for example, with the Glasgow Coma Scale or similar tool)

        a. Alert, wakeful state

        b. Lethargic state

        c. Obtunded state

        d. Stuporous state

        e. Deep coma

      2. Orientation to time, place, person

      3. Motor function

        a. Involuntary movements

        b. Motor response to stimuli

        c. Strength testing

        d. Muscle tone

      4. Reflexes

      5. Sensory function

      6. Coordination

  VI. Drainage output

    A. Monitor drainage from chest tube, naso- or orogastric tube, surgical drains, and incision.

TABLE 9-11

■ Normal Hemodynamic Parameters[12, 47, 48]

Parameter	Definition/Description	Normal Range	Increased in:	Decreased in:
Cardiac output	Amount of blood ejected by the LV in 1 minute	4–8 L/min	Sepsis	LV failure ↓ preload ↑ afterload ↓ contractility Dysrhythmias
Cardiac index	Cardiac output adjusted for body size; Cardiac output divided by body surface area	2.5–4.0 L/min/m²	Sepsis	LV failure ↓ preload ↑ afterload ↓ contractility Dysrhythmias
Stroke volume	Amount of blood ejected by the LV in one contraction	60–130 mL/beat		HF
Stroke volume index	Stroke volume adjusted for body size; Stroke volume divided by body surface area	36–48 mL/beat/m²		HF
Pulmonary artery pressures	PA systolic pressure: reflects pressure produced by RV	20–30 mm Hg	Hypertension Pulmonary hypertension	
	PA diastolic pressure: reflects LV end-diastolic pressure	5–10 mm Hg	Pulmonary emboli	
	PA mean	10–20 mm Hg	LV failure Volume overload Ischemia Mitral stenosis or regurgitation	
Pulmonary capillary wedge pressure	Reflects left atrial pressure	4–12 mm Hg	Fluid overload LV failure Ischemia Mitral stenosis Mitral regurgitation Cardiac tamponade Constrictive pericarditis	Hypovolemia Hypovolemic shock Septic shock Vasodilator therapy
Pulmonary vascular resistance	Measurement of flow resistance in the lung from pulmonary artery to left atrium	50–250 dynes/sec/cm⁵ (0.625–3.12 Wood units)	Large pulmonary embolism Pulmonary hypertension Hypoxemia	Use of pulmonary vasodilators
Pulmonary vascular resistance index	Pulmonary vascular resistance divided by body surface area	80–240 dynes.sec/cm⁵m²		

(Continued next page.)

Parameter	Definition/Description	Normal Range	Increased in:	Decreased in:
Central venous pressure or RA pressure	Reflects right atrial filling pressure and mean pressure of systemic veins	2–8 cm H_2O or 2–6 mm Hg	Pulmonary hypertension Pulmonary embolism Cardiac tamponade Cardiogenic shock Pulmonary stenosis Right-sided HF RV infarct	Hypovolemia (may be secondary to diuretics, blood loss, vomiting, etc) Hypovolemic shock Vasodilatation
RV pressure	Systolic Diastolic	15–30 mm Hg 2–6 mm Hg	Pulmonary hypertension Left-sided failure LV ischemia LV infarct Pulmonary embolism Hypoxemia Mitral stenosis or regurgitation	Hypovolemia (may be secondary to diuretics, blood loss, vomiting, etc.) Hypovolemic shock Vasodilatation
Systemic vascular resistance	Vascular resistance across arterial and venous circuits	800–1300 dynes/sec/cm⁵	Hypovolemia Hypothermia Vasoconstriction Cardiac tamponade	Vasodilator drugs Cardiogenic shock Septic shock
Systemic vascular resistance index	Systemic vascular resistance divided by body surface area	1200–2500 dynes/sec/cm⁵m²		
SvO_2	Mixed venous oxygen saturation	60%–80%	Sepsis Anesthesia	Hypovolemia Hemorrhage Cardiac tamponade MI Dysrhythmias Tachycardia HF Pulmonary edema Anemia Fever Respiratory failure

HF = heart failure; LV = left ventricle; MI = myocardial infarction; PA = pulmonary artery; RA = right atrial.

TABLE 9-12

■ Response of Denervated Cardiac Allograft to Medications

Medication	Action	Response in Cardiac Allograft[23, 42]
Aminophylline FC: Spasmolytic	↑ HR	Unchanged; not mediated by CNS
Atropine FC: Parasympathetic blocking agent	↑ HR	No effect on AV conduction; does not ↑ ventricular HR in setting of bradycardia, sudden heart block, or asystole
Dobutamine FC: β_1-adrenergic agonist	Catecholamine ↑ contractility, SV and CO, coronary blood flow ↓ SVR	Unchanged inotropic and chronotropic effect; not mediated by CNS
Dopamine FC: β_1- and α-adrenergic agonist	Vasopressor High dose (> 10 micrograms/kg/min): ↑ CO; ↑ peripheral vasoconstriction, ↑ SVR; Low dose (2.5 micrograms/kilogram/minute): may be used to ↑ renal blood flow, particularly in setting of cyclosporine-induced nephrotoxicity	↓ inotropic response
Ephedrine FC: β-adrenergic agonist	↑ HR and contractility	↓ inotropic response
Epinephrine FC: β-adrenergic agonist	↑ SVR	Unchanged inotropic and chronotropic effect; not mediated by CNS
Isoproterenol FC: β-adrenergic agonist	↑ HR (dose titrated upward until HR is typically 100–120 bpm); ↓ pulmonary vascular resistance; ↑ CO	Unchanged or ↑ inotropic effect or ↑ chronotropic effect
Norepinephrine FC: β-adrenergic agonist	↑ SVR	Unchanged inotropic and chronotropic effect; no reflex bradycardia with ↑ in BP
Milrinone FC: Inotropic/vasodilator agent	Phosphodiesterase inhibitor Positive inotrope that ↑ contractility without ↑ HR Vasodilator properties ↓ preload and afterload by relaxing vascular smooth muscle	Unchanged; not mediated by CNS
Nitroglycerine FC: Coronary vasodilator	Relaxes arteries and veins; ↓ preload and afterload	Unchanged; not mediated by CNS
Sodium nitroprusside FC: Antihypertensive; vasodilator	Afterload reducer; improves LV function by dilating arteries; ↓ afterload; ↑ venous capacitance; ↓ preload; ↓ BP; ↑ CO; ↓ SVR; ↓ PCWP; ↑ SV with little ↑ in HR	Unchanged; not mediated by CNS
Terbutaline FC: Selective β_2-agonist	Catecholamine ↑ HR	Unchanged; not mediated by CNS
Theophylline FC: Spasmolytic	↑ HR	Unchanged; not mediated by CNS

AV = atrioventricular; BP = blood pressure; CNS = central nervous system; CO = cardiac output; FC = functional class; HR = heart rate; PCWP = pulmonary capillary wedge pressure; SV = stroke volume; SVR = systemic vascular resistance.

TABLE 9-13
■ **Normal Adult Blood Gases**[50]

Parameter	Arterial	Mixed Venous
pH	7.40 (7.35–7.45)	7.36 (7.31–7.41)
PO_2	80–100 mm Hg	35–40 mm Hg
SaO_2	95% or >	70%–75%
PCO_2	35–45 mm Hg	41–51 mm Hg
HCO_3	22–26 mEq/L	22–26 mEq/L
Base excess	–2 to +2	–2 to +2

From Ellstrom K. The pulmonary system. In Alspach JG (Ed.). *Core Curriculum for Critical Care Nursing*, 6th ed. Philadelphia: Elsevier, 2006, pp. 45-183.

    B. Report chest tube drainage that exceeds hospital protocol parameters (for example, >100 mL/hr).

    C. Observe quality of chest tube drainage.

        1. Bright red blood can be indicative of active arterial bleeding.

        2. Old dark blood is usually not indicative of active bleeding.

    D. Assess patency of chest tubes; maintain patency per hospital protocol; inadequate chest tube drainage can lead to tamponade.

    E. A soft surgical drainage catheter may be inserted in the posterior pericardial space to decrease the incidence of pericardial effusions.[52]

        1. This catheter is connected to a drainage bulb.

        2. The drainage bulb is compressed to induce negative pressure.

        3. This drain may remain in place for 3 or 4 days following the removal of chest tubes.

        4. This drain is typically removed once the drainage is less than hospital protocol parameters (for example, <40 mL/24 hr).

  VII. Telemetry monitoring and epicardial pacemaker

    A. Dysrhythmias may be an indication of rejection or irritability secondary to ischemia and manipulation of the heart.[40]

    B. β-adrenergic agonists and/or atrial or atrioventricular sequential pacing may be required to increase intrinsic HR.

    C. Preoperative administration of amiodarone may blunt sinus node and/or AV node function.[27]

    D. Epicardial pacemaker wires may be placed on the surface of the right atrium and ventricle.[27]

        1. In early postoperative period, atrial pacing or atrioventricular sequential pacing may be required.

        2. In some centers, pacing wires are left in place until after first endomyocardial biopsy.

 VIII. Fluid balance[42]

    A. Measure and record weight daily.

    B. Measure and record intake and output per protocol.

    C. Fluid management

        1. Maintenance IV fluid administration may not be necessary during the first 24–48 hours due to:

      a. Extravascular fluid accumulation during CPB

      b. IV fluids given with IV medications or to monitor CO

   D. Observe for clinical manifestations of hyper- or hypovolemia (see sections on hypervolemia and hypovolemia).

IX. Pain management[41, 52]

   A. Postoperative pain management is vital not only for the comfort of the patient but also to facilitate the patient's ability to participate in activities (for example, coughing, turning, deep breathing, ambulation) that help to prevent atelectasis and pneumonia.

   B. Review chart to determine if patient is allergic to any pain medication(s).

   C. Assess for pain frequently; administer pain medications in a timely manner.

   D. While the patient is intubated, continuous morphine or fentanyl infusions may be used to control pain.

   E. Following extubation and tolerance of oral intake, oral pain medications are administered (for example, acetaminophen/oxycodone).

   F. Pain control should be such that patient is able to ambulate at least two to three times per day.

   G. Encourage patient to splint sternal incision with pillow while coughing and ambulating.

X. Laboratory test results

   A. Baseline laboratory studies upon arrival in ICU typically include complete blood cell count with differential, platelet count, serum electrolytes, creatinine, glucose, coagulation studies (fibrinogen, partial thromboplastin time, prothrombin time), and arterial blood gas.

   B. Laboratory tests following transfer to intermediate care unit typically include complete blood cell count with differential, platelet count, serum electrolytes, carbon dioxide, renal function panel, liver function panel, serum glucose, albumin, total protein, prealbumin, cyclosporine, tacrolimus, or sirolimus level (trough level [C0] or 2 hours post-dose [C2]), mycophenolate mofetil levels, urinalysis cultures (if infection is suspected).

   C. Potential complications and associated laboratory test results are shown in Table 9-14.[53, 54]

MONITOR GRAFT FUNCTION FOR POTENTIAL COMPLICATIONS: REJECTION

Graft rejection has been classified in a number of ways. For the purposes of this discussion, rejection is classified on the basis of time of occurrence and primary mediators.

I. Hyperacute and acute graft rejection

   A. Types of rejection

      1. Hyperacute rejection[29, 55, 56]

         a. A catastrophic antibody-mediated immune response that occurs within minutes to hours upon initiation of blood flow to the graft

         b. Primary mediators:

TABLE 9-14
■ Potential Complications and Associated Laboratory Test Results[53, 54]

Complication	Other Abnormal Findings		Comment/Potential Cause
Left ventricular failure ↑ Serum creatinine ↑ Blood urea nitrogen ↑ Liver function tests ↑ BNP	↓ CO ↓ SV ↑ Ventricular diastolic pressure ↓ EF ↓ Tissue perfusion		See sections on ventricular dysfunction below
Bleeding ↓ Hemoglobin ↓ Hematocrit ↓ Red blood cells ↓ Platelet count (↑ in acute hemorrhage) ↓ Iron ↓ Total iron binding capacity	↓ Serum albumin ↑ Total bilirubin ↓ Total protein		Bleeding from anastomoses Effects of CPB Hepatomegaly secondary to HF (↓ ability of hepatocytes to produce coagulation factors) Splenomegaly (thrombocytopenia)

Infection
↑ White blood cell count
↑ Sedimentation rate
+ C-reactive protein
Positive cultures (serum, wound, sputum, stool, etc.)
	↑ Neutrophils
	  Acute infection
	  Empyema
	  Endocarditis
	  Inflammation
	  Pancreatitis
	  Septicemia
	↑ Eosinophils
	  Coccidioidomycosis
	  Thrombophlebitis
	↑ Basophils
	  Sinusitis
	↑ Lymphocytes
	  Cytomegalovirus
	  Endocarditis
	  Hepatitis
	  Mononucleosis
	  Toxoplasmosis
	↑ Monocytes
	  Epstein-Barr virus
		↓ Neutrophils
		  Infectious hepatitis
		  Mononucleosis
		  Influenza
		  Pneumonia
		  Septicemia
		
		↓ Eosinophils
		  Coccidioidomycosis
		  Mononucleosis
		↓ Basophils
		  Acute infections
			Continuation of pretransplant infection
			Transmission of infection from allograft
			Surgical technique
			Iatrogenic sources
			Reactivation of viral infections
			Note: Corticosteroid therapy may blunt inflammatory response

Rejection	There are no biomarkers for rejection; ↑ BNP levels may indicate development of heart failure.		Indications of dysfunction or failure of other organ systems may be indirect markers of decreased perfusion (e.g., ↑ serum creatinine level; ↑ liver function tests)

BNP = brain natriuretic peptide; CO = cardiac output; CPB = cardiopulmonary bypass; EF = ejection fraction; HF = heart failure; SV = stroke volume.

        i. The recipient's circulating, preexisting, cytotoxic antibodies bind to antigens found on the endothelium of the donor heart and activate the complement pathway.

        ii. Complement activation initiates a cascade of subsequent events that lead to thrombosis and ultimately necrosis of the graft.

        iii. The heart dilates rapidly and turns dark red with damage to the capillary wall structure; hemorrhage and fibrillation ensue.[55]

  c. Risk factors for hyperacute rejection include:

        i. Blood group mismatching

        ii. Preexisting antibodies to donor cells

        iii. Presensitization associated with multiple blood transfusions, multiparity, long-term VAD support, and prior organ transplants[55, 57]

  d. The prognosis is poor. Fortunately, the incidence of hyperacute rejection is < 1% due to careful screening of preformed recipient antibodies and careful blood group matching.

  e. Report clinical manifestations of hyperacute rejection (similar to clinical manifestations of cardiogenic shock).[12]

        i. Hypotension (systolic blood pressure <80 mm Hg; mean arterial pressure <60 mm Hg)

        ii. Decreased cardiac output

        iii. Decreased cardiac index (<2.0 L/min/m²)

        iv. Increased central venous pressure

        v. Elevated pulmonary capillary wedge pressure (>18 mm Hg)

        vi. Elevated systemic vascular resistance

        vii. Pulmonary congestion

        viii. Peripheral edema

        ix. Auscultation of S_3, S_4

  f. Report results of retrospective cross-match

  g. Intervene as ordered by physician; administer inotropes; prepare patient for plasmapheresis, mechanical circulatory support (for example, extracorporeal membrane oxygenation, ventricular assist device), and emergent relisting for retransplantation

  h. Collaborate with multidisciplinary team: physicians (surgeon, cardiologist, intensivist), operating room staff, transplant coordinator (for emergent relisting), social worker, and chaplain (for support to patient's family)

2. Acute humoral (or vascular) rejection

  a. Generally refers to rejection that is associated with severe hemodynamic compromise accompanied by low-grade cellular rejection[57]

  b. Primary mediator:

        i. B cell antibodies

        ii. Characterized by vascular inflammation and damage

  c. Diagnosis of acute humoral rejection

        i. Immunofluorescence stains of endomyocardial biopsy tissue that reveal vascular immunoglobulin deposits (typically IgM; may include IgG) and complement deposits with or without fibrin deposits.[58]

ii. Antibodies to donor-specific antigens
3. Acute cellular rejection[58]
   a. Primary mediators
      i. Characterized by infiltration of T lymphocytes and macrophages into myocardium
      ii. In severe form: polymorphonuclear cell accumulation and myocyte necrosis
   b. T-cell response is the primary target for prevention and treatment via:
      i. Suppression of cytokine production (for example, corticosteroids, calcineurin inhibitors such as cyclosporine or tacrolimus)
      ii. Prevention of clonal expansion of lymphocytes (for example, immunosuppressive antimetabolites such as azathioprine or mycophenolate mofetil)

B. Signs and symptoms of acute rejection
   1. Successful treatment of rejection depends on the early recognition of signs and symptoms.
      a. Prompt treatment may mean the difference between a successful recovery from a rejection episode and damage that leads to morbidity and mortality.
   2. Because rejection is a natural process of the body's immune system, many of the signs and symptoms can mimic those of:
      a. A generalized flu-like infection (for example, malaise, nausea, vomiting, diarrhea)
      b. Heart failure: Rejection in the cardiac transplant population involves irritation, damage or destruction of cardiac myocytes that reduce the pumping ability of the heart—thus essentially causing heart failure. Many of the objective signs and symptoms of graft rejection can mimic those of heart failure
   3. The mnemonic "REJECTION EPISODE" may be useful for remembering the signs and symptoms of rejection (Box 9-2).[59]
   4. Because of the potentially serious consequences of rejection, patients experiencing these signs and symptoms must be promptly evaluated by the transplant team.
   5. If rejection is suspected, an endomyocardial biopsy is performed and treatment is initiated as soon as possible in order to control the rejection process, prevent further damage to the myocardium, and reverse the symptoms.

C. Diagnosis of acute rejection: Endomyocardial biopsy
   1. Unlike other types of solid organ transplantation (liver, kidney, pancreas), there are currently no serum biochemical markers that can assess for the presence of cardiac rejection.
      a. New methods of evaluating rejection via serum biomarkers are currently under investigation; however, the endomyocardial biopsy remains the gold standard for evaluating rejection in cardiac transplantation.[60, 61]
   2. Endomyocardial biopsy procedure
      a. The biopsy procedure typically takes approximately 10–15 minutes and is generally done on an outpatient basis.

BOX 9-2

■ **Mnemonic for Signs and Symptoms of Rejection**

R	Rub (pericardial friction)*
E	Electrocardiogram voltage decreased*
J	Jugular venous distention*
E	Edema (new onset, peripheral)*
C	Cardiac dysrhythmias (atrial dysrhythmias; bradydysrhythmias)*
T	Tiredness, fatigue
I	Intolerance of exercise*
O	Onset of low-grade fever
N	New S_3 or S_4*
E	Enlarged cardiac silhouette*
P	Pulmonary crackles, wheezes*
I	Increase in weight* (particularly sudden weight gain of $\geq$ 1 pound/day)
S	Shortness of breath*
O	Onset of hypotension*
D	Disturbances in mood
E	Echocardiogram findings: decreased systolic function, change in left ventricular mass and wall thickness, decreased in left ventricular chamber size*

* May indicate severe rejection

Adapted from Cupples SA. Heart transplantation. In Cupples SA, Ohler, L (Eds.). *Transplantation Nursing Secrets.* Philadelphia: Hanley & Belfus, 2003, pp. 85-105.

      b. Intravenous access for endomyocardial biopsies is typically obtained via the right internal jugular (IJ) vein using local anesthetic. The right subclavian vein or femoral vein may be used as alternate access sites.[62]

      c. With access achieved, the bioptome is advanced into the RV and small tissue samples are obtained. These samples are examined under the microscope and assigned a rejection grade (Figure 9-6).

   3. Endomyocardial biopsy grading

      a. Humoral (vascular rejection)

         i. Former (1992) guidelines for the histologic diagnosis of humoral rejection included the following:[63-65]

            a) Endothelial cell swelling

            b) Immunoglobulin (IgM or IgG) deposition in perivascular spaces (with or without deposition of complement or fibrin)

            c) Cellular infiltrates may be absent

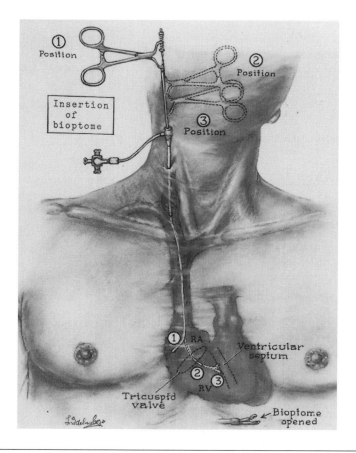

Figure 9-6. Positioning of bioptome for endomyocardial biopsy. From Baughman KL. History and current techniques of endomyocardial biopsy. In Baumgartner WA, Reitz B, Kasper E, Theodore J, (Eds.). *Heart and Lung Transplantation,* 2nd ed. Philadelphia: Saunders, 2002; pp. 267-281, Figure 25-4.

      ii.   2005 grading system for acute antibody-mediated rejection (AMR) is shown in Table 9-15.[66]

   b. Cellular rejection

     i   Former (1990) grading system for acute cellular rejection: Biopsies graded according to the classification system in Table 9-16.[60]

     ii. Revised (2005) grading system: International Society for Heart and Lung Transplantation Standardized Cardiac Biopsy Grading: Acute Cellular Rejection is shown in Table 9-17.[66]

4. Post-procedure activity depends on the biopsy approach:[62]

   a. IJ or subclavian vein approach: patients may resume normal activities; maintaining an upright position decreases risk of venous oozing or bleeding

   b. Femoral venous approach: Bed rest for 2–4 hours to facilitate venous plugging and endothelial repair

5. Common (minor) side effects of the procedure are:

   a. Pain or discomfort at the puncture site

TABLE 9-15

■ 2005 Grading System for Acute Antibody-Mediated Rejection

AMR 0   Negative for acute antibody mediated rejection (AMR)

No histologic or immunologic features of AMR

AMR 1   Positive for AMR

Histologic features of AMR

Positive immunofluorescence or immunoperoxidase staining for AMR (positive CD68, C4d)

Adapted from Stewart S, Winters GL, Fishbein MC, et al. Revision of the 1990 Working Formulation for the Standardization of Nomenclature in the Diagnosis of Heart Rejection. *J Heart Lung Transplant.* 2005; 24: 1710-1720.

TABLE 9-16

Former Grading System for Acute Cellular Rejection

Grade	Interpretation
0	No rejection
1A	Focal (perivascular or interstitial) infiltrates without necrosis; no myocyte injury
1B	Diffuse but sparse infiltrate without necrosis; no myocyte injury
2	One focus only with aggressive infiltrate and/or myocyte damage
3A	Multifocal aggressive infiltrates and/or myocyte injury
3B	Diffuse inflammatory infiltrates with necrosis; myocyte injury
4	Diffuse aggressive polymorphous infiltrate with necrosis; with or without edema, hemorrhage, vasculitis

Adapted from Billingham MR, Cary NR, Hammond ME, et al. A working formulation for the standardization of nomenclature in the diagnosis of heart and lung rejection: Heart rejection study group. *J Heart Lung Transplant*, 1990; 9: 587-593.

TABLE 9-17

■ **International Society for Heart and Lung Transplantation Standardized Cardiac Biopsy Grading**

Grade	Description	Interpretation
0 R*	No acute rejection	No evidence of mononuclear inflammation or myocyte damage
Grade 1 R	Mild Low-grade	Manifested in one of two ways: • Presence of perivascular and/or interstitial mononuclear cells • Up to 1 focus of mononuclear cells with myocyte damage
Grade 2 R	Moderate Intermediate-grade	2 or more foci of infiltrate with associated myocyte damage Foci may be present in 1 or more biopsy fragment Areas of uninvolved myocardium are present between rejection foci Low-grade rejection (1 R) may be present in other biopsy fragments
Grade 3 R	Severe High-grade	Diffuse inflammatory process that involves multiple biopsy fragments Majority of biopsy fragments are typically involved Involves multiple areas of myocyte damage Edema, interstitial hemorrhage and vasculitis may or may not be present

*"R" denotes revised grade

Adapted from Stewart S, Winters GL, Fishbein MC, et al. Revision of the 1990 Working Formulation for the Standardization of Nomenclature in the Diagnosis of Heart Rejection. *J Heart Lung Transplant,* 2005; 24: 1710-1720.

      i.   Pain may become more noticeable as the effect of the local anesthetic wears off.
      ii.   Pain is typically managed with acetaminophen or with prescription analgesics if needed
    b.   Small hematoma and bruising at the puncture site (typically resolves within 24–48 hours)
  6.   Complications of endomyocardial biopsy include:[62]
    a.   RV perforation and pericardial tamponade (see section on Cardiac Tamponade below)
    b.   Malignant ventricular dysrhythmias
    c.   Transient complete heart block
    d.   Pneumothorax
    e.   Carotid artery puncture
    f.   Supraventricular dysrhythmias
    g.   Nerve paresis (vocal cord paresis, temporary diaphragmatic weakness)
    h.   Venous hematoma

7. Baseline (preprocedure) and postprocedure monitoring includes assessment of the following parameters:
   a. Blood pressure and heart rate and rhythm
   b. Respiratory rate and quality of respirations
      i. Increased respiratory rate or difficulty breathing may indicate cardiac tamponade, pneumothorax or hemothorax and must be reported immediately
   c. Bruising or hematoma at puncture site
   d. Bleeding from puncture site
      i. If bleeding occurs, apply pressure to the site for a minimum of 5 minutes (or more as per protocol) and then apply an occlusive dressing.
   e. In the event of cardiac tamponade[12] (see "Cardiac Tamponade")
      i. Notify physician immediately.
      ii. Administer oxygen as ordered.
      iii. Obtain echocardiogram.
      iv. Prepare patient for emergency pericardiocentesis or subxiphoid pericardial window.
8. Patient education regarding endomyocardial biopsy procedure
   a. Instruct patient to monitor the biopsy site and report:
      i. Severe pain at the site of the puncture wound
      ii. Chest pain
      iii. Shortness of breath
      iv. Increased bruising, swelling, or bleeding at puncture site
   b. Outpatients: instruct patient to remove dressing after 12–24 hours unless bleeding or oozing continues
   c. Educate patient about potential interventions based on abnormal biopsy findings; for example:
      i. Increase in immunosuppression dose
      ii. Prednisone "pulse" (for example, prednisone 50 mg twice daily for 3 days; may be followed by prednisone taper)
      iii. Administration of intravenous corticosteroids at home
      iv. Hospitalization for administration of more potent antirejection agents
9. In some centers, endomyocardial biopsies are repeated approximately 2–4 weeks after treatment.
   a. Waiting approximately 2–4 weeks allows the edema and inflammation associated with myocyte damage to recede enough to allow for accurate grading of rejection.
10. Once rejection has been successfully treated, close monitoring of follow-up biopsy results, the immunosuppressive regimen, dose adjustments, and immunosuppressant levels must be continued in an attempt to prevent recurrent episodes of rejection.
11. Other factors that may have contributed to the episode of rejection should be assessed such as:
    a. Tapering of corticosteroid therapy
    b. Change in immunosuppressant medications
    c. Patient noncompliance
12. Collaborate with multidisciplinary team:
    a. Rejection monitoring and treatment may require collaboration among the following multidisciplinary team members: physicians (surgeon, cardiologist, pathologist, intensivist), transplant

pharmacist, immunologist, nurse practitioner, physician's assistant, and dietitian.

b. Depending upon the immunosuppressant side effects the patient may develop, collaboration with the following specialists may also be necessary: endocrinologist, neurologist, infectious disease physician, nephrologist, pulmonologist, gastroenterologist, ophthalmologist, and social worker, psychologist, or psychiatrist.

D. Treatment of acute rejection
   1. Treatment strategies are based on a number of factors including:
      a. Histological grade of rejection
      b. Type of rejection (for example, cellular vs. humoral)
      c. Time elapsed since transplantation
      d. Effectiveness of previous rejection treatment strategies
      e. Patient's current hemodynamic status
      f. Patient's prior rejection pattern
      g. Patient's current immunosuppression regimen
      h. Patient's current comorbidities
   2. Treatment options for humoral rejection include:
      a. Plasmapheresis
      b. Intravenous immunoglobulins (IVIG)
      c. Photopheresis
      d. Corticosteroids
      e. Anti-B cell agents such as cyclophosphamide (Cytoxan®)
      f. Total lymph node irradiation
      g. Antithymocyte globulin
   3. Treatment options for cellular rejection include:
      a. Treatment regimens vary among transplant centers, but typically the first line treatment is high-dose intravenous or oral steroid pulses followed by a tapering oral course, for example:
         i. Intravenous corticosteroid therapy (for example, 500 to 1000 mg of methylprednisolone [Solu-Medrol®] daily for 3 days)
         ii. Increase in oral corticosteroid therapy (for example, 50 mg of prednisone twice daily for 3 days followed by a gradual wean back to baseline prednisone dose)
      b. Other treatment options include the following:
         i. Antilymphocyte antibody (Muromonab-CD3 [OKT®3])[45, 55, 64]
         ii. Antithymocyte globulin (Thymoglobulin®)
         iii. Anti-CD25 antibodies (e.g., basiliximab [Simulect®]; dacluzimab [Zenapax®])
         iv. Cyclophosphamide
         v. Methotrexate
         vi. Photopheresis
         vii. Total lymph node irradiation

E. Monitoring of rejection therapy
   1. The improvement or deterioration of the patient's hemodynamic parameters, clinical status, and follow-up test results (for example, endomyocardial biopsy, immunofluorescence stains, antibodies to donor-specific antigens) are important indications of the effectiveness of antirejection therapy.
   2. Rejection therapy is administered cautiously and requires close monitoring for side effects including bone marrow suppression and opportunistic infections.

        a.   Antimicrobial agents may be administered during periods of rejection therapy (for example, sulfamethoxazole/trimethoprim, clotrimazole, and valganciclovir)

     3.   Potential side effects of major rejection therapies are shown in Table 9-18.

II. Chronic rejection: Coronary artery vasculopathy (CAV)

   A. Description of CAV:

     1.   A rapid and progressive form of coronary artery disease (CAD) characterized by concentric diffuse intimal proliferation and luminal stenosis, progressing to total occlusion of the smaller coronary arteries[67]

     2.   Thought to be a form of chronic graft rejection

     3.   A major impediment to long-term survival following heart transplantation

     4.   Remains the most common reason for retransplantation

   B. Prevalence of CAV[26]

     1.   The cumulative prevalence of CAV in heart transplant survivors at 1 year post-transplant is 7.9% (follow-ups between January 2001 and June 2005).

     2.   The cumulative prevalence of CAV in heart transplant survivors at 5 and 8 years post-transplant is 32.1% and 44.3%, respectively (follow-ups between April 1994 and June 2005).

   C. Characteristics of CAV:

     1.   CAV is an unusual form of CAD that affects both epicardial and myocardial vessels. It differs from CAD as shown in Table 9-19.

   D. Etiology of CAV

     1.   Both immunological and nonimmunological processes play a role in the development of CAV. Etiologic factors of note are shown in Table 9-20.

   E. Clinical manifestations of CAV

     1.   Unlike classic CAD, angina is rarely associated with CAV because the allograft is denervated.

     2.   Clinical manifestations may include:

        a.   Increasing fatigue

        b.   Exertional dyspnea or dyspnea at rest

        c.   Elevated left ventricular filling pressures

        d.   Clinical manifestations of graft failure

           i.   Congestive heart failure

          ii.   Dysrhythmias

         iii.   Sudden death

   F. Diagnosis of CAV

     1.   Noninvasive tests such as exercise electrocardiography and myocardial nuclear imaging generally lack sufficient sensitivity to be reliable screening tools.

     2.   CAV causes diffuse, concentric narrowing of arteries; focal stenoses are rare. Therefore, conventional coronary arteriography also lacks sensitivity and can underestimate the presence of this disease.

     3.   Intravascular ultrasound (IVUS) has been shown to be an effective imaging modality. IVUS permits:

        a.   Delineation of the actual lumen diameter

        b.   Assessment of vessel wall morphology

        c.   Quantification of the stenosis

TABLE 9-18

■ Side Effects of Major Rejection Therapies

Rejection Therapy	Potential Side Effects		Monitor
Corticosteroids	**Masking of infection** **Endocrine:** ↓ glucose tolerance Hyperglycemia Hypercholesterolemia Glycosuria ↑ insulin or sulfonylurea requirements Cushingoid appearance **Fluid and electrolyte balance:** Hypokalemia alkalosis Hypokalemia Hypocalcemia **CV:** Hypotension or hypertension Thromboembolism Thrombophlebitis Dysrhythmias ECG changes **Hematologic:** Leukocytosis **Dermatologic:** Impaired wound healing Thinning of skin Petechiae Ecchymoses Erythema Urticaria	**Ophthalmic:** Glaucoma Cataract formation Exophthalmos **GI:** Nausea, vomiting ↑ appetite (occasionally, anorexia) Diarrhea or constipation Abdominal distention Pancreatitis Gastric irritation Peptic ulcers **CNS:** Headache Vertigo Insomnia Restlessness Seizures Mood swings, personality changes	Blood glucose level Serum electrolytes Complete blood cell count with differential Impaired wound healing Cardiovascular status Gastrointestinal status Neurologic status Signs and symptoms of infection Patient's response to therapy
Antilymphocyte antibody (Muromonab-CD3 [OKT®3]) Patient may be premedicated with methylprednisolone to attenuate cytokine release syndrome	Anaphylaxis Opportunistic infection Cytokine release syndrome: Fever Chills Dyspnea Nausea, vomiting Chest pain Diarrhea Tremor Wheezing Headache Tachycardia Hypertension Rigor **Neuropsychiatric:** Seizures Encephalopathy Cerebral edema Aseptic meningitis **Respiratory:** Dyspnea Pulmonary edema Wheezing Tachypnea Hypoxemia Respiratory failure, arrest ARDS **GU:** Oliguria Anuria	**Hematologic:** Neutropenia Leukopenia Thrombocytopenia Lymphopenia Leukocytosis **Musculoskeletal:** Arthralgia Myalgia Arthritis **Hepatic:** Hepatomegaly Splenomegaly Hepatitis **Ophthalmic:** Blurred vision Diplopia Photophobia Conjunctivitis **Dermatologic:** Rash Urticaria Pruritus Erythema Flushing Diaphoresis **Other:** ↓ hearing Tinnitus Vertigo Otitis media PLTD	Muromonab-CD3 levels CD3 level Complete blood cell count, differential Renal function Hepatic function Vital signs Signs and symptoms of infection, particularly: Herpes Fungal CMV Patient's response to therapy

Rejection Therapy	Potential Side Effects		Monitor
Antithymocyte globulin (Thymoglobulin®)	Fever Chills Leukopenia Abdominal or other pain	Headache Thrombocytopenia Dyspnea Malaise Dermatologic reactions	Temperature Complete blood cell count Platelet count Respiratory status Patient's response to therapy
Basiliximab (Simulect®)	Infection **Respiratory:** Pulmonary edema Dyspnea Wheezing Cough **CV:** Cardiac failure Chest pain Hypotension Hypertension Edema **CNS:** Pyrexia Chills Tremors Headache Weakness Insomnia	**Electrolytes:** Hyperkalemia Hypokalemia Hypocalcemia Hypophosphatemia **Endocrine:** Hypercholesterolemia **GI:** GI bleeding Hepatotoxicity Nausea, vomiting Diarrhea Constipation Abdominal pain Stomatitis Gingival hyperplasia **Dermatologic:** Acne **Other:** Acidosis Hyperuricemia	Temperature Complete blood cell count, differential Liver function Electrolytes Uric acid Symptoms of hepatotoxicity (dark urine, jaundice, itching, light-colored stools) Patient's response to therapy
Dacluzimab (Zenapax®) Have corticosteroids, epinephrine available in case of anaphylactic reaction	**Respiratory:** Pulmonary edema Dyspnea Wheezing Atelectasis Cough **CV:** Tachycardia Hypertension Thrombosis Bleeding **CNS:** Chills Tremors Headache	Impaired wound healing **GI:** Nausea, vomiting Diarrhea Abdominal pain Constipation **GU:** Renal tubular necrosis Oliguria Dysuria Hydronephrosis	Complete blood cell count, differential Liver function Renal function Wound healing Symptoms of hepatotoxicity (dark urine, jaundice, itching, light-colored stools) Patient's response to therapy
Cyclophosphamide (Cytoxan®)	Opportunistic infections Leukopenia Nausea, vomiting Alopecia Urinary bladder fibrosis	Hemorrhagic cystitis Renal tubular necrosis Sterility (males and females) Oligospermia Azoospermia	Complete blood cell count, differential Platelet count Renal function Hepatic function Urinalysis Patient's response to therapy

(Continued next page.)

Rejection Therapy	Potential Side Effects		Monitor
Rituximab (Rituxan®)	**During infusion**: Fever Chills Rigor Nausea Urticaria Fatigue Headache Pruritus Bronchospasm Hypotension Angioedema Dyspnea Rhinitis Vomiting Flushing **General:** Asthenia Arthralgia Pain Malaise **CV:** Dysrhythmias Hypotension or hypertension Angina Peripheral edema **Hematologic:** Thrombocytopenia Anemia Neutropenia Leukopenia Coagulation disorders	**Respiratory:** Angioedema Bronchospasm Dyspnea Cough Rhinitis Hypoxia Asthma Sinusitis Bronchitis **Dermatologic:** Pruritus Rash Urticaria Flushing **CNS:** Headache Paresthesia, hyperesthesia Anxiety, agitation Insomnia **GI:** Abdominal pain Nausea, vomiting Dyspepsia Impaired taste Anorexia	Complete blood cell count, differential Vital signs Respiratory status Cardiovascular status Neurologic status Renal function Patient's response to therapy
Plasmapheresis	Hypotension		Patient's response to therapy
Photopheresis	Fever Myalgia Nausea, vomiting	Hypotension Infection	Serum electrolytes Complete blood cell count Patient's response to therapy
Total lymphoid irradiation	Leukopenia Thrombocytopenia		Complete blood cell count Platelet count Clinical manifestations of infection Patient's response to therapy

CMV = cytomegalovirus; CNS = central nervous system; GI = gastrointestinal; GU = genitourinary; PTLD = post-transplant lymphoproliferative disease

TABLE 9-19

■ **Difference Between Natural CAD and Transplant CAV**

Natural CAD	Transplant CAV
Asymmetrical lesions	Concentric intimal lesions
Involves focal lesions	Diffuse process, affects entire length of vessel
Affects small branches	Typically does not affect small branches
Internal elastic lamina disrupted	Internal elastic lamina intact
Does not affect intramyocardial vessels	Affects intramyocardial vessels
Calcification common	Calcification rare
Develops slowly over years	Develops rapidly (may develop over months)
Development of collaterals common	Development of collaterals rare

TABLE 9-20

■ **Etiologic Factors in Development of CAV**

Immunological Factors	Nonimmunological Factors
Human leukocyte antigen mismatching	Donor characteristics: age, sex, ischemic time, preexisting CAD
Suboptimal immunotherapy	Recipient characteristics: age, sex, obesity, hypertension, hyperlipidemia, diabetes mellitus, cytomegalovirus infection, smoking, oxidative injury
Acute rejection	

G. Treatment of CAV
  1. Revascularization procedures such as percutaneous transluminal coronary angioplasty (PTCA) or coronary artery bypass graft surgery are limited treatment options because of the diffuse, concentric nature of CAV.
  2. For those recipients with focal lesions in epicardial vessels, PTCA has been somewhat successful; however, follow-up angiography demonstrated that restenosis occurs in 50%–60% of these patients within 6 months.
  3. The only definitive treatment for CAV is retransplantation.
III. An at-a-glance summary of the key characteristics of the major types of rejection is shown in Table 9-21.[26, 30, 55, 56, 68]

TABLE 9-21

■ **Key Characteristics of Major Types of Rejection**[26, 30, 55, 56, 68]

Type of Rejection	Hyperacute	Acute Humoral (Vascular)	Acute Cellular	Chronic Rejection (Coronary Artery Vasculopathy)
Timing	Within minutes to hours of reestablishment of circulation to allograft	1 to 12 months post-transplant (but can occur later)	1 to 12 months post-transplant (but can occur later)	Median time to CAV development: 562 days (for transplants performed between April 1994 and June 2003)*
Occurrence	Rare (≤ 1%)	Common. Between 28% - 44% of recipients were treated for rejection during the first post-transplant year (transplants performed between January 2000 and June 2004)†*. Number of rejection episodes during first post-transplant year ranges from 1.6 to 2.0 (for transplants performed between January 2000 and June 2004) †*		Cumulative prevalence in survivors at 1 year post-transplant = 7.9% (follow-ups between January 2001 and June 2006)*. Cumulative prevalence in survivors at 5 and 8 years post-transplant = 32.1% and 44.3%, respectively (follow-ups between April 1994 and June 2005)*
Primary mediators	Preformed circulating cytotoxic antibodies against donor antigens (ABO group antigens, major histocompatibility antigens and endothelial antigens). Complement	B cells	Leukocytes (T cells and macrophages). Cytokine activation (tumor necrosis factor; interleukin-2; gamma-interferon, alpha-interferon, interleukin-4)	Alloantibodies. T cell products. Tissue growth factors
Pathophysiology	Antibody-antigen binding; activation of complement pathway; endothelial cell damage, platelet aggregation, vascular thrombosis, tissue infarction	Deposition of immunoglobulin (typically IgM) and complement components in capillary walls. HLA-DR expressed on endothelium following endothelial injury.	Activation and proliferation of T lymphocytes; subsequent infiltration of lymphocytes and destruction of allograft tissue	Tissue-remodeling response (vascular occlusion) secondary to peri- and post-transplant vascular trauma to endothelia associated with ischemia, reperfusion injury, immunosuppressants, vascular stress, acute rejection, and the production of donor-reactive alloantibodies. Neointimal formation results in luminal occlusion of arteries and veins.

Type of Rejection	Hyperacute	Acute Humoral (Vascular)	Acute Cellular	Chronic Rejection (Coronary Artery Vasculopathy)
Diagnosis	Clinical manifestations	Immunofluorescence stains Donor specific antibodies	Endomyocardial biopsy	Intravascular ultrasound (gold standard) Coronary angiography
Therapeutic options	Inotropic therapy Plasmapheresis Mechanical circulatory support Retransplantation	Plasmapheresis Photopheresis Total lymph node irradiation Corticosteroids Anti-B cell agents such as cyclophosphamide Antithymocyte globulin	Immunosuppressive agents that (1) inhibit clonal expansion (e.g., azathioprine) and cytokine production (e.g., steroids, cyclosporine); (2) deplete circulating T lymphocytes (monoclonal and polyclonal antilymphocyte antibodies)	Revascularization procedures are of limited utility due to the diffuse, concentric nature of CAV Retransplantation is the only definitive treatment

* ISHLT Registry Data 2006.

† Based on type of immunosuppressant therapy.

MONITOR PATIENT FOR POTENTIAL COMPLICATIONS: VENTRICULAR DYSFUNCTION/FAILURE

I. Right ventricular dysfunction/failure[69]
   A. RV failure is one of the leading causes of morbidity early in the post-transplant period.[70]
   B. Etiology: RV failure can result from:
      1. Loss of contractility in the allograft (may be associated with changes in the donor myocardium following brain death)
      2. Increased pulmonary vascular resistance in the recipient
         a. Patients with HF often develop pulmonary hypertension as the disease progresses.
         b. RV failure occurs when the donor right ventricle fails due to the recipient's elevated pulmonary vascular resistance.
         c. If a donor heart is transplanted into a recipient with severe pulmonary hypertension, the new RV is at high risk for failure as it may be unable to pump against the increased pressure found in the recipient's pulmonary vasculature.
         d. Because the RV is a thin-walled chamber, it is compliant and able to accommodate increased amounts of blood volume; however, because the RV consists of only a thin wall of myocardium, it is unable to pump against a high-pressure system.
         e. RV dysfunction can occur in the setting of a normal PVR.
      3. Ischemic injury; inadequate donor organ preservation
      4. Reperfusion injury
      5. Effects of cardiopulmonary bypass
      6. Donor/recipient size mismatch (considerably smaller donor heart implanted into larger recipient)
      7. Obstruction at site of pulmonary artery anastomosis
   C. Report clinical manifestations of RV dysfunction/failure:[71]
      1. Hypotension
      2. Tachycardia
      3. S_3, S_4 gallop
      4. Elevated central venous pressure in the setting of decreased LV filling pressures and decreased CO[30]
      5. Increased right ventricular diastolic pressure
      6. Decreased CO: RV failure leads to RV dilation, ischemia, decreased contractility, decreased pulmonary blood flow, and shift of the interventricular septum towards the LV. These physiologic changes subsequently result in decreased LV filling and CO.
      7. Echocardiogram findings:
         a. RV dilatation and hypokinesis
         b. Shift of interventricular septum towards the LV
   D. Intervene as ordered by physician[30, 41, 42]
      1. The goals of therapy are to:[71]
         a. Optimize RV preload
         b. Decrease RV afterload by decreasing PVR
         c. Decrease pulmonary pressures via pharmacologic management
         d. Decrease pulmonary vasoconstriction by ventilating with high inspired oxygen concentrations and/or increasing tidal volume

       e. Maintain systemic blood pressure and thus preserve coronary perfusion

  2. Potential interventions include:[30, 41, 42]

       a. Inhaled nitric oxide

           i. Action: lowers pulmonary vascular resistance without affecting SVR

           ii. Administered in setting of persistent, elevated PA pressure ($\geq$45 mm Hg) and severe RV dysfunction

       b. Intravenous medications: sodium nitroprusside, nitroglycerine, isoproterenol, milrinone, dobutamine, prostaglandin E-1, prostacyclin

           i. In setting of normal or near normal PA pressures: administer/titrate inotropic agents as ordered to support RV contractility; adjust RV preload as needed.

           ii. In setting of elevated PA pressures and transpulmonary gradient: administer/titrate vasodilators as ordered (e.g., nitroglycerin).

           iii. In setting of systemic hypotension: administer/titrate inotropic agents and optimize RV preload via volume resuscitation.

       c. Mechanical circulatory support (intraaortic balloon pump; ventricular assist device)

           i. For persistent isolated RV failure: prepare patient for return to operating room for implantation of a RV assist device.

       d. Prepare patient for return to operating room if etiology is due to obstruction at site of pulmonary artery anastomosis

 E. Follow-up monitoring: Monitor patient's response to therapy.

  1. Hemodynamic parameters: With effective interventions:

       a. CVP should decrease as right atrial filling pressure and mean pressure of systemic veins decrease.

       b. CO should increase as RV contractility improves.

       c. Pulmonary vascular resistance should decrease with improvement in CO.

       d. RV end-diastolic pressure should decrease as RV contractility improves.

  2. Blood pressure: With effective interventions, systemic hypotension should resolve as LV filling and CO improve.

 F. Collaborate with multidisciplinary team: physicians (surgeon, cardiologist, pulmonologist, intensivist), critical care pharmacist, OR staff; if patient's condition is critical: social worker, chaplain.

II. Left ventricular systolic dysfunction/failure[41, 42, 57]

 A. Etiology of LV systolic dysfunction/failure

  1. Ischemic injury

  2. Reperfusion injury

  3. Damage to allograft due to trauma

  4. Poor preservation techniques

 B. Report clinical manifestations of LV systolic dysfunction/failure:

  1. $\downarrow$ CO

  2. $\downarrow$ CI (severe LV dysfunction: CI $\leq$2.0/min/m^2)

  3. $\downarrow$ SV

  4. $\uparrow$ ventricular diastolic pressure

5. ↓ EF (severe LV dysfunction: EF = ≤30% or EF has decreased 25% from post-transplant baseline)
6. Need for resumption or increased dose of inotropic therapy (severe LV dysfunction)
7. ↓ tissue perfusion
8. Renal failure (↑ serum creatinine; ↑ blood urea nitrogen)
9. Liver failure (↑ bilirubin and liver enzymes)
10. Evidence of HF: dyspnea, fatigue, orthopnea, palpitations

C. Intervene as ordered by physician; potential interventions for LV systolic dysfunction/failure include:
1. Administration/titration of agents to augment CO without increasing SVR (for example, milrinone, low-dose dopamine, dobutamine)
2. Administration/titration of isoproterenol to increase HR
3. Atrial pacing
4. Volume correction to maintain PA diastolic pressure 15–20 mm Hg
5. Preparation of patient for one of the following:
   a. Intraaortic balloon pump counterpulsation
   b. Extracorporeal membrane oxygenation
   c. Implantation of a left ventricular assist device

D. Monitor patient's response to therapy; with effective interventions:
1. Hemodynamic parameters
   a. CO, SV, and EF should increase as LV contractility improves
   b. LV diastolic pressure should decrease as LV contractility improves and volume status is optimized
2. Tissue perfusion should improve as CO increases
3. Renal function test results: Elevated BUN and creatinine should decrease as CO improves and blood flow to the kidney increases.
4. Liver function test results: Elevated bilirubin and liver enzymes should decrease as CO improves and blood flow to the liver increases.

E. Collaborate with multidisciplinary team: physicians (surgeon, cardiologist, intensivist), critical care pharmacist, OR staff; if patient's condition is critical: social worker, chaplain.

III. Left ventricular diastolic dysfunction/failure[42]
A. Etiology of LV diastolic dysfunction/failure:
1. Ischemic injury
2. Reperfusion injury
3. Poor preservation techniques

B. Report clinical manifestations of LV diastolic dysfunction/failure (ventricle becomes stiff)
1. Elevated left atrial and left-ventricular end-diastolic pressures as a consequence of poor LV compliance
2. Pulmonary congestion/edema secondary to elevated left atrial and left ventricular end-diastolic pressures

C. Intervene as ordered by physician: Potential interventions for LV diastolic dysfunction/failure include:
1. Administration/titration of IV nitroglycerine or nitroprusside (to decrease afterload)
2. Administration of diuretics to decrease preload
3. Restriction of IV fluids to decreased preload

D. Monitor patient's response to therapy; with effective interventions:
1. Hemodynamic parameters

      a.   LA pressures should decrease as afterload is decreased.

      b.   LV end-diastolic pressure should decrease as afterload is decreased.

   2.   Oxygen saturation should improve as pulmonary congestion resolves.

E.   Collaborate with multidisciplinary team: physicians (surgeon, cardiologist, intensivist, critical care pharmacist).

MONITOR PATIENT FOR OTHER COMPLICATIONS

I.   Bleeding[41]
   A.   Potential etiology of bleeding:
      1.   Preoperative liver dysfunction secondary to HF
      2.   Hypothermia induced during surgery
      3.   Administration of heparin during cardiopulmonary bypass (CPB)
      4.   CPB-associated platelet destruction and fibrinolysis
      5.   Surgical trauma
   B.   Report clinical manifestations of bleeding:
      1.   Excessive chest tube drainage (for example, >100 mL/hr; check hospital protocol)
      2.   Decreasing hematocrit and hemoglobin
      3.   Tachycardia (HR >110–120 bpm)
      4.   Low CO and CI (<3.0 L/min/m^2)
      5. SvO_2 <65%
      6.   Hypotension (<90 mm Hg systolic)
      7.   Increasing O_2 requirements
   C.   Intervene as ordered; potential interventions for bleeding may include:
      1.   Administration of blood products (e.g., packed red cells, platelets, fresh frozen plasma)[52]
         a.   Cytomegalovirus (CMV) is carried in the leukocytes that are in red cell and platelet transfusions; therefore:
            i.   Platelets should be administered through a leukocyte filter
            ii.   Packed red cells should be leukocyte-reduced if possible and infused via a leukocyte filter
         b.   Cytomegalovirus (CMV)-negative recipients should receive CMV-negative blood products.
      2.   Administration of medications such as protamine or aprotinin
      3.   If needed, preparation of patient for return to operating room for subxiphoid pericardial window or mediastinal reexploration
   D.   Follow-up monitoring:
      1.   Continue to monitor hemoglobin, hematocrit, platelet count, prothrombin time, partial thromboplastin time to assess the patient's response to therapy.
      2.   Monitor patient for signs of cardiac tamponade.
   E.   Collaborate with multidisciplinary team: physicians (surgeon, cardiologist, intensivist), blood bank personnel, operating room staff (if needed).
II.   Cardiac tamponade
   A.   Overview[12, 41]

1. Cardiac tamponade is a serious and life-threatening complication that occurs when the accumulation of blood and clots in the pericardial space is so severe that it compresses the heart and impairs its ability to fill and/or pump effectively, thereby severely diminishing the CO and causing massive hemodynamic compromise.
2. Can occur with as little as 150 mL of fluid in the pericardial space
3. May occur suddenly or gradually over time
4. Without immediate treatment, cardiac tamponade will ultimately lead to cardiac arrest and death.

B. Etiology of cardiac tamponade
   1. Trauma (for example, catheter or bioptome perforation, contusion during cardiopulmonary resuscitation [CPR])
   2. Laceration during pericardiocentesis
   3. Aortic dissection
   4. MI with myocardial rupture

C. Report clinical manifestations of cardiac tamponade: Notify physician immediately as this is a life-threatening complication.
   1. Patient's symptoms: shortness of breath, chest or arm pain, unexplained apprehension or anxiety
   2. Marked decrease in chest tube drainage (typically occurs suddenly)
   3. Increased CVP
   4. Increased PCWP
   5. Equalizing right- and left-sided heart pressures (RA mean, RV end-diastolic pressure, PA diastolic pressure, PCWP: within 5 mm Hg)
   6. Decreased CO
   7. Decreased CI (<3.0 L/min/m^2)
   8. Hypotension (systolic pressure < 80 mm Hg or mean arterial pressure < 60 mm Hg)
   9. Narrowed pulse pressure
   10. Pulsus paradoxus (drop of 10 to 15 mm Hg during inspiration; only valid in nonventilated patients)
   11. Decreased mixed venous oxygen saturation (SvO_2)
   12. Compensatory tachycardia (may subsequently progress to bradycardia)
   13. Echocardiogram: presence of fluid in pericardial space
   14. Chest radiograph: widened mediastinum
   15. Distant heart sounds
   16. Weak peripheral pulses
   17. Decreased urinary output
   18. Altered level of consciousness

D. Intervene as ordered by physician; potential interventions for cardiac tamponade include:
   1. Administration of oxygen
   2. Volume and/or inotropic support to improve CO
   3. Preparation of patient for emergent pericardiocentesis

E. Monitor:
   1. Hemodynamic parameters
   2. Vital signs
   3. Oxygen saturation
   4. Patient's response to intervention(s); with effective therapy and improvement in heart's ability to fill and pump effectively:

      a. Patient's symptoms should improve (decreased shortness of breath, chest or arm pain, anxiety).

      b. Elevated CVP and PCWP should decrease.

      c. Right- and left-sided heart pressures should normalize.

      d. CO and CI should increase.

      e. Blood pressure should increase.

      f. Pulse pressure should widen.

      g. Pulsus paradoxus should resolve.

      h. SvO_2 should increase.

      i. Weak peripheral pulses should become stronger.

      j. Chest tube drainage should normalize.

      k. Urine output should increase.

F. Collaborate with multidisciplinary team: physicians (surgeon, cardiologist, intensivist, radiologist), echocardiographer, radiology technician, cardiac catheterization laboratory or operating room personnel (for pericardiocentesis).

III. Pericardial effusion[12]

  A. Etiology of pericardial effusion

    1. Transplant-specific

      a. The recipient's native heart dilates as HF progresses and the pericardium stretches in order to accommodate the enlarging heart.

      b. During transplantation, a normal-sized heart is placed into the space that was once occupied by an enlarged heart. The "unfilled" space is a potential site of fluid accumulation or effusion.

    2. General

      a. Infection

        i. Viruses: for example, adenovirus, enterovirus, influenza, varicella virus

        ii. Bacteria: for example, streptococci, staphylococci, pneumococci, *Pseudomonas* species, *Mycobacterium tuberculosis*

        iii. Fungi: for example, *Histoplasma, Aspergillus, Candida*

      b. Postcardiotomy syndrome

      c. Chest trauma: for example, pacemaker insertion; fractured ribs secondary to CPR

      d. Systemic disease: for example, severe hypothyroidism, uremia

  B. Report clinical manifestations of pericardial effusions promptly as large effusions can result in cardiac tamponade.

    1. Clinical manifestations can be subtle until the effusion becomes quite large and begins to cause hemodynamic compromise. At that point the symptoms can be identical to that of tamponade (see "Cardiac Tamponade"). Pericardial effusions can also be seen on echocardiogram and by chest radiography (enlarging cardiac silhouette).

  C. Intervene as ordered by physician; potential interventions for pericardial effusions may include:

    1. Withholding anticoagulants or substitution of heparin for other anticoagulants such as warfarin

    2. Aspiration of pericardial fluid via pericardial catheter

    3. Pericardiocentesis

    4. Subxyphoid pericardiotomy

    5. Pericardial window

D. Monitor:
1. Hemodynamic parameters
2. Vital signs
3. Oxygen saturation
4. Patient's response to intervention(s)
E. Collaborate with multidisciplinary team: physicians (surgeon, cardiologist, intensivist), operating room or cardiac catheterization lab staff if pericardial window, pericardiotomy or pericardiocentesis is required).

IV. Low cardiac output
A. Potential etiology of low CO[72]
1. ↓ HR
2. Hypovolemia (due to bleeding, diuresis)
3. Hemorrhage
4. Fluid shift (third spacing)
5. Elevated SVR (due to hypothermia, circulating catecholamines, hypovolemia)
6. Graft failure (see sections on left and right ventricular dysfunction)
7. Cardiac tamponade (see "Cardiac Tamponade")
8. Dysrhythmias
9. Rejection
B. Report clinical manifestations associated with low CO.[12, 72]
1. Cardiovascular
a. Hemodynamic changes: decreased blood pressure; increased heart rate
b. Dysrhythmias
c. Decreased peripheral pulses
d. Jugular venous distention
e. Cyanosis
f. Pallor
g. Cold, clammy skin
h. Slow capillary refill
2. Renal
a. ↑ serum creatinine level
b. ↑ BUN
c. Oliguria (typically <0.5 mL/kg/hr)
d. Anuria
3. Respiratory
a. Dyspnea
b. Crackles
c. Shortness of breath
d. Tachypnea
e. Metabolic acidosis
4. Neurologic
a. Mental status changes (decreased mentation; confusion; agitation, etc.)
b. Loss of consciousness
C. Intervene as ordered by physician; depending on cause, potential interventions for low CO may include:[27]
1. Atrial or AV sequential pacing to achieve an adequate HR
2. Volume infusion to increase PCWP to 15–20 mm Hg with SVR between 1000 to 1400 dynes/sec/cm[5]
3. Blood products

4. Vasopressors or vasodilators (depending on SVR)
5. Increased dose of inotropes if CI is less than 2 L/min/m²
6. Agents to treat rejection
7. IABP or other type of mechanical circulatory support for graft failure

D. Monitor response to intervention(s):
1. Hemodynamic status: CO, PAWP, SVR, heart rate/rhythm, blood pressure
2. Perfusion status: skin temperature, capillary refill, presence of cyanosis or pallor
3. Fluid status: intake and output; weight
4. Respiratory status (pulse oximetry, breath sounds, respirations)
5. Neurologic status
6. Perfusion

E. Collaborate with multidisciplinary team: physicians (surgeon, cardiologist, neurologist, nephrologist, pulmonologist), social worker, chaplain (if patient's condition is critical).

V. Alterations in blood pressure
A. Hypertension
1. Hypertension is a fairly common complication after transplantation with a cumulative prevalence of 94% and 97% within 5 and 8 years post transplant, respectively.[26]
2. Pathophysiology
   a. Early postoperative period: hypertension increases myocardial oxygen demand and increases the risk of postoperative bleeding.
   b. Hypertension is a known risk factor for the development of cardiac allograft vasculopathy (CAV).
3. Potential etiology of hypertension:
   a. Side effect of immunosuppressant medications (particularly corticosteroids, cyclosporine)
   b. Renal dysfunction
4. Report clinical manifestations of hypertension (note: hypertension may be asymptomatic)
   a. Headache
   b. Visual disturbances
   c. Nausea, vomiting
   d. Seizures: Recipients who had been hypotensive prior to transplantation may be at risk for seizures post-transplant, even though they are normotensive or slightly hypertensive. Recipients who complain of a headache and have a systolic blood pressure >140 mm Hg in the first weeks post-transplant require immediate antihypertensive therapy.
5. Intervene as ordered by physician
   a. Early postoperative period:
      i. Warming lights or blankets
      ii. IV antihypertensive agents (e.g., sodium nitroprusside, nitroglycerine) (see "Response of Denervated Cardiac Allograft to Medications")
      iii. Sedation, analgesia
      iv. Optimize ventilation and oxygenation
   b. Long-term management:

         i. May require multi-drug therapy consisting of a combination of calcium channel blockers, ACE inhibitors, alpha-2 adrenergic agonists and angiotensin receptor blockers.

         ii. Persistent hypertension may require a change in immunosuppressant medications (for example, from cyclosporine to sirolimus).

6. Monitor
   a. Blood pressure
   b. Hemodynamic parameters
   c. Serum immunosuppressant levels
   d. Renal function tests
   e. Patient's response to therapy
7. Collaborate with multidisciplinary colleagues: physicians (surgeon, cardiologist, intensivist, nephrologist, etc.), transplant pharmacist.

B. Hypotension
   1. Hypotension in the early postoperative phase decreases end-organ perfusion and places the recipient at risk of end-organ damage.
   2. Potential etiology of hypotension
      a. Decreased myocardial contractility due to:
         i. Myocardial ischemia
         ii. Allograft rejection
         iii. Other causes such as acidosis
      b. Cardiac tamponade
      c. Dysrhythmias
      d. ↓ SVR (due to sepsis, transfusion reaction, drug reaction, etc.)
      e. Pneumothorax
      f. Pulmonary embolus
      g. Bleeding
      h. Hypovolemia (see section on hypovolemia)
      i. Excessive use of diuretics
      j. Impaired metabolism of antihypertensive medications
   3. Report clinical manifestations of hypotension (vary with etiology)
      a. Low blood pressure (systolic pressure ≤80–90 mm Hg)
      b. Lightheadedness, dizziness
      c. Weakness
      d. Syncope
      e. Blurred vision
      f. Mental status changes
   4. Intervene as ordered by physician; potential interventions depend on the etiology and severity of the hypotension and may include:
      a. Placement of patient in Trendelenberg position
      b. Administration of oxygen
      c. IV fluid bolus
      d. Administration of dopamine (or increase in dopamine dose to obtain pressor effect (15–20 micrograms/kg/min)
      e. Optimize preload, afterload, contractility (See "Response of Denervated Cardiac Allograft to Medications")
      f. Treatment of primary cause
   5. Monitor
      a. Blood pressure
      b. Hemodynamic parameters
      c. Patient's mental status

    d.   Patient's response to therapy

   6.   Collaborate with multidisciplinary team members: physicians (surgeon, cardiologist, intensivist), transplant pharmacist.

VI. Disturbances of cardiac rate and/or rhythm

   A. Sinus node dysfunction[42]

     1. 25%–50% of recipients have sinus node dysfunction.

     2. Etiology of sinus node dysfunction

        a.   Surgical trauma to the sinoatrial node

        b.   Inadequate myocardial preservation

        c.   Cardiac denervation

        d.   Sinus node dysfunction in donor heart

     3. Report clinical manifestations of sinus node dysfunction.[42]

        a.   Sinus bradycardia (<70–80 bpm) has been linked to prolonged ischemic time, direct injury to the sinoatrial node, and preoperative use of amiodarone.[73]

        b.   Junctional bradycardia

     4. Intervene as ordered by physician; potential interventions for sinus node dysfunction include:

        a.   Preparation of patient for atrial pacing via epicardial wires that were placed during surgery

        b.   Administration/titration of isoproterenol if atrial pacing wires are nonfunctional

        c.   If bradycardia persists (>4–5 days), administration of aminophylline, theophylline, or terbutaline to increase HR

        d.   Preparation of patient for implantation of a temporary or permanent pacemaker (dual chamber) in the setting of persistent symptomatic bradycardia associated with decreased CO, persistent junctional escape rhythms, or persistent sinus bradycardia

     5. Monitor

        a.   ECG

        b.   HR

        c.   Patient's response to therapy

     6. Collaborate with multidisciplinary team: physicians (surgeon, cardiologist, intensivist, electrophysiologist), electrophysiology lab staff (if pacemaker is required).

   B. Atrial dysrhythmias

     1. Transient, asymptomatic atrial dysrhythmias are fairly common, occurring in approximately 25% of recipients while hospitalized.[42]

     2. Etiology of atrial dysrhythmias

        a.   Rejection (particularly atrial fibrillation and flutter)

        b.   Electrolyte imbalances (hypokalemia and hypomagnesemia)

        c.   Preoperative use of amiodarone

        d.   Biatrial surgical technique

     3. Report clinical manifestations of atrial dysrhythmias

        a.   Premature atrial complexes (most common type of atrial dysrhythmias)

        b.   Atrial flutter

        c.   Atrial tachycardia

        d.   Atrial fibrillation

     4. Intervene as ordered by physician; potential interventions for atrial dysrhythmias include:

      a. Administration of antirejection agents if dysrhythmias are due to rejection

      b. Atrial pacing (especially for atrial flutter)

      c. Administration of electrolyte replacements where necessary; consider other possible causes of atrial dysrhythmias

      d. Administration of beta-blockers or calcium channel blockers with caution

      e. *Note:* Digoxin is not used to treat atrial dysrhythmias because its effects are vagally mediated; therefore, it has no effect on the denervated sinoatrial or atrioventricular nodes[23]

      f. Preparation of patient for cardioversion if atrial dysrhythmias do not respond to pharmacologic therapy or if they lead to hemodynamic instability

  5. Monitor

      a. ECG

      b. HR and rhythm

      c. Patient's response to therapy

  6. Collaborate with multidisciplinary team: physician (surgeon, cardiologist, electrophysiologist), electrophysiology or cardiac catheterization lab staff (if cardioversion is required).

C. Ventricular dysrhythmias[42, 74]

  1. Potential etiology of ventricular dysrhythmias:

      a. Electrolyte imbalances (hypokalemia or hypomagnesemia)

      b. Rejection

      c. Increased sensitivity of the heart to catecholamines

      d. Reperfusion injury

      e. Prolonged ischemic time

      f. Manipulation of donor heart

  2. Report clinical manifestations of ventricular dysrhythmias:

      a. Premature ventricular complexes

      b. Ventricular tachycardia (rare)

      c. Ventricular fibrillation (rare)

  3. Intervene as ordered by physician; potential interventions for ventricular dysrhythmias include:

      a. Administration of intravenous lidocaine

      b. Electrolyte replacement therapy

      c. Advanced cardiac life support for malignant dysrhythmias

  4. Monitor:

      a. ECG

      b. Serum electrolytes

      c. Patient's response to intervention(s)

  5. Collaborate with multidisciplinary team: physicians (surgeon, cardiologist, intensivist, electrophysiologist), transplant pharmacist.

VII. Fluid imbalance

A. Hypovolemia: fluid volume deficit; loss of isotonic fluid and solutes from extracellular space)[41, 59, 75]

  1. Potential etiology of hypovolemia:

      a. Effects of cardiopulmonary bypass (movement of fluid into interstitial space; increased capillary permeability)

      b. Administration of diuretics during or after surgical procedure

      c. Increase in intravascular space during rewarming

      d Excessive urine output

       e.   Excessive bleeding or drainage

       f.   Diabetes mellitus

       g.   Vomiting, diarrhea

       h.   GI tube drainage

       i.   Third space fluid shifts

2.   Report clinical manifestations of hypovolemia (Box 9-3).[12, 75]

3.   Intervene as ordered by physician; potential interventions for hypovolemia include:

       a.   Insuring that patient has a central line and/or two patent, large-bore IV lines available

       b.   Administration of fluids to expand circulating volume and replace urine output with volume

          i.   Crystalloids (for example, normal saline)

          ii.   Colloids (for example, albumin; Hespan®)

          iii.   Electrolyte solutions (for example, Plasma-lyte®)

       c.   Replacement of electrolytes

       d.   Oxygen therapy to enhance tissue perfusion

       e.   Administration of vasopressors

       f.   Meticulous skin care to prevent breakdown

4.   Monitor patient's response to interventions:

       a.   Vital signs at least hourly; more often if indicated

       b.   Hemodynamic parameters (MAP, CVP, PCWP) to assess patient's response to therapy

       c.   Lab tests; for example:

          i.   Hematocrit: should decrease as hypovolemia is reversed.

          ii.   Electrolytes: should normalize with the administration of electrolyte solution and as diarrhea, vomiting, excessive urine loss resolve.

          iii.   BUN level: should decrease as hypovolemia is reversed.

       d.   Intake and output (hourly or per protocol)

       e.   Weight (daily)

       f.   Mental status; changes in level of consciousness

       g.   Skin: color, turgor, temperature

       h.   Patient's response to sedatives and narcotic pain medications

       i.   Clinical manifestations of volume overload and pulmonary edema (crackles, increased oxygen requirements) (see section on hypervolemia).

5.   Collaborate with multidisciplinary team: physicians (surgeon, cardiologist), dietitian, physical therapist, wound care nurse, ancillary nursing staff.

B.   Hypervolemia: Excess of isotonic fluid (water and sodium) in extracellular (interstitial or intravascular) compartment[75]

   1.   Potential etiology of hypervolemia:

       a.   Fluid accumulation secondary to CPB

       b.   Administration of IV fluids: normal saline or lactated Ringer's solution; fluids used to administer medications or perform monitoring procedures (for example, CO)[52]

       c.   Renal dysfunction

       d.   Excessive oral fluid intake

       e.   High intake of dietary sodium

       f.   Blood or plasma replacement

BOX 9-3
■ Manifestations of Hypovolemia[12, 75]

Hypotension or labile blood pressure

Tachypnea

↓ CI

↓ PAP/CVP

↑ HR; weak pulse

↓ urine output

↑ hematocrit

Increasing serum BUN/creatinine levels

↑ serum sodium levels

↑ urine specific gravity

Subnormal body temperature (unless there is a concurrent infectious process)

Poor skin turgor

Pallor

Dry skin and mucous membranes

Flat jugular veins

Weakness

Mental status changes (restlessness, anxiety, irritability, ↓ level of consciousness)

Exaggerated response (hypotension) to sedatives or narcotic pain medication

Weight loss

Thirst

Delayed capillary refill

Cool, pale skin over arms and legs

Negative intake and output balance (output > intake)

Postural hypotension (Drop in systolic blood pressure > 15 mm Hg or increase in heart rate > 15 bpm when patient changes from supine to upright position)

Hypovolemic shock:

Low CVP (< 5 to 10 cm H_2O)

Low PCWP < 6 to 12 mm Hg)

Low PAP (< 10 to 20 mm Hg)

Low CO (< 4 to 8 L/minute)

High SVR

BUN = blood urea nitrogen; CI = cardiac index; CVP = central venous pressure; HR = heart rate; PAP = pulmonary artery pressure; PCWP = pulmonary capillary wedge pressure; SVR = systemic vascular resistance.

       g. Fluid or sodium retention secondary to heart failure, liver failure, nephrotic syndrome, corticosteroid therapy, low dietary protein intake

       h. Use of plasma proteins (for example, albumin)

2. Report clinical manifestations of hypervolemia (Box 9-4).[12, 75]
3. Intervene as ordered by physician; potential interventions for hypervolemia include:

       a. Administration of diuretics

       b. Restriction of fluid and sodium intake

       c. Administration of oxygen

       d. Good skin care to prevent breakdown of edematous areas

---

BOX 9-4

■ **Manifestations of Hypervolemia**[12, 75]

↑ CVP

↑ PAP

↑ PCWP

Hypertension

Dependent edema (legs and feet when patient is standing; sacrum and buttocks when patient is lying down)

Anasarca (severe generalized edema)

Distended veins in neck and hands

Rapid, bounding pulse

S_3 gallop (in heart failure)

Pulmonary edema: crackles, shortness of breath, tachypnea, frequent frothy (pink) sputum, cough

Pulmonary congestion on chest radiograph

Dyspnea

Ascites

Weakness

Weight gain

Mental status changes

Intake exceeds output

Lab values:

   ↓ hematocrit (secondary to hemodilution)

   ↓ or normal serum sodium

   ↓ serum osmolality

BUN = blood urea nitrogen; CO = cardiac output; CVP = central venous pressure; PAP = pulmonary artery pressure; PCWP = pulmonary capillary wedge pressure

      e. If pulmonary edema develops: administration of medications to dilate blood vessels (e.g., nitroglycerine, morphine), aggressive diuresis, bilevel positive airway pressure (BiPAP)

      f. Hemodialysis

      g. Continuous renal replacement therapy for hemodynamically unstable patients

    4. Follow-up monitoring

      a. Volume status and filling pressures (CVP, PCWP, and other hemodynamic parameters)

      b. Respiratory rate and pattern

      c. Neck vein distention

      d. Heart sounds

      e. Breath sounds (presence of crackles or rhonchi)

      f. Arterial blood gases

      g. Weight (daily trends)

      h. Intake and output (hourly or per protocol)

      i. Lab results; for example:

        i. Potassium may decrease with diuretic therapy

        ii. Hematocrit may increase

      j. Clinical manifestations of hypovolemia (see section on hypovolemia)

    5. Collaborate with multidisciplinary team: physicians (surgeon, cardiologist nephrologist), transplant pharmacist, dietitian, physical therapist, ancillary nursing staff.

VIII. Renal dysfunction

    A. Potential etiology of renal dysfunction:

      1. Preoperative factors: HF, prolonged diuretic therapy, decreased perfusion

      2. Intraoperative factors: abnormal renal perfusion with CPB

      3. Postoperative factors: low CO, nephrotoxic effects of immunosuppressive agents, particularly calcineurin inhibitors[42]

    B. Report clinical manifestations of renal dysfunction

      1. Oliguria (typically <0.5 mL/kg/hr)

      2. Anuria

      3. Elevated serum creatinine level

    C. Intervene as ordered by physician; potential interventions for renal dysfunction include:[41, 42, 52]

      1. Placement of Foley catheter to urimeter with gravity drainage

      2. Administration of low-dose dopamine (2-3 μg/kg/min) to increase renal blood flow

      3. Administration of medications to maintain mean arterial pressure between 60 to 80 mm Hg (for example, epinephrine, vasopressin, inotropes)

      4. Cautious volume administration if oliguria (urine output < approximately 50 mL/hr) occurs early after transplantation

        a. Augment preload to increase CVP or LA pressure to 12–13 mm Hg

      5. Optimizing CO

      6. Administration of diuretics (for example, furosemide) for persistent oliguria

a. If blood urea nitrogen is elevated and/or serum creatinine is elevated, it is important to maintain intravascular volume.

b. If diuretic therapy results in brisk diuresis, urine output replacement may be useful (replacing hourly urine output with an equal volume of normal or half-normal saline solution until LA pressure or CVP reaches 13–14 mm Hg).

7. Delaying initiation of cyclosporine therapy in setting of oliguria and rising serum creatinine level

   a. If renal function fails to improve within 48 hours, other cytolytic therapy may be initiated (for example, antilymphocyte antibodies, anti-CD25 antibodies).

8. Changing administration of cyclosporine from oral to IV administration

   a. In the setting of increasing renal dysfunction, IV administration of cyclosporine may ameliorate renal dysfunction by preventing the peaks in serum concentration levels that result from oral administration.[51]

9. Decreasing immunosuppressive dose

10. Changing immunosuppressive medications

11. Avoiding other nephrotoxic drugs, especially antibiotics

12. Initiating dialysis or continuous hemofiltration

D. Follow-up monitoring:

1. Urine output per ICU protocol (for example, hourly)

   a. As with other types of cardiac surgery patients, a urine output of at least 1ml/kg/hour is generally an indication of adequate cardiac output, blood volume, and peripheral perfusion.[76]

2. Renal function (serum creatinine, blood urea nitrogen)

3. Serum electrolytes

4. Hemodynamic parameters

5. Serum immunosuppressant levels

E. Collaborate with multidisciplinary team members: physicians (surgeon, cardiologist, nephrologist), critical care pharmacist.

IX. Pleural effusions

A. Potential etiology of pleural effusions[77]

1. Postoperative bleeding into pleural space

2. Increased hydrostatic pressure associated with a positive fluid balance

3. Increased vascular permeability associated with certain infections such as pneumonia

4. Decreased osmotic pressure associated with a low protein state

5. Increased intrapleural negative pressure associated with atelectasis

B. Report clinical manifestations of pleural effusions:

1. Patients with pleural effusions may not become symptomatic until the effusion becomes quite large.

2. Clinical manifestations vary with the cause of the effusion and may be vague.[4]

   a. Infection: fever; signs of inflammation

   b. Shortness of breath due to decrease in lung volume on affected side

   c. Tachypnea

   d. Diminished breath sounds

e. Percussion: dullness or flatness

f. Pleuritic pain (associated with inflammatory process)

g. Visualization of effusion on chest radiograph (typically observed when there is an accumulation of 250 mL or more of fluid)

h. Mediastinal shift towards contralateral side (with large, acute effusion)

C. Intervene as ordered by physician

1. Definitive therapy is directed to the cause of effusion

2. Potential interventions include:

a. Preparation of patient for thoracentesis (for diagnostic and therapeutic purposes)

b. Administration of antimicrobial agents if infection is the cause of the effusion

X. Infection: General[40, 52] (see Chapter 5 for additional information)

A. Immunosuppression places transplant recipients at risk for:

1. Nosocomial infections (particularly at surgical incisions and sites of vascular lines and percutaneous tubes)

2. Emergence of latent endogenous infections

3. Infections transmitted via allograft or blood products

4. Opportunistic infections

5. Community-acquired infections

B. Incidence of infection

1. Non-CMV infections account for 13% of deaths in the first 30 days after heart transplantation. The incidence of fatal non-CMV infection increases to 33% within 2-12 months post transplantation.[26]

2. Approximately 25% of patients have one or more major infections during the first two post-transplant months.[52]

3. Bacterial infections are the most frequently occurring type of infection during the transplant hospitalization; the peak risk is during first postoperative week.[52]

4. During the immediate postoperative period, the lung is the most common site of infection and the pulmonary infection is typically bacterial.[27]

C. Prevention of infection

1. Implement neutropenic protocol per physician's order.

a. For neutropenic patient: limit room traffic and place a visitor restriction sign on the door.

2. Maintain protective isolation status per hospital policy.

a. Protocols differ widely among transplant centers.

b. Most centers place patients in an ICU room that has been specially cleaned, observe strict hand-washing technique and use gloves; some centers use complete reverse isolation.

c. Proper hand-washing technique is the single most important and successful intervention aimed at decreasing the incidence of nosocomial infections.

3. Administer appropriate blood products based on CMV sero-status as ordered by physician.

a. Leukocyte-poor blood products

b. CMV-negative blood for CMV-negative recipient

4. Strictly adhere to hospital protocol regarding care of indwelling lines and catheters, for example:

      a.   Changing vascular access monitoring line dressings per protocol

      b.   Changing IV tubing, transducers, and flush solutions per protocol[27]

      c.   Removing Foley catheter within 24 hours, if possible (per physician's order)

      d.   Discontinuing all drains, arterial lines, and large caliber central venous lines within 3 to 4 days, if possible (per physician's order)

   5.   Administer antimicrobial agents per protocol; examples of prophylactic antimicrobial agents include:[78]

      a.   Ganciclovir for CMV-negative recipients who receive an allograft from a CMV-positive donor

      b.   Sulfamethoxazole/trimethoprim for prophylaxis against pneumocystis

      c.   Nystatin for prophylaxis against *Candida* infections

   6.   Extubate as soon as possible (per physician's order).

   7.   Maintain meticulous pulmonary toilet (frequent coughing, deep breathing, turning, chest physiotherapy).

   8.   Facilitate mobility per physician's order.

      a.   Get patient out of bed to chair on first postoperative day or as soon as possible.

      b.   Ambulate patient as soon as possible.

      c.   Increase ambulation as tolerated by patient.

   9.   Instruct family members and other visitors in infection control techniques, particularly hand-washing.

D.   Recognize and report clinical manifestations of infection.[40, 41]

   1.   General (Box 9-5)[40, 41]

   2.   Site-specific (Table 9-22)

   3.   It is important to note that the anti-inflammatory effects of steroid therapy may:

BOX 9-5

■ **General Manifestations of Infection**[40, 41]

Fever (38° Celcius/100.4° Fahrenheit)

Tachycardia

Tachypnea

Hypotension

↑ CO/CI

↓ SVR

↑ Oxygen requirements

Chills

Leukocytosis

C-reactive protein (positive)

↑ sedimentation rate

TABLE 9-22

■ **Site-Specific Manifestations of Infection**

Site	Example of Clinical Manifestations
Ear, nose, throat	Sinus drainage, rhinitis, cough, sneeze, ear ache, pruritus, fever, thrush, mouth sores, lesions, dental caries, swollen lymph glands
Respiratory tract	Cough, wheezing, change in color and quantity of sputum, shortness of breath
Gastrointestinal tract	Diarrhea, nausea, vomiting, abdominal pain, bleeding, loss of appetite
Urinary tract	Frequency, burning, urgency, dysuria, flank pain, cloudy urine, urine with foul odor
Skin	Purulent drainage from any surgical or line site; erythema; lesions, rash, pruritus, foot ulcers
Neurologic system	Mental status changes, neck pain, headache
Musculoskeletal system	Joint pain, muscle aches, fever

      a. Blunt the patient's ability to produce pyrogens. As a consequence, the recipient's body temperature may be lower than would be expected.
         i. Even small increases in body temperature should be noted and reported.
      b. Mask symptoms of infection (for example urinary tract infections may be asymptomatic)
   E. Anticipate physician's order for cultures for evidence of infection—particularly in response to a fever; obtain samples and test results in a timely manner
     1. A thorough fever workup (for example, pan cultures [culture of blood, urine, sputum], urinalysis, CBC with differential, etc.) should be initiated for temperature $\geq$38° Celsius ($\geq$100.4° F).[51]
   F. Intervene as ordered by the physician; potential interventions include:
     1. Administration of antimicrobial therapy
     2. Preparation of patient for additional diagnostic tests (for example, chest radiograph, CT scan, bronchoscopy with bronchoalveolar lavage)
     3. Preparation of patient for surgical exploration/debridement (for example, for mediastinitis)
   G. Monitor patient's response to therapy; depending on site and nature (local versus systemic) of infection, with effective therapy:
     1. Test results should return to normal (for example, CBC, cultures, chest radiograph, CT scan)
     2. Hemodynamic parameters
       a. Elevated CO/CI should decrease
       b. Decreased SVR should increase
     3. Vital signs; for example, body temperature should return to normal

4. Oxygen requirements; with effective therapy, oxygen requirements should decrease
5. Surgical incisions, drainage, and access lines: for example, drainage should decrease
6. Pain: should decrease
7. Patient's mental status: should improve

H. Collaborate with multidisciplinary team members: physicians (surgeon, cardiologist, infectious disease specialist), wound-care nurse, transplant pharmacologist; home health care nurse (for example, if postdischarge intravenous antibiotics and wound monitoring are required).

XI. Wound infection
A. Types
1. Suprasternal soft tissue infection
a. Treatment options: antibiotic therapy, wound care, drainage, debridement
2. Deep wound infection that causes mediastinitis

B. Mediastinitis[54]
1. Incidence: <5%
2. Etiology of mediastinitis:
a. Colonization of recipient
b. Less common: microbial colonization from donor
3. Potential causative organisms
a. Most common: Gram-positive bacteria (*Staphylococcus aureus*, coagulase-negative *S. aureus*)
b. Gram-negative bacteria
c. Fungal pathogens: *Aspergillus fumigatus; Candida* spp.
4. Report clinical manifestations of mediastinitis
a. Purulent wound drainage
b. Mobile sternal fragments
c. Wound edge separation
d. Sternal pain or tenderness
e. Fever
f. Leukocytosis
g. Erythema
h. Increasing wound drainage
5. Treatment options (based on severity of infection)
a. Antimicrobial agents
b. Wound drainage
c. Surgical debridement
d. Tissue flap wound closure
6. Monitor patient's response to therapy; with effective therapy:
a. Test results should normalize: for example
i. White blood cell count should decrease
ii. Cultures should be negative
b. Temperature should normalize
c. At site of wound infection:
i. Drainage and redness should decrease
ii. Drainage should become less purulent
iii. Sternal mobility should decrease
iv. Wound edges should begin to approximate
v. Pain or tenderness should decrease

7. Collaborate with multidisciplinary team members: physicians (surgeon, cardiologist, infectious disease specialist, plastic surgeon) wound-care nurse, transplant pharmacologist; home health care nurse (for example, if postdischarge intravenous antibiotics and wound monitoring are required).

XII. Impaired wound healing

    A. Potential etiology of impaired wound healing:

        1. Corticosteroid therapy

           a. Decreases collagen content in dermis; as a result, skin becomes thin and easily damaged and wound healing is impaired[42]

           b. Increases risk of infection

        2. Use of proliferation inhibitors (for example, sirolimus, everlimus)

        3. Poor nutritional status

        4. Poor blood glucose control

    B. Report clinical manifestations of impaired wound healing at any incisional or cannulation site

        1. Purulent drainage; excessive drainage

        2. Wound edge separation

        3. Erythema

        4. Swelling

        5. Necrosis

        6. Dehiscence

    C. Intervene as ordered by physician; potential interventions for impaired wound healing may include:

        1. Meticulous sterile wound care; dressing changes per protocol

        2. Enzymatic debridement

        3. Medications

           a. Antimicrobial therapy

           b. Medications to improve blood glucose control

           c. Changing immunosuppressant therapy from proliferation inhibitors to other agents

        4. Dietary changes to enhance nutritional status

        5. Return to operating room for surgical debridement

    D. Monitor patient's response to interventions:

        1. Incisions, IV access, and cannulation sites:

           a. Drainage, wound edges, swelling, erythema

        2. Serum glucose level

        3. Nutritional status (prealbumin; calorie counts)

    E. Collaborate with multidisciplinary team: physicians (surgeon, cardiologist, intensivist, plastic surgery specialist, infectious disease specialist, endocrinologist), wound care nurse, dietitian, physical therapist, home health care nurse.

XIII. Neurologic complications

    A. Etiology of neurologic dysfunction[42]

        1. Ischemic stroke

           a. The manipulation of the diseased native heart along with the cannulation, clamping, and unclamping of the aorta may dislodge material such as thrombus and atheromatous plaque that has the potential to embolize to the brain.[79, 80]

        2. Cerebral emboli from dilated LV with thrombus

        3. Low CO with hypotension and watershed infarction

        4. Encephalopathy secondary to:

a. Operative or postoperative global hypoxic-ischemic insult (within first 48 hours)

b. Metabolic abnormalities (within first 48 hours)

c. Calcineurin inhibitor (cyclosporine or tacrolimus) toxicity (headache, depression, obtundation, cortical blindness)

d. Muromonab-CD3 [OKT®3]: aseptic meningitis: fever, headache, photophobia

e. High-dose steroids: psychosis

5. Side effects of pre- and post-transplant medications (may be more pronounced in the setting of renal and/or hepatic dysfunction)

6. Metabolic abnormalities

B. Clinical manifestations of neurologic complications (depend on etiology)

1. Ischemic insult: hemiparesis, aphasia, visual deficits, severe delirium, and coma[79]

2. Medication side effects:

a. β-blockers: depression, confusion

b. Calcium channel blockers: headache, confusion, vertigo, tremor

c. Amiodarone: neuropathy, ataxia, tremor

d. Corticosteroid therapy: convulsions, vertigo, headache

e. Calcineurin inhibitors: tremor, headache

3. Encephalopathy: may range from mild confusion to coma

4. Focal cerebral abnormalities: typically associated with embolic events

5. Seizures: typically associated with drug toxicity (for example, cyclosporine, tacrolimus, Muromonab-CD3 [OKT®3])

C. Intervene as ordered by physician; potential interventions depend on etiology and may include:

1. Initiating seizure precautions

2. Optimizing CO

3. Decreasing dose of immunosuppressant medications

4. Changing immunosuppressant agents or other medications

5. Correcting metabolic abnormalities

6. Administering anticonvulsants

a. It is important to note that certain anticonvulsants (for example, phenytoin, phenobarbital, carbamazepine) may increase the metabolism of calcineurin inhibitors (cyclosporine and tacrolimus); this may result in low serum levels of these immunosuppressants.

b. Monitor serum levels of calcineurin inhibitors carefully; dose of calcineurin inhibitor may have to be adjusted.

D. Monitor patient's response to therapy:

1. Neurologic status

2. Cognitive status

3. Mood state

4. Serum anticonvulsant levels (for example, phenytoin [Dilantin®] level)

E. Collaborate with multidisciplinary team members: physicians (surgeon, cardiologist, neurologist, neuropsychologist, psychologist), transplant pharmacist, physical therapist, occupational therapist.

XIV. Electrolyte imbalance
    A. Potential etiology:
        1. Intra- and postoperative IV fluid administration
        2. Renal dysfunction; decreased excretion of electrolytes
        3. Inadequate intake or supplementation of electrolytes through intravenous solutions, diet, enteral feedings, total parenteral nutrition
        4. Increased or decreased absorption of electrolytes in GI tract
        5. Excessive loss of electrolytes through vomiting, diarrhea, gastric suctioning, severe diaphoresis, wound drainage
        6. Excessive intake of electrolytes
        7. Adverse effects of medications (for example, antibiotics, diuretics, corticosteroids)
        8. Infection
        9. Rhabdomyolysis
       10. Insulin deficiency
       11. Acid-base imbalances
       12. Lack of vitamins that promote absorption of electrolytes
       13. Comorbidities (for example, hypoalbuminemia, hyperparathyroidism)
    B. Report clinical manifestations of electrolyte imbalance (see Appendix A)
    C. Intervene as ordered by physician (see Appendix A)
    D. Monitor:
        1. Serum electrolytes
        2. Associated lab tests
        3. Patient's response to intervention(s)
    E. Collaborate with multidisciplinary team: physicians (surgeon, cardiologist, intensivist, nephrologist, gastroenterologist, endocrinologist), dietitian, transplant pharmacist.

XV. Disorders of glucose metabolism
    A. Hyperglycemia (fasting blood glucose level ≥126 mg/dL or ≥6.9 μmol/L)
        1. Potential etiology of hyperglycemia
            a. Preexisting diabetes mellitus
                i. Insulin dependent
                ii. Non-insulin dependent
            b. Side effects of medications such as corticosteroids and tacrolimus
        2. Clinical manifestations of hyperglycemia (Table 9-23)
        3. Intervene as ordered by physician:
            a. Serum blood glucose monitoring
            b. Capillary blood glucose monitoring
            c. Administration of insulin (subcutaneous or IV insulin drip)
            d. Oral hypoglycemic agents
            e. American Diabetic Association diet
            f. Diabetes education for patient and family
        4. Monitor patient's response to interventions
            a. Serum and capillary blood glucose level
            b. Hemoglobin A_{1C}
            c. Patient's and family's knowledge of diabetes

TABLE 9-23

■ **Manifestations of Hyperglycemia**

Clinical Manifestation	Pathophysiology
Glycosuria	Amount of glucose molecules filtered by kidney exceeds amount of glucose that can be reabsorbed by renal tubules
Polyuria	Osmotic diuresis
Polydipsia	Intracellular dehydration as blood glucose levels ↑ and water is pulled out of cells, particularly those in thirst center
Polyphagia	In IDDM: cellular starvation and ↓ in carbohydrate, fat, and protein stores
Weight loss (particularly in IDDM)	Loss of fluid secondary to osmotic diuresis; Loss of body tissue as body uses fat and protein stores for energy
Obesity (particularly in uncomplicated NIDDM)	Altered metabolism
Recurrent blurred vision	Exposure of lens and retina to hyperosmolar fluid
Weakness, fatigue	Lowered plasma volume
Paresthesias	Dysfunction of peripheral sensory nerves
Skin infections	Growth of yeast organisms

IDDM = insulin dependent diabetes mellitus; NIDDM = non-insulin dependent diabetes mellitus.

    5. Collaborate with multidisciplinary team: physicians (surgeon, cardiologist, intensivist, endocrinologist), dietitian, ancillary nursing staff, diabetes educator, home health care nurse).
  B. Hypoglycemia (serum glucose level ≤50 mg/dL or ≤2.77 μmol/L)
    1. Potential etiology of hypoglycemia
      a. Insulin dose that exceeds patient's metabolic requirements
      b. Oral hypoglycemic agents
      c. Insufficient caloric intake
      d. Strenuous activity or increased exercise that is not accompanied by appropriate increase in food intake or decrease in insulin dose
      e. Factors that potentiate the action of hypoglycemic medications:
        i. Renal insufficiency
        ii. Medications (e.g., sulfonamides)
      f. Weight loss
      g. Decrease in corticosteroid dose
      h. Comorbidities (for example, liver disease)
    2. Report clinical manifestations of hypoglycemia (Table 9-24)
    3. Intervene as ordered by physician; potential interventions include
      a. Administration of oral or IV glucose

TABLE 9-24

■ **Manifestations of Hypoglycemia**

Clinical Manifestation	Pathophysiology
Impaired cerebral function:	Results from ↓ availability of glucose for brain metabolism
Headache	
Slurred speech	
Motor dysfunction	
Impaired problem solving	
Feeling of vagueness	
Change in emotional behavior	
Convulsions	
Coma	
Parasympathetic nervous system:	Compensatory changes due to activation of autonomic nervous system
Hunger	
Nausea	
Hypotension	
Bradycardia	
Sympathetic nervous system:	
Anxiety, irritability	
Diaphoresis	
Cool, pale skin	
Tachycardia	

        b. Discontinuation of IV insulin
        c. Decrease in dose of insulin or oral hypoglycemic agent
    4. Monitor
        a. Serum glucose level (keep between 80–110 mg/dL or 4.44–6.1 μmol/L)
        b. Capillary glucose levels
        c. Patient's mental status
        d. Patient's response to intervention(s)
    5. Collaborate with multidisciplinary team: physicians (surgeon, cardiologist, endocrinologist), diabetes educator, dietitian, home health care nurse.
  XVI. Altered bowel function
    A. Constipation
      1. Potential etiology
        a. Effects of general anesthesia, especially the opioid component; the smooth muscles of the gastrointestinal tract are often temporarily paralyzed and peristalsis may be impaired[81]
        b. Narcotic analgesics that may suppress peristalsis and lead to constipation or obstruction

       c.   Reduced mobility: inactivity slows progression of materials through the GI tract

  2.   Report clinical manifestations of constipation
      a.   Infrequent bowel movements
      b.   Difficult defecation
      c.   Passage of unduly hard and dry fecal material
      d.   Abdominal distention
      e.   Abdominal pain or tenderness
      f.   Abnormal abdominal radiograph, ultrasound or CT scan results

  3.   Intervene as ordered by physician; potential interventions may include:
      a.   Increasing patient's level of activity (ambulation, scheduled exercise)
      b.   Administration of medications to relieve constipation (e.g., prokinetic agents, stool softeners, suppositories, laxatives)
          i.   Note: Aluminum-based laxatives may decrease absorption of medications in the gut.
      c.   Enemas
      d.   Nasogastric tube for decompression
      e.   Increasing patient's intake of fluid and fiber
      f.   Changing type and/or frequency of pain medication

  4.   Monitor:
      a.   Bowel sounds (absent, hypoactive, hyperactive)
      b.   Abdominal pain, tenderness, distention
      c.   Patient's response to intervention(s):
          i.   Bowel movements (e.g., frequency, quantity)
          ii.   Observe trend via stool charts

  5.   Collaborate with multidisciplinary team members: physicians (surgeon, cardiologist, intensivist, gastroenterologist), dietitian, physical therapist, ancillary nursing personnel.

B. Diarrhea
  1.   Potential etiology
      a.   Medications that irritate the bowel and precipitate ulcerations, bleeding, and diarrhea
          i.   Mycophenolate mofetil
          ii.   Antiplatelet agents
          iii.   Antibiotics that alter the normal flora of the bowel and subsequently cause diarrhea
      b.   Opportunistic infections (for example, CMV may cause gastritis or colitis)
      c.   Hospital-acquired infections such as *Clostridium difficile*

  2.   Report clinical manifestations of diarrhea
      a.   Frequent passage of unformed, watery stool
      b.   Positive stool cultures
      c.   Weight loss
      d.   Abnormal test results (for example, positive stool cultures); abnormal abdominal radiograph, ultrasound or CT scan)

  3.   Intervene as ordered by physician; potential interventions may include:

   a. Altering medication time schedule (for example, administering mycophenolate mofetil 500 mg three times daily instead of 750 mg twice daily)
   b. Treatment of infection (e.g., metronidazole or oral vancomycin for *Clostridium difficile*)
   c. Administration of binding agents for diarrhea caused by non-toxin secreting organisms (for example, loperamide)
4. Monitor:
   a. Bowel sounds (absent, hypoactive, hyperactive)
   b. Abdominal pain, tenderness, distention
   c. Laboratory test values (for example, electrolytes)
   d. Patient's response to intervention(s):
      i.   Bowel movements (frequency, quantity, characteristics)
      ii. Observe trend via stool charts
5. Collaborate with multidisciplinary team members: physicians (surgeon, cardiologist, intensivist, gastroenterologist), dietitian, physical therapist, ancillary nursing personnel.

XVII. Altered nutrition
   A. The patient's nutritional status at the time of transplantation may influence post-transplant nutrition
      1. Heart transplant recipients are at risk for malnutrition due to pre-transplant:[82]
         a. Anorexia (secondary to gastric compression from ascites)
         b. Gastrointestinal symptoms (nausea, vomiting, diarrhea, constipation)
         c. Dysgeusia (impaired taste)
         d. Dysphagia
         e. Hypermetabolism (increase in resting energy expenditure)
         f. Drug-nutrient interactions
         g. Malabsorption (secondary to engorgement of viscera with fluid)
         h. Poor nutrient delivery to tissues
         i. Early satiety
         j. Restricted diets
         k. Impaired ability to prepare food
         l. Altered mental status
   B. The goal of pretransplant care is to optimize the candidate's weight and nutritional status.
   C. Following transplantation, the energy expended by the body through the healing and recovery process is increased from basal levels and a greater amount of protein is required for tissue repair and regeneration.
   D. Pretransplant heart failure dietary restrictions (e.g., sodium and fluid restrictions) are typically relaxed in the immediate postoperative period, thereby expanding the patient's food choices.
      1. For the long term, however, patients are encouraged to follow a heart healthy (e.g. low fat, low salt, low cholesterol) diet and maintain ideal body weight to prevent or reduce the severity of complications such as obesity, hypertension, diabetes mellitus, etc.
   E. Nutrition remains an area that requires close monitoring as there is some evidence that cachexia and obesity increase the risk of poor post-transplant outcomes.[83] In addition, obesity may increase the risk of other post-transplant complications.[82]

F. Report:
1. Patient's baseline and current appetite
2. Patient's baseline and current weight
3. Low serum albumin level
   a. Normal values: adults: 3.5–5.5 g/dL or 35–55 g/L
   b. Normal values: adults >60 years of age: 3.4–4.8 g/dL or 34–48 g/L
4. Low prealbumin level
   a. Normal values: 10–40 mg/dL or 100–400 mg/L
5. Result of calorie counts
6. Nausea, vomiting (may be associated with general anesthesia)
7. Diarrhea, constipation
8. Absent bowel sounds, increasing abdominal girth and tension or reflux of feedings (may indicate hypomotility or the presence of a bowel obstruction or ileus)

G. Intervene as ordered by physician; potential interventions include:
1. Calorie counts to assess patients' ability to meet their nutritional needs
2. Small, frequent feedings if patients continue to have early satiety
3. Nutritional supplements
4. Enteral feedings
   a. Confirm correct placement of feeding tube prior to initiating feeding
   b. Monitor for aspiration: increased ventilator resistance, increased temperature, changes on chest radiograph, or the presence of tube feed in the secretions of intubated patients
   c. Early postoperative feeding must be initiated slowly due to the effects of general anesthetics on the motility of GI tract
5. Total parenteral nutrition (TPN) if the patient does not tolerate enteral feedings
   a. Monitor nutritional status, electrolyte and mineral levels, blood glucose level; triglycerides, liver function tests
6. Administration of medications to control nausea, vomiting, diarrhea

H. Monitor:
1. Lab test results
   a. Serum albumin
   b. Serum prealbumin
   c. Electrolytes
   d. Liver function tests
2. Appetite
3. Bowel sounds
4. Activity level
5. Patient's response to interventions:
   a. Weight gain or loss
   b. Calories consumed
   c. Presence or absence of nausea, vomiting, diarrhea, constipation
   d. Tolerance of nutritional supplements, enteral feedings, or TPN

I. Collaborate with multidisciplinary team: physicians (surgeon, cardiologist, intensivist), dietitian, physiotherapists, social worker (for psychological etiology of altered nutrition), ancillary nursing personnel.

1. Collaboration with the dietitian is of particular importance as this clinician can:[82]
   a. Conduct a pretransplant nutrition screening and assessment (history, physical assessment, analysis of laboratory test results)
   b. Implement strategies to correct pretransplant malnutrition and/or optimize candidate's pretransplant weight, particularly with respect to requirements of calories, protein, vitamins, minerals and electrolytes
   c. Develop a plan of post-transplant nutritional support and monitor patient's progress (particularly if the recipient requires enteral or parenteral feedings)
   d. Identify medication side effects that can interfere with post-transplant nutrition
   e. Provide continuity of care with respect to potential chronic post-transplant problems such as obesity, hyperlipidemia, diabetes mellitus, and hypertension
   f. Serve as a resource regarding food safety issues

XVIII. Altered mobility and/or self-care deficit
   A. Early mobility is an important factor in preventing postoperative complications and facilitating recovery.
   B. Potential etiology of altered mobility and/or self-care deficit:
      1. Pain or anticipatory pain
      2. Pre- or post-transplant deconditioning
      3. Altered mood state (for example, depression, anxiety)
   C. Clinical manifestations:
      1. Inability or unwillingness to participate in self-care
      2. Inability or unwillingness to ambulate
   D. Interventions
      1. Administer adequate pain medication prior to self-care activities or ambulation
         a. Assess effectiveness of pain medication before patient engages in self-care activities or ambulation
      2. Establish mutual goals for self-care, ambulation, and exercise
      3. Instruction in sternal precautions
      4. Physical therapy
         a. Establishment of mutual goals
         b. Development of exercise program (in hospital and at home)
      5. Occupational therapy
         a. Establishment of mutual goals
      6. Involve family in patient's care
      7. Referral for home physical and/or occupational therapy, if needed
      8. Referral to outpatient Phase II cardiac rehabilitation program upon discharge
      9. Referral for mental health services, if needed
   E. Monitor
      1. Effectiveness of pain medication
      2. Patient's ability to perform self-care activities
      3. Patient's progress with physical and occupational therapy
   F. Collaborate with multidisciplinary colleagues: physicians (surgeon, cardiologist, intensivist); physical therapist; occupational therapist; home health care nurse; mental health provider.

REFERENCES

1. Hunt SA, Abraham WT, Chin MH, et al. *American College of Cardiology/American Heart Association 2005 guideline update for the diagnosis and management of chronic heart failure in the adult: A report of the American College of Cardiology/American Heart Association Task Force on Practice Guidelines (Writing Committee to Update the 2001 Guidelines for the Evaluation and Management of Heart Failure)*. 2005.

2. Braunwald E. Heart failure. In: Fauci AS, Braunwald E, Isselbacher KJ, et al., (Eds). *Harrison's Principles of Internal Medicine*, 14th ed. New York: McGraw Hill, 1998, p. 1287-1298.

3. Carelock J, Clark AP. Heart failure: Pathophysiological mechanisms. *Am J Nurs,* 2001; 101: 26-33.

4. Porth CM. *Pathophysiology: Concepts of Altered Health States*, 3rd ed. Philadelphia: Lippincott, 1990.

5. Anderson EL. Arrhythmogenic right ventricular dysplasia. *Am Fam Physician,* 2006; 73: 1391-1398.

6. Colucci WS, Braunwald E. Pathophysiology of heart failure. In Zipes DP, Libby P, Bonow RO, et al. (Eds). *Braunwald's Heart Disease: A Textbook of Cardiovascular Medicine*, 7th ed. Philadelphia: Elsevier Saunders, pp. 509-538.

7. ONeill JO, Ng K. Heart failure with preserved systolic function. In: Griffin BP, Topol E. (Eds). *Manual of Cardiovascular Medicine*, 2nd ed. Philadelphia: Lippincott, Williams, & Wilkins, 2004, pp. 119-130.

8. Pinney SP, Mancini DM. Myocarditis and specific cardiomyopathies—Endocrine disease and alcohol. In: Fuster V, Alexander RW, O'Rourke RA, et al. (Eds.). *Hurst's The Heart*, 11th ed., Vol 2. New York: McGraw-Hill, 2004, pp. 1949-1974.

9. Tang WHW. Heart failure with systolic dysfunction. In: Griffin BP, Topol EJ. (Eds.). *Manual of Cardiovascular Medicine*, 2nd ed. Philadelphia: Lippincott, Williams, & Wilkins, 2004, pp. 101-118.

10. Chatterjee K. Physical examination in heart failure. In: Hosenpud JD, Greenberg BH (Eds.). *Congestive Heart Failure: Pathophysiology, Diagnosis, and Comprehensive Approach to Management,* 2nd ed. Philadelphia: Lippincott, Williams, & Wilkins, 2000, pp. 615-627.

11. Greenberg BH. The medical management of chronic congestive heart failure. In: Hosenpud JD, Greenberg BH. (Eds). *Congestive Heart Failure: Pathophysiology, Diagnosis, and Comprehensive Approach to Management,* 2nd ed. Philadelphia: Lippincott, Williams, & Wilkins, 2000, pp. 673-693.

12. Lessig ML.The cardiovascular system. In: Alspach JG. (Ed.). *Core Curriculum for Critical Care Nursing*, 6th ed. St. Louis: Elsevier Saunders, 2006, pp. 185-380.

13. Heart Failure Society of America. *The Stages of Heart Failure – NYHA Classification,* 2006. Heart Failure Society of America.

14. American College of Cardiology / American Heart Association, *ACC/AHA Guidelines for the Evaluation and Management of Chronic Heart Failure in the Adult*. 2001.

15. Grady KL, Drakup K, Kennedy G, et al. Team management of patients with heart failure: A statement for healthcare professionals from the Cardiovascular Nursing Council of the American Heart Association. *Circulation,* 2000; 102: 2443-2456.

16. Tokarczyk TR. Cardiac transplantation as a treatment option for the heart failure patient. *Crit Care Nurs Q,* 2003; 26: 61-68.

17. Gibbs RC, Davies MK, Lip GYH. ABC of heart failure: Management: Digoxin and other inotropes, B blockers, and antiarrhythmic and antithrombotic treatment. *Br Med J,* 2000; 320: 490-498.

18. Davies MK, Gibbs CR, Lip GYH. ABC of heart failure. Management. Diuretics, ACE inhibitors, and nitrates. *Br Med J,* 2000; 320: 428-431.

19. Ammon S. Managing patients with heart failure. *Am J Nurs,* 2001; 101: 34-40.

20. Barnard CN. Human cardiac transplantation: An evaluation of the first two operations performed at the Groote Schuur Hospital, Cape Town. *Am J Cardiol,* 1968; 22: 584-596.

21. Caves PK, Stinson EB, Graham AF, et al. Percutaneous transvenous endomyocardial biopsy. *J Am Medical Assoc,* 1973; 225: 288-291.

22. Borel JF, Feurer C, Gubler HU, et al. Biological effects of cyclosporine A: A new antilymphocytic agent. *Agents Actions*, 1976; 6: 468-475.

23. Horvath KA, Fullerton DA. Heart transplantation. In: Stuart FP, Abecassis MM, Kaufman DB. (Eds). *Organ Transplantation*, 2nd ed. Georgetown, TX: Landes Bioscience, 2003. pp. 261-279.

24. Mehra MR, Kobashigawa J, Starling R, et al. Listing criteria for heart transplantation: International Society for Heart and Lung Transplantation Guidelines for the Care of Cardiac Transplant Candidates - 2006. *J Heart Lung Transplant*, 2006; 25: 1024-1042.

25. Cupples SA, Boyce SW, Stamou SC. Heart transplantation. In: Cupples SA, Ohler L, (Eds.). *Solid Organ Transplantation: A Handbook for Primary Health Care Providers*. New York: Springer, 2002; pp. 146-188.

26. Taylor DO, Edwards LB, Boucek MM, et al. Registry of the International Society for Heart and Lung Transplantation: Twenty-second Official Adult Heart Transplant Report – 2006. *J Heart Lung Transplant*, 2006; 25: 869-879.

27. Borkon AM, Stuart RS. Heart. In: Baumgartner WA, Reitz B, Kasper EK, et al. (Eds.). *Heart and Lung Transplantation*, 2nd ed. Philadelphia: Saunders, 2002. pp. 219-224.

28. Bakr M. Induction therapy. *Exp Clin Transplant*, 2005; 3: 320-328.

29. Szeto WY, Rosengard BR. Basic concepts in transplantation immunology and pharmacologic immuosuppression. In: Baumgartner WA, Reitz B, Kasper EK, et al. (Eds.). *Heart and Lung Transplantation*, 2nd ed. Philadelphia: Saunders, 2002. pp. 15-25.

30. Hoffman FM. Outcomes and complications after heart transplantation: A review. *J Cardiovasc Nurs*, 2005; 20: 531-542.

31. Lower RR, Stofer RC, Shumway NW. Homovital transplantation of the heart. *J Thorac Cardiovasc Surg*, 1961; 41: 196-204.

32. Rees AP, Milani RV, Lavie CJ, et al. Valvular regurgitation and right-sided cardiac pressures in heart transplant recipients by complete Doppler and color flow evaluation. *Chest*, 1993; 104: 82-87.

33. Aziz TM, Burgess MI, El-Gamel A, et al. Orthotopic cardiac transplantation techniques: A survey of current practice. *Ann Thorac Surg*, 1999; 68: 1242-1246.

34. Miniati DN, Robbins RC. Techniques in orthotopic cardiac transplantation: A review. *Cardiol Rev*, 2001; 9: 131-136.

35. El Gamel A, Yonan NA, Grant S, et al. Orthotopic cardiac transplantation: A comparison of standard and bicaval Wythenshawe techniques. *J Thorac Cardiovasc Surg*, 1995; 109: 721-729.

36. Deleuze PH, Benvenuti C, Mazzucotelli JP, et al. Orthotopic cardiac transplantation with direct caval anastomosis: Is it the optimal procedure? *J Thorac Cardiovasc Surg*, 1995; 109: 731-737.

37. Barnard CN, Losman JG. Left ventricular bypass. *S Afr Med J*, 1975; 49: 303-312.

38. Newcomb AE, Esmore DS, Rosenfeldt FL, et al. Heterotopic heart transplantation: An expanding role in the twenty-first century? *Ann Thorac Surg*, 2004; 78: 1345-1350.

39. Peck EA, Redmond JM. Heterotopic heart transplantation. In: Baumgartner WA, Reitz B, Kasper E, et al. (Eds.). *Heart and Lung Transplantation*, 2nd ed. Philadelphia: Saunders, 2002. pp. 5113-5120.

40. Augustine S, Ohler L. Postoperative care and immunosuppressive monitoring—Nursing care. In: Baumgartner WA, Reitz B, Kasper EK, et al. (Eds.). *Heart and Lung Transplantation*, 2nd ed. Philadelphia: Saunders, 2002. pp. 233-245.

41. Wade CR, Reith KK, Sikora JH, et al. Postoperative nursing care of the cardiac transplant recipient. *Crit Care Nurs Q*, 2004; 27: 17-28.

42. Kirklin JK, Young JB, McGiffin DC. *Heart Transplantation*. New York: Churchill Livingstone, 2002.

43. Kobashigawa JA. Physiology of the transplanted heart. In: Norman DJ, Turka LA (Eds). *Primer on Transplantation*, 2nd ed. Mt. Laurel, NJ: American Society of Transplantation, 2001. pp. 358-362.

44. Bernardi L, Bianchini B, Spadacini G, et al. Demonstrable cardiac reinnervation after human heart transplantation by carotid baroreflex modulation of RR interval. *Circulation*, 1995; 92: 2859-2903.

45. Cotts WG, Oren RM. Function of the transplanted heart: Unique physiology and therapeutic implications. *Am J Med Sci,* 1997; 314: 164-174.

46. Wilson RF, Christensen BV, Olivari MT, et al. Evidence for structural sympathetic reinnervation after orthotopic cardiac transplantation in humans. *Circulation,* 1991; 83: 1210-1220.

47. Marino PL. *The ICU Book.* Philadelphia: Lea Febiger, 1991.

48. Vitello-Cicciu J, Eagan JS. Data acquisition from the cardiovascular system. In: Kinney MR, Packa DR, Dunbar SB. (Eds.). *AACN's Clinical Reference for Critical-Care Nursing.* New York: McGraw-Hill, 1988. pp. 530-570.

49. Tolman DE, Taylor DO, Olsen SL, et al. Heart transplantation. In: Makowka L, Sher L. (Eds.). *Handbook of Organ Transplantation.* Austin, TX: Landes, 1995. pp. 107-131.

50. Ellstrom K. The pulmonary system. In: Alspach JG (Ed.). *Core Curriculum for Critical Care Nursing,* 6th ed. St. Louis: Saunders Elsevier, 2006. pp. 45-183.

51. Augustine S, Baumgartner WA, Stuart RS, et al. Heart and lung transplantation and cardiomyoplasty for end-stage cardiopulmonary disease. In: Baumgartner WA, Owens SG, Cameron DE, et al. (Eds.). *The Johns Hopkins Manual of Cardiac Surgical Care,* 1994. St. Louis: Mosby. p. 461-484.

52. Kirklin JK. Immediate postoperative management of the heart transplant recipient. In: Norman DJ, Turka LA (Eds.). *Primer on Transplantation,* 2nd ed. Mt. Laurel, NJ: American Society of Transplantation, 2001. pp. 352-357.

53. Chernecky CC, Berger BJ. *Laboratory Tests and Diagnostic Procedures,* 2nd ed. Philadelphia: Saunders, 1997.

54. Tucker PC. Infectious complications. In: Baumgartner WA, Reitz B, Kasper E, et al. (Eds.). Heart and lung transplantation 2nd ed., Philadelphia. Saunders, 2002. pp. 355-71.

55. Berry GJ, Billingham ME. Pathology of human cardiac transplantation. In: Baumgartner WA, Reitz B, Kasper EK, et al. (Eds.). *Heart and Lung Transplantation,* 2nd ed. Philadelphia: Saunders, 2002. pp. 286-306.

56. VanBuskirk AM, Pidwell DJ, Adams PW, et al. Transplantation immunology. *J Am Medical Assoc,* 1997; 278: 1993-1999.

57. Eisen H. Left ventricular dysfunction after cardiac transplantation: Etiologies, diagnosis and treatment. In: Norman DJ, Turka LA (Eds.). *Primer on Transplantation,* 2nd ed. Mt. Laurel, NJ: American Society of Transplantation, 2001. pp. 366-369.

58. Cotts WG, Johnson MR. The challenge of rejection and cardiac allograft vasculopathy. *Heart Failure Reviews,* 2001; 6: 227-240.

59. Cupples SA. Heart transplantation. In: Cupples SA, Ohler L, (Eds.). *Transplantation Nursing Secrets.* Philadelphia: Hanley & Belfus, 2003. pp. 85-105.

60. Billingham ME, Cary NR, Hammond ME, et al. A working formulation for the standardization of nomenclature in the diagnosis of heart and lung rejection: Heart Rejection Study Group. The International Society for Heart Transplantation. *J Heart Transplant,* 1990; 9: 587-593.

61. Mehra M. The emergence of genomic and proteomic biomarkers in heart transplantation. *J Heart Lung Transplant,* 2005; 2005: S213-S218.

62. Baughman KL. History and current techniques of endomyocardial biopsy. In: Baumgartner WA, Reitz B, Kasper DL, et al. (Eds.). *Heart and Lung Transplantation,* 2nd ed. Philadelphia: Saunders, 2002. pp. 267-281.

63. Hammond EH, Yowell RI, Price GD, et al. Vascular rejection and its relationship to coronary artery disease. *J Heart Lung Transplant,* 1992; 11(3 Pt 2): 111-119.

64. Koransky ML, Robbins RC. Additional strategies in immunosuppression. In: Baumgartner WA, Reitz B, Kasper E, et al. (Eds.). *Heart and Lung Transplantation,* 2nd ed. Philadelphia: Saunders, 2002. pp. 341-351.

65. McNamara D, Di Salvo T, Mathier M, et al. Left ventricular dysfunction after heart transplantation: Incidence and role of enhanced immunosuppression. *J Heart Lung Transplant,* 1996; 15: 506-515.

66. Stewart S, Winters GL, Fishbein MC, et al. Revision of the 1990 working formulation for the standardization of nomenclature in the diagnosis of heart rejection. J *Heart Lung Transplant,* 2005; 24: 1710-1720.

67. Valantine H. Cardiac allograft vasculopathy after heart transplantation. *J Heart Lung Transplant,* 2004; 23(5 Suppl): S187-S193.

68. Fishbein MC. Pathologic findings of cardiac dysfunction. In: Norman DJ, Turka LA (Eds.). *Primer on Transplantation,* 2nd ed. Mt. Laurel, NJ: American Society of Transplantation, pp. 370-374.

69. Kirklin J. Management of the recipient during the transplant hospitalization. In: Kirklin JK, Young JB McGiffin DC. (Eds.). *Heart Transplantation,* New York: Churchill Livingstone, 2002. pp. 375-389.

70. Bittner HB, Chen EP, Biswas SS, et al. Right ventricular dysfunction after cardiac transplantation: Primarily related to status of donor heart. *Ann Thorac Surg,* 1999; 68: 1605-1611.

71. Stobierska-Dzierzek B, Awad H, Michler RE. The evolving management of acute right-sided heart failure in cardiac transplant. *J Am Coll Cardiol,* 2001; 38: 923-931.

72. Fleischer KJ, Stuart RS. Postoperative hemodynamics. In: Baumgartner WA, Owens SG, Cameron DE, et al. (Eds.). *The Johns Hopkins Manual of Cardiac Surgical Care.* St. Louis: Mosby, 1994. pp. 119-160.

73. Traill TA. Physiology and function of the transplant cardiac allograft. In: Baumgartner WA, Reitz B, Kasper E, et al. (Eds.). *Heart and Lung Transplantation,* 2nd ed. Philadelphia: Saunders, 2002. pp. 456-466.

74. Scott CD, Dark JH, McComb JM. Arrhythmias after cardiac transplantation. *Am J Cardiol,* 1992; 70: 1061-1063.

75. Brady CL. *Fluids and Electrolytes Made Incredibly Easy.* Philadelphia: Lippincott, Williams, & Wilkins, 2005.

76. Heitmiller ES. Monitoring the cardiac surgery patient. In: Baumgartner WA, Owens SG, Cameron DE, et al. (Eds.). *The Johns Hopkins Manual of Cardiac Surgical Care.* St. Louis: Mosby, 1994. pp. 95-118.

77. Husain AN, Kumar V. The lung. In: Kumar V, Abbas AK, Fausto N. (Eds.). *Robbins and Cotran Pathologic Basis of Disease.* Philadelphia: Elsevier Saunders, 2004. pp. 711-772.

78. Cupples SA. Infectious disease. In: Cupples SA, Ohler L, (Eds.). *Transplantation Nursing Secrets.* Philadelphia: Hanley & Belfus, 2003. pp. 247-270.

79. Bojar RM. Manual of *Perioperative Care in Adult Cardiac Surgery,* 4th ed. Malden, MA: Blackwell Sciences, 1999.

80. Jarquin-Valdivia AA, Wijdicks EF, McGregor C. Neurologic complications following heart transplantation in the modern era: Decreased incidence, but postoperative stroke remains prevalent. *Transplant Proc,* 1999; 31: 2161-2162.

81. Mythen MG. Postoperative gastrointestinal tract dysfunction. *Anesth Analg,* 2005; 100: 196-204.

82. Hasse J. Nutritional issues in adult organ transplantation. In: Cupples SA, Ohler L. (Eds.). *Solid Organ Transplantation: A Handbook for Primary Health Care Providers.* New York: Springer, 2002. pp. 64-87.

83. Grady KL, Naftel D, Pamboukian SV, et al. Post-operative obesity and cachexia are risk factors for morbidity and mortality after heart transplant: Multi-institutional study of post-operative weight change. *J Heart Lung Transplant,* 2005; 24: 1424-1430.

REVIEW QUESTIONS

1. You are caring for a 55-year-old female heart transplant recipient who had severe liver dysfunction prior to transplantation. On postoperative day 2, you assume care of this patient at 7 AM and you observe the following trends that occurred on the night shift: Decreasing hemoglobin and hematocrit; decreasing cardiac output and cardiac index, increasing chest tube output, and increasing oxygen requirements. During your first assessment, you note the following: Cardiac index: 2.8 L/min/m², systolic pressure: 88 mm Hg, HR: 140 bpm, chest tube output: 200 mL/hour. You notify the physician and anticipate orders for:
   1. Anti-rejection therapy
   2. Blood products
   3. Protamine
   4. Stripping of chest tubes
   5. Increased immunosuppression
   6. Preparation of patient for return to OR

   a. 1, 2, and 3
   b. 1, 4, and 5
   c. 2, 3, and 6
   d. 2, 3, and 4

2. A 56-year-old male transplant recipient develops metabolic acidosis secondary to hyperkalemia. His symptoms of hyperkalemia would likely include:
   a. Skeletal muscle weakness, irregular pulse, inverted T waves on ECG
   b. Increased deep tendon reflexes, nausea, vomiting
   c. Constipation, small muscle hypoactivity, irregular pulse
   d. Skeletal muscle weakness, tall peaked T waves on ECG, nausea, and vomiting

3. Immediately following heart transplantation, the nurse notices the following vital signs:

Time	Urine Output	CVP	Blood Pressure	Heart Rate
11 AM	200 cc/hour	12 mmHg	150/100	110 bpm
12 noon	150 cc/hour	10 mm Hg	140/98	90 bpm
1 PM	100 cc/hour	8 mm Hg	128/78	88 bpm
2 PM	25 cc/hour	4 mm Hg	98/70	100 bpm

The nurse should anticipate an order for:

a. A diuretic
b. An IV fluid bolus
c. A vasodilator
d. A pacemaker

4. A 56-year-old male transplant candidate is admitted to the hospital for worsening heart failure. His signs and symptoms would likely include:
    a. Rising serum creatinine level, decreasing serum sodium level, and increasing brain natriuretic peptide level
    b. Rising serum creatinine level, increasing serum sodium level, and decreasing brain natriuretic peptide level
    c. Heart rate > 85 bpm, systolic blood pressure < 80 mm Hg, and decreasing brain natriuretic peptide level
    d. Increasing peripheral edema, decreasing abdominal fullness, and increased responsiveness to diuretics

5. You are caring for a 44-year-old male heart transplant recipient in the step-down unit who suddenly becomes bradycardic. You should anticipate an order for:
    a. Atropine
    b. Isoproterenol
    c. Nitroprusside
    d. Digoxin

6. Absolute contraindications to heart transplantation would be:
    1. History of carcinoma within the last year
    2. History of alcohol abuse
    3. Recent pulmonary infarction
    4. Positive cytomegalovirus IgG antibody

    a. 1 and 3
    b. 1 and 4
    c. 2 and 4
    d. 3 and 4

7. The clinical manifestations of rejection are likely to include:
    1. Hypertension
    2. Fever >101° F
    3. Hypotension
    4. Atrial dysrhythmias

    a. 1 and 2
    b. 3 and 4
    c. 2 and 4
    d. 1 and 4

8. Your patient is 5 days post–heart transplantation and has just had his first endo-myocardial biopsy. When he returns to the step-down unit, you notice the following vital signs:

Time	CVP	Blood Pressure	Heart Rate	Urine Output
11 AM	6 mm Hg	110/90	110 bpm	200 cc/hour
12 noon	8 mm Hg	100/86	90 bpm	150 cc/hour
1 PM	12 mm Hg	90/84	72 bpm	100 cc/hour
2 PM	15 mm Hg	80/62	68 bpm	25 cc/hour

You suspect that the patient has:

a. Rejection
b. Acute renal failure
c. Cardiac tamponade
d. Sepsis

9. Clinical manifestations of infection in a heart transplant recipient may include:
1. Fever ($\geq$ 38° Celcius/100.4° Fahrenheit)
2. Negative C-reactive protein
3. Leukocytosis
4. Elevated sedimentation rate

a. 1, 2, and 3
b. 1, 2, and 4
c. 2, 3, and 4
d. 1, 3, and 4

10. Premature atrial or ventricular contractions in a heart transplant recipient are most often due to:
a. Hypokalemia and/or hypomagnesemia
b. Hypercalcemia and/or hypophosphatemia
c. Hyponatremia and/or hyperphosphatemia
d. Hypophosphatemia and/or hypernatremia

11. As a result of denervation of the donor heart, heart transplant recipients are likely to:
1. Have a higher resting heart rate
2. Have a lower resting heart rate
3. Experience angina
4. Have an altered response to certain cardiac drugs
5. Have an altered diurnal variation in blood pressure

a. 2, 3, and 5
b. 1, 3, and 5
c. 1, 4, and 5
d. 2, 4, and 5

12. In your discharge teaching, you would tell patients to report which of the following signs and/or symptoms that might indicate complications after an endomyocardial biopsy?
    1. Severe pain at site of puncture wound
    2. Nausea or vomiting
    3. Shortness of breath
    4. Chest or arm pain

    a. 1, 2, and 4
    b. 2, 3, and 4
    c. 1, 2, and 3
    d. 1, 3, and 4

13. Coronary artery vasculopathy is thought to be a form of:
    a. Chronic graft rejection
    b. Hyperacute rejection
    c. Acute humoral rejection
    d. Acute cellular rejection

14. In a heart transplant recipient, the clinical manifestations of a myocardial infarction *typically* may include:
    1. Fatigue
    2. Dyspnea
    3. Angina
    4. Dysrhythmias

    a. 1, 2, and 3
    b. 1, 2, and 4
    c. 2, 3, and 4
    d. 1, 3, and 4

15. Clinical manifestations of mediastinitis include:
    a. Increasing and/or purulent wound drainage
    b. Separation of wound edges
    c. Sternal pain or tenderness
    d. All of the above

Correct answers:

1. c	5. b	9. d	13. a
2. d	6. a	10. a	14. b
3. b	7. b	11. c	15. d
4. a	8. c	12. d	

10 Lung and Heart-Lung Transplantation

CONNIE WHITE-WILLIAMS

CHRISTIANE KUGLER

BRIAN WIDMAR

INTRODUCTION

I. Lung transplantation has evolved to become a treatment option for patients with end-stage pulmonary disease.

II. It has been over 40 years since the first successful human lung transplant was performed by Dr. James Hardy and his team at the University of Mississippi in 1963.[1]

A. That patient died 18 days later of renal failure. Similar to the experiences of other solid organ transplant pioneers, dismal outcomes resulted in slow progress.[2-4]

B. It took another 20 years when in 1986, the Stanford group performed the first successful heart-lung transplant.[5]

C. Also in 1986, the Toronto Lung Transplant Group reported the first successful single lung transplant.[6]

D. These noteworthy events led to a series of clinical advances in the area of lung transplantation, including advancements in immunosuppression, avoidance of steroids immediately postoperatively, utilization of the bronchial wrap, and improved selection criteria.[7-11]

III. Two decades later, lung transplantation has become an established treatment choice for selected patients with different end-stage lung diseases, leading to increased survival, and undoubted improvements in quality of life.

A. Remarkable progress has occurred through refinements in surgical techniques and improved understanding of transplant immunology and microbiology.

B. Estimated 1-year survival is 74%, and the 5-year survival is 47%.[12]

C. Despite these improvements in short- and intermediate-term survival, prolonged survival following lung transplantation is reduced in comparison to other solid organ transplantation results. It is limited by the prevalence of chronic allograft rejection, known as bronchiolitis obliterans syndrome (BOS), and by the worldwide shortage of donor organs, which unfortunately leads to mortality rates on the waiting list of approximately 20%.[13]

RECIPIENT EVALUATION AND SELECTION

I. Indications for lung transplantation
  A. Lung transplantation is indicated when other options (medical and surgical) of therapeutic interventions are exhausted and the predicted life expectancy is less than 24 months.
  B. Lung transplant candidates typically:
    1. Are oxygen-dependent
    2. Experience severe exercise intolerance
    3. Are younger than 65 years of age
    4. Report a poor quality of life
  C. Table 10-1 lists diseases currently accepted as indications for lung transplantation (single or bilateral) or a combined heart and lung transplantation at most transplant centers.
    1. The most common indications for lung transplantation are:
      a. Chronic obstructive pulmonary disease (COPD)
      b. Idiopathic pulmonary fibrosis (IPF)
      c. Pulmonary hypertension
      d. Cystic fibrosis
  D. Contraindications for lung transplantation
    1. In 1998, selection criteria were published and endorsed by leading societies in the field to standardize the selection process and to provide evidence-based practice quidelines.[11]
    2. Detailed criteria concerning medical conditions that may have an impact on transplant selection eligibility and contraindication of lung transplantation can be seen in Tables 10-2 and 10-3.
    3. Currently, the International Society for Heart and Lung Transplantation (ISHLT) is adopting these guidelines.[14]
    4. Despite the recommended guidelines, controversial issues with respect to the candidate selection appear in the literature.
    5. Those include handling of upper age limits, selection of patients colonized or infected with antibiotic-resistant organisms, history of noncompliance, and limitations due to physical conditions.[15-17]

PATIENT REFERRAL AND EVALUATION OF POTENTIAL CANDIDATES

I. Patients are usually referred to the lung transplant program by their local pulmonologist or primary care physician.
  A. Medical information is sent to the transplant center for review.
  B. The patient is then scheduled for a clinic visit to determine:
    1. Whether the patient does indeed have end-stage disease
    2. If the patient has any conditions that may preclude lung transplantation
  C. Timing of the referral is one of the most important aspects in lung transplantation.
    1. Referring too late may result in the patient being too sick for transplantation or unable to survive the long waiting times.

TABLE 10-1
■ Diseases Treated by Lung Transplantation

Single Lung Transplantation

- Chronic obstructive pulmonary diseases

    Emphysema with or without alpha$_1$-antitrypsin deficiency

- Interstitial lung diseases

    Idiopathic interstitial pulmonary fibrosis
    Sarcoidosis
    Eosinophilic granuloma
    Lymphangioleiomyomatosis

- Pulmonary vascular diseases

    Primary pulmonary hypertension
    Eisenmenger's syndrome with cardiac repair

Bilateral Sequential Lung Transplantation

- Infectious lung diseases

    Cystic fibrosis
    Bronchiectasis

- Chronic obstructive pulmonary disease

    Emphysema

- Pulmonary vascular diseases

    Primary pulmonary hypertension
    Eisenmenger's syndrome with cardiac repair

- Bronchoalveolar carcinoma (at some centers)

Heart-Lung Transplantation

- Pulmonary vascular diseases

    Primary pulmonary hypertension
    Eisenmenger's syndrome with cardiac repair

TABLE 10-2
■ Medical Conditions Impacting Lung Transplantation Eligibility

- Severe osteoporosis (e.g., symptomatic compression fractures)

- Severe musculoskeletal disease

- Current use of corticosteroids: dose > 20 mg daily

- Malnutrition: < 70% or > 130% of ideal body weight

- Substance abuse or addiction

- Cigarette smoking within 4-6 months of activation on the waiting list

- Psychosocial problems that place patient at high risk of poor outcome

- Requirement of mechanical ventilation

- Colonization of respiratory tract with fungi or atypical mycobacterium

- Previous thoracotomy, sternotomy, pneumonectomy, or extensive pleural scarring

TABLE 10-3

■ **Contraindications to Lung Transplantation**

General Contraindications

Presence of any condition that would itself shorten life expectancy or increase the risk of death from rejection or complications of immunosuppression

General—Absolute Contraindications for Organ Transplantation

- Active infection
- Malignant disease—patients should be tumor-free for at least 5 years prior to consideration for transplantation
- HIV
- Active peptic ulcer disease
- Active drug, tobacco, or alcohol abuse
- Severe, irreversible organ system damage other than organ to be transplanted
- Inability to understand the procedure or the risks involved or comply with follow-up care
- History of failure to comply with medical regimen
- History of marked depression or emotional instability
- Lack of functional psychosocial support system
- Lack of financial resources to pay for surgery, hospitalizations, medications, and follow-up care
- History of smoking within last 6 months
- Inability to make strong commitment to transplantation
- Cognitive impairment severe enough to limit comprehension of medical regimen
- Psychiatric instability severe enough to jeopardize incentive for adherence to medical regimen
- Failure of established stable address or telephone number

Lung Transplant-Specific Absolute Contraindications

- Age: >65 for single-lung, >55 for bilateral lung, >45 for heart-lung
- Corticosteroid dependency: >20 mg of prednisone or equivalent per day
- Significant, untreatable coronary artery disease: greater than one vessel coronary artery disease
- Cardiac insufficiency: right or left ventricular ejection fraction <20%
- Dependent on mechanical ventilation and clinically unstable
- Significant infection present outside the lungs and upper respiratory tract
- Obesity: body weight > 140% predicted
- Cachexia: body weight < 80% predicted
- Active, systemic collagen vascular disease
- Nonrehabilitative pulmonary disability
- Six-minute walk < 150 meters at some centers
- Creatinine clearance < 50mg/ml/min
- Bleeding diathesis
- Surgically remediable chronic thromboembolic disease
- Complicated or uncontrolled diabetes mellitus
- Significantly impaired hepatic function with persistent marked elevation of liver function tests (AST, ALT, total bilirubin)
- Hepatitis B virus antigen positive
- Hepatitis C virus infection with biopsy-proven evidence of liver disease

2. Careful consideration of the natural history and prognosis of the underlying primary disease is crucial in this decision process.
3. Measures of quality of life with and without transplant must be weighed.[18]
4. Attention should be given to:
   a. The candidate's age at time of referral
   b. Associated consequences of the lung disease on other organ systems
   c. Current physical condition
5. Waiting time for donor lungs and for combined heart and lungs needs to be factored in the time of referral and listing for transplantation.[19]

TRANSPLANT EVALUATION

I. The transplant evaluation consists of a number of medical tests and consultations.
   A. Ensures that the individual is an appropriate candidate
   B. Minimizes the risk associated with the transplant surgery
   C. Consists of objective measures of end-stage organ failure (Table 10-4) and a psychosocial assessment including cognitive functioning, history of psychiatric disorders, compliance issues, history of substance abuse, and status of social support.[20-21]
II. The transplant evaluation consists of a series of tests, procedures, and assessments that may take 3-5 days to complete.
III. The evaluation (Table 10-5) is usually completed on an outpatient basis unless the patient is acutely ill.
IV. Lung transplant candidates undergo a complete medical history and physical assessment including the following:
   A. Vital signs
   B. Hemodynamic parameters
   C. Skin testing
   D. Physical conditioning
   E. Body weight
V. Full laboratory work assessment is performed with special attention to:
   A. Blood type and antibody screening
   B. Hematology
   C. Chemistry
   D. Virology
   E. Immunopathology
VI. Radiology tests
   A. Chest x-ray
   B. Computed tomography scan (CT) with high-resolution images
   C. Magneto-resonance tomography scan (MRT)[22-26]
VII. The evaluation process can be a very stressful time for the patient and family.
   A. Many patients experience feelings of anxiety, ambivalence, and hopelessness during this process.
   B. The needs of the patient should be addressed by providing educational and emotional support to the patient and family.

TABLE 10-4
■ Objective Measures of Deteriorating Medical Condition

Primary Disease	Clinical Criteria
COPD/emphysema	$FEV_1 < 20$ % predicted
	$pCO_2 \leq 50$ mm Hg
	$pO_2 < 50$ mm Hg (rest)
	PAPm > 25 mm Hg
	Hypercapnia; pulmonary hypertension
Cystic fibrosis	$FEV_1 < 30$ % predicted
	$pCO_2 \leq 50$ mm Hg
	$pO_2 < 50$ mm Hg (rest)
	Rapid decline in FEV_1
	Frequent hospitalization, recurring hemoptysis, pneumothoraces, loss of body weight
Pulmonary fibrosis	VC or TLC < 60% predicted
	DLCO < 50%-60% predicted
	PAPm > 25 mm Hg
	Resting hypoxemia
	Pulmonary hypertension
	Progression of disease despite steroid therapy
Pulmonary hypertension	NYHA class III or IV
	Right arterial pressure > 10 mm Hg
	Pulmonary arterial pressure > 50 mm Hg
	Cardiac index < 2.5 L/min/m²
	Uncontrolled syncope, hemoptysis, or right heart failure

Abbreviations: FEV_1 = forced expiratory volume in one second; pCO_2 = carbon dioxide tension; PAPm= pulmonary arterial pressure by mean; VC= vital capacity; TLC= total lung capacity; DLCO= diffusing capacity of carbon monoxide; NYHA= New York Heart Association

TABLE 10-5
■ Evaluation Protocol for Lung Transplantation

GENERAL

Lab Tests/Blood Chemistries

- liver and renal profiles (bilirubin, SGOT [AST])
- alkaline phosphatase
- BUN
- creatinine
- calcium
- phosphorus
- magnesium
- serum electrolytes
- lipid profile
- stool for heme (x3)
- prostate-specific antigen (PSA)*

Hematology and Coagulation Profile

- complete blood cell count, differential
- platelet count
- prothrombin time (or International Normalized Ratio)
- partial thromboplastin time
- fibrinogen

Urine Tests

- urinalysis
- 24-hour urine for creatinine clearance
- 24-hour urine for protein if diabetic or if urinalysis positive for protein*

Scans

- nuclear renal scan with measurement of effective renal plasma flow (ERPF)
- ventilation-perfusion scan (V-Q scan)*
- C-T scan

Radiology and Ultrasound

- mammography*
- sinus films*
- chest x-ray
- abdominal ultrasound study (liver, pancreas, gallbladder, and kidney evaluation)
- carotid ultrasound*

(Continued next page.)

CONSULTATIONS AND PHYSICAL EXAMINATIONS

- complete history and physical examination
- respiratory therapist
- pulmonologist
- cardiologist
- transplant coordinator
- surgeon
- Infectious disease
- nutritional status evaluation
- social evaluation
- psychiatric evaluation
- neuropsychiatric evaluation (neurocognitive evaluation)
- dental evaluation

CARDIOVASCULAR

- electrocardiogram
- two-dimensional echocardiogram with Doppler study
- right heart catheterization with detailed hemodynamic evaluation
- left heart catheterization with coronary angiography*

IMMUNOLOGY

- ABO blood type and antibody screen
- panel reactive antibody (PRA) screen
- human leukocyte antigen (HLA) typing (if listed for transplantation)

PULMONARY

- chest x-ray (PA and lateral)
- pulmonary function testing with arterial blood gases
- six-minute walk at some centers

INFECTIOUS DISEASE SCREENING

Serologies for:

- hepatitis A, B, and C
- herpes virus
- human immunodeficiency virus (HIV)
- cytomegalovirus (CMV)
- toxoplasmosis
- varicella
- rubella
- Epstein-Barr virus
- venereal disease research laboratory (VDRL)
- lyme titers*
- histoplasmosis
- coccidioidomycosis complement fixing antibodies*

Cultures

- throat swab for viral cultures (CMV, adenovirus, herpes simplex virus)*
- urine culture and sensitivity*
- stool for ova and parasites*
- skin swabs for MRSA

Skin Test

- PPD (purified protein derivative) skin test with controls (i.e., mumps, dermatophytin, histoplasmosis, and coccidioidomycosis)*

Vaccinations

- hepatitis series
- pneumovax
- influenza each fall

*Only performed if appropriate or indicated.

LISTING PATIENTS FOR LUNG TRANSPLANTATION

I. When the evaluation is complete, the results are compiled and presented at a multidisciplinary transplant team meeting to review the information. Members of the transplant team requested to be present at the transplant evaluation include:
   A. Pulmonologists
   B. Cardiothoracic surgeons
   C. Cardiologists
   D. Respiratory therapists
   E. Dietitians
   F. Nurse coordinators
   G. Social workers
   H. Psychiatrists or psychologists
   I. Ethicists
II. The patient may fall into one of the following categories:
   A. Ready for transplantation and listing
   B. Defer a final decision
   C. Reassess after addressing unresolved issues
   D. Refuse the patient as a candidate
III. If the decision is made to list the patient as a candidate for transplant, this is discussed with the patient who ultimately decides if he/she wants to be placed on the waiting list for a donor organ.
IV. Candidates for lung transplantation are listed on a national computerized waiting list maintained by the United Network for Organ Sharing (UNOS), a private organization contracted by the federal government to allocate organs according to sharing policies.[27]
   A. Listing information consists of
      1. Patient name
      2. Age
      3. Sex
      4. Race

5. Social Security number
6. Blood group
7. Acceptable donor weight range
8. Whether a donor-specific crossmatch will be needed at the time of transplant
9. In addition, the medical severity of the candidate is indicated by lung allocation scores (LAS) to prioritize patients during the donor-recipient selection process.
B. Candidates are generally required to remain within a 2-hour drive of the transplant center.
   1. However, transplant centers may assist patients and families by making arrangements for air transportation when a donor organ becomes available.
   2. This allows patients at a greater distance from the transplant center the opportunity to wait for their transplant at home.

MANAGEMENT OF PATIENTS AWAITING LUNG TRANSPLANTATION

I. During the waiting period, the health status of the lung transplant candidate is monitored regularly.
II. Stable patients are usually followed in an outpatient clinic every 6-8 weeks.
III. It is important to impress upon the patient and family that the transplant team must be notified of any hospitalizations or deterioration in pulmonary or general health status.
IV. Many transplant centers require patients to participate in cardiopulmonary rehabilitation 2-3 times a week while they are awaiting their donor organ.

SIGNS OF DETERIORATION

I. Many investigations have explored the accompanying burdens of end-stage lung failure within the psychological and social dimensions.
A. Subjective complaints may include:
   1. Symptoms of increased anxiety and depression
   2. Fear of dying
   3. Increased shortness of breath
   4. Decreased exercise tolerance
   5. Increased dependence on others
   6. Weight loss
   7. These factors are multidimensional influences and may be interrelated.

EDUCATION OF THE PATIENT AWAITING LUNG TRANSPLANTATION

I. Patient and family education is an essential component of solid organ transplantation (see Chapter 3).
II. Educational issues begin to arise as soon as the patient is referred for transplant evaluation and becomes a potential candidate for a transplant.

III. Pretransplant education requires special attention to educating critically ill individuals.

A. They may be restricted in abilities to concentrate and learn due to poor oxygenation and anxiety.

B. Family members may be an important resource and may benefit from the education.

C. Topics that should be covered while the patient is awaiting transplant include:

    1. Waiting for a transplant
       a. Self-care
       b. Follow-up care with the transplant center
       c. Exercise program[28]
       d. Nutrition and weight management
          i. Cachectic patients may require nutritional supplements.
          ii. Obese patients require weight loss counseling.
       e. Support groups
       f. Communication with the transplant center
          i. Admission to other hospitals during the waiting period
          ii. Deterioration of condition

    2. Surgical procedure
       a. Type of incision

    3. Immediate postoperative course
       a. Education concerning the post-operative course
       b. Important topics to cover are the following:[22, 23, 25]
          i. Length of stay
          ii. Postoperative routines
          iii. Family and significant others visitation
          iv. Lines, tubes, and devices
          v. Pain management
          vi. Medications

    4. Long-term follow-up care post-transplantation
       a. Compliance
       b. Quality of life and realistic expectations
       c. Strategies to prevent respiratory infections
          i. Wearing a mask during a specified time after surgery
          ii. Good hand hygiene
          iii. Pet care
          iv. Construction projects at home or work
             a) Pulling up carpet
             b) Working with walls/ceilings
       d. Daily use of a spirometry device to monitor the lung function
       e. Immunosuppressive therapy is a key component for successful organ transplantation.
          i. Intended effect of medication
          ii. Compliance regarding timing, exact dosing, and intervals
          iii. Potential side effects
          iv. Management of symptom distress
          v. Monitoring medications
          vi. Potential drug interactions
             a) Over-the-counter medications
             b) Prescription drugs
             c) Food/drug interactions such as those with grapefruit/grapefruit juice

          f. Coverage of health care costs for the post-transplant treatment and expensive immunosuppressant medications can be one of the greatest concerns for patients and health care professionals.
              i. Without prescription benefits as part of their health insurance plan, transplant recipients face a significant challenge.
              ii. Refer to social worker or to transplant financial coordinator.
                  a) Identify potential resources
                  b) Apply for pharmacy assistance programs
          g. Returning to work after lung transplantation should be encouraged.
              i. Social worker may assist patients and families with return to work issues.
                  a) Insurance coverage concerns
                  b) Potential loss of Medicare benefits
          h. When to call the transplant center or coordinator on call.
          i. Frequency of follow-up visits to transplant center.

DONOR SELECTION

    I. Successful lung transplantation is dependent on optimal donor selection.[29, 30]
   II. Guidelines for the identification and management of potential lung donors have been reported by UNOS.
  III. Characteristics of optimal lung donors:
        A. Usually younger than 55 years of age
        B. No long history of smoking or pulmonary disease
        C. Clear chest radiograph
        D. $PaO_2 > 300$ mm Hg on 100% oxygen and 5 cm positive end expiratory pressure for 5 minutes
        E. No previous surgery, pulmonary contusions, or trauma
        F. Bronchoscopy should demonstrate clear airways
            1. Free of purulent or aspirated material
  IV. Donor and recipient size match is also an important factor considered during the selection process.

SURGICAL PROCEDURE

    I. Several types of lung procedures are utilized.
        A. Single lung transplantation, either left or right
        B. Bilateral sequential
        C. Double lung en bloc
        D. Heart-lung transplantation
        E. Living donor lobar transplant
   II. Determining the type of surgery depends on:[31-35]
        A. Underlying disease
        B. Recipient age
        C. Recipient anatomy
        D. Surgeon's preference (to some degree)
  III. Patients who are candidates for deceased donor lung transplantation may be considered for living donor lobar transplantation at select centers.
        A. Procedure requires two living donors.

B. Each donates a lower lobe of a lung to the recipient.
C. This procedure is usually reserved for cystic fibrosis patients.

IMMEDIATE POSTOPERATIVE CARE

I. Monitoring and maintenance of the lung transplant recipient begins as transport is completed from the operating room (OR) to the intensive care unit (ICU).
II. Communication and collaboration between intraoperative and postoperative teams is essential to a seamless transition.
III. Role of the nurse during this phase of recovery is:
   A. Ensure physiologic stability
      1. Obtain and document baseline measurements[34]
         a. Vital signs
            i. Vital signs fluctuate due to a physiological response to thoracic surgery and immunosuppressive therapy during the initial postoperative period.
            ii. Core body temperature will gradually increase with rewarming but might remain slightly hypothermic due to corticosteroid therapy.
            iii. During the early postoperative period, a decrease in blood pressure generally presents as a response to vasodilatation secondary to rewarming.
            iv. Regulation of blood pressure is generally achieved by vasopressor administration and gentle use of colloid fluids if necessary.[32]
            v. Heart rate will vary according to:
               a) Fluid volume status
               b) Vasopressor and inotropic therapy
               c) Body temperature
               d) Pain experienced by the patient
            vi. Respirations should remain within standard normal limits as ventilatory support is weaned.
               a) Oxygen saturation should remain within 90 to 100%.
   B. Telemetry monitoring
      1. Tachycardia may present initially as a response to:
         a. Fluid loss
         b. Bleeding
         c. Diuretic therapy
         d. Nebulizers
         e. Corticosteroids
         f. Pain
         g. Catecholamine release with stress response to surgery
      2. Cardiac dysrhythmia is fairly common after surgery, most often including:
         a. Atrial flutter or fibrillation
            i. Atrial flutter may be due to circus electrical movement related to inflammation near pulmonary vein and atrial cuff suture lines.[35]
            ii. Initial management of atrial dysrhythmias includes:
               a) Rate-controlling drugs such as diltiazem or verapamil

           b) Chronic anticoagulation therapy might be necessary should sinus rhythm not be restored.[37]
     b. Supraventricular tachycardia (SVT)[36]
     c. Dysrhythmias may be associated with electrolyte imbalances post-surgery.

C. Hemodynamic monitoring
    1. Hemodynamic status is closely monitored via a pulmonary artery catheter.[36]
       a. Maintaining a normal PAP is essential.
          i. Protects anastomosis sites
          ii. Prevents pulmonary edema in the early postoperative period
          iii. PAP pressures are maintained by diuretic administration or by inhaled nitric oxide therapy.[35]
              a) If fluid administration is necessary, gentle administration of colloid fluids are preferred over crystalloid due to increased capillary permeability common in transplanted lung tissue.[36]
       b. CI and mixed venous oxygen saturation (SvO$_2$) trends should be followed to ensure adequate tissue perfusion and oxygenation to end-organs.[38]
       c. Due to en bloc and sequential anastomoses of lung transplantation, pulmonary artery wedge pressures (PAWP) are usually not measured.
          i. Increase in arterial pressure may precipitate rupture of the pulmonary artery anastomosis.[36]
          ii. If measured, maintain PAWP at low normal level.

D. Maintain fluid and electrolyte balance
    1. Minimize edema formation
       a. Monitor urine output
       b. Intravenous (IV) fluid therapy
    2. Physiological or systemic responses to therapy should be included in the baseline examination of the patient.[35]
    3. Monitor electrolytes that may contribute to cardiac dysrhythmias

E. Identify and report potential complications
    1. Bleeding
    2. Acute or hyperacute rejection

F. Prevent infections
    1. Ensure strict hand hygiene for all caregivers and visitors

G. Neurologic assessment and pain control
    1. Neurologic assessment is crucial to determining arousal from anesthesia and assessment of levels of comfort.
       a. Neurologic assessment becomes especially important as serum immunosuppressant drug trough levels rise.
          i. Calcineurin inhibitors such as cyclosporine and tacrolimus have been associated with encephalopathy and vasculitis when serum drug levels become too elevated.
          ii. These conditions subsequently manifest as seizure activity, visual disturbances, headaches, confusion, or neuropathies.[35]
    2. Pain management:
       a. Allows earlier physical therapy, rehabilitation, ambulation
       b. Maximizes ventilation and decreases risk for atelectasis[35]

    c.   Current efforts to control pain have trended towards use of epidural catheters and patient-controlled analgesia (PCA), with gradual transition to oral medications for pain management.

    d.   Nonsteroidal anti-inflammatory drugs are generally avoided due to the concomitant nephrotoxic effects when combined with immunosuppressant drugs and antibiotics.[35]

H. Surgical site care

  1. Surgical site care is especially important in the postoperative care phase.

    a.   Immunosuppressive therapy can leave any invasive line or wound a potential source for infection.

       i.   Bacterial infection is typically the most common infection in the transplant recipient within the first month after surgery.[35]

    b.   Wound care and invasive line site care is part of daily routine management.

       i.   Most health care organizations have preestablished protocols especially created for transplant patients.

      ii. Most invasive lines are removed as soon as possible to prevent catheter-borne infections.

     iii. Assessment of surgical wounds should be done frequently to monitor for the beginnings of infective process.

         a) Early signs of infection should be reported immediately.

I. Monitor lab results

  1. Laboratory data and trends should be followed closely.

    a.   Monitor for complications of immunosuppressive therapy such as hepatotoxicity or acute renal insufficiency.

    b.   Daily complete blood counts (CBC) with differential

       i.   Assess for marrow depression related to medications

      ii. Assess for infections

    c.   Determine efficacy of immunosuppressive therapy

       i.   Trough levels (i.e., cyclosporine or tacrolimus)

      ii. Assess therapeutic levels

J. Monitor for complications

  1. Hyperacute rejection is an antibody-mediated process which can be seen immediately post-implantation or within hours of transplant.

    a.   Routine screening for preformed or panel-reactive antibodies (PRA) prior to transplantation has made hyperacute rejection a relatively uncommon occurrence.[35]

    b.   May present as acute desaturation and tissue hypoxia, or by noticeable radiographic changes

  2. Acute or cellular-mediated rejection

    a.   Immune response occurs within the first 12 weeks post-transplant in as many as 60%-75% of recipients.[39]

    b.   Symptoms of acute rejection are generally nonspecific and may include one or more of the following:

       i.   Fatigue

      ii. Malaise

     iii. Dyspnea

     iv. Fever

      v. Chest pressure[35]

c. The attending physician or house officer should be notified immediately upon assessment of any of these symptoms postoperatively, and prompt intervention should be anticipated.

d. Symptoms may be similar to those seen with infection.

   i. Must differentiate between infection and rejection.

3. Primary graft dysfunction (PGD)

   a. Also known as reperfusion injury or implantation response

   b. Major cause of morbidity and mortality in lung transplant recipients

   c. Comparable to acute respiratory distress syndrome (ARDS)

   d. Possible causes are related to:

      i. Increased capillary permeability of transplanted lung tissue

      ii. Interrupted lymphatic drainage from transplant and cardiopulmonary bypass (CPB)

      iii. Edema from an extended ischemic time

      iv. Overall change in compliance and vascular resistance in donor and recipient[35]

   e. Potential warning signs for graft dysfunction that should be reported promptly[36]

      i. General malaise

      ii. Increased work of breathing

      iii. Activity intolerance

      iv. Frequent oxygen desaturation

   f. Current treatment options for PGD are similar to those for ARDS

      i. Generous oxygen concentrations

      ii. Lower tidal volumes

      iii. Positive pressure ventilation

      iv. For extubated patients:

         a) Generous oxygen supplementation

         b) Aggressive pulmonary toileting is essential to prevent further complications

   g. Current research strategies investigate the use of complement inhibitors

      i. Nitric oxide (NO) inhalation

      ii. Prostaglandin infusions to prevent primary graft dysfunction[34]

   h. Patients may exhibit persistent PGD refractory to the interventions listed above. In this instance:

      i. Extracorporeal membranous oxygenation (ECMO) may provide a temporary support and allow for lung rest.

      ii. Long-term efficacy of this intervention remains controversial.[34]

4. Inadequate bronchial anastomosis

   a. Along with primary graft dysfunction, inadequate bronchial anastomosis remains a major cause of increased morbidity during the early postoperative period following lung transplantation.[35]

      i. Bronchial dehiscence and stenosis are the two major airway complications seen.

      ii. Improved organ preservation and surgical anastomosis techniques have greatly diminished the occurrence of dehiscence.

   iii. Tracheal stenosis most often occurs concurrently with acute allograft rejection.

    a) Symptoms commonly reported are stridor; palpable tracheal rumble on examination; and intermittent hypoxemia resolved by expectoration of secretions

    b) Urgent bronchoscopy is done to determine diagnosis.

    c) Treatment for this complication generally includes high-dose corticosteroids, balloon dilatation of the stenotic area, and bronchial stenting.[35]

5. Pleural complications: pneumothorax

 a. Resolution of pneumothorax occurs within 1-2 days postoperatively.

  i. Two thoracostomy drains are placed into the anterior and posterior pleura during surgery.

  ii. A small but persistent air leak is commonly noted.

   a) Often related to undersized donor lungs[35]

  iii. Presence of subcutaneous air should be assessed daily.

 b. Reexpansion of the transplanted lung should be evaluated.

  i. Daily chest radiographs

  ii. Following reexpansion, the chest tube suction system is generally placed to water seal.

   a) Allows serous and sanguineous drainage to occur by gravity

   b) Chest tube drains are removed sequentially.[35]

    1) Fluid typically drains from anterior to posterior in the supine position.

     i) The anterior tube is usually discontinued first.

     ii) The posterior tube is generally removed after there is no further evidence of persistent pneumothorax, air leak, or drainage.

 c. Indications of airway compromise that should be reported immediately are stridor, dyspnea, hoarseness, and dysphonia.

6. Monitor for chylothorax: chylothorax occurs more commonly in pediatric transplant recipients.

 a. It may occur in adults if trauma or manipulation of the thoracic duct occurs during surgery.

 b. It appears as a milky white discharge of lipid-rich lymphatic drainage in pleural fluid.

 c. Definitive diagnostic testing includes pleural fluid analysis for triglycerides and cholesterol levels.[40]

 d. A rapidly reaccumulating chylothorax should be addressed and treated, as this may inhibit lung expansion and oxygenation.

 e. Chest tube drains remain in place until the chylous drainage resolves.

 f. Standard treatment options include:

  i. Restriction of dietary fat

  ii. Hyperalimentation therapy and transthoracic duct ligation may be required.[40]

7. Pleural effusions are common within the first month of transplantation.

 a. Causes of pleural effusions:

  i. An interrupted bronchial lymphatic drainage

ii. Low serum albumin related to poor nutrition prior to transplantation

iii. Rejection or infection

    a) If the effusion is related to rejection or infection (empyema), a diagnosis is typically yielded by bronchoscopy with bronchoalveolar lavage (BAL) and transbronchial biopsy (TBBx).

    b) Further treatment strategies can be determined when diagnosis is confirmed.[35]

b. Effusions often respond to diuretic therapy and restoration of protein stores.

c. Occasionally pleural effusions require therapeutic thoracentesis to drain accumulated fluid.

8. Impaired wound healing

a. May occur as a result of poor nutritional status prior to transplantation, general deconditioning, or immunosuppression.

b. Meticulous assessment and care of surgical sites is crucial to prevention and management of infections.[36]

c. Wounds typically noted upon assessment include:

  i. Posteriolateral thoracotomy in single lung transplants (SLT)

  ii. Transverse "clamshell" thoracosternotomy in bilateral lung transplants (BLT)

  iii. These incisions should be assessed daily to monitor for dehiscence, erythema, edema, and tissue necrosis.

  iv. In most hospitals, prophylactic antibiotic therapy is utilized post-transplantation to prevent skin or wound infections.[36]

    a) Antibiotics may be administered over a predetermined amount of time, or until chest drains have been removed.

9. Fluid and electrolyte balance

a. Fluid volume status is critical in the early postoperative phase.

  i. With interrupted lymphatic drainage and hemodynamic changes from surgery, the risk of primary graft dysfunction is high due to increased capillary permeability.

  ii. After hemodynamic stability and improved oxygenation is assured, fluid volume status becomes especially important.

  iii. Renal clearance of nephrotoxic medications such as immunosuppressant drugs and antibiotics is vital to long-term tolerance of medication therapy.

    a) At higher serum levels, calcineurin inhibitors may induce vasoconstriction of the afferent arterioles in the glomerular units of the kidney, reducing renal blood flow and glomerular filtration rate.[35]

    b) Mobilization of secretions is essential to tolerance of effective pulmonary rehabilitation.

  iv. Monitoring for ineffective fluid management includes:

    a) Reporting hypotension, tachycardia, dry mucous membranes, weakness, altered mental status, oliguria, decreased urine output

    b) Trending of metabolic indicators of acute renal failure, such as rising blood urea nitrogen (BUN) and creatinine levels.

      c) Treatment to anticipate for fluid volume deficit (FVD) includes urine output replacement by crystalloid fluids, electrolyte replacement as needed, and daily weights.

      d) Fluid volume overload predisposes transplant recipients to pulmonary and peripheral edema. Signs to report include ventricular gallop (S_3 sound), jugular venous distention (JVD), rales, and generalized edema or ascites.[36]

      e) A varying degree of anemia will occur as a result of bone marrow suppression from immunosuppressive drugs.

         1) Intravenous fluid boluses or blood product administration might be necessary.

            i) Maintain adequate hemoglobin levels necessary for oxygen transport.

            ii) Maintain urine output within normal limits.

10. Glycemic monitoring and control

  a. Patients may develop diabetes secondary to:

    i. Chronic corticosteroid therapy

    ii. Diabetogenic impact of calcineurin inhibitors

    iii. Frequently resolves as steroids are tapered to a daily maintenance dose

      a) Patients may require oral hypoglycemic agents or insulin therapy to control blood glucose levels.[35]

      b) Glucose levels are checked regularly in the early postoperative phase, as corticosteroid dosages are higher.

      c) Patients should be instructed to track their glucose monitoring.[41]

  b. Nurses should collaborate with social workers, case managers, dietitians, pharmacists, and physicians.

    i. Ensure patients have access to educational materials, diabetes educators, and monitoring supplies and medications

    ii. Goal: prevent long-term end-organ damage resulting from poorly controlled diabetes

  c. Patients should be familiar with signs and symptoms of:

    i. Hyperglycemia

      a) Polyuria, polydipsia, and polyphagia

    ii. Hypoglycemia

      a) Cool and clammy skin, diaphoresis, fatigue

  d. With the assistance of a clinical dietitian and home health nursing, patients and families should be able to address these warning signs appropriately.

11. Blood pressure monitoring and regulation

  a. Hypotension generally presents early in the surgical recovery phase as the body temperature returns to normal and vasodilatation occurs from the response to warmth.

    i. Vasopressor therapy is titrated to maintain mean arterial pressure and adequate end-organ perfusion until hemodynamic stability is achieved.[36]

    ii. As the body equilibrates and stability is maintained, hypotension may occur due to a fluid volume deficit and increased drainage from the surgical site.

      iii. Frequent vital sign monitoring is essential to evaluating efficacy of interventions to support blood pressure.

        a) Hypertension may develop as immunosuppressant serum drug levels rise to therapeutic limits.

        b) Chronic use of beta-agonists and preexisting essential hypertension will resume once hemodynamic stability is established.

        c) Patients should resume antihypertensive medications.

          1) Dosages should be adjusted to reflect other causative factors.

          2) Patients should report symptoms of worsening hypertension, including headache, nausea and vomiting, chest pain, dyspnea, and palpitations.[36,41]

          3) Patients must monitor and document their blood pressure at home.

12. Altered bowel functioning

  a. Gastrointestinal (GI) complications occur in the lung transplant recipient more often than with any other type of organ transplantation.[42]

    i. Gastroesophageal reflux disease (GERD) is commonly encountered and may be treated with histamine-2 (H_2) antagonists such as famotidine, proton-pump inhibitors (PPI) such as omeprazole, or drugs to help stimulate gastric motility, such as metoclopramide.[3]

    ii. Diarrhea is common, but in many cases the etiology is hard to determine.

      a) Mycophenylate mofetil may contribute to GI upset and diarrhea.

      b) Dose regimens may need to be adjusted to promote GI tolerance.

      c) Magnesium supplementation may also cause diarrhea.

      d) Prophylactic antibiotic therapy may predispose the immunocompromised patient to diarrhea related to *Clostridium difficile*.

        1) Infectious causes of GI upset should be ruled out prior to administering medications to decrease gastric and intestinal motility.

    iii. Other notable GI complications seen after lung transplantation may include colonic perforation due to glucocorticoid therapy, ischemic bowel, and cytomegalovirus (CMV) colitis.

    iv. Assessment should result in prompt reporting of symptoms experienced by the patient.[42]

      a) Abdominal distention and pain

      b) Absence of bowel sounds

      c) Abdominal rigidity or guarding

      d) Frequency and consistency of bowel movements

      e) Fever

    v. Malabsorptive GI complications may stem from primary disease processes.

a) Cystic fibrosis (CF) involves abnormal chloride transport across epithelial cells.
1) Causes dehydration of secretions and exocrine gland dysfunction
2) Results in fluid shift
3) Predisposes patients to relative gut dehydration and distal intestinal obstructions[43]
b) CF patients who are transplanted are especially at risk for small bowel obstructions.
1) Early postoperative dehydration, anesthesia, and delayed ambulation slow gastric motility.
c) Bowel prophylaxis for this patient population should include:
1) Advancement to a high fiber, low-fat diet
2) Increased oral fluid intake
3) Regular stool softeners

13. Altered nutrition
a. Deconditioning and cachexia prior to transplantation can impede rehabilitation efforts after surgery.[36]
i. Intercostal muscle wasting can lead to difficulty weaning from mechanical ventilation and poor pulmonary toileting postoperatively.
ii. Serum albumin, prealbumin levels, electrolytes, and calorie counts should be followed carefully.
iii. Enteral feedings or hyperalimentation may be initiated to meet the caloric needs essential for proper rehabilitation and wound healing.
iv. Nutritional support is a multidisciplinary effort in developing a nutritional plan that includes collaboration with pharmacy, clinical nutrition, social worker, and family members.
v. Close attention should be paid to the special nutritional needs of patients with malabsorptive disease processes, such as CF.
a) Many CF patients must supplement oral intake with pancreatic enzymes and fat-soluble vitamins to assure that dietary daily vitamin and mineral requirements are met.[43]

14. Altered mobility and self-care deficit
a. One of the major goals of lung transplantation is to restore adequate oxygenation to vital organs.
i. For most patients and families this is expressed as an ability to perform activities and self-care practices.
a) Activity and level of independence are markers of progression of health for many patients and families.
b) Reassurance and support should be given liberally, to motivate and nurture.
c) Patients should be taught to monitor their activity levels and progress.

d) The importance of monitoring these levels lies in the early detection and reporting of signs of allograft rejection.[36]

e) Self-care practices and rehabilitation are a multidisciplinary effort: occupational and physical therapy, respiratory therapy, pharmacy, and nursing.

f) These disciplines collaborate to restore the highest level of function and independent self-care behaviors possible.

g) Social workers may be consulted as needed if home care equipment such as ambulation assistive devices and portable oxygen is needed.

IV. Immunosuppression

   A. The goal of immunosuppressive therapy is to:
      1. Maintain optimal drug levels within a therapeutic range
      2. Achieve a balance of suppressing the immune system
      3. Prevent rejection
      4. Prevent adverse side effects
      5. Prevent complications of the agents

   B. The immunosuppressive regimen for lung transplant patients is individualized and varies from center to center.
      1. Therapy consists of a triple drug regimen:
         a. Calcineurin inhibitor (cyclosporine or tacrolimus)
            i. More centers are utilizing tacrolimus as the primary calcineurin inhibitor agent.
            ii. Data suggests a potential role in retarding the development of bronchiolitis obliterans syndrome (BOS).
         b. Corticosteroids
         c. Mycophenolate mofetil or azathioprine
         d. Induction therapy with a monoclonal or polyclonal antibody may also be used to prevent rejection.
         e. See Chapter 4 for a complete description of immunosuppressive drug therapies.

V. Rejection

   A. Most lung transplant recipients will experience at least one acute rejection episode during the early postoperative period.

   B. Early acute rejection is characterized by one or more of the following symptoms:
      1. Low-grade fever
      2. Hypoxemia
      3. Pulmonary infiltrates
      4. Pleural effusions
      5. Dyspnea
      6. Fatigue
      7. Decreased exercise tolerance

   C. Diagnosis is made by:
      1. Clinical presentation
      2. Objective findings on chest radiograph
      3. Pulmonary function tests

    4.   Transbronchial biopsies[47-51]

D. Treatment is based on the severity of the rejection and clinical symptoms.

    1.   Acute rejection is usually treated with:

        a. High-dose corticosteroids

        b. Optimizing maintenance immunosuppression

        c. Adding another agent

    2.   Recurrent acute rejection has been associated with the development of chronic rejection or BOS.

        a. Current emphasis is placed on the prevention, early diagnosis, and complete eradication of acute rejection episodes to assure optimal short- and long-term outcomes.

E. Formulated in 1990 and revised in 1995, the grading schema for pulmonary allograft rejection was developed by leading lung transplant specialists.[44-46]

    1.   Acute rejection is reported with the presence of perivascular and interstitial mononuclear infiltrates.

    2.   Characterization of each grade includes the presence and intensity of coexisting airway inflammation.

    3.   Chronic rejection is categorized as BOS either active or inactive, and vascular atherosclerosis.

        a. BOS is used to describe lung allograft deterioration secondary to progressive airway disease for which there is no other cause.

        b. Alloimmune and nonalloimmune factors have been shown to produce the fibroproliferative airway response seen in patients with obliterative bronchiolitis (OB).

        c. The final common pathway is the release of proinflammatory cytokines and growth factors that cause fibrous scarring and airway obliteration.[51-56]

    4.   BOS is the principal manifestation of chronic rejection in lung allografts.

        a. Compared with chronic rejection in other vascularized allografts, chronic rejection is a particularly pervasive problem in lung transplantation.

            i.   It develops in about 40% of survivors by the second year post-transplant.[56]

            ii. BOS is the most significant obstacle to long-term, morbidity-free survival.

               a) Equally affects single-lung, double-lung, and heart-lung transplant recipients

               b) OB or BOS can occur within months after transplantation, but the median onset is 16-20 months.[56-62]

        b. Symptoms of BOS include:

            i.   Progressive shortness of breath

            ii. Decreased exercise tolerance

        c. The characteristic physiologic hallmarks of BOS are:

            i.   Airflow limitation

            ii. Progressive decline in the FEV_1 to values $< 80\%$ of post-transplantation baseline

d. The International Society for Heart and Lung Transplantation classified BOS based on a comparison of the patient's current FEV_1 with his/her best post-transplant FEV_1:[54]
   i. Grade 0: FEV_1 is > 80% of baseline
   ii. Grade 1: FEV_1 equals 66% to 79% of baseline
   iii. Grade 2: FEV_1 equals 51% to 65% of baseline
   iv. Grade 3: FEV_1 is < 50% of baseline
e. OB is the pathologic entity believed to be due to chronic lung allograft rejection.
   i. OB is the principal histopathologic manifestation of chronic rejection in lung allografts.
      a) Recognized by the findings of inflammation and fibrosis (via a mechanism of organizing fibrin)
         1) Occur predominantly in the walls and contiguous tissues of membranous and respiratory bronchioles
            i) Cause narrowing of their lumens[57-63]
   ii. The terms BOS and OB are often used synonymously.
      a) BOS does not necessarily require histologic confirmation.
         1) BOS is the physiological entity defined by a 20% reduction in forced expiratory volume from a previous documented baseline.
            i) The clinical and functional aspects of BOS are not always consistent with the typical pathology.
            ii) Due to sampling problems related to small transbronchial biopsies
      b) Risk factors for OB include:[59-63]
         1) HLA mismatching
         2) Elevated panel-reactive antibodies
         3) Acute rejection, particularly frequent episodes during the first month
         4) Late-onset acute rejection
         5) Inadequate immunosuppression
         6) CMV mismatching (seropositive donor in seronegative recipient)
         7) Lung infection
         8) Organizing pneumonia.
   iii. Strategies to prevent OB may include:
      a) Aggressive prophylaxis and management of acute rejection and CMV infection
      b) Management of OB/BOS should be individualized for each patient based on current immunosuppressive regimen and severity of disease and symptoms.
         1) Decreased pulmonary function associated with chronic rejection is generally irreversible.
            i) Warrants close monitoring of pulmonary function and early intervention
      c) Immunosuppression regimen is optimized by switching

1) Cyclosporine-based therapy to tacrolimus
2) Azathioprine to mycophenolate mofetil
3) High-dose corticosteroid therapy
4) Additional agents such as sirolimus may be instituted.
5) Other drug therapies such as antithymocyte globulin, thymoglobulin, or OKT3 may be given.
6) Photopheresis, a leukapheresis-based therapy that removes and treats lymphocytes with 8-methoxypsoralen and ultraviolet A irradiation, has been shown to stabilize symptoms of BOS.

VI. Infection
  A. Infection is one of the major complications of immunosuppression therapy after transplantation.
  B. See Chapter 5 for a detailed discussion of transplant infections.
  C. The lung is the most common site of infection in all organ solid transplantation and the leading cause of morbidity in lung transplantation.
  D. The transplanted lung is particularly susceptible due to the impairment of mucociliary clearance and the cough reflex response which occurs during surgery.[64]
  E. The risk for developing all types of infection is highest during the first months after transplantation and decreases subsequently thereafter.
    1. Bacterial and fungal infections comprise the majority of infections that occur in the transplanted lung in the first months after transplant.
    2. Viral infections are most prevalent during the second to third post-transplant months.[65]
      a. Cytomegalovirus (CMV) infection is the most common and debilitating viral infection after lung transplantation.
      b. CMV can be a primary or secondary infection.
        i. Primary infections occur when a CMV seronegative recipient is exposed to a CMV seropositive donor organ.
        ii. Secondary infections develop as a result of reactivation of the disease in the recipient who has been exposed to CMV (patient is seropositive) in the past.
        iii. The most common sites for CMV infections are blood, lungs, gastrointestinal tract, and retina.
        iv. CMV pneumonitis is associated with a 50% mortality in lung transplant patients.
          a) Most transplant centers have an aggressive prophylactic protocol with ganciclovir, valganciclovir, or immune globulin after transplantation.

VII. Outcomes and quality of life
  A. As lung transplantation becomes an accepted therapy for select patients with end-stage pulmonary disease, results are still plagued by complications that make long-term survival suboptimal.
  B. According to the International Society for Heart and Lung Transplantation, 1-year survival is 74% and 5-year survival is 47%.[12]
  C. Over 40% of patients will develop BOS by 2 years post-transplant.[57]
  D. For these reasons, quality of life research is needed in this population.

1. Quality of life research has been extensive in other solid organ transplants.
   a. Research examining quality of life outcomes in lung transplant patients has been steadily increasing.
   b. Smeritschnig and colleagues studied health related quality of life in 94 patients who were greater than 3 months post-transplant.[66]
      i. They found 76% of patients were happy with transplant outcome.
         a) Those with cystic fibrosis as a pretransplant diagnosis reported the most satisfaction with their quality of life.
      ii. Side effects of medications were found to be a major factor influencing quality of life.
      iii. Patients who had developed BOS grade ≥ 1 had significantly poorer quality of life than those with a BOS = 0.
   c. Vermeulen and colleagues examined 29 lung transplant patients who had developed BOS for at least 18 months.[67]
      i. After the onset of BOS, restrictions with mobility and energy were reported.
      ii. Patients had more difficulty with activities of daily living and more difficulty with dyspnea after on the onset of BOS.
   d. Vermeulen and colleagues also examined long-term quality of life in patients surviving greater than 55 months.
      i. After 43 months, patients began to experience more dyspnea, depression, and a lowered sense of well-being.[68]
   e. In a study of 61 patients before and 1 year after lung transplant, Kugler and colleagues reported that health-related quality of life improved significantly until about 6 months after transplant.[69]
      i. There was no difference seen in social or emotional functioning.
   f. Lanuza and colleagues examined functional status in 10 lung transplant patients before and at 3 months post-transplant.[70]
      i. Patients reported improvement in physical strength, current health, and quality of life.
      ii. As in other studies, psychological functioning did not significantly change.
         a) 90% of patients reported satisfaction with their transplant decision.
   g. De Vito Dabbs and colleagues studied the effect of psychosocial vulnerability on physical limitations in 50 lung transplant recipients between 2 and 17 months post-transplant.[71]
      i. Patients with more psychological distress significantly reported more physical symptoms and limitations.
   h. Most studies found patient quality of life significantly improved from before to after transplantation.[66-72]

VIII. Summary
   A. Lung transplantation is an alternative therapy for select patients with end-stage pulmonary disease.
      1. Long-term survival is limited by the development of BOS.
      2. Patients do enjoy an improved quality of life.

B. The future of lung transplantation will be defined by:
1. New immunosuppressive therapies to prevent long-term complications
    a. Inhaled cyclosporine
2. Refinement of selection criteria
3. Increasing the availability of donor organs

REFERENCES

1. Hardy JD, Webb WR, Dalton ML, Walker GR. Lung homotransplantation in man. *JAMA*, 1963; 186: 1065-1074.
2. Nelems JMB, Rebuck AS, Cooper JD. Human lung transplantation. *Chest*, 1980; 78: 569-573.
3. Kamholz SL, Veith FL, Mollenkopf FP, et al. Single lung transplantation with cyclosporine immunosuppression. *J Thorac Cardiovasc Surg*, 1983; 86: 537-542.
4. Derom F, Barbier F, Ringoir S. Ten-month survival after lung transplantation in man. *J Thorac Cardiovasc Surg*, 1971; 61: 835-846.
5. Reitz BA, Wallwork JL, Hunt SA, et al. Heart-lung transplantation: Successful therapy for patients with pulmonary vascular disease. *N Engl J Med*, 1982; 306: 557-564.
6. Toronto Lung Transplantation Group. Unilateral lung transplantation for pulmonary fibrosis. *N Engl J Med*, 1986; 314: 1140-1145.
7. Dubois P, Chiniere L, Cooper JD. Bronchial omentopexy in canine lung allotransplantation. *Ann Thorac Surg*, 1984; 38: 11-14.
8. Cooper JD, Pearson FG, Patterson GA, et al. Technique of successful lung transplantation in humans. *J Thorac Cardiovasc Surg*, 1987; 93: 173.
9. Morgan WE, Lima O, Goldberg M, Ferdman A, et al. Improved bronchial healing in canine left lung reimplantation using omental pedicle wrap. *J Thorac Cardiovasc Surg*, 1983; 85: 134-139.
10. Lima O, Cooper JD, Peters WJ, et al. Effect of methylprednisolone and azathioprine on bronchial healing following lung autotransplantation. *J Thorac Cardiovasc Surg*, 1981; 82: 211-215.
11. American Society for Transplant Physicians, Thoracic Society, European Respiratory Society, International Society for Heart and Lung Transplantation. International guidelines for the selection of lung transplant candidates. *Am J Respir Crit Care Med*, 1998; 158: 335-339.
12. Trulock EP, Eswards LB, Taylor DO, Boucek MM, et al. The Registry of the International Society for Heart and Lung Transplantation: Twenty-first Official Adult Lung and Heart-Lung Report—2004. *J Heart Lung Transplant*, 2004; 23 (7): 804-815.
13. Glanville AR, Estenne M. Indications, patient selection and timing of referral for lung transplantation. *Eur Respir J*, 2003; 22: 845-852.
14. Maurer JR, Frost AE, Estenne MM, Higenbottam T, et al. International guidelines for the selection of lung transplant candidates. *J Heart Lung Transplant*, 1998; 17: 703-709.
15. Studer SM, Levy RD, McNeil K, Orens JB. Lung transplantation outcome: A review of survival, graft function, physiology, health-related quality of life and cost-effectiveness. *Eur Respir J*, 2004; 24: 674-685.
16. Egan JJ. The clinical practice of lung transplantation in North America. *Chest*, 2004; 125(4): 1183-1184.
17. Gottlieb J, Simon A, Welte T. Lung Transplantation. *Pneumologe*, 2005; 2: 131-141.
18. Fischer S, Strueber M, Haverich A. Current status in lung transplantation: Patients, indications, techniques, and outcome. *Medizinische Klinik*, 2002; 97 (3): 137-143.
19. Glanville AR, Estenne M. Indications, patient selection and timing of referral for lung transplantation. *Eur Respir J*, 2003; 22: 845-852.
20. Nathan SD. Lung transplantation: Disease-specific considerations for referral. *Chest*, 2005; 127 (3): 1006-1016.
21. Charman SC, Sharples LD, McNeil KD, Wallwork J. Assessment of survival benefit after lung transplantation by

patient diagnosis. *J Heart Lung Transplant,* 2002; 21 (7): 226-232.

22. Manzetti, JD. Lung transplantation. in Cupples SA, Ohler L, (Eds.). *Transplantation Nursing Secrets.* Philadelphia: Hanley & Belfus, 2003. pp. 75-83.

23. White-Williams C. Lung Transplanation. In Smith S. Organ Transplant, 2002; www.medscape.com. Accessed 4/17/06.

24. Anyanwu AC, McGuire A, Rogers CA, Murday, AJ. An economic evaluation of lung transplantation. *Journal of Thoracic and Cardiovascular Surgery,* 2002; 123: 411-420.

25. Dumas-Hicks, DH. In Cupples SA, Ohler L, (Eds.). *Transplantation Nursing Secrets.* Philadelphia: Hanley & Belfus, 2003. pp. 67-74.

26. Levine SM. On behalf of the Transplant/Immunology Network of the American College of Chest Physicians. A Survey of Clinical Practice of Lung Transplantation in North America. *Chest,* 2004; 125 (4): 1224-1238.

27. United Network for Organ Sharing. 1999 Annual Report of the U.S. Scientific Registry of Transplant Recipients and the Organ Procurement and Transplantation Network: Transplant Data 1989-1998. (February 21, 2000). Rockville, MD, and Richmond, VA: HHS/HRSA/OSP/DOT and UNOS. Available at: http://www.unos.org/Data/anrpt_main.htm. Accessed April, 2005.

28. Manzetti JD, Hoffman LA, Serika SM. Exercise, education, and quality of life in lung transplant candidates. *J Heart Lung Transplant,* 1994; 13: 297-305.

29. Calhoon JH, Grover FL, Gibbons WJ, et al. Single lung transplantation: Alternative indications and technique. *J Thorac Cardiovasc Surg,* 1991; 101: 816-824.

30. Snell GI, Griffiths A, Macfarlane L, et al. Maximizing thoracic organ transplant opportunities: The importance of efficient coordination. *J Heart Lung Transplant,* 2000; 19: 401-407.

31. Weill D, Keshavjee S. Lung transplantation for emphysema: Two lungs or one. *J Heart Lung Transplant,* 2001; 20: 739-742.

32. Pasque MK, Cooper JD, Kaiser LR, Haydock DA, et al. An improved technique for bilateral lung transplantation: Rationale and initial clinical experience. *Ann Thorac Surg,* 1990; 49: 785-791.

33. Meyer BF, Sundaresan RS, Cooper JD, Patterson GA. Bilateral sequential lung transplant without sternal division eliminates post transplant sternal complications. *Thorac Cardiovasc Surg,* 1999; 117: 358-364

34. Pierre A, Keshavjee S. Lung transplantation: Donor and recipient critical care aspects. *Curr Op Crit Care,* 2005; 11: 339-344.

35. Nicolls M, Zamora, M. Lung transplantation. In Hanley ME, Welsh CH (Eds.). *Current Diagnosis and Treatment in Pulmonary Medicine.* New York: McGraw-Hill, 2003. pp. 173-186.

36. Ochoa L. The current status of lung transplantation: A nursing perspective. *AACN Clinical Issues,* 1999; 10(2): 229-239.

37. Clark S. Vascular complications of lung transplantation. *Ann Thoracic Surg,* 1996; 61: 1079.

38. Meyer S, Bass M, Ash R, Duffy S, et al. Postoperative care of the lung transplant recipient. *Crit Care Nurs Clin North Am,* 1996; 8: 239-252.

39. Meyers B, de la Morena M, Sweet S, Truloc, E, et al. Primary graft dysfunction and other selected complications of lung transplantation: A single-center experience of 983 patients. *J Thoracic Cardiovasc Surg,* 2005; 129(6): 1421-1429.

40. Suratt B. (2003). Pleural effusions, excluding hemothorax. In Hanley ME, Welsh CH (Eds.). *Current Diagnosis and Treatment in Pulmonary Medicine.* New York: McGraw-Hill, 2003. pp. 222-232.

41. Martin R. Organ transplantation: The role of the acute care nurse practitioner across the spectrum of health care. *AACN Clinical Issues,* 1999; 10(2): 285-292.

42. Smith P, Slaughter M, Petty M, Shumway S. Abdominal complications after lung transplantation. *J Heart Lung Transplant,* 1995; 14: 44-51.

43. Saavedra M, Nick J. (2003) Cystic fibrosis and bronchiectasis. In Hanley ME, Welsh CH (Eds.). *Current Diagnosis and Treatment in Pulmonary Medicine.* New York: McGraw-Hill, 2003. pp. 92-104.

44. Cooper JD, Billlingham M, Egan T. A working formulation for the standardization of nomenclature and for clinical staging of chronic dysfunction in lung allografts. *J Heart Lung Transplant*, 1993; 12: 713-716.

45. Yousem SA, Berry GJ, Cagle PT, et al. Revision of the 1990 working formulation for the classification of pulmonary allograft rejection: Lung Rejection Study Group. *J Heart Lung Transplant*, 1996; 15: 1-15.

46. Transplant pathology Internet services. Revised Working Formulation for Classification and Grading of Lung Allograft Rejection—1995. Available at: http://tpis.upmc.edu/tpis/schema/LungRej.html. Accessed April 2005.

47. Gorman JH III, Gorman RC, Kaiser L. Appropriate indications for single and bilateral lung transplantation. *Curr Op Organ Transplant*, 2001; 6: 243-247.

48. Eagan TM, Westerman JH, Lambert J, et al. Isolated lung transplantation for end stage lung disease: A viable therapy. *Ann Thorac Surg*, 1992; 53: 590.

49. Resnikoff PM, Ries AL. Pulmonary rehabilitation for chronic lung disease. *J Heart Lung Transplant*, 1998; 17: 643-650.

50. Garrity ER Jr, Villanueva J, Bhorade SM, Husain AN, et al. Low rate of acute lung allograft rejection after the use of daclizumab, an interleukin 2 receptor antibody. *Transplantation*, 2001; 71: 773-777.

51. Sundaresan S, Trulock EP, Mohanakumar, Cooper JD, et al. Prevalence and outcome of bronchiolitis obliterans syndrome after lung transplantation. *Ann Thorac Surg*, 1995; 60: 1341-1347.

52. Kroshus TJ, Kshettry VR, Savik K, John R, et al. Risk factors for the development of bronchiolitis obliterans syndrome after lung transplantation. *J Thorac Cardiovasc Surg*, 1997; 114: 195-202.

53. Boehler A, Estenne M. Obliterative bronchiolitis after lung transplantation. *Curr Opin Pulm Med*, 2000; 6: 133-139.

54. Cooper JD, Billingham M, Egan T, et al. A working formulation for the standardization of nomenclature and for clinical staging of chronic dysfunction in lung allografts. *J Heart Lung Transplant*, 1993; 12: 713-716.

55. Kroshus TJ, Kshettry VR, Savik K, John K, et al. Risk factors for the development of bronchiolitis obliterans syndrome after lung transplantation. *J Thorac Cardiovasc Surg*, 1997; 114: 195-202.

56. Heng D, Sharples LD, McNeil K, Stewart S, et al. Bronchiolitis obliterans syndrome: Incidence, natural history, prognosis and risk factors. *J Heart Lung Transplant*, 1998; 17: 1255-1263.

57. Nathan S. Bronchiolitis obliterins syndrome. www.medscape.com. Accessed April 2005.

58. Boehler A, Kesten S, Weder W, Speich R. Bronchiolitis obliterans after lung transplantation: A review. *Chest*, 1998; 114: 1411-1426.

59. Boehler A, Estenne M. Post-transplant bronchiolitis obliterans. *Eur Respir J*, 2003; 22: 1007-1018.

60. Belperio JA, Lake K, Tazelaar H, Keane MP, et al. Bronchiolitis obliterans syndrome complicating lung or heart-lung transplantation. *Semin Respir Crit Care Med*, 2003; 24: 499-530.

61. Burke CM, Theodore J, Dawkins KD, et al. Post-transplant obliterative bronchiolitis and other late lung sequelae in human heart-lung transplantation. *Chest*, 1984; 86: 824-829.

62. Sharples LD, McNeil K, Stewart S, Wallwork J. Risk factors for bronchiolitis obliterans: A systematic review of recent publications. *J Heart Lung Transplant*, 2002; 21: 271-281.

63. Markopoulo KD, Cool CD, Elliot TL, et al. Obliterative bronchiolitis: Varying presentations and clinicopathological correlation. *Eur Respir J*, 2002; 19: 20-30.

64. Maurer JR, Tullis DE, Grossman RF, Velland H, et al. Infectious complications following isolated lung transplantation. *Chest*, 1992; 101: 1056-1059.

65. Ettinger NA, Bailey TC, Trulock EP. Cytomegalovirus infection and pnuemonitis: Impact after isolated lung transplantation. *Am Rev Respir Dis*, 1993; 147: 1017-1023.

66. Smeritschnig B, Jaksch P, Kocher A, Seebacher G, et al. Quality of life after lung transplantation: A cross-sectional study. *J Heart Lung Transplant*, 2005; 24: 474-480.

67. Vermeulan KM, Groen H, van der Bij W, Erasmus ME, et al. The effect of bronchiolitis obliterans syndrome on health related quality of life. *Clin Traansplant*, 2004 Aug; 18 (4): 377-383.

68. Vermeulan KM, Ouwens JP, van der Bij W, Koeter GH, et al. Long-term quality of life in patients surviving at least 55 months after lung transplantation. *Gen Hosp Psychiatry*, 2003; 25(2): 95-102.

69. Kugler C, Strueber M, Tegrbur U, Niedermeyer J, et al. Quality of life 1 year after lung transplantation. *Prog Transplant*, 2004 Dec; 14(4): 331-336.

70. Lanuza DM, McCabe M, Farcas GA, Garrity E. Prospective study of functional status and quality of life before and after lung transplantation. *Chest*, 2000 Jul; 188(1): 115-22.

71. De Vito Dabbs A, Dew MA, Stiley CS, Manzetti H, et al. Psychosocial vulnerability, physical symptoms and physical impairment after lung and heart-lung transplantation. *J Heart Lung Transplant*, 2003; 22(11): 1268-1275.

72. Rodrigue J, Baz M, Kanasky W, MacNaughton K. Does lung transplantation improve health-related quality of life? The University of Florida experience. *J Heart Lung Transplant*, 2005; 24: 755-763.

REVIEW QUESTIONS

1. The rationale for maintaining the pulmonary artery pressure within normal limits in the immediate post-operative period following lung transplantation is to:
   a. Protect anastomosis sites
   b. Prevent immediate graft dysfunction
   c. Prevent pulmonary edema
   d. a and c
   e. All of the above

2. Pulmonary artery pressures are maintained within normal limits with which of the following?
   a. Diuretic administration
   b. Administration of inhaled nitric oxide
   c. Intravenous administration of nipride
   d. All of the above
   e. a and b

3. If additional fluids must be administered to the immediate post-op lung recipient, it should be done cautiously due to:
   a. High fluid volumes that would tear the anastomosis
   b. Increased capillary permeability in transplanted lung tissue
   c. Nephrotoxicity of anesthesias
   d. Hyporesponsiveness of alveoli in the immediate post-operative phase

4. Cardiac dysrhythmias are not uncommon in the immediate post-operative period following lung transplantation. Atrial dysrhythmias are often associated with which of the following?
   a. Systemic inflammatory processes related to chest surgery
   b. Inflammation near pulmonary vein and atrial cuff suture lines
   c. Early signs of hyperacute rejection
   d. Low levels of sodium related to dehydration

5. Tachycardia may be present in the immediate post-operative stages due to which of the following problems?
   a. Bleeding, use of nebulizers
   b. Pain, catecholamine release with stress
   c. Fluid loss, diuretic therapy
   d. All of the above
   e. a and b

6. With en bloc and sequential anastomoses of lung transplantation, pulmonary artery wedge pressures are usually not performed due to which of the following rationales?
   a. Increase in arterial pressure may precipitate rupture of the anastomoses sites.
   b. Increase in venous pressure may precipitate rupture of the anastomoses sites.
   c. Increases in atrial pressures may precipitate rupture of the anastomoses sites.
   d. Increases in ventricular pressures may precipitate rupture of the anastomoses sites.

7. Warning signs of primary graft dysfunction include which of the following symptoms?
   a. Sudden rise in potassium levels
   b. Frequent oxygen desaturation
   c. Increased work of breathing
   d. All of the above
   e. b and c

8. Possible causes of primary graft dysfunction include which of the following?
   a. Decreased capillary permeability
   b. Change in compliance and vascular resistance between donor and recipient
   c. Edema from extended ischemic time
   d. All of the above
   e. a and c

9. Acute rejection symptoms include which of the following?
   a. Dyspnea
   b. Elevation in temperature
   c. Decrease in FEV_1
   d. All of the above
   e. a and c

10. Two major airway complications of lung transplantation are:
   a. Bronchial dehiscence and tracheal stenosis
   b. Alveolar collapse and rejection
   c. Loss of surfactant and infections
   d. Increased production of CO_2 and an increase in reperfusion injury

Correct answers:

1. d
2. e
3. b
4. b
5. d
6. a
7. e
8. d
9. d
10. a

11 Liver Transplantation

SALLY BUFTON

KAREN EMMETT

ANNE-MARIE BYERLY

PRETRANSPLANT CARE: OBJECTIVES OF END-STAGE LIVER FAILURE

I. End-stage liver disease is a major health problem causing more than 25,000 deaths each year in the United States.[1]

II. Although medical management may be effective for a period of time, liver transplantation is a recognized form of treatment with excellent results worldwide, but it is not without significant risk.

A. The leading indication for liver transplantation is hepatitis C.

B. Approximately 3% of the world's population is infected with the virus and in the United States this is not expected to peak until 2015.

C. Table 11-1 includes a list of common diseases for which liver transplantation is an option.

III. The development of cirrhosis has placed a significant burden on liver transplant waiting lists; one of the main problems faced by clinicians is that of a shortage of organs available for transplantation.

A. Selection of appropriate patients is vital to ensure the best use of a scarce resource.

B. Timing of when to list the patient is paramount.

IV. The overall aim of liver transplantation is to prolong life and improve the patient's quality of life.

V. As of June 2007, 16,857 patients were waiting for liver transplants in the United States.

A. 6,650 liver transplants were performed in 2005.

B. During the same period, 1,650 patients were removed from the waiting list because of death.[2]

DISEASES THAT MAY LEAD TO HEPATIC FAILURE

I. Hepatitis A is an acute, necroinflammatory disease of the liver from infection by the hepatitis A virus.

A. The virus is detectable in blood or feces for 2 weeks before the onset of jaundice and for up to 8 days afterwards.

TABLE 11-1

■ **Common Liver Diseases: Acute and Chronic**

Disease	Total
Hepatitis C	1525
Alcohol	704
Acute liver disease	492
Alcohol/Hepatitis C	411
Cryptogenic	407
Hepatoma—cirrhotic	361
Pediatric liver diseases	244
Primary sclerosing cholangitis—with or without inflammatory bowel	271
Nonalcoholic steatohepatitis	207
Primary biliary cirrhosis	194
Hepatoma—noncirrhotic	176
Autoimmune	165
Sarcoidosis, granulomatous, histiocytosis	165
Hepatitis B	115
Alpha-1 antitrypsin	83
TPN induced liver disease	80
Hemachromatosis	34
Cholangiocarcinoma	33
Hepatoblastoma	30
Wilson's disease	23
Polycystic liver disease	13
Trauma	8
Miscellaneous*	703*
Total	6444

Main indications for liver transplantation in the U.S. in 2005.[2]

*All other liver diseases and multiple diseases with small numbers being transplanted.

    B.   It is acquired through the oral-fecal route or by ingestion of contaminated food or water.

    C.   Symptoms may include malaise, fatigue, anorexia, low-grade fever, nausea, and vomiting.

    D.   Most patients will have full biochemical recovery within 3 months.

    E.   Acute liver failure occurs rarely and chronic infection is never seen.

II. Hepatitis B is transmitted by contact with blood or body fluids of an infected person.
   A. Most infections occur in the following instances:
      1. From mother to child
      2. Unprotected sexual contact
      3. Blood transfusions
      4. Sharing infected needles
   B. Hepatitis B may lead to acute infection which usually resolves, although liver failure can occur.
      1. A small number of patients fail to clear the virus and develop chronic infection which leads to cirrhosis and/or liver cancer.
III. Hepatitis C is a slow, progressive disease that can be transmitted by infected blood products, sharing of needles in IV drug abuse, sexual contact, or from needlestick injuries.
   A. More commonly seen in males.
   B. Clinical presentation of acute hepatitis is rare.
   C. Most cases progress asymptomatically and present with cirrhosis or liver cancer.
   D. Main indication for liver transplantation.
IV. Hepatitis D infection occurs only in the presence of concurrent or underlying chronic hepatitis B.
   A. Spread by sexual contact or intravenous drug use.
   B. Chronic hepatitis D may be completely asymptomatic or present with nonspecific symptoms like fatigue.
   C. Acute hepatitis D may lead to fulminant liver failure.
V. Hepatitis E may occur in epidemics or sporadic cases.
   A. Acquired similarly to hepatitis A and thought to be waterborne.
   B. More serious to pregnant mothers and fetuses.
VI. Postnecrotic cirrhosis secondary to alcohol (PNC-E) (Alcoholic liver disease)
   A. Alcohol is one of the main causes of liver disease.
   B. Women have increased susceptibility to progress to liver disease, but this mechanism is poorly understood.
   C. May present as alcoholic hepatitis, fibrosis, or cirrhosis.
   D. No particular quantity of alcohol consumption predictably results in PNC-E[3] but risk increases with the amount consumed.
VII. Hepatocellular carcinoma (HCC)
   A. HCC is a malignant cancer of the liver cells.
   B. Risk factors include male gender, cirrhosis, chronic hepatitis B and C.
   C. Liver transplantation is an option in select patients.
VIII. Primary biliary cirrhosis (PBC) is a chronic, progressive cholestatic (retention of bile) disorder, which mainly affects middle-aged women.
   A. There is a gradual destruction of the interlobular bile ducts which leads to the development of cirrhosis.
   B. PBC is associated with itching (pruritus).
IX. Primary sclerosing cholangitis (PSC) is a chronic progressive disease of unknown etiology.
   A. Multiple fibrosing inflammatory strictures of the extra- and intrahepatic bile ducts.
   B. Progresses to cirrhosis, liver failure, and sometimes cholangiocarcinoma.
   C. Closely associated with inflammatory bowel disease, predominantly ulcerative colitis.

X. Autoimmune hepatitis is a chronic inflammatory disease of the liver of unknown cause.
 A. High percentages of patients with this diagnosis are female.
 B. 50% of these are under 50 years old.
 C. Some patients respond to steroid treatment.

XI. Hemachromatosis is an inherited disease in which an excessive amount of iron is absorbed and cannot be excreted from the body and is deposited in the liver and other organs.
 A. Eventually cirrhosis may develop.

XII. Wilson's disease is an autosomal recessive disorder of copper metabolism.
 A. Copper is a component of many enzymes and plasma proteins such as ceruloplasmin.
 B. Biliary excretion of copper, as well as ceruloplasmin synthesis, is impaired in Wilson's disease leading to the accumulation of copper in the liver and other organs.
 C. Wilson's disease can present as chronic liver disease or acute liver failure.

XIII. Alpha 1-antitrypsin deficiency (A1AT): A1AT is an enzyme made by the liver which helps to break down trypsin and other tissue proteases.
 A. A1AT deficiency is a common inherited disorder; structural abnormalities of the protein may disrupt normal cellular transport of A1AT in hepatocytes, and accumulation of the defective protein results in potentially severe liver disease.
 B. The lungs can also be affected, leading to emphysema.

XIV. Nonalcoholic Steatohepatitis (NASH) is a condition being diagnosed more frequently.
 A. It involves the development of fatty changes (steatosis) and lobular infiltration in the absence of alcohol excess, which leads to fibrosis and cirrhosis.
 B. It is associated with obesity and diabetes.

XV. Cryptogenic cirrhosis is a term given to patients with liver disease where no diagnosis can be established.

XVI. Drug-induced cirrhosis is a syndrome in which hepatotoxicity is caused by drugs, toxins, or other foreign chemicals.
 A. Sometimes this may cause fibrosis and cirrhosis over many years, or it may be acute.
 B. In the United States, United Kingdom, and Australia, acetaminophen (paracetamol) is one of the most common causes of acute liver failure, often resulting from deliberate or inadvertent overdosing.
 C. Other selected common drugs that cause hepatotoxicity include:
  1. Isoniazid
  2. Antiseizure medication
  3. Nonsteroidal anti-inflammatory drugs
  4. Some herbs and health food supplements
  5. Lipid-lowering drugs

XVII. Budd-Chiari syndrome is thrombosis of the hepatic veins, and patients present with abdominal pain, ascites, and hepatomegaly.
 A. This process can occur in patients with underlying thrombotic conditions.
 B. When occlusion of the hepatic veins is more gradual, collateral vessels form and fibrosis develops leading to cirrhosis.

C. However, when thrombosis occurs rapidly, acute liver failure may develop.

XVIII. Acute fatty liver of pregnancy (AFLP) is a rare disorder.
  A. Diffuse centrilobular fatty infiltration of hepatocytes is seen.
  B. Patients usually present in their third trimester of pregnancy.
  C. Symptoms are varied from none to acute liver failure.
  D. Nausea, vomiting, abdominal pain, and jaundice may be the presenting complaints.
  E. Prompt recognition and delivery is necessary to save the fetus and mother.

XIX. Acute liver failure
  A. In patients with acute liver failure, time is an important indicator of prognosis, and the term has been further subdivided into:
    1. Hyperacute liver failure, which is development of encephalopathy within 7 days.
    2. Acute liver failure includes those with jaundice-to-encephalopathy progression within 8 to 28 days.
    3. Subacute liver failure is suggested in patients with jaundice-to-encephalopathy progression from 5 to 12 weeks.[4]

XX. Subjective complaints of candidates: signs of worsening failure
  A. Patients should be referred for transplant assessment when they develop or experience their first major complication, for example:
    1. Ascites
    2. Variceal bleed
    3. Spontaneous bacterial peritonitis
    4. Hepatic encephalopathy
    5. Malnutrition[5]

XXI. Clinical manifestations of chronic liver disease
  A. Early symptoms include the following:
    1. Anorexia
    2. Indigestion
    3. Nausea and vomiting
    4. Fatigue
    5. Fever
    6. Constipation or diarrhea
    7. General weight loss

XXII. Signs and symptoms of worsening liver failure include:
  A. Jaundice, which occurs because the liver fails to metabolize bilirubin normally
  B. Bilirubin levels and jaundice increasing in patients with progressive liver disease
  C. Bleeding tendencies: the liver is the principal site of synthesis and regulation of coagulation proteins
  D. In worsening failure there is increased prothrombin time and decreased platelets, which results in easy bruising to significant bleeding when trauma or invasive procedures occur
  E. Pruritus, caused by increased concentration of bile salts or other chemicals in the blood
  F. Peripheral and ankle edema, caused by low albumin (usually below 30 g/L SI units or 3 g/dL conventional units) and/or massive ascites blocking venous return

G. Prominent abdominal wall veins (caput medusa): collateral vessels bypass the scarred liver to carry portal blood to the superior vena cava

H. Hemorrhoids—internal veins dilate with pressure of portal hypertension

I. Anemia due to:
1. GI blood losses
2. Erythrocyte destruction by pooling in enlarged spleen
3. Decreased folic acid due to dietary deficiency

J. Infection—leukopenia (low white cells) due to enlarged overactive spleen

K. Emaciation—caused by malnutrition and hypoalbuminemia

L. Fatigue

M. Most patients are generally hemodynamically compensated while exhibiting some symptoms of volume overload.

XXIII. Complications of worsening liver failure include:

A. Portal hypertension—defined as the elevation of hepatic venous pressure gradient (HVPG) to greater than 5 mm Hg.
1. This is caused by increased resistance to the passage of blood flow through the liver and increased splanchnic blood flow secondary to vasodilation within the splanchnic vascular bed.[5]

B. Ascites—accumulation of fluid in the peritoneal cavity caused by portal hypertension and low albumin, leading to excess formation of fluid within congested hepatic sinusoids

C. Spontaneous bacterial peritonitis (SBP)—this is infection in the ascites that can be induced when a patient has a paracentesis (ascites drained)

D. Esophageal and gastric varices—collateral veins in the esophagus and stomach bypass scarred liver cells to carry portal blood to the superior vena cava

E. Encephalopathy and coma
1. Ammonia and other toxins are no longer removed by the liver and accumulate to severe toxic levels in the brain causing confusion.
   a. This is usually treated with Lactulose and in some cases Neomycin.
   b. Normal ammonia levels are less than 40 μmol/L.
2. Grades of encephalopathy
   a. Grade 1—Slowing of consciousness
   b. Grade 2—Drowsiness
   c. Grade 3—Confusion, reactive only to vocal stimuli
   d. Grade 4—Presence of deep coma with absence of reaction to vocal stimuli

F. Hepatorenal failure involves rapidly failing renal function
1. Occasionally precipitated by volume depletion
2. Often seen in patients with advanced liver disease

LIVER TRANSPLANT ASSESSMENT

I. Patients with chronic end-stage liver disease will have to undergo a thorough assessment before they are accepted to go onto a liver transplant list.

II. This assessment includes:
A. Laboratory tests
B. Radiology and other clinical investigations

C. Consultations with members of the transplant team including:
   1. Surgeon
   2. Physician
   3. Anesthetist
   4. Dietitian
   5. Nurses
   6. Social worker
   7. Transplant coordinator
   8. Psychiatric liaison alcohol nurse
   9. Psychiatrist
   10. Meeting other patients who have undergone liver transplantation (see also Chapter 1).
D. Evaluation of the patient's family/social situation is also of major importance.
   1. Different centers will have different ways to do this, but it is often the role of the social worker and transplant coordinator.
   2. Identifying who will be the key caregiver for the patient both pre- and post-transplant is necessary in order to ensure compliance with attending hospital appointments and also to ensure quick and effective discharge from hospital.
   3. Chronic illness and having to give up employment, as well as patients often living long distances from the transplant unit can also have major financial implications for individuals.
   4. Input from social workers is needed to deal with these issues.
E. In many centers, patients being transplanted for alcoholic cirrhosis will undergo a thorough assessment by an alcohol team which may consist of an alcohol liaison nurse, psychiatrist, and/or social worker.
   1. Data suggest that long-term post-transplant survival for alcoholic cirrhosis is no different from other types of cirrhosis.[7, 8]
   2. In the U.S., many centers will follow the guidelines laid down by the American Society of Transplant Physicians with the American Society for the study of Liver Disease,[9] which states that patients should have refrained from drinking for a minimum of 6 months prior to liver transplantation.
   3. In the UK, a strict 6-month rule is not in place; however, it is very clear that patients need to be abstinent from alcohol from the time that they have been informed by a medical doctor to stop drinking.
      a. This, of course, could be less than six months.
      b. Centers will also have different rules about getting patients to sign a contract or agreement that states they will not go back to drinking post-transplant.
III. Due to the sudden deterioration of patients in acute liver failure, these patients can be listed very quickly and do not go through the same process of assessment.
A. Often family members are spoken with to gather a history and further information about the patient.
B. This is especially important for patients who have taken acetaminophen (paracetamol), deliberately, to establish whether they really want to survive with transplantation.
IV. The medical assessment of the patient for transplantation includes:
A. Basic laboratory tests
   1. Liver function tests (LFT)

2. Creatinine and electrolytes or blood urea nitrogen (BUN)
3. Full blood count (FBC)/complete blood count (CBC)
4. Clotting prothrombin time (PT), International Normalized Ratio (INR), and partial thromboplastin time (PTT)
5. Antinuclear antibody (ANA), antimitochondrial antibody (AMA)
6. Alpha-fetoprotein (cancer marker)
7. Blood type
8. Alcohol and drug levels
9. Virology screen, including:
   a. Hepatitis A virus
   b. Hepatitis C virus
   c. Hepatitis B virus
   d. HIV
   e. Cytomegalovirus (CMV), IgG/IgM
   f. Epstein-Barr virus (EBV)
   g. Varicella zoster
10. Other tests
    a. Liver biopsy or review of liver histology slides from local hospital may be needed
    b. Chest x-ray (CXR)
    c. Electrocardiogram (ECG/EKG)
    d. Echocardiogram (ECHO)
    e. Pulmonary artery pressure and ejection fraction should be assessed
    f. Ultrasound scan of liver (USS/US)
       i. To assess patency of portal and hepatic veins and mass lesions
          a) If patency of portal vein cannot be documented on Doppler ultrasound, computed tomography (CT) imaging or magnetic resonance imaging (MRI) should be conducted.
          b) There is also often significant variation in normal anatomy of both the vascular and biliary trees in the liver.
          c) This dictates the specific surgical approaches in transplantation; it is therefore important to map out these variations.
          d) Individual transplant centers will decide the best investigation to map these variations, CT versus MRI/MRA.
    g. Spirometry tests are usually an adequate screen.
       i. If readings are abnormal or lung function abnormality is suspected (for example, alpha-1 antitrypsin or pulmonary fibrosis) formal lung function tests are required.
    h. Endoscopy is done to observe for esophageal varices.
    i. Colonoscopy is done in patients with:
       i. Primary sclerosing cholangitis, as they are more at risk of colon cancer
       ii. Crohn's disease or colitis, to look at severity of disease in the bowel, polyps, or cancer.
V. Multidisciplinary team consultations and education
   A. Each transplant service will have an individualized transplant assessment process for their patients.
   B. This may be done purely in an outpatient setting or in some centers, while the patient is in the hospital.

1. Either way, the process is similar and involves key team members.
C. Education and information provision to patients and their families is a major focus in the assessment process.
   1. This is best done by both written and verbal means.
   2. Many patients will not remember everything that is said during the assessment process.
   3. Some will need time to take the information in (see also Chapter 3, Patient Education).

VI. Transplant meeting
  A. In many centers, there is a multidisciplinary transplant meeting in which patients are discussed by the team and either accepted or turned down for liver transplantation.
  B. Reasons for not accepting a patient for transplant by individual centers include:
    1. Hepatoma size too large
    2. Active substance abuse
    3. Extra hepatic malignancy
    4. Advanced cardiac or pulmonary disease
    5. Unacceptable psychological situation such as homelessness or absence of family/social network

VII. Listing and preparing the patient for transplantation
  A. In liver transplantation, due to the regenerative capacity of the liver cells, splitting or reducing a liver is a possibility.
    1. This means that an adult patient can receive either a split or whole liver.
    2. Pediatric patients can receive either a whole, split, or reduced-size graft (see Chapter 15).
  B. When a patient has been placed onto the transplant waiting list in the United States, he or she is awarded a priority based on the UNOS organ allocation scheme.
    1. This is based on the current Model for End-stage Liver Disease (MELD).
      a. The MELD score is calculated on serum creatinine, serum bilirubin, and International Normalized Ratio.
      b. The score range is 6-40.
      c. The MELD gives each patient a score based on how urgently he/she needs a liver transplant.
      d. Other countries will have different ways of organ allocation and do not necessarily use the MELD scoring system.
  C. Once an organ becomes available, the transplant coordinator will contact the hospital unit if the patient is hospitalized and standing orders are implemented to begin preoperative laboratory testing.
    1. If the patient is at home waiting:
      a. Directions are given to the patient regarding the time and place to report for admission.
      b. The charge nurse is contacted to ensure bed availability.
    2. Patients can react in different ways when they are called in for their transplant.
      a. Some are happy and excited and look forward to the surgery.
      b. Others can be an exceptionally distressed, emotional, and frightened.

VIII. On admission to the hospital
    A. The patient should have all vital signs taken, including temperature, blood pressure, and pulse.
    B. Any sign of infection could prevent transplantation, and a fever should be discussed with the physician.
    C. Weight should be recorded as a baseline for drug dose calculations.
    D. Patients and their families need psychological/emotional support, and they may need questions answered and reassurance.
    E. Some patients may want the opportunity to speak to a hospital chaplain.

  IX. Preparation for the surgery includes:
    A. Laboratory tests
        1. Full blood count to check for raised white cell count, platelet, and hemoglobin (HB) levels.
        2. Clotting screen—to check INR
        3. Full chemistry panel to check sodium and creatinine
        4. Crossmatch (see chapter on Transplant Immunology)
        5. A set amount of blood products will be ordered for the surgery
            a. Centers may differ in the amount ordered.
        6. Glucose
            a. If a patient is diabetic, a sliding scale insulin regimen and fluids should be given before surgery when patients are taking nothing by mouth.
        7. Other investigations
            a. CXR—to look for any infection or new changes
            b. ECG—to look for any cardiac changes
            c. If febrile, blood cultures should be taken
            d. If gross ascites is present, a diagnostic tap should be done to exclude spontaneous bacterial peritonitis.
            e. Consent for the operation may have already been obtained by the transplant surgeon at listing
                i. If not, this will be done on admission

   X. Transplant operation
    A. The liver transplant procedure will last for 6-12 hours and consists of:
        1. The hepatectomy (removal of the liver)
        2. Implantation of the new liver which involves:
            a. Anastomosis of the inferior vena cava, portal vein, hepatic artery, and the biliary connection via a duct-to-duct anastomosis (choledochocholedochostomy).
            b. Some centers excise the vena cava with the native liver, though others preserve it and suture the donor cava and recipient cava as a piggyback.
            c. Some centers may use a T tube which is placed in the bile duct before the anastomosis.
            d. However, if a Roux-en-Y choledochojejunostomy is performed where the bile duct is connected to the bowel, a T tube is not needed (Fig. 11-1).

  XI. Post-transplant monitoring and maintenance in Intensive Care (ICU)
    A. Intra-operative mortality remains very rare.
    B. Patients will return to an ICU post-transplant, and many patients will be fully ventilated for the first 12-24 hours.

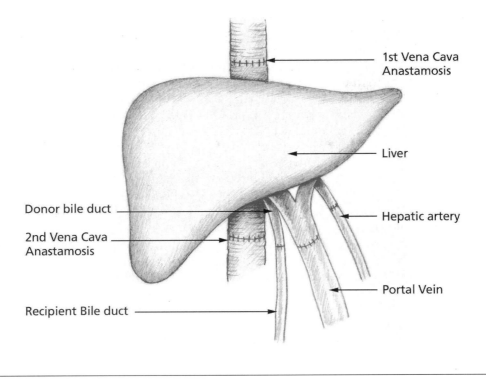

1st Vena Cava
Anastamosis

Liver

Donor bile duct

Hepatic artery

2nd Vena Cava
Anastamosis

Portal Vein

Recipient Bile duct

Figure 11-1. Standard liver transplant.

    C. Those with good clotting and platelet counts preoperatively and no significant portal hypertension may have had an epidural.

    D. Some units will "fast-track" patients using a rapidly acting opioid such as remifentanil as part of the anesthetic technique.

        1. This will allow extubation in the operating room before returning to the ICU.

    E. The immediate postoperative course can vary greatly, and each patient will have a different recovery.

    F. Patients with chronic liver disease may experience hyperdynamic circulation, a low systemic vascular resistance (SVR), and high cardiac output (CO) and cardiac index (CI), and this can often continue post-transplant in the early stages.

        1. May be treated with fluid management, but can also require inotrope support.

        2. Adequate perfusion is necessary for the transplanted liver and other vital organs.

        3. As the liver function improves, the cardiac output and index will fall and the systemic vascular resistance will return to normal.

XII. Monitoring immediately post-transplant includes:

    A. Hemodynamic monitoring may be done via a pulmonary artery catheter, central venous catheter, and an arterial line.

    B. A pulmonary artery catheter allows for measurements of:

        1. CO

        2. CI

        3. SVR

    4. Pulmonary artery wedge pressure (PAW)
        a. The pulmonary artery catheter is the only accurate way to measure PAW pressure.
        b. Use of pulmonary artery catheters is decreasing and patients are now often monitored with a transesophageal echo probe (TEE) instead.
            i. This probe is inserted via the esophagus and gives a picture of the heart.
                a) Enables the anesthetist to see the chambers dilating
                b) Demonstrates how well the heart is beating
           ii. There is software with the TEE which can generate cardiac output measurements based on dimensions.
    C. Blood pressure is monitored via an arterial line.

XIII. Hypovolemia associated with rewarming
    A. Post-transplant, as the patient warms up, hypotension and a drop in CVP may take effect due to hypovolemia.
        1. This is treated with colloid or blood or if a patient has a low albumin, an infusion of albumin 20%.
        2. Occurs less frequently with active patient warming.

XIV. Bleeding can be seen in the first 48 hours.
    A. Can result from an underlying coagulopathy, which can be seen with a poorly functioning graft.
    B. Hemoglobin (Hb) and CVP measurements should be monitored.
        1. Ideally, Hb should be kept between 11-14 mg/dl (U.S.) 8-10 g/L (U.K.)
        2. CVP should be maintained around 6-8 cm H_2O.
    C. INR and hematocrit should also be monitored.

XV. Hypovolemia due to bleeding should be corrected with blood as appropriate and FFP or platelets to correct abnormal coagulation.
    A. Observation of the surgical drain to monitor extent of output and a swollen abdomen can also reveal signs of bleeding.
    B. Tachycardia and pallor of the patient will be observed if he or she is bleeding.
    C. If the coagulopathy cannot be corrected and bleeding continues, re-exploration may be necessary.

XVI. Renal function
    A. Urine output should be > 30 ml/hr or 1–2 ml/kg/hr.
    B. If a patient has persistent oliguria and an adequate CVP > 6 cm H_2O, dialysis may be required.
    C. There are three main indications for renal dialysis:
        1. Elevated serum urea or potassium
           a. No absolute values, but serum urea (BUN) > 40 μmol/L (SI units) or hyperkalemia are common indicators.
        2. Acidosis
        3. Volume overload management

XVII. Laboratory tests
    A. Laboratory blood tests will include:
        1. Urea and creatinine
        2. Liver function tests
           a. Aspartate transaminase (AST) should steadily decline over the first few days.
           b. Bilirubin levels will decline initially.

          i.   This is not a sign of graft function but hemodilution.

    c. Alkaline phosphatase (ALP) can often be seen with normal values in the early postoperative period.

        i.   However, a rise in ALP can be a sign of biliary complications or cholestasis.

        ii. In a nonfunctioning graft, a high AST and ALT will be seen.

        iii. AST elevations will be more pronounced and occur earlier than elevated ALT.

        iv. These high values are a sign of liver parenchymal injury.

  3. Complete blood count (CBC)

  4. Clotting screen

    a. PT/INR should be measured every 8 hours.

    b. A decline in PT is a sign of returning hepatic function.

    c. FFP may be given to correct clotting, and low platelets may be supported with a platelet infusion.

    d. A PT which is elevated >25 seconds and that continues to rise with vitamin K or FFP is a sign of a nonfunctioning liver.

  5. Glucose

    a. Glucose levels should return to normal quickly after transplant if the liver is functioning.

        i.   The liver is the primary source of blood glucose.

        ii. High glucose levels should be treated with insulin.

        iii. In a nonfunctioning liver, glucose levels will be low and support will be necessary with 50% dextrose.

  6. Arterial blood gases (ABGs)

    a. ABGs will be monitored every 8 hours if the patient is stable but may need to be done every 2-4 hours in an unstable patient.

    b. Acid-base disturbances should resolve rapidly in a functioning liver transplant.

        i.   The lactate will decline.

        ii. A high lactate and acidosis is a sign of poor function.

XVIII. Maintenance fluid

  A. For all transplant patients with liver failure, IV maintenance fluid is generally necessary and should be titrated according to BP, CVP, and urine output.

  B. Some centers may use $D_{10}W$ as maintenance to provide adequate glucose for the new stabilizing liver until good gluconeogenesis and glycolysis can occur.

  C. Bowel sounds should be monitored closely and should be present before oral fluids are commenced.

XIX. Drainage output

  A. Nasogastric (NG) drainage

    1. All patients will return to the Intensive Care unit with an NG tube in place.

      a. This can be used to give medication or be aspirated if vomiting occurs.

    2. Once patients are able to tolerate oral fluids, the tube is removed.

  B. A urinary catheter will be in place to enable close monitoring of urine output.

    1. A low urine output could be a sign of dehydration.

    2. If output does not improve with fluid or diuretics, dialysis may be necessary.

3. The catheter is generally removed once a patient has been transferred to the ward and is able to void.
C. A surgical drain or drains are inserted at the end of the transplant.
    1. Different transplant centers will have different practices, but in the U.S., Jackson-Pratt drains are used.
    2. There can be three drains:
        a. Two in the right lower quadrant
        b. One in the left
        c. Other centers may only insert one drain in the right side
        d. The color and consistency of the drainage should be monitored for signs of bleeding.
            i. If the drainage is green, this could be a sign of a bile leak.
    3. T-tube drains are used routinely in some centers, but in other centers T-tubes are used only if the transplant was performed using a split liver.
        a. Amount and consistency of bile drainage can be monitored.
        b. They can stay in for up to 3 months.
        c. T tube cholangiograms can be performed to assess the extra hepatic bile ducts.
XX. Pain management
    A. Pain is initially controlled by giving intravenous morphine or fentanyl in the first 24-48 hours.
    B. Pain medication is weaned to help patients to breathe spontaneously and wean from the ventilator.
    C. When the dose is lower, oral analgesic agents like acetaminophen or oxycodone are commenced.
XXI. Fever
    A. Fever can be seen post-transplant.
    B. A patient's temperature should be measured peripherally and centrally.
    C. In the first few days, a fever is probably due to infection which can lead to sepsis if not treated.
        1. In immunocompromised patients, a fever is typically defined at 38.2° C (lower than for other patients).
        2. Hypothermia can also be suggestive of sepsis.
    D. Blood cultures should be sent.
    E. C reactive protein (CRP) should be monitored.
        1. This is a protein present in acute inflammatory conditions and sepsis.[10]
    F. White blood cell count should be evaluated.
    G. Fever can also be present in acute rejection, which can be seen from day 6.
        1. Rejection is discussed later in the chapter.
XXII. Daily weights
    A. Daily weights are important to assess fluid accumulation or loss, malnutrition, and for drug calculations for immunosuppression.
XXIII. Neurologic assessment
    A. Post-transplant neurologic complications can be seen.
        1. A decreased level of consciousness can be due to the anesthetic agents used.
            a. The rate of recovery may depend on the function of the new liver.
        2. Hepatic encephalopathy seen in a patient pretransplant can also take time to resolve post-transplant.

3. Renal failure or sepsis post-transplant may lead to metabolic encephalopathy.
4. Significant perioperative hypotension may lead to hypoxic ischemic encephalopathy.
5. Transplant patients with acute liver failure who have encephalopathy and cerebral edema pretransplant, may also have a period of diminished consciousness level postoperatively.
6. In recipients who have initial normal postoperative neurologic course and then a sudden deterioration, an intracranial bleed needs to be ruled out.[5]
7. *De novo* seizures can occur after liver transplant, and these can be caused by:
   a. Electrolyte imbalances
      i. Magnesium, phosphate, sodium, and calcium levels should be checked.
   b. Reaction to cyclosporine or tacrolimus
   c. Intracerebral abcesses
   d. Intracranial hemorrhage or cerebral infarction
8. EEG and CT/MRI brain scans should be considered.
9. Figure 11-2 demonstrates complications reported in the U.K. post liver transplantation.

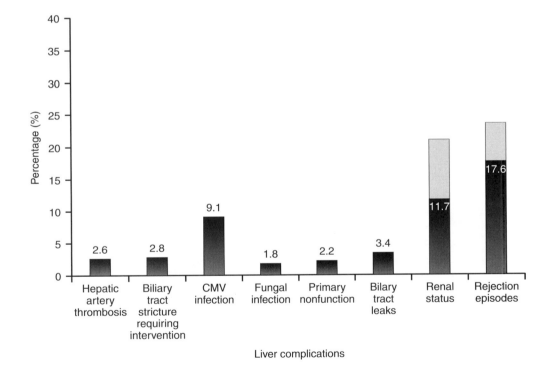

Figure 11-2. Complications within 3 months of liver transplant from 504 adult liver only transplants in the U.K. in 2005.[11] Note: Figure shows percentage of complications that occurred in patients where reported. Five other liver-only transplants occurred in this period but have no follow-up data.

XXIV. Primary nonfunction and early dysfunction
  A. Graft function can be seen at the time of reperfusion.
  B. Early indicators of nonfunction
      1. The quantity and quality of bile production
      2. Extreme edema of the organ
      3. Abnormal color
      4. Lack of reperfusion
      5. Mottled reperfusion
      6. Adequacy of urine output
      7. Hemodynamic instability
      8. Absence of increased temperature
      9. Glucose, potassium, and lactate abnormalities, and coagulopathy
  C. One of the causes for primary nonfunction is preservation injury which prevents the organ from recovery.
      1. Causative factors include:
          a. Donor steatosis
          b. Donor age (older donors)
          c. Prolonged donor hospital stay
          d. Prolonged cold ischemic time
      2. Primary nonfunction leads to multiorgan failure.
          a. Without retransplantation, death occurs.
      3. Although the incidence of primary nonfunction will vary in different centers, the risk is about 2%-5%.
  D. In cases of initial poor function, recovery is usually seen by the third post-transplant day.
XXV. Early hepatic artery thrombosis
  A. Elevated AST and ALT can also be due to a thrombosed hepatic artery.
  B. This is more commonly seen in children than adults.
      1. If no action is taken, this can progress to:
          a. Parenchymal infarction
          b. Necrosis
          c. Sepsis
  C. Hepatic artery thrombosis can be seen as early as day 1 post-transplant.
      1. There is no clear cause of this thrombosis, but it must always be excluded if primary nonfunction occurs.
      2. Retransplantation may be necessary.
  D. Figure 11-3 demonstrates the rise in AST that can be seen in primary graft nonfunction and hepatic artery thrombosis.

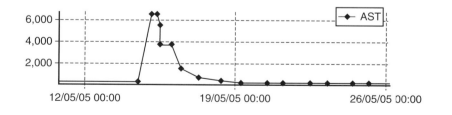

Figure 11-3. The rise in AST that can be seen in primary graft nonfunction and hepatic artery thrombosis. Following retransplantation, the AST resolves to normal range.

XXVI. Bleeding
    A. Bleeding is generally seen in the first 48 hours and can be due to an underlying coagulopathy or technical problems.
    B. Observation of the surgical drains to monitor extent of output and color of drainage, as well as observing for a swollen abdomen, are necessary to assess for signs of bleeding.
    C. If bleeding cannot be controlled with blood and clotting factors, reexploration may be necessary.

XXVII. Infection
    A. Infections in post liver transplant patients can be common.
    B. This is related to suppression of the immune system by medications used to prevent rejection.
    C. In the first few weeks, infections are usually nosocomial gram-negative bacteria from lines, wound, blood, urinary, respiratory, or biliary tract.
    D. Fungal infections can also occur.
        1. This is more frequently seen in high-risk patients, acute liver failure patients, retransplantation, those with renal support pretransplant, and those on high doses of immunosuppression.[12]
    E. Temperature, CRP, and white cell counts should be monitored and appropriate antibiotics should be commenced if elevated.
    F. Sending of specimens of urine, sputum, wound swabs, and blood cultures should be done to locate the area of infection.
    G. Cytomegalovirus (CMV) can also be seen post liver transplant.
        1. CMV is carried in approximately 50% of the population and can be passed on through the donor liver.
        2. CMV infection rarely occurs before 21 days, and can be seen 1-4 months post-transplant.
        3. Patients may experience high temperatures, rigors, body aches, and night sweats.
        4. In immunocompromised patients, it can also cause pneumonia, hepatitis, gastrointestinal infection, pancreatitis, and retinitis.
        5. Treatment is with intravenous ganciclovir until the virus has cleared (see also Chapters 5 and 6).

XXVIII. Renal dysfunction
    A. Renal dysfunction can be seen pretransplant as hepatorenal failure, but can also be seen in the postoperative phase.
    B. Causes for postop renal dysfunction can be:
        1. Hypotensive episodes
        2. Blood loss
        3. High renal vein pressure intraoperatively and postoperatively due to:
            a. Hemodynamic instability
            b. Sepsis
            c. Immunosuppressive drugs and other drugs such as vancomycin
        4. Although some patients may require dialysis for a period of time, once the liver function improves, the renal function recovers and dialysis may be discontinued.

XXIX. Ascites
    A. Patients with preoperative ascites may continue to have this postoperatively; the problem is not immediately resolved.
    B. Diuretics may be required in some cases.
    C. Good nutrition and high-protein diet are the best treatment.

    D. It is important to ensure the patient is aware that the ascites will decline as liver function improves.

XXX. Pleural effusions

    A. Pleural effusions are very common post liver transplant.

       1. They occur on the right side due to the trauma of the surgical retractors during surgery.

       2. Small effusions are not necessarily treated; but if breathing is affected, then drainage of the effusion may be needed.

          a. Before this is done, a complete blood count and clotting screen should be taken and any underlying coagulopathy corrected.

       3. Treatment for pleural effusion may include a thoracentesis, antibiotics, or chest tube drainage depending on the severity of this complication.

XXXI. Cholestasis

    A. Cholestasis may develop and is usually associated with rejection, sepsis, drug toxicity, or preservation injury.

    B. If preservation injury is the causative factor, liver function tests start to normalize after 3-4 days.

    C. There is no specific treatment for cholestasis.

       1. Some centers may use ursodeoxycholic acid (Actigall, URSO 250).

          a. A pharmaceutical agent used to dissolve gallstones and prevent liver disease.

          b. Used to promote bile flow in cholestatic conditions.

XXXII. Bile duct complications

    A. A rise in alkaline phosphatase, and sometimes bilirubin, gamma glutamyltransferase (GGT), and transaminase levels can be signs of biliary tract problems.[14]

    B. Biliary complications can be seen at any time post liver transplant.

    C. There are two types: biliary leaks and biliary obstructions

       1. Biliary leaks

          a. Bile leaks can occur in the following locations:

             i. At the site of anastomosis

             ii. T tube exit site

             iii. Along the T tube tract at the time of removal

             iv. Within the liver as a result of bile duct destruction (bile lake)

             v. From the cut surface in a split liver or after a liver biopsy.[14]

          b. Anastomotic leak

             i. If there is an anastomotic leak, bile-stained fluid may be seen in the surgical drain.

             ii. In severe cases, frank bile may even leak through the surgical wound.

             iii. The patient may develop peritonitis with signs of systemic sepsis.

             iv. Blood tests frequently show elevated bilirubin and white cell count.

             v. In duct-to-duct anastomoses (Figure 11-4), small leaks may be treated with internal stents placed percutaneously or via endoscopic retrograde cholangiopancreatography (ERCP).

             vi. Bile collections can be drained percutaneously and a Pigtail drain inserted.

             vii. Large leaks should be surgically repaired with construction of a Roux-en-Y choledochojejunostomy (Figure 11-5).

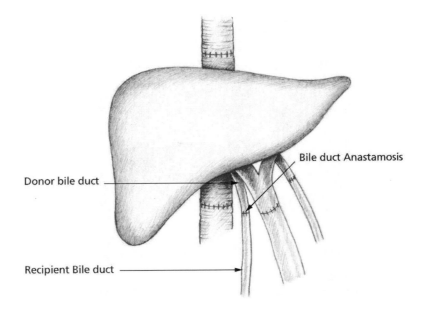

Figure 11-4. Duct-to-duct anastomosis.

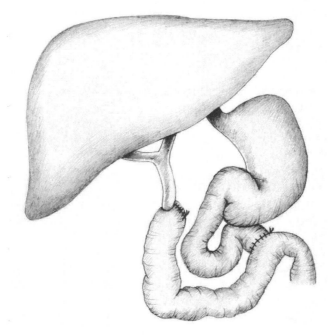

Figure 11-5. Roux-en-Y choledochojejunostomy.

    c. T tube leaks
        i. A transient leak at the exit site of a T tube is quite common after T-tube removal and usually settles spontaneously.
       ii. Rarely, T-Tube removal results in bile leaking into the peritoneal cavity, causing biliary peritonitis.
          a) This requires urgent radiological or surgical drainage.
      iii. Delaying the removal of T-tubes for up to 3 months post-transplant allows for the biliary tract to mature, but even after this time leaks can occur.

2. Biliary obstruction
    a. Bile duct obstruction is usually associated with technical complications at the anastomosis.
    b. The earliest sign is an elevated serum alkaline phosphatase, followed by a rising bilirubin.
    c. An ultrasound scan will show biliary dilatation and a cholangiogram will demonstrate the site of obstruction.

XXXIII. Anastomotic strictures
    A. An anastomotic stricture is a narrowing at the point where the donor bile duct has been sewn onto the recipient bile duct.
    B. This may be seen due to faulty surgical technique, local ischemia, scar tissue formation, or hepatic artery thrombosis.
    C. Anastomotic strictures can be treated with ERCP, balloon dilatation, and a biliary stent.
    D. Recurrent strictures often require surgical correction.[14, 15]

XXXIV. Nonanastomotic strictures
    A. Strictures which form at other sites are usually secondary to ischemia, and are associated with hepatic artery thrombosis, prolonged cold ischemic time of the donor organ, livers from non-heart beating donors, and recurrent cholangitis.

XXXV. Intestinal perforation
    A. Perforations of the intestinal tract can be related to intra-operative events and can be seen in the first 10 days post-transplant.
    B. The use of steroids for immunosuppression can also delay healing and assist development of a perforation.
    C. In children, intestinal perforation can be spontaneous.
    D. Patients usually present with abdominal pain and distension together with fever and systemic sepsis.

XXXVI. Portal vein thrombosis
    A. Portal vein thrombosis is a very rare postoperative complication.
    B. If it occurs in the early postoperative period, it is usually a technical complication; or it can be seen in patients who had a preoperative thrombosis and inadequate restoration of the portal flow.
    C. It manifests with abnormal liver function tests and can lead to variceal hemorrhage, intestinal ischemia, and ascites.[14]
    D. Diagnosis is made by doppler ultrasound scan. In the late post-transplant course, a patient may present with variceal hemorrhage due to portal hypertension caused by thrombosis.

XXXVII. Hepatic vein strictures and thrombosis
    A. Strictures and thrombosis of the hepatic vein are rare but may be associated with a hypercoaguable state, particularly in patients with preoperative Budd-Chiari syndrome.

B. It may also be caused by anastomotic strictures or kinking at the caval anastomosis.

C. Patients usually present with severe ascites and leg edema.

    1. Diagnosis is made with a doppler ultrasound but may also need venography.

    2. Partial hepatic vein thrombosis can be tolerated or the patient may even be asymptomatic.

    3. Complete venous outflow obstruction may require stenting, angioplasty, or even retransplantation.[13, 14]

XXXVIII. Other complications and appropriate interventions

A. Impaired wound healing

    1. Transplant recipients are at risk of impaired wound healing due to their immunosuppressant drugs and poor nutritional status.

    2. Daily skin assessments should be done on every patient.

    3. Complete inspection of incisions, tube sites, and pressure areas help to prevent complications.

    4. Patients will often have an inverted Y incision which is commonly called a Mercedes incision.

    5. The skin is held together by surgical clips or staples and will typically be removed 3 weeks post-op.

    6. Incisions should be well-approximated without any signs of edge separation, necrosis, or dehiscence.

    7. If a wound should break down, a saline dressing should be applied and a surgeon notified immediately.

    8. There should be no sign of redness, swelling, or purulent drainage. If an infection does occur, some incisions may need to have staples removed and be left open.

        a. Wet-to-dry dressings and/or a wound culture and antibiotics may be warranted.

        b. Depending on the wound appearance, a wound care nurse may be consulted for recommendations which might include an enzymatic debridement.

    9. Daily incision care should include cleaning the wound with normal saline or soap and water.

        a. No lotions or powder should be applied directly to the incision.

        b. Those patients with extra fluid on board immediately postoperatively, may require a dry dressing over the incision until drainage ceases.

   10. For patients with Jackson-Pratt (JPs) and/or a T-tube drains in place, these sites need to be monitored for signs of redness, swelling, or purulent drainage.

        a. Once a drain is pulled, the site should still be cleaned daily and covered with a dry dressing until the site is healed.

        b. Generally, the T-tube, whether it is open or capped off, remains for 3-4 months.

   11. Patient education is a primary key to preventing wound infections.

        a. Patients and their families must be instructed on the importance of proper incision and drain care.

        b. A home health nurse may be consulted as needed upon discharge from hospital.

            i. Collaboration with the multidisciplinary team is also an integral part of the patient recovery.

     ii. The physical therapist and occupational therapist help to mobilize the patient to prevent pressure ulcers, which in turn helps to promote wound healing.

     iii. The nutritionist may be needed to make recommendations to ensure the patient is receiving adequate nutrition which goes hand in hand with promoting wound healing.

12. Fluid and electrolyte imbalances
   a. Fluid and electrolyte imbalances are another possible complication post liver transplant.
   b. Careful monitoring of fluid imbalances, such as overload or dehydration, is imperative on a daily basis.
   c. Routine assessment for fluid overload and dehydration should include observing for:
      i. Dyspnea
      ii. Dry mucous membranes
      iii. Poor skin turgor
      iv. Decreased urine output
      v. Dizziness
      vi. Lightheadedness
      vii. Distended neck veins
      viii. Mental status changes
      ix. Edema (commonly seen in the extremities and scrotum)
      x. Ascites
      xi. Muscle aches and/or weakness
      xii. Abnormal laboratory values
   d. Interventions as ordered by the physician may include:
      i. Fluid replacement or fluid restriction
      ii. Daily weights
      iii. Strict intake and output measurements
      iv. Diuretics with/without salt poor albumin replacement
      v. Electrolyte replacement as needed
      vi. In regard to electrolyte imbalance, daily laboratory assessment should include:
         a) Sodium
         b) Potassium
         c) Magnesium
         d) Chloride
         e) Bicarbonate
         f) Creatinine
         g) Blood urea nitrogen
         h) Glucose
      vii. Any abnormalities may be treated with oral or intravenous electrolyte replacements.
      viii. A nutritionist may need to be consulted for recommendations for dietary restrictions or supplements as well.

13. Hypoglycemia and hyperglycemia
   a. Hypo- and hyperglycemia can be seen post liver transplant.
   b. If the new liver is able to convert glucose into glycogen and store it, the transplanted liver is functioning.
      i. Therefore, some degree of hyperglycemia is evident.

    ii. Hyperglycemia is also commonly related to the patient's immunosuppressant regimen, which may include tacrolimus and steroids.

   iii. In a nonfunctioning liver, the patient may experience hypoglycemia.

   iv. Signs and symptoms of hypoglycemia include:
- a) Cool clammy skin
- b) Diaphoresis
- c) Mental status changes
- d) Fatigue
- e) Palpitations
- f) Tremors

   v. Any of the mentioned signs or symptoms, should be reported immediately if noted.

   vi. Signs and symptoms of hyperglycemia include:
- a) Polyuria
- b) Polydipsia
- c) Polyphagia
- d) Blurred vision
- e) Poor wound healing
- f) Recurrent infections

   vii. The following interventions would be expected for each complication:
- a) Measurements of capillary blood glucose levels, administration of glucose or insulin, and offering of limited carbohydrates
- b) Collaborating with the members of the multidisciplinary team as necessary
- c) Recommendations on dietary changes given by the nutritionist
- d) Better management of the specific complication, as elaborated on by a diabetes educator
- e) Reinforcement of the patient's education in the home setting by a home health nurse

14. Hypo- and hypertension
   a. Hypo- and hypertension can be seen in post liver transplant patients.
   b. Patients need to be monitored for vital sign changes and level of consciousness.
   c. Hypotension can be due to dehydration, bleeding, or sepsis.

    i. Signs of hypotension include:
- a) Decreased blood pressure
- b) Increased pulse
- c) Dizziness
- d) Lightheadedness
- e) Any signs and symptoms of bleeding

   ii. Hypotension is usually treated with fluid boluses or blood transfusions and in sepsis, inotrope therapy.

   iii. Patients may need to be placed on bed rest until vital signs stabilize.

    iv. Patients also need to have electrolyte and blood counts checked every morning and appropriate antibiotic regimens commenced if septic.

  d. Hypertension may be due to too much fluid, to pain, or to calcineurin inhibitors and/or corticosteroids used for antirejection regimen.

    i. Signs of hypertension may include:

      a) Increased blood pressure and pulse

      b) Headaches

    ii. Pain control should be optimized; then treatment with diuretics or by administering oral/IV vasoactive drugs may be needed if hypertension persists.

      a) This must be done with careful observation because calcium channel blockers such as diltiazem or verapamil may increase cyclosporine or tacrolimus levels and doses may need to be adjusted accordingly.

      b) Patients need to be monitored with frequent vital signs and evaluated for a response to any interventions performed.

      c) Patient and family education should include:

        1) Signs and symptoms of hypo- and hypertension

        2) Instructions about blood pressure medications

        3) Instructions on monitoring blood pressure everyday and recording readings

        4) Instructions on when to contact the postoperative coordinator

15. Altered bowel function

  a. Constipation can be a common problem post-transplant.

  b. The nurse should assess and document daily whether the patient has a bowel movement.

  c. If a patient complains of abdominal pain and distention, the physician should be notified.

  d. Encouraging an increase in fluid and fiber intake, in addition to increasing activity, may help the patient move his/her bowels.

    i. However, if the discomfort is too severe, it is unlikely that the patient can tolerate the mobility.

    ii. In such a case, the physician may prescribe a stool softener such as docusate sodium (Colace).

    iii. If that is ineffective, a suppository may be needed (glycerin or dulcolax are most commonly used).

    iv. An enema may be needed.

  e. Diarrhea may also develop.

    i. The frequency and consistency of the bowel movement should be assessed and documented.

    ii. The physician should be notified and a specimen may need to be collected to rule out infection as the cause.

    iii. A watery, foul-smelling stool may indicate *Clostridium difficile*.

      a) Isolation may be required.

      b) Oral metronidazole may be started until *Clostridium difficile* is ruled out.

        c) Dehydration should be of concern in a patient with diarrhea.

           1) Administer IV hydration if necessary.

        d) A review of the patient's medications should be done as some of the post liver transplant medications can cause diarrhea.

           1) If applicable, those medicines should be reduced or stopped.

16. Altered nutrition
    a. During the initial post-transplant period, it is not uncommon for a patient to be unable to meet nutritional requirements.
        i. In the liver transplant recipient, oral intake is usually started 1-3 days postoperatively with a clear liquid diet, advancing to solids as tolerated.
        ii. Those patients who have had a Roux-en-Y anastomosis may take longer to start oral fluids and diet.
    b. Appetite should be assessed with each meal to ensure adequate intake of dietary needs.
        i. If there is any question of altered nutrition, consult the nutritionist who in turn may recommend a calorie count to measure caloric intake.
        ii. Patients should be assessed for low serum albumin levels and weight changes.
        iii. Ideally, oral diets are the preferred methods of nutrition for the patient.
        iv. If patients are unable to tolerate large meals, small, frequent, and high-calorie meals should be encouraged.
        v. If nutritional goals are unable to be met, it may be beneficial to start oral nutritional supplements.
            a) If the goals are still not met, a nutritionist may recommend a physician to order enteral tube feedings via a feeding tube.
            b) In extreme cases where the gut is nonfunctioning, parenteral nutrition supplements may be instituted.
        vi. With collaborative teamwork, patient's nutritional needs can be met.
            a) This ultimately will help to prevent infection, promote adequate wound healing, and provide the metabolic support the patient requires.

17. Altered mobility/self-care deficit
    a. Liver transplant recipients will have some degree of altered mobility or self-care deficit initially.
    b. Advancement will require the efforts of the extended multidisciplinary team including physical therapy, occupational therapy, respiratory, and, in extreme cases, speech therapy.
    c. Early assessment of level of independence with activities of daily living is essential for setting goals for discharge from the hospital setting.
    d. The patient's pretransplant strength and activity may influence post-transplant recovery.
        i. Usually, the stronger the patient is going into the transplant, the quicker and easier the recovery should be.

ii. Once a patient is off the ventilator and the organ is functioning, physical therapy should be initiated and respiratory therapy continued.

iii. Patients should be encouraged on a daily basis to increase their progression to an independent level.

    a) When goals are unable to be met, patients sometimes need to be referred to an outpatient setting for further rehabilitation.

    b) Along with the multidisciplinary team, families are a vital part to the patient's recovery.

    c) They should be included in the patient's hospital care to assist in preparing the patient for discharge home.

18. Rejection

  a. Patients are monitored on a daily basis for signs and symptoms of rejection while in hospital.

  b. Liver function tests, total bilirubin levels, and tacrolimus or cyclosporine levels are checked every morning and monitored for any increased or abnormal levels that may indicate rejection.

  c. There are three different types of rejection: hyperacute, acute, and chronic.

    i. Hyperacute rejection is rare and occurs within minutes to days post-transplant.

    ii. The most common rejection is acute rejection. This can occur as early as 6 days or any time in the first 3 months post-transplant and needs to be confirmed by biopsy.

    iii. Up to 40% of patients may suffer acute rejection, which generally resolves after treatment.

    iv. Chronic rejection occurs less frequently and over a longer period of time and may lead to the need for retransplantation.

19. Post-biopsy monitoring

  a. Some centers may routinely biopsy patients on day 7, however most centers will only biopsy when there is a rise in liver function tests, indicating a possible rejection.

  b. Liver biopsies may be done in interventional radiology or on the ward.

    i. A small piece of liver tissue is extracted.

    ii. Patients need to be monitored in the post-biopsy period for any changes in vital signs such as low blood pressure or tachycardia that may be due to bleeding.

    iii. Hematoma and/or severe pain at the biopsy site should be reported to the physician.

      a) Patients are usually kept on bed rest for 4-6 hours with bathroom privileges only.

      b) They should also be instructed to notify staff immediately of severe abdominal pain, dizziness, lightheadedness, shortness of breath, and/or bleeding from the biopsy site.

      c) If the patient has a T-tube, the nurse must monitor for any blood in the bile.

d) A hemoglobin and hematocrit is usually checked 4 hours after the procedure and compared to the previously drawn one to assess for any decreases in the level.

e) Patient education should include:

1) Why the biopsy is being done

2) The different levels of acute rejection—mild, moderate, severe

3) Possible interventions that may occur if there is any rejection

i) Immunosuppressants are often increased and high dose steroids given.

ii) The need for longer hospitalization should be discussed.

20. Signs and symptoms of graft rejection

a. Patients must be monitored for signs and symptoms of graft rejection on a daily basis.

i. Liver enzymes, bilirubin, and coagulation studies are drawn every morning.

ii. A rise in AST, ALT, and bilirubin could be a sign of rejection.

iii. T tube drainage should be golden brown.

a) Any changes in the bile, such as a lighter color, the presence of sludge, or the thinning of bile, should be reported to the physician.

iv. Assess for any light-colored stools, dark-colored urine, or jaundice of the sclera or skin.

v. Patients must also be monitored for fever, right upper quadrant pain, fatigue, malaise, and pruritus.

b. Patient education is very important for patients and families.

i. They need to be able to recognize these signs and symptoms and call the physician or postoperative coordinator if they occur.

ii. It is also important to instruct patients about the importance of having labs drawn as ordered since rejection is often asymptomatic.

21. Medication for immunosuppression post liver transplant

a. Immunosuppression regimens will vary from patient to patient and also among centers.

b. Patients need to be taught about their drug regimen and understand that these are lifelong drugs.

c. The primary aim of immunosuppression is to prevent rejection while minimizing side effects.[13]

d. Triple therapy may include a combination of:

i. Tacrolimus (Prograf) or cyclosporine (Neoral): a calcineurin inhibitor

ii. Azathioprine (Imuran) or mycophenolate mofetil (Cellcept) or mycophenolate sodium (Myfortic)

iii. Corticosteroid—prednisolone/SoluMedrol IV

e. Double therapy may include:

i. Tacrolimus (Prograf) or cyclosporine (Neoral): a calcineurin inhibitor

ii. Corticosteroid—prednisolone/SoluMedrol IV

f. Monotherapy

    i.   Some patients will be maintained on one immunosuppressant only; this is called monotherapy.

22. Other agents

  a. Sirolimus (Rapamycin)

    i.   Sirolimus (Rapamycin) is now being used in some patients and does not have nephrotoxic side effects of calcineurin inhibitors.

    ii.   It is used for continuing rejection and has been shown to prevent chronic rejection; however, some centers are evaluating its use as a baseline immunosuppressor.

  b. Induction agents

    i.   Induction agents, in the form of antilymphocyte preparations (OKT3 or ATG), have not been so widely used in liver transplantation.

    ii.   However, there are some newer humanized induction agents now being used in some patients. These include:

      a) Basiliximab (Simulect)

      b) Daclizumab (Zenepax)

      c) Alemtuzumab (Campath)

    iii. Induction agents are to be given pre or intraoperatively to decrease the incidence of acute rejection, delay first rejection and/or delay the use of calcineurin inhibitors (Tacrolimus/Neoral), due to the potential of renal toxicity.

    iv. The long-term results of these newer agents still have to be seen in liver transplantation.

  c. Side effects of immunosuppression

    i.   The side effects of immunosuppression need to be monitored carefully at follow-up post liver transplant examinations and are the reason for such close monitoring in the early discharge period.

    ii.   Tacrolimus (Prograf) and cyclosporine (Neoral) (calcineurin inhibitors) have side effects that include:

      a) Tremors

      b) Headaches

      c) High blood pressure

      d) Nephrotoxicity

      e) Elevated blood sugars

      f) Hair growth or loss and a higher risk of developing cancer

      g) Tacrolimus has a narrow therapeutic range and absorption may vary.

        1) Tacrolimus levels need to be checked daily in the early postop phase.

    iii. Corticosteroid (prednisolone) has side effects which include:

      a) Diabetes

      b) Hypertension

      c) High cholesterol

      d) Weight gain

      e) Fluid retention

      f) Indigestion

    iv. It is due to these side effects that some centers now prefer to use steroid-sparing regimens.

v. Azathioprine (Imuran)—side effects include low white cell count, aching joints, vomiting, dizziness, and stomach upset.

vi. Sirolimus (Rapamycin)—side effects include leukopenia, thrombocytopenia, anemia, hypertension, rash, acne, diarrhea, and poor wound healing.

vii. Mycophenolate mofetil (Cellcept)—side effects include low white cell count (especially low neutrophils), diarrhea (this may be helped by splitting the dose), vomiting, headaches, and elevated blood pressure.

viii. Basiliximab (Simulect)—side effects include abdominal pain, sore throat, shaking, vomiting, swelling of ankles, body, face, lower legs, and loss of energy.

ix. Daclizumab (Zenepax)—side effects include dizziness, nausea, vomiting, rapid heart rate, chest pain, shaking, swelling of feet or lower legs.

x. Alemtuzumab (Campath)—side effect include fever, chills shortly after infusion.

d. Other medications post liver transplant

i. The following medications are used post liver transplantation, as preventative treatments for potential complications that can be seen due to the immunosuppressive regimen.

a) *Pneumocystis carinii* pneumonia (PCP) prophylaxis
1) Bactrim, Septrin, Clotrimoxazole

b) Candida prophylaxis
1) Nystatin

c) Herpes prophylaxis
1) Acyclovir

d) CMV prophylaxis
1) Valganciclovir (Valcyte) (oral)
2) Ganciclovir (IV)

e) Antacids—due to steroid use
1) Axid
2) Pepcid
3) Lansoprazole

f) (See Chapters 2 and 4)

ACKNOWLEDGMENTS

Professor James Neuberger, Professor of Hepatology, Liver Unit, University Hospital Birmingham NHS Trust, Edgbaston, Birmingham, England

Medical Illustration, University Hospital Birmingham NHS Trust, Edgbaston, Birmingham, England

REFERENCES

1. Rockey DC. Selection of patients and timing of liver transplantation. In Killenberg P, Clavien P (Eds.). *Medical Care of the Liver Transplant Patient*, second edition. Williston, VT: Blackwell Science, 2001.
2. www.unos.org. Accessed June 10, 2007.
3. Diehl AM. Alcoholic liver disease: Natural history. *Liver Transplantation and Surgery*, 1997; 3(3): 206-211.
4. O'Grady JG, Schalm S, Williams R. Acute liver failure: Redefining the syndromes. *Lancet*, 1993; 342: 373-375.
5. Humar A. *Manual of Liver Transplant Medical Care*. Minneapolis: Fairview Publications, 2002.
6. Bacon BR, O'Grady J, Di Bisceglie AM, Lake JR. *Comprehensive Clinical Hepatology*, second edition. Philadelphia: Elsevier Mosby, 2006.
7. Keefe EB. Assessment of the alcoholic patient for liver transplantation: Comorbidity, outcome and recidivism. *Liver Transplant Surg*, 1996; 2: 12-20.
8. Pereira SP, Williams R. Liver transplantation for alcoholic liver disease at King's College Hospital: Survival and quality of life. *Liver Transplant Surg*, 1997; 3: 245-250.
9. Consensus conference on indications of liver transplantation. *Hepatology*, 1994; 20 (supplement): 1s-685.
10. Their M, Ronnholm K, Sairanen H, Holmberg C, et al. Serum C-reactive protein in pediatric kidney and liver transplant patients. *Ped Transplant*, Apr 2002; 6(9): 153-160.
11. http://www.uktransplant.org.uk/. Accessed May 2006.
12. Flynn B. Liver transplantation. In Cupples SA, Ohler L (Eds.). *Transplantation Nursing Secrets*. Philadelphia: Hanley & Belfus; 2003.
13. Molmenti EP, Klintmalm GB. *Atlas of Liver Transplantation*. Philadelphia: Saunders; 2002.
14. Branch MS, Clavien PA. Biliary complications following liver transplantation. In Killenberg PG, Clavien PA (Eds.). *Medical Care of the Liver Transplant Patient*, second edition. Williston, VT: Blackwell Science, 2001.
15. Buckels JAC, de Ville de Goyet J. Innovative techniques in liver transplant surgery. In Forsythe JLR (Ed.). *Transplantation Surgery: Current Dilemmas*. London: WB Saunders Ltd.; 2001.

SUGGESTED READINGS

Al Knawy B, Shiffman ML, Wiesner RH. *Hepatology: A Practical Approach*. San Diego: Elsevier, Inc., 2004.

Cupples S, Ohler L (Eds.). *Solid Organ Transplantation*. New York: Springer Publishing Company, 2002.

Killenberg PG, Clavien PA. *Medical Care of the Liver Transplant Patient*, second edition. Williston, VT: Blackwell Science, 2001.

REVIEW QUESTIONS

1. Following liver transplantation, some patients will receive a drug such as remifentanil. This will allow for which of the following actions prior to admission to the ICU?
   a. Early withdrawal of pain medications
   b. Quick withdrawal of biliary drains in the OR
   c. Removal of urinary catheter in the OR
   d. Extubation in the OR
   e. Removal of inotropic drips in OR

2. Patients with chronic liver disease may demonstrate which of the following hemodynamic changes in the immediate postoperative period?
   a. Elevated cardiac output
   b. Low systemic vascular resistance
   c. Elevated cardiac index
   d. All of the above
   e. a and b only

3. Transesophageal echo probes are being used more often to monitor patients post liver transplantation. This probe is inserted into the esophagus and gives a picture of:
   a. Diaphragmatic excursion
   b. All contents of the duodenum
   c. Any dilation of the heart chambers
   d. How well the heart is beating
   e. c and d

4. Bleeding may occur in the first 48 hours post liver transplantation due to which of the following factors?
   a. Poor functioning graft with underlying coagulopathy
   b. Improperly functioning drains
   c. Ascites developing from fluid mismanagement
   d. Poor renal function

5. Green-colored drainage post liver transplantation may be a sign of:
   a. Bleeding into the GI tract
   b. Bile leakage
   c. The development of a fistula to the gallbladder
   d. Ruptured gallbladder

6. *De novo* seizures may occur post liver transplant and may be related to which of the following factors?
   a. Electrolyte imbalances
   b. Cyclosporine or tacrolimus
   c. Intracerebral abcesses
   d. All of the above
   e. b and c only

7. Early indicators of primary non-function of the new liver may include which of the following?
   a. The quantity and quality of bile production
   b. Extreme edema of the organ
   c. Hemodynamic instability
   d. All of the above
   e. a and b only

8. The risk for primary nonfunction of a liver is:
   a. 10-15%
   b. 15-20%
   c. 1-2%
   d. 2-5%

9. Factors related to primary nonfunction of a new liver include which of the following?
   a. Prolonged ischemic time
   b. Donor age
   c. Prolonged donor management/hospital stay
   d. All of the above
   e. a and c only

10. The most reliable indicators of liver rejection post-transplantation include which of the following?
    a. A rise in AST, ALT, and bilirubin
    b. A rise in WBC, a decrease in INR
    c. Golden brown drainage from T-tube
    d. All of the above
    e. b and c

11. Hyperglycemia in the first few days post liver transplantation may be related to which of the following?
    a. Calcineurin inhibitors
    b. Steroids
    c. A normal functioning liver that is converting glucose into glycogen
    d. All of the above
    e. a and b only

12. In the immediate postoperative period, hypovolemia may be associated with rewarming. The patient may present with which of the following changes associated with hypovolemia?
    a. Hypertension and elevated urine output
    b. Hypotension and a decrease in CVP
    c. Increased urine output and drop in AST and ALT levels
    d. All of the above

12 Intestine Transplantation

BEVERLY KOSMACH-PARK

MARIA DE ANGELIS

I. Introduction
  A. Intestine transplantation has evolved into an accepted treatment for adults and children with permanent intestinal failure.
  B. Total parental nutrition (TPN) provides caloric and nutritional requirements for patients with intestinal failure but places patients at high risk for life-threatening complications:
    1. TPN-induced liver disease
    2. Recurrent sepsis
    3. Loss of venous access
II. History
  A. Intestine transplants were first performed over 40 years ago, but clinical success has only recently been achieved.
  B. 1964-1972: Eight transplants performed with the longest survival being only 6 months.[1] This poor survival rate was attributed to:
    1. Technical complications
    2. Infection
    3. Inability of available immunosuppressive protocols to control and treat rejection
  C. 1984-89: attempts to renew this procedure were motivated by the success of cyclosporine as the primary immunosuppressant for kidney, liver, and heart transplantation.
    1. Mean survival of the second era of patients (n=6) improved to 25.7 months.[2]
    2. Cyclosporine did not have the significant impact on survival in intestine transplantation that it had in the other solid organs.
    3. One surviving patient from cyclosporine era, currently over 16 years post-transplant; immunosuppression changed to tacrolimus after episode of rejection in 1998.[3]
  D. Since 1990, significantly improved patient and graft survival has been achieved with introduction of tacrolimus as the primary immunosuppressant medication.
III. Current results
  A. Intestine Transplant Registry data (Table 12-1)[4]
    1. 44% have received isolated intestine transplants.
    2. 38% have received combined liver and intestine grafts.

        a. Adults more commonly receive isolated intestine while pediatric patients usually require composite graft.

    3. 65 centers in 20 countries

    4. Less than 25% of these centers perform 75% of the procedures.[4]

B. Survival

    1. One-year graft survival ranged from 30% in 1990 to over 80% in patients receiving transplants from 2003 to 2005.[4]

    2. Factors significantly affecting improved survival[4]:

        a. Use of tacrolimus as primary immunosuppressive therapy

        b. Transplant center size (performing ≥10 transplants)

        c. First transplant procedure

        d. Being at home when called for transplant

    3. Sepsis is most common cause of death

IV. Pretransplant care: Objective measures of end-stage short gut syndrome

A. Short gut syndrome (SGS) is a disorder in which the small intestine is unable to maintain an adequate nutritional status and/or fluid and electrolyte balance.

B. SGS may be structural or functional.

    1. Structural disorders are a consequence of extensive surgical resection.

        a. Etiologies include Crohn's disease, trauma, or vascular insufficiency or an anatomic loss related to congenital anomalies such as gastroschisis.

    2. Functional disorders are due to absorptive, secretory, or motility disorders that lead to varying levels of malabsorption and TPN dependency.

C. Malabsorption results in an inability to gain or sustain weight, maintain fluid balance, and in children, affects growth and development.

D. Intestinal failure defined as not enough gut mass to maintain fluid and nutrition in the adult and/or growth in the child[5]

E. Common causes of intestinal failure (Table 12-2)[6, 7]

    1. Massive surgical resection

    2. Dysmotility disorders

    3. Congenital enteropathy

    4. Tumors

F. Depending on the length of healthy intestine and absorption, some patients with SGS can be managed on a combination of enteral and parenteral nutrition with the goal of discontinuing TPN as the intestine adapts.

G. Surgical intervention through bowel lengthening may be helpful in some cases.

    1. Serial transverse enteroplasty (STEP) procedure

    2. Bianchi intestinal lengthening procedure

H. Treatment for intestinal failure

    1. Total parental nutrition (TPN) via central venous lines (CVL)

        a. Fluid, electrolyte, and nutritional replacement therapy via daily infusions

        b. Requires long-term venous access

        c. Places patient at great risk for developing life-threatening complications

            i. TPN-induced liver disease

            ii. Sepsis

TABLE 12-1

■ **Interntional Transplant Registry 1985-2005**

Intestine transplant recipients	1210
Intestine transplants	1292
Surviving patients	658
Lost to follow-up	14

TABLE 12-2

■ **Common Causes of Intestinal Failure**

Adult	Pediatric
• Ischemia	• Midgut volvulus
• Crohn's disease	• Necrotizing entercolitis
• Desmoid tumor	• Gastroschisis
• Trauma	• Congenital atresias
• Volvulus	• Hirschsprung's disease
• Pseudo-obstruction	• Pseudo-obstruction
• Gardner's disease	• Microvillus inclusion disease

      iii. Loss of venous access
  2. TPN cycling with enteral feedings
    a. May be helpful to preserve liver function
    b. Patients with normal intestinal motility of existing gut should receive enteral nutrition to avoid intestinal stasis, the most important intervention for preventing and treating TPN-induced cholestasis[8]
  3. Surgical interventions
    a. Intestines exhibiting normal motility should be reconnected, closing all stomas, whenever possible
    b. Dysmotile segments, when reanastomosed, increase the risk of bacterial translocation due to intestinal stasis[8]
  4. Interventions to improve or preserve intestinal function
    a. Decrease dextrose and lipid load of TPN solution when possible
    b. Promote bile flow by treatment with ursodiol
    c. Intervene with timely surveillance and treatment for bacterial overgrowth
    d. Provide attentive care of indwelling catheters to avoid catheter-related sepsis and loss of venous access
 H. Types of intestine transplants
  1. Depends on indication for intestinal failure and extent of deterioration and dysfunction of other abdominal organs
  2. Isolated intestinal transplant

a. Recommended for patients with intestinal failure without associated liver disease

b. Indications include extreme short gut, motility disorders, malabsorption syndromes, gastrointestinal neoplasms

3. Composite intestine and liver transplant

a. Performed for patients with irreversible intestinal and hepatic failure

4. Multivisceral transplant

a. Various combinations of intestine, liver, stomach, and pancreas

i. Modified multivisceral without the liver performed if minimal cholestasis with good liver function

b. Recommended based on the etiology of short gut and associated organ dysfunction

c. Indications include massive gastrointestinal polyposis, mesenteric desmoid tumors, hollow visceral myopathy, and extensive splanchnic vascular thrombosis

5. Isolated liver transplantation in children with TPN-induced liver disease

a. An isolated liver transplant may be performed in patients who have a sufficient bowel length to expect adaptation with increasing enteral feedings and eventual weaning of parenteral nutrition

b. Strategy is controversial, although short-term outcomes have improved[9]

V. Pretransplant care: Objective measures of intestinal failure

A. Vital signs: Temperature

1. Monitor routinely as indicated and more frequently with complaints of illness and malaise

2. Fever is usually a symptom of infection which requires immediate attention

3. Increased risk for sepsis

a. Central venous lines

b. Intestinal stasis due to impaired motility of the residual intestine which contributes to bacterial overgrowth and translocation

B. Vital signs: Blood pressure/heart rate

1. Hypotension and tachycardia may indicate:

a. Dehydration

b. Sepsis

c. Bleeding in patients with impaired synthetic function

2. Hypertension may occur with impaired renal function secondary to prolonged and frequent administration of aminoglycosides and antifungals in patients with recurrent sepsis

C. Lab values (Table 12-3)

1. Vary in patients with intestinal failure depending on:

a. Indication for transplant

b. Effect on other organ systems

c. Organ deterioration

d. Infection history

e. TPN solution

2. Infection should be considered with an increase in the white blood count, sedimentation rate (ESR), and platelets

a. If infection is suspected, blood cultures should be obtained to identify the specific organism causing infection

TABLE 12-3

■ **Electrolyte Imbalances in Intestinal Failure and Post-Intestinal Transplantation**

Electrolyte	Alteration	Cause	Symptoms	Treatment
Sodium	Hypernatremia Na >150 mEq/L	• Water loss secondary to diarrhea and vomiting • Increased evaporative water loss: fever • Excess sodium intake: increased oral or IV source	Nonspecific: thirst, irritability, lethargy, increased deep tendon reflexes, seizures	• Reduce serum sodium slowly through administration of appropriate IV fluids and volumes
	Hyponatremia Na <130 mEq/L	• Edema-associated states: hepatic failure leading to third spacing of fluid • Hyperglycemia • GI losses: vomiting, ostomy losses, tube drainage, diarrhea • Diuresis; thiazides and loop diuretics	Nonspecific: headache, lethargy, nausea weakness, encephalopathy, seizures	Dependant on cause • Restore intravascular volume • Edematous state (low albumin)—do not restrict water intake but restrict NA intake • Hyperglycemia: resolve hyperglycemia
Potassium	Hyperkalemia K+>5.5 mEq/L	• Metabolic acidosis • Increased K+ intake: supplements, blood transfusions • Decreased renal excretion: K+ sparing diuretics, calcineurin immunosuppression • Increased tacrolimus levels post-transplant	Cardiac arrhythmias (V fib and asystole) Muscle weakness, decreased tendon reflexes, ileus, anorexia, tingling of mouth and extremities, malaise, tetany	Dependant on cause and severity. May include administration of: • Kayexelate • Lasix • Sodium Bicarbonate • Insulin • Salbutamol • Dialysis • Calcium gluconate
	Hypokalemia K+ <3.5 mEq/L	• Increased GI losses: vomiting, diarrhea, ostomies, tube drainage • Increased renal losses: drug-related aminoglycoside toxicity	Cardiac arrhythmias (bradycardia, V tac, AV block, premature atrial and ventricular beats), fibrillation, muscle paralysis, ileus, tetany, confusion, hypotension, polyuria, polydipsia	• Administer K+ supplementation (oral /IV)
Magnesium	Hypermagnesemia Mg >2.5 mEq/L	• Excess magnesium intake (i.e., oral prep, via TPN) • Decreased renal excretion; assess GFR	Decreased deep tendon reflexes; weakness, confusion, lethargy and hypotension with levels >7 mEq/L), bradycardia	• Remove excess source • Administer calcium • Dialysis

(Continued next page.)

Electrolyte	Alteration	Cause	Symptoms	Treatment
	Hypomagnesemia Mg <1.5 mEq/L	• GI losses: diarrhea, prolonged NG drainage • Malnutrition: ↓ calories, ↓ protein • Fat malabsorption • Increased renal losses: renal tubular acidosis, diuretic therapy, drugs (aminoglycosides, amphotericin, calcineurin inhibitors) • Pancreatitis • Refeeding	Weakness, tremors, anorexia, seizures, cardiovascular manifestations (widening QRS complex, prolonged PR interval, ventricular arrhythmias), increased susceptibility to digitalis toxicity	• Administer magnesium supplement (IV/PO)
Phosphate	Hypophosphatemia (varies by age)	• Decreased intestinal absorption (diarrhea, vitamin D deficiency, antacid abuse, fat malabsorption) • Internal redistribution (recovery from malnutrition, sepsis, rickets) • Decreased phosphate intake • Hyperventilation	Muscle weakness, bone pain, arthalgias, hemolytic anemia, anorexia, nausea, vomiting, confusion, rhabdomylosis	• Low phosphate associated with hypercalcemia; treating high calcium often resolves low phosphate • Administer phosphate once calcium and renal function assessed
	Hyperphosphatemia (varies by age)	• Increased external load (IV/oral) • Increased endogenous load (bowel infarction) • Reduced renal excretion (Mg deficiency, bisphosphonate therapy) • Hypocalcemia	With associated hypocalcemia, tetany can occur. Ectopic calcification in vessels and wall tissues	• Restrict phosphate intake • Administer phosphate binding salts (aluminum, calcium, magnesium) • Saline diuresis if normal renal function
Calcium	Hypocalcemia (varies by age)	• Low albumin • High phosphate • Low magnesium • Vitamin D deficient rickets • Pancreatitis	Muscle weakness, numbness and tingling in extremities, cramps, hyper reflexes, tetany, seizures, prolonged QT interval	• Correct other electrolyte imbalances • Administer calcium (IV/oral) • Vitamin D therapy

Electrolyte	Alteration	Cause	Symptoms	Treatment
	Hypercalcemia	• Excess vitamin D administration • Thiazide drug therapy	Renal etiology: polyuria, polydipsia, nephrocalcinosis, renal insufficiency Nonrenal etiology: fatigue, weakness, nausea, vomiting, constipation, symptoms of pancreatitis, headache, pruritus, bone pain, hypotonia, hypertension, arrhythmias, short QT interval, heart block	• Correct dehydration • Saline diuresis • Loop diuretics • Steroids • Calcitonin • Biphosphonates
Metabolic Acidosis	Assessed on blood gas • Low pH • Reduced HCO_3	• GI losses: diarrhea, intestinal fluid loss from ileostomy, NG drainage • Excess acid via TPN • Renal losses: drugs (spironolactone, amphotericin)	Vomiting, nausea, diarrhea, hyperventilation, headache, lethargy	• Treat underlying cause • Bicarbonate • Correct fluid balance
Metabolic Alkalosis	Assessed on blood gas • High pH • Elevated HCO_3	• GI losses: vomiting, NG drainage, chloride losing diarrhea • Renal losses: diuretics, penicillins • Low chloride intake • Refeeding syndrome • Hypocalcemia • Hypokalemia • Massive blood transfusions (excessive citrate)	Related to underlying cause. Refer to hypokalemia. Refer to hypocalcemia. If volume depleted: thirst, lethargy, muscle cramps, irritability.	• Treat underlying cause • Correct K+ deficit • Correct calcium deficit • Correct chloride deficit • Correct fluid imbalances

    b.   Stool, sputum, and/or urine cultures obtained as indicated

    c.   Liver function monitored by serial liver function tests (ALT, AST, GGTP, and bilirubin), markers for synthetic function (PT/PTT and INR), platelets, hemoglobin, and serum albumin

3.   Patients are at risk for increased fluid losses with electrolyte imbalances

    a.   Fluid losses from the intestine are due to the development of a hypersecretory state, bacterial overgrowth, infection, and/or intrinsic deficits

    b.   There may be interruptions in ability to provide optimal TPN because of venous access problems

    c.   Labs obtained weekly or every other week to monitor abnormalities and to make appropriate adjustments in contents of TPN solution and volume

      d.   Lab tests commonly obtained include electrolyte panel (calcium, magnesium, phosphorus, sodium, potassium, carbon dioxide, chloride); renal function tests (blood urea nitrogen, creatinine); vitamins A, D, E, K, and B_{12}; trace elements; zinc; and cholesterol and triglycerides

      e.   Albumin and total protein obtained to assess nutritional status

      f.   Ammonia levels obtained in patients with liver disease

      g.   D-xylose testing and fecal fat testing may be obtained to assess absorption of existing intestine

D. Radiology tests

   1.   Completed during the evaluation for intestine transplantation or as complications arise related to the original disease

   2.   Upper and lower barium studies of the gastrointestinal tract

      a.   Reveal existing anatomy and any abnormalities

         i.   Observe for dilated loops of bowel, strictures, or narrowing of the bowel

        ii.   Short gut leads to decreased absorption of fluids, nutrients, and electrolytes

      b.   Provide estimates of bowel length and transit time

      c.   Structural etiologies

         i.   Short bowel length (<20 cm in pediatric etiologies)

      d.   Functional etiologies

         i.   Normal or near-normal length

        ii.   Transit time is usually fast or delayed

       iii.   May have distended loops of bowel

       iv.   Motility testing and gastric emptying tests are performed

   3.   Vascular patency

      a.   Important to identify occlusion of common central venous access sites because access may be required for or a year or more post-transplant

      b.   Evaluation completed through an ultrasound of the great vessels to assess the splanchnic venous anatomy and internal jugular, subclavian, and iliac veins

      c.   Angiography may be indicated in some cases.

      d.   An MRI is used to confirm any reported occlusions of the primary vasculature

   4.   Abdominal ultrasound evaluation

      a.   Hepatomegaly and/or splenomegaly

      b.   Patency of the hepatic vasculature and blood flow

      c.   Patency of the biliary system

      d.   Presence of varices

   5.   Liver biopsy

      a.   Performed in patients with deteriorating liver function to determine the extent and severity of liver disease

      b.   Evidence of bridging fibrosis or cirrhosis is an indication for liver transplantation

      c.   The extent of liver disease, rate of progression, and estimated waiting time to transplant are also considered in listing for liver transplant

   6.   Cardiology testing

      a.   To rule out cardiac anomalies and any contraindications for surgery

b. Tests include an electrocardiogram (ECG), ECHO, and chest radiograph (CXR)

c. CXR used to assess for any respiratory complications, particularly in pediatric candidates with history of bronchopulmonary dysplasia (BPD) or cystic fibrosis

E. Physical assessment
  1. Widely variable from relatively healthy to critically ill
  2. Nursing assessment to identify symptoms and prioritize nursing care
     a. Symptoms of electrolyte and fluid imbalances
     b. Infection
     c. Malabsorption
     d. Skin breakdown
     e. Liver or kidney dysfunction
     f. Mental status changes
     g. Mood disorders
  3. General overview
     a. Will vary by age, indication for transplant, severity and duration of intestinal failure, and associated complications
     b. Observe for the general state of health or distress, skin color, height/weight, mobility, and mood
  4. Skin
     a. Jaundice and bruising in patients with concomitant liver disease
     b. Lesions secondary to scratching from pruritus, particularly in pediatric patients
     c. Decreased skin turgor or edema due to nutritional deficits and fluid imbalances
     d. Dry, scaling skin that lacks elasticity
     e. Poor nail growth or thin nails
     f. Thinning, dull hair
     g. Potential for ulcers, rash, and skin breakdown around catheter sites, drainage or feeding tube sites, stomas, mucous fistulas, and around the buttocks/diaper area.
     h. Assess scarring from previous surgeries for any breaks in skin integrity or keloid formations
  5. HEENT
     a. Abnormalities occur based on the indication for intestinal failure and complications
     b. Sclerae usually jaundiced in liver disease
     c. Hearing deficits should be evaluated for patients who have received repeated courses of parenteral aminoglycosides
        i. Aminoglycosides are associated with ototoxicity
        ii. Related to duration of treatment and amount of drug administered
        iii. Infants are particularly at risk and often have high-range hearing deficits
     d. Cervical lymphadenopathy may be associated with infection
     e. Dentition is affected by nutritional status
        i. Assess for the presence\absence of teeth, staining, obvious caries, gingivitis, and gum integrity

a) Tooth eruption may be delayed in nutritionally impaired infants.

f. Dehydration assessed through decreased or absent tearing, sunken eyes, a dry oral mucosa, and cracked lips

g. A smooth red tongue, without the normal rough appearance may indicate a vitamin deficiency.

6. Cardiac
    a. There are no specific cardiac abnormalities directly related to intestinal failure
    b. Cardiac-related symptoms can occur as a result of complications related to intestinal failure
    c. Baseline cardiac assessment is completed to determine any baseline cardiac illness or anomaly that may be a contraindication to transplant
    d. Signs and symptoms may include:
        i.   Tachycardia due to blood loss and/or volume depletion
        ii. Arrhythmias secondary to electrolyte imbalances
        iii. Murmurs from anemia or fluid imbalance
        iv. Hypotension may be associated with bleeding, volume depletion, and sepsis
        v.   Skin mottling may be a sign of sepsis

7. Respiratory
    a. Abnormalities are secondary to the consequences of intestinal failure
        i.   Tachypnea can be associated with metabolic acidosis, hypoglycemia, fever, and/or anxiety
        ii. Rales and tachypnea may be present with fluid overload related to hypoalbuminemia
        iii. Decreased breath sounds may be due to atelectasis, effusions, and/or pneumonias

8. Gastrointestinal
    a. GI examination determines the extent and function of the existing bowel and any associated abdominal anomalies
    b. Abdominal assessment
        i.   Observation
             a) Surgical scars
             b) Enteral tubes: gastrostomy tube, jejunostomy tube, combined gastrojejunostomy tube
             c) Fistulas
             d) Ostomies
             e) Protuberance suggests ascites and/or organomegaly
             f) Distended abdominal veins and spider angioma are indicative of liver disease with vascular obstruction
             g) Herniations
        ii. Auscultation
             a) Hyperactive bowel sounds may be indicative of diarrhea or an early obstruction
             b) Hypoactivity, then absent bowel sounds may indicate an ileus and/or peritonitis
        iii. Palpation
             a) Assess the size of the liver and spleen

        b)   Hepatomegaly in patients with TPN-induced liver disease can be evaluated by palpating in the right upper quadrant and assessing the size of liver below the coastal margin.

        c)   In splenomegaly, the spleen may be palpated well below the costal margin due to portal hypertension; tenderness may be present.

        d)   Epigastric and rebound tenderness are associated with pancreatitis.

        e)   Generalized discomfort may be indicative of peritonitis.

9. Musculoskeletal assessment
   a. Fractures
      i. Malabsorption of fat soluble vitamins, specifically vitamin D, may cause rickets, leading to fractures.
   b. Joint abnormalities
      i. Assess for swollen, painful, and reddened joints
      ii. May indicate arthritis-associated liver disease
10. Neurologic and mental status
    a. Neurologic changes associated with high serum ammonia levels
       i. Altered sleep patterns (day-night reversal)
       ii. Extreme lethargy
       iii. Behavioral changes
       iv. Confusion
       v. Obtundation
       vi. Ataxia
       vii. Astrexis
       viii. Clonus
11. Growth and development
    a. Infants and young children usually display significant growth and developmental delay because the onset of intestinal failure occurred in utero or early infancy.
       i. Height and weight curves are often less than the 25th percentile and growth along the curve is not commonly achieved with early-onset disease.
       ii. Developmental milestones may not be achieved due to frequent illnesses, poor nutrition, decreased muscle mass and strength, repeated hospitalizations with impaired socialization, and isolation from the family environment.
       iii. Oral aversion common in children who have been limited in oral intake or who have had frequent periods of nothing by mouth.
    b. Adults and children display weight loss and decreased muscle mass.
    c. Growth and development closer to the norm in children or adults with a later onset of short gut, such as a spontaneous volvulus or trauma, or with diseases having a slower, chronic impact, such as Crohn's disease or pseudo-obstruction
VI. Pretransplant care: Subjective complaints of candidates
    A. Subjective complaints are also variable, depending on patient age and duration of illness, the severity of intestinal failure, and associated complications.

    B. Common subjective complaints related to short gut include:
1. Weight loss
2. Poor growth
3. Intractable diarrhea
4. Dry, scaling skin
5. Skin breakdown
6. Thinning hair
7. Abdominal distention
8. Flatus
9. Malaise
10. Lethargy
11. Weakness
12. Abdominal pain
13. Complaints related to mental status and mood changes

    C. Additional complaints of patients with concomitant liver disease
1. Bruising
2. Extreme tiredness
3. Confusion, mood changes
4. Abdominal distention
5. Bleeding
6. Abdominal pain
7. Pruritus
8. Acholic stools

    D. Emotional struggles
1. Time-consuming nature of care
2. Activity and social limitations
3. Frequent hospitalizations
4. Inability to work or attend school
5. Social isolation
6. Impaired family support
7. Fear of dying before an organ is available
8. Symptoms related to anxiety, depression, and/or sleep disturbances

VII. Preparing the pretransplant patient for surgery
    A. Transplant evaluation (Table 12-4)
1. Center-specific
2. 3-5 day inpatient stay or several days outpatient

    B. Nursing interventions
1. Provide patients and families with schedule for the evaluation with a listing of tests and consultations
2. Provide education regarding test procedures and examinations
3. Support the patient and family throughout the evaluation by answering questions to clarify information and reinforce information and results presented by the transplant team
4. Facilitate discussions with the associated transplant team members for specific information and results
    a. A smaller group may be responsible for providing an overview of the results, the immediate plan for listing and medical management, longer-term management, and reinforcement of teaching
    b. Core group usually includes the transplant surgeon, GI physician, transplant coordinator, advanced practice nurse (CNS or CRNP), and/or the social worker

TABLE 12-4

■ **Evaluation for Intestinal Transplantation**

Assessment	Testing/Procedures
Routine assessment	Complete history and physical
	CXR
	ABO compatibility
Gastrointestinal assessment	Upper and lower barium studies to assess bowel length, anatomy, and abnormalities
	Motility testing and gastric emptying for functional indications
	D-xylose testing and fecal fat testing to assess absorption
Nutritional assessment	Laboratory testing: electrolytes, blood urea nitrogen, creatinine, calcium, magnesium, phosphorus, zinc, trace elements, cholesterol, triglycerides, vitamin levels (A, D, E, K, B_{12})
	Feeding history to assess tolerance, absorption, weight gain, growth (children)
	Caloric intake: enteral and parenteral
	Growth parameters: height, weight, skin folds, head circumference (infants)
	Assess for oral aversion, abnormal eating behaviors, pica
Hepatic function	Liver function tests including ALT, AST, GGT, direct and indirect bilirubin, albumin, prothrombin time, partial thromboplastin time, alpha-fetoprotein, platelets, ammonia, and Factors V and VII
	Physical exam to assess for hepatomegaly, splenomegaly, ascites, caput medusae
	Liver ultrasound to further assess liver size, vasculature, and any evidence of portal hypertension
	Liver biopsy if indicated to establish baseline hepatic injury
Vascular patency	Catheter history with number of line placements, location, duration, and reason for replacement
	Ultrasound of the great vessels to assess vascular access and to evaluate the splanchnic venous anatomy and internal jugular, subclavian, and iliac veins
	Angiography if indicated
	MRI to confirm any reported occlusions of the primary vasculature

(Continued next page.)

Assessment	Testing/Procedures
Infection history and immunology assessment	History of infections to assess etiology and frequency of infection, pathogens, response to treatment, resistant organisms
	Screening cultures of blood, urine, stool, throat, or ascitic fluid for bacterial, fungal or viral organisms as indicated
	Complete blood count and differential
	Tissue typing and cross-match
	Screening for Hepatitis B and C and HIV
	IgG and IgM titers for CMV, EBV, herpes zoster, and MMR
	Quantitative immunoglobulins in patients with intestinal atresia
Cardiac assessment	EKG, ECHO
	Rule out cardiac anomalies and contraindications for surgery
Respiratory assessment	CXR
	Obtain pulmonology consult for patients with a history of BPD, cystic fibrosis or other respiratory complications
Neurologic assessment	Obtain neurology consult in patients with seizure disorders or neurologic impairments
Development and physical functioning	Further evaluation as indicated for developmental delays, impairments in physical functioning, oral aversion, behavioral issues
	Consults may include physical therapy, speech therapy, occupational therapy, and neurodevelopment
	Child life, child development in pediatrics
Psychological evaluation	To assess patient (age-appropriate) and parent/family's psychological status and history for psychopathology, coping skills, responses to stress, family support
	Assess for alcohol or substance abuse in adults, adolescent patients, and parents
	Compliance history
	Referrals for psychotherapy, counseling
Social work evaluation	Assess patient and family psychosocial functioning
	Provide psychosocial care and support during the evaluation and in preparation for transplant
	Guide families in referrals for financial assistance programs and Supportive services
	Assist in referrals to volunteer pilot associations if needed for transport to the transplant center when organs are available
	Assist family in preparing for temporary relocation needs to the transplant center

Assessment	Testing/Procedures
Clinical nurse specialist	Addresses the educational needs of the patient and family pre- and post-transplant
	Provides information and psychosocial support during the transplant process
	Consultation to assess developmental needs, patient or family psychosocial functioning, compliance
Transplant coordinator	Maintains outpatient communication with candidate and referring physician following evaluation
	Lists patient according to UNOS requirements
	Provides information to the patient and family about the transplant process
	Maintains updated medical information on the candidate during the waiting period
	Follows patient post-transplant to facilitate medical management and follow-up; with physician, assesses for problems/complications through lab testing and procedures; communicates medication changes and assesses for medication compliance
Financial counselor	Works with the family and insurer to obtain insurance coverage for transplantation
	Provides guidance in fund-raising for personal expenses related to relocation

Adapted from *Progress in Transplantation*, 12(2); 2002.

C. The evaluation process
   1. Thorough medical assessment of the candidate
      a. History
         i. Previous surgeries
         ii. Infection history
         iii. Nutritional history
      b. Physical examination
   2. Focus of evaluation
      a. Anatomy of the GI tract
      b. Nutritional status
      c. Liver function
      d. Venous access and patency
      e. Infection history
      f. Cardiovascular system
   3. Patient-specific consultations
      a. Anesthesia
      b. Neurology
      c. Immunology
      d. Respiratory
      e. Child development
      f. Nephrology
   4. Psychosocial evaluation

      a. To assess psychological status, history of psychopathology, coping skills, responses to stress, and family support

      b. Completed by psychiatrist/psychologist, social worker, clinical nurse specialist/nurse practitioner, and/or child development specialist

   D. Pretransplant education (Table 12-5)

   E. The waiting period

     1. Candidates managed by the referring physician in the home area

     2. May return to the transplant center as requested for intermittent follow-up, educational needs, and local support services

     3. Extremely stressful time as the patient deteriorates and fears that organs may not become available

     4. Nursing interventions

       a. Supportive role

         i. Develop a supportive relationship with patient and family during repeated hospitalizations

         ii. Increased fear and anxiety as waiting period extends

         iii. Fear of death due to organs not being available, complicated surgery, postoperative complications, and anesthesia

       b. Identify patient's fears and clarify misconceptions

       c. Encourage patients to verbalize concerns to alleviate anxiety

       d. Facilitate referral for psychological and/or spiritual counseling

       e. Be aware of patient and family's cultural needs and religious practices

         i. Acknowledge and discuss cultural considerations regarding coping methods, diet, blood products, and religious practices

         ii. Facilitate care conferences to better understand cultural differences and to design appropriate supportive interventions

VIII. Preparation for surgery

   A. Preoperative orders are center-specific

   B. Vary according to the patient's medical status prior to intestine transplant, organs transplanted, and concurrent complications

   C. Standard preoperative orders (Table 12-6)

     1. Ensure that informed consent has been given and consent forms signed

     2. Escort family to an assigned waiting area so they are available if needed during the surgery and can be updated on how the surgery is progressing

     3. Reinforce previous teaching

       a. Duration of surgery

       b. What to expect when seeing the patient in the ICU

       c. Provide a brief summary of the early postoperative period and possible complications

IX. Surgical procedure

   A. Operative time ranges from 6-18 hours depending on:

     1. Type of transplant (isolated intestine versus liver/intestine or multivisceral)

     2. Amount of abdominal adhesions

     3. Recipient's current health status

     4. Concomitant complications

TABLE 12-5
■ Educational Topics Pretransplant

Basic anatomy and physiology of the intestine

Organ donation and listing

Waiting period:
- Patient responsibilities
- Coping and stress
- Staying healthy
- Communicating with the transplant center

Surgical procedure

What to expect in the intensive care unit:
- Unit routines
- Tubes and drains
- Procedures

Pain:
- Current pain status
- Pain control
- Postoperative pain
- Treatment

Surgical complications

Immune system basics

Rejection

Infection

Medications

Life after transplant:
- Care needs
- Follow-up care
- Labs
- Development (pediatrics)
- Returning to work/school
- Sexuality
- Exercise
- Nutrition

Family support and psychosocial stressors

TABLE 12-6
■ **Preoperative Orders**

Maintain NPO status

Obtain vital signs, height, weight, abdominal girth, subxyphoid girth

Obtain labs: complete blood count and differential, liver function tests, calcium, magnesium, phosphate, urea, BUN, creatinine, glucose, electrolytes, PT/PTT, INR, protein, albumin

Type and cross for specified amount of packed red blood cells and fresh frozen plasma

Obtain viral serologies for cytomegalovirus (CMV), Epstein Barr Virus (EBV)

Chest X-ray

Infuse fluids and/or TPN as ordered

Administer preoperative broad spectrum antibiotics

Administer methylprednisolone

Administer induction immunosuppression per center protocol

B. Total cold and warm ischemia time for the donor intestine should be less than 6 hours.[10]
C. Patients are prepared in the usual fashion, sedated and intubated
D. Tubes and lines placed
   1. Several peripheral intravenous lines in addition to the existing central line catheter
   2. Arterial line
   3. Nasogastric drainage tube
   4. Urinary catheter
E. Midline abdominal incision with unilateral or bilateral transverse extensions as needed
   1. Variants of the surgery for isolated intestine transplantation depending on the indication for transplant and the amount of viable intestine
F. Isolated intestine transplant (Figures 12-1 and 12-2)
   1. Diseased intestine removed proximally from the ligament of Treitz and distally to the ileocecal valve or ileocolic anastomosis in patients with functional disorders[10]
   2. Healthy residual intestine is usually preserved in patients with structural disorders
      a. Patient may present with previous enterectomy of native residual intestine related to pretransplant complications
   3. Donor intestine is implanted using the appropriate vascular anastomoses
      a. Vascular anastomoses vary based on the patient's anatomy and usable vessels
      b. Preferred vessels are the recipient superior mesenteric artery and vein
      c. Infrarenal aorta is used for arterial input and the portal vein or inferior mesenteric vein are used for venous drainage[10] if SMA and SMV are not appropriate for anastomoses

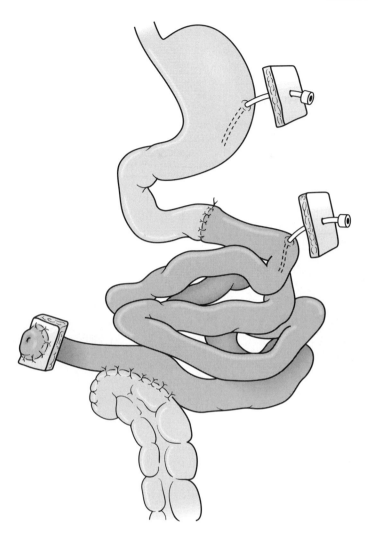

Figure 12-1. Isolated intestine transplant. *Adapted from the Department of Transplant Surgery, Children's Hospital of Pittsburgh of the University of Pittsburgh Medical Center.*

        d.   The inferior vena cava is used for venous drainage if the portal venous system can not be accessed

        e.   Proximal end of the donor intestine is anastomosed to the most distal segment of the recipient's residual intestine, usually at or distal to the ligament of Treitz[10]

G. Liver and intestine transplant (Figure 12-3)

    1. Native liver is removed and organs are implanted in the standard piggy-back fashion, preserving the vena cava

    2. Recipient portal vein is anastomosed to the recipient vena cava or to the donor portal vein

    3. Aortic segment including the celiac and superior mesenteric artery trunks is anastomosed to the infrarenal aorta[10]

    4. Healthy residual intestine is usually preserved in patients with structural disorders

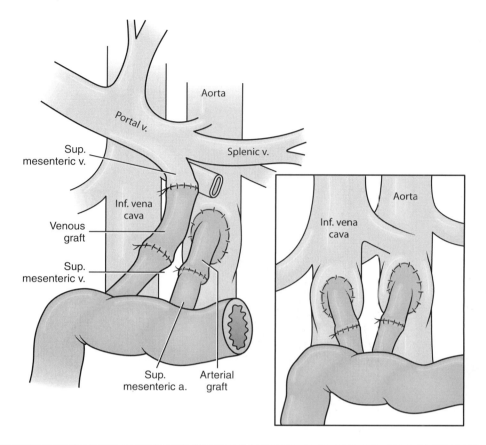

Figure 12-2. Vascular implantation of an isolated intestine graft using vascular conduits to the mesenteric vessel or to the aorta and IVC. *Adapted from the Department of Transplant Surgery, Children's Hospital of Pittsburgh of the University of Pittsburgh Medical Center.*

H. Multivisceral transplant (Figures 12-4 and 12-5)
    1. Several variants depending upon organs transplanted and recipient anatomy
    2. Regardless of the variant, the corresponding native organs are removed
I. Colon anastomosis
    1. Proximal end of the native colon is anastomosed to the distal end of the donor intestine if recipient has a healthy, intact colon
    2. Transplantation of the colon considered in patients with a minimal length or absence of the colon
        a. Procedure is controversial
        b. Colon may help alleviate fluid and electrolyte imbalances in the early postoperative period but has been associated with a higher incidence of bacterial translocation and infections[11]
J. Reperfusion
    1. Donor organs reperfused following completion of all vascular anastomoses
K. Ileostomy

1. Created following completion of intestinal anastomoses and reperfusion
2. Provides direct access for surveillance endoscopies in the early postoperative period
3. Usually closed between 3 to 6 months post-transplant depending on the function of the graft and complications

L. Feeding tube placement
   1. Feeding tubes placed because oral intake is not dependable in the early post-operative period
   2. Common tubes
      a. Feeding gastrostomy (GT)
      b. Jejunostomy (JT) and/or
      c. Gastrojejunostomy (G-JT)

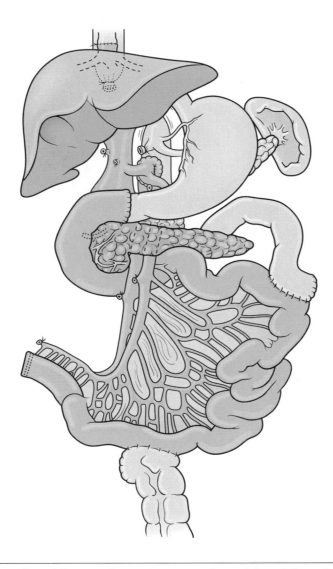

Figure 12-3. Combined liver and intestine transplant. *Adapted from the Department of Transplant Surgery, Children's Hospital of Pittsburgh of the University of Pittsburgh Medical Center.*

    i. Passes into the native stomach and then into the transplanted proximal jejunum

  3. Patients frequently have a well cannulated GT so an additional JT is placed into the transplanted jejunum

  4. Nasogastric tube and enteral tubes provide for decompression

  5. Jackson-Pratt drainage tubes

   a. 2-4 tubes

   b. Placed in the abdominal cavity to promote drainage of residual fluid

M. Closure

  1. Fascia

  2. Muscle layer

   a. May not be able to close initially if abdominal cavity compromised related to the size of the donor organs

  3. Abdomen is closed with sutures or staples

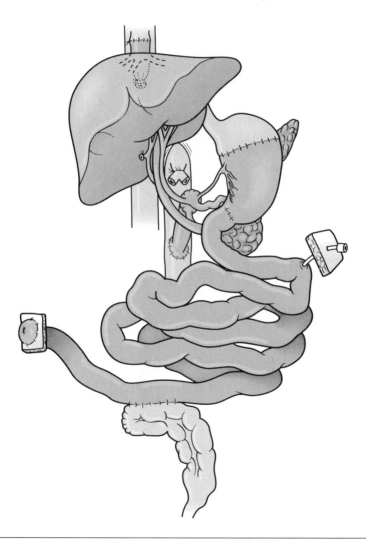

Figure 12-4. Complete multivisceral transplant. *Adapted from the Department of Transplant Surgery, Children's Hospital of Pittsburgh of the University of Pittsburgh Medical Center.*

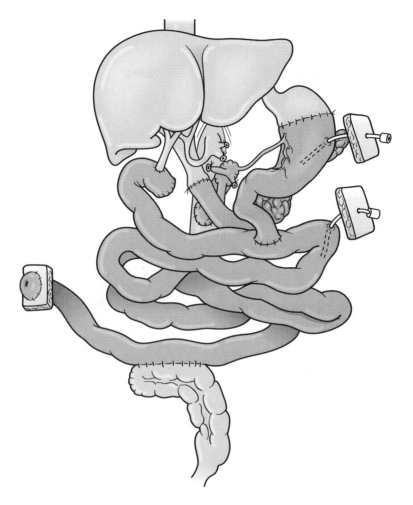

Figure 12-5. Modified multivisceral transplant. *Adapted from the Department of Transplant Surgery, Children's Hospital of Pittsburgh of the University of Pittsburgh Medical Center.*

        a.   Usually removed within 2-3 weeks depending on complications and wound healing

X. Post-transplant monitoring

   A. Challenging period

   B. Requires an in-depth understanding of the patient's responses to the surgical procedure, potential complications, and effects of immunosuppression

      1. Detail management essential

      2. Quick and appropriate response to signs and symptoms of infection, rejection, or fluid and electrolyte imbalance

   C. Patients transferred directly from the operating room to intensive care

      1. Length of stay ranges from a few days to weeks depending on center-specific protocols and complications

   D. Transfer to a transplant or general surgical unit when stable for further recovery and monitoring of graft function, rejection, infection, and electrolyte balance

1. Length of stay ranges from 1-2 weeks to several months depending on center-specific protocols and complications

E. Surgical complications
  1. Incidence
    a. Complications associated with surgical technique is less than 10%[12]
    b. A rate of nearly 50% has been reported in pediatric recipients[13]
  2. Postoperative hemorrhage
    a. Usually a technical problem from an anastomotic leak, peritoneal bleeding, or vascularized adhesions from previous surgeries[14]
      i. Pre-existing coagulopathy and portal hypertension may predispose patients with hepatic dysfunction to bleed
    b. Symptoms
      i. Pallor
      ii. Tachycardia
      iii. Hypotension
      iv. Increased serosanguineous drainage through Jackson-Pratt drains
      v. Reduction in serial hemoglobin levels
      vi. Abnormal serum pH and lactate levels may indicate intestinal ischemia or tissue injury
    c. Treatment
      i. Surgical re-exploration and repair
      ii. Improved liver function following liver transplantation and administration of blood products contributes to the resolution of bleeding
  3. Vascular thromboses
    a. Rare complication but can significantly compromise the graft and result in necrosis of the organs provided by that arterial supply
    b. Symptoms are usually acute and patient presents with general clinical deterioration
      i. Thrombosis of intestinal vasculature
        a) Stoma may become pale or dusky
        b) Function of the graft deteriorates
      ii. Complete obstruction
        a) Can lead to ascites and infarction of the mesentery
        b) Requires enterectomy of graft
      iii. Thromboses affecting the liver vasculature
        a) Results in significantly elevated liver function tests
        b) May lead to fulminant hepatic failure
    c. Diagnosis confirmed through vascular radiologic testing
    d. Prevention/treatment
      i. Anticoagulant therapy standard to decrease the risk of thrombus
        a) Protocols vary by center
        b) Most commonly used medications include various combinations of heparin, aspirin, persantine, and enoxaparin

ii.   Abdominal ultrasounds obtained routinely in early post-operative period to assess for thrombus formation and increased pressure

iii. Surgical intervention and/or

iv.   Dilatation

4. Gastrointestinal complications
    a. Hemorrhage
        i.   Early
             a) Usually occurs due to a technical problem
             b) May require surgical intervention
        ii. Later bleeding
             a) May be a consequence of rejection or infection
        iii. Symptoms
             a) Sanguineous ileostomy drainage or rectal bleeding
             b) Tachycardia
             c) Hypotension
             d) Abdominal pain
             e) Decreasing hemoglobin levels
        iv. Definitive diagnosis through endoscopy and biopsy to determine an infectious etiology versus rejection
        v.   Treatment
             a) Surgical intervention for technical complications
             b) Increased immunosuppression if etiology is rejection
             c) Antimicrobials and reduced immunosuppression if etiology is infection

5. Gastrointestinal leaks
    a. Etiology
        i.   Technical complications
        ii. Poor wound healing due to malnutrition and/or the effect of immunosuppressive medications
    b. Symptoms
        i.   Abdominal distention
        ii. Fever
        iii. Peritonitis
    c. Diagnosis
        i.   Confirmed through CT scans with contrast
    d. Prevention/treatment
        i.   Important to maintain decompression of the stomach and intestine through the jejunostomy, ileostomy, and nasogastric tube to minimize risk of leaks
        ii. Exploratory laparotomy performed to revise the affected segment of intestine and remove the infected peritoneal fluid
        iii. Intravenous antibiotics and/or antifungal agents administered as indicated

6. Motility of the transplanted intestine
    a. Extrinsic innervation to the transplanted intestine is absent following procurement
    b. Peristalsis begins when the intestine is reperfused but can be erratic
    c. Hypermotility is common

      d. Fluid and electrolyte balance must be accurately maintained by monitoring intake and output, daily weight, and serum electrolytes

  7. Absorption of the transplanted intestine

      a. Generally absorbs well post-transplant as seen through monitored immunosuppressive levels, particularly tacrolimus

          i. Tacrolimus levels may also be affected by NPO status, dysfunction of the intestine, vomiting, drug interactions, and adherence

      b. Carbohydrate absorption

          i. Determined by D-xylose testing

          ii. Appears to normalize within the first several months post-transplant[15]

      c. Protein absorption

          i. Appears to be adequate in the early post-transplant period

          ii. Measured by pre-albumin levels

      d. Fat absorption

          i. Fats commonly malabsorbed due to surgical disruption of the lymphatic drainage of the donor intestine

          ii. May take several months for the intestinal lymphatic drainage to be reestablished allowing for better absorption of medium chain triglycerides[10]

F. Vital signs

  1. Continually monitored during the intensive care phase to assess for complications

  2. Obtained less frequently, every 4-8 hours, when the patient is on the transplant unit

  3. Taken more frequently, per individual hospital protocol, during certain medication administrations, or procedures such as infusions of immunoglobulin, blood products, or post-biopsy

  4. Temperature

      a. Temperature elevation related to infection

          i. $\geq 38.5°C/101°$ F in early postoperative period

          ii. Usually related to surgical interventions, the patient's pre-transplant status, or postoperative complications

          iii. Source of fever must be identified quickly through pan cultures (blood, urine, sputum, wound, stool), chest x-ray, and/or CT scan

          iv. Appropriate broad-spectrum antimicrobial administered until the source of infection and sensitivity of the organism is identified

          v. Aggressive pulmonary toilet required in patients with atelectasis and pneumonia

          vi. Antipyretics are usually ordered for comfort

          vii. Cooling blankets may be used adjunctively with high fevers

      b. Temperature elevation related to rejection

          i. Less common in the very early post-transplant period

          ii. The first episode of rejection is most commonly observed around 14-21 days post-transplant

        iii. Fever is present but usually in conjunction with a change in stool output and consistency, and/or abdominal pain and distention

5. Tachycardia
   a. Usually related to fluid imbalance
   b. Can also be present with fever
   c. Can be a symptom of pain or anxiety
   d. Other differential diagnoses
      i. Hypernatremia
      ii. Anemia
      iii. Hypoglycemia
      iv. Hyperthyroidism
      v. Effect of medications: albuterol, pseudoephedrine, antiarrhythmics
   e. A sustained heart rate greater than the upper limits of normal for age or subjective complaints of palpitations should be reported
   f. Treatment
      i. Tachycardia as a result of dehydration is corrected by administration of IV fluids to achieve the desired response
      ii. If arrhythmias are suspected, an EKG should be obtained
      iii. Tachycardia due to postoperative pain is controlled through administration of pain medications and supportive nursing care

6. Bradycardia
   a. A low heart rate sustained at less than the lower limits of normal for age
   b. Associated with a disruption of the electrical impulses generated by the sinoatrial or atrioventricular node
   c. Etiology
      i. Present in patients with other cardiac conditions including coronary artery disease and myocarditis
      ii. Hypothyroidism
      iii. Hyperkalemia
      iv. As a potential side effect of narcotics
      v. Side effect of some cardiac medications including beta-blockers, calcium channel blockers, antiarrhythmics, and digoxin

7. Hypotension
   a. Etiology
      i. Fluid imbalance
      ii. Electrolyte abnormalities
      iii. Sepsis
      iv. Bleeding
      v. Narcotics
      vi. Other medications associated with hypotension include diuretics, beta-blockers, calcium channel blockers, angiotensin-converting enzyme (ACE) inhibitors, nitrates, antipsychotics, anti-anxiolytics, tricyclic antidepressants
   b. Symptoms
      i. Sustained low systolic blood pressure for age/height
      ii. Weak pulse
      iii. Decreased capillary refill
      iv. Output greater than intake

       v. Fever

      vi. Signs/symptoms of bleeding and/or

     vii. Decreased hematocrit

  c. Treatment

    a). Dehydration corrected through administration of IV fluids

    b). If bleeding is suspected, the source of blood loss is identified with appropriate treatment/intervention

8. Hypertension

  a. Etiology

    i. Nephrotoxicity from immunosuppressant medications (primarily corticosteroids and calcineurin inhibitors)

    ii. Fluid and electrolyte imbalance

    iii. Hepatorenal syndrome

    iv. Pre-existing diabetes

    v. Postoperative pain

  b. Symptoms

    i. Sustained high blood pressure >95th percentile for age and sex

    ii. Decreased urinary output

    iii. Increasing renal function tests

    iv. Rarely have subjective complaints, but headache may be present

  c. Treatment

    i. Varies based on etiology

    ii. Scheduled or PRN antihypertensive medications

    iii. If hypertension related to nephrotoxicity from high levels of tacrolimus or steroids, dosage may be decreased while balancing risk of rejection

    iv. Fluid and electrolyte imbalances corrected by balancing intake and output, infusing or restricting fluids, and ordering electrolyte additives in fluids

9. Tachypnea

  a. Patients ventilated until able to sustain a normal respiratory rate and appropriate oxygenation

  b. Seen with fever and infection, particularly pneumonias and septicemia

  c. Pain

10. Hypoxia

  a. Usually related to the effects of anesthesia and/or narcotics

  b. Symptoms

    i. Decreased respiratory rate and effort

    ii. Decreased oxygen saturation

    iii. Need for supplemental oxygen

    iv. Decreased PaO_2 and/or increased $PaCO_2$

  c. Treatment

    1. Supportive oxygenation as needed

    2. Decrease or discontinue narcotics

11. Neurologic assessment

  a. Assess neurologic status every 2 hours in early postoperative period, then less frequently as patient recovers

b.   Assess pupils and reaction to light, facial symmetry, reflexes, response to stimuli, speech, and bilateral strength of the extremities related to the patient's level of consciousness

c.   Neurotoxic side effects may be related to the tacrolimus level

d.   Tacrolimus has been associated with headache, tremor, insomnia, photophobia, confusion, and seizures

   i.   Monitor tacrolimus trough levels

   ii.   Observe for side effects related to a high trough level

   iii. Higher tacrolimus levels generally are associated with increased symptoms

e.   Neurotoxicities vary by patient

f.   Other conditions that increase seizure risk include hyperglycemia, hypomagnesemia, and hyponatremia.

XI. Postoperative appliances and drains

A.   Venous/arterial access

1.   Substantial venous access required due to fluid needs

2.   1-2 central lines

a.   Preferably double lumens

b.   Access via the internal/external jugular veins, subclavians, or inguinal veins

c.   Patients with a paucity of sites may have a transhepatic line

3.   Additional peripheral intravenous lines for increased access

a.   Intravenous tacrolimus must be administered through a dedicated line not used for lab draws

4.   Arterial line

a.   Inserted to monitor blood gases and central venous pressure

b.   Discontinued following extubation

5.   Meticulous nursing care of central lines is essential

a.   Minimize entry when possible to prevent infection

b.   Maintain patency to save access for possible long-term intravenous needs

B.   Appliances for respiratory support

1.   Ventilated for 12-24 hours or more depending on the length of surgery, pre-transplant status, and post-operative complications

a.   Monitor blood gases and central venous pressure while intubated

2.   Supportive oxygenation as needed following extubation

a.   Via cannula or face mask

b.   Oxygenation monitored through continual pulse oximetry readings

C.   Gastrointestinal appliances (prefeeding)

1.   Imperative to decompress the stomach and intestine to avoid gastric or intestinal perforation at the anastomotic lines or within the intestine

2.   Decompression through suction and drainage from nasogastric tube, gastrostomy tube and/or jejunostomy tube, and ileostomy

D.   Enteral feeding appliances

1.   Enteral feedings begun after upper gastrointestinal contrast study confirms absence of any intestinal leaks

2.   Feedings administered through a gastrostomy tube (GT), jejunostomy tube (JT) or gastrojejunostomy tube (G-JT)

a. G-JT used to avoid complications from an insertion site in the graft

E. Abdominal drainage appliances
1. Jackson-Pratt drains
   a. Remove residual fluid in peritoneum
   b. Pediatric recipients have 1-2 drains
   c. Adults may have up to 4 drains
   d. Drainage emptied and recorded every 4 hours
   e. Fluid initially serosanguineous, becoming less serous over the first 3-5 days post-transplant
      i. Increased serous drainage may be a sign of bleeding from vascular anastomoses
      ii. Hematocrit of the fluid may be obtained to assess bleeding
      iii. Site of bleeding determined through abdominal ultrasound or CT scan
   f. Drains usually removed within 7 days after surgery as drainage decreases
2. Biliary drain or percutaneous transhepatic catheter (PTC)
   a. Uncommon in patients receiving a composite liver and intestine graft
   b. Inserted in patients with bile duct complications to dilate the occluded bile duct and maintain bile flow
3. Urinary catheter
   a. Accurate measurement of intake and output is imperative in the early postoperative period
   b. Urinary catheter provides a drainage method to accurately assess urinary output
   c. To avoid infection, the urinary catheter is removed as soon as the patient is continent
4. Ileostomy
   a. Created to provide easy access to the transplanted intestine for routine surveillance for rejection
   b. Bulk of stool output will drain from the ileostomy
   c. Patients with an intact large intestine may pass some stool from the rectum
   d. Drainage is emptied and recorded every 4 hours or as needed
   e. Stool assessed for amount, color, and consistency
   f. Stool output when motility stabilizes
      i. 1-2 liters/day for adults
      ii. 40-60 cc/kg/day for pediatric patients
   g. Stomal output can be inconsistent
   h. Stool color ranges from yellow to brown
   i. Stool consistency
      i. Watery because the large intestine is bypassed, particularly in the early period
      ii. Thicker consistency achieved depending on diet, the addition of fiber, and less rapid motility
5. Abdominal incision
   a. Closed with staples or sutures
   b. Dressing over site for the first 12 hours post-transplant, then left open to air
   c. Steri-strips may be applied to the suture line

        d.   Staples removed 2-3 weeks post-operatively depending on complications

XII. Fluid and electrolyte balance (see Table 12-3)

    A. Fluid imbalance and related complications are common

    B. Intravenous fluids administered at two-thirds maintenance to maintain a CVP of 6-10 cm H_2O and a urine output of 0.5-1.5 ml/kg/hour

    C. Intravascular volume depleted while retaining fluids

        1. Result of increased interstitial fluid accumulation in the peripheral tissue, the intestinal graft, and lungs due to leakage of the mesenteric lymphatics

    D. Hypermotility is common until the graft adapts due to the disruption of extrinsic innervation

        1. Increased transit time

        2. Decreased enteral absorption

        3. Increased output with subsequent electrolyte imbalance

    E. Nursing interventions

        1. Maintain strict record of intake and output.

        2. Observe for symptoms of electrolyte imbalance, fluid overload, or dehydration (see Table 12-3)

        3. Obtain electrolytes and renal function tests as ordered

        4. Notify the physician with abnormal levels

        5. Administer IV fluids to correct imbalances as ordered

        6. Obtain repeat lab values to evaluate resolution of imbalance or lab value

    F. Alterations in blood glucose levels

        1. Hyperglycemia

            a. Presents as a complication of calcineurin inhibitors and high doses of steroids

           b. Monitor blood glucose levels as ordered, usually four times daily

           c. Administer insulin as ordered

           d. Provide education regarding the signs and symptoms of hyper- and hypoglycemia and treatment

    G. Daily weights

        1. Important element to assess fluid overload and absorptive capacity of graft

        2. Weigh patient at approximately the same time every day, in the same manner, and on the same scale

        3. Weight gain

            a. Gain with edema may be a sign of fluid overload and/or renal dysfunction

        4. Weight loss

            a. May occur in early postoperative period as TPN and enteral feedings are adjusted to meet the patient's caloric needs

           b. Occurs in longer term as result of inadequate calories, poor absorption, and hypermotility with a high output

XIII. Pain management

    A. Most patients experience some degree of postoperative pain.

    B. Goal is satisfactory control of pain

    C. Pain management education is essential part of preoperative teaching for transplant nurses

        1. Help patients prepare for postoperative pain

2. Facilitate understanding of their ability to control their own pain
3. Know and understand the patient's beliefs and attitudes about pain
4. Explain use of 0-10 pain scale and be sure patients understand how to report their level of pain
5. Investigate other methods for coping with pain
    a. Deep breathing
    b. Relaxation techniques
    c. Imagery
6. Be aware of any sociocultural factors that affect coping, pain, and pain management

D. Pain control
1. Early postoperative period
    a. Intravenous bolus and/or continuous administration of narcotics such as morphine, fentanyl, and dilaudid[-6]
2. Later postoperative period
    a. Intravenous patient-controlled anesthesia (PCA)
        i.   Provides patient with ability to control pain
        ii. Gives more sustained pain relief
    b. Oral narcotics prescribed when patients are tolerating enteral feeds
    c. Transitioned to nonnarcotic analgesics for any residual discomfort
3. Pain Service consultation helpful for further or prolonged pain management
4. Nursing considerations in administering narcotics
    a. Assess patient for excessive sedation, respiratory depression, bradycardia, and hypotension
    b. Assess the graft for dysmotility
        i.   Constipation is a side effect of narcotics and motility of the transplanted intestine may be further compromised with prolonged narcotic use
5. Dependency on pain medications
    a. Some intestine transplant candidates have pain control issues prior to transplant depending on etiology of short gut and complications
    b. Concerns of dependency must be investigated prior to transplant
    c. Establish a plan with the patient for pain control and narcotic weaning post-transplant

XIV. Graft function
A. Extrinsic innervation to the graft is absent
B. Peristalsis begins immediately but motility may be intermittent and/or rapid
C. Early graft nonfunction (postoperative day 1-3) is rare and is usually a result of a surgical complication
D. Monitoring graft function (Table 12-7)
1. Clinical surveillance through endoscopy with biopsy
2. Performed frequently during the first 3 months post-transplant to assess graft status
3. Monitoring protocols
    a. Vary by center

TABLE 12-7

■ Nursing Assessment of Graft Function

Observe for abdominal distention and signs of discomfort or pain

Auscultate for hypoactive bowel sounds

Palpate to assess any firmness or abdominal rigidity

Assess stoma output for changes in:

- Volume—a trend or acute increase in stoma output
- Color—from yellowish-brown to melena and/or frank blood
- Consistency—increased watery fluid with little consistency

Observe for presence of blood

---

   b. Usually twice weekly for 4-6 weeks, weekly for 4-6 weeks, then every other week until the risk of rejection is minimal
   c. Subsequent surveillance completed when clinically indicated
   d. Long term stable patients assessed on an annual basis per transplant center protocol
4. Monitoring nutritional status
   a. Goal is for the patient to obtain full nutritional needs from oral and/or enteral nutrition
   b. Carbohydrate absorption normalizes within the first few months post-transplant as measured by D-xylose testing
   c. Protein absorption normalizes within the first several months as measured by pre-albumin levels
   d. Fat absorption is monitored through 24-72 hour fecal fat studies
      i. Fat malabsorption is common until the intestinal lymphatic drainage is reestablished[15]
   e. Nursing interventions
      i. Obtain stool for D-xylose testing or fecal fat collection per laboratory protocol as ordered
      ii. Assess for fat malabsorption
         a) Observe for increased stool output
         b) Change in stool consistency
         c) Presence of oily stool
         d) Weight loss
         e) Abdominal pain
   f. Treatment for fat malabsorption
      i. Low fat diet
      ii. Administration of pancreatic enzymes
      iii. Short-term lipid infusions in cases of severe and/or prolonged fat malabsorption with weight loss and/or poor growth
XV. Immunosuppression
   A. Immunosuppressant protocols vary by center
   B. Multiple agents may be used
      1. Induction therapy

        a.   Induction therapy significantly improves graft survival[4, 18]
           i.   Antithymocyte globulin
           ii.   Alemtuzumab
           iii.   Daclizumab
           iv.   Muromonab-CD3
           v.   Basiliximab

2. Tacrolimus is the primary immunosuppressant agent in intestine transplantation
   a. If using induction therapy, oral tacrolimus is begun on the first postoperative day[17]
   b. Intravenous tacrolimus is rarely used in the early post-operative period because of the effect of the induction agent
   c. Intravenous tacrolimus is sometimes used for brief periods to optimize a low tacrolimus level or to maintain adequate levels if GI absorption is compromised
   d. Minimum trough levels in the *early* postoperative period are usually maintained at 15-18 ng/ml in whole blood.[10,17] Trough levels vary based on:
      i. Use of induction therapy
      ii. Renal function
      iii. Concomitant nephrotoxic medications
      iv. Time post-transplant
      v. Presence of rejection or infection
      vi. Center-specific protocols
3. Corticosteroids
   a. Steroid therapy varies by center
   b. Long-term vs. short-term need
   c. Used in treatment of rejection if patient on monotherapy
   d. Some centers prefer to wean and discontinue steroids when possible
4. Adjunctive agents
   a. Mycophenolate mofetil
   b. Sirolimus
   c. Azathioprine

XVI. Rejection
   A. Common complication following intestine transplantation because of the large amount of lymphoid tissue associated with the graft
   B. Incidence of rejection
      1. Rates vary by center
      2. Overall incidence[18] (Intestine Transplant Registry)
         a. 57% for intestine grafts
         b. 39% for combined intestine and liver grafts
         c. 48% for multivisceral grafts
   C. Timing
      1. First episode most commonly seen within 6-12 months post-transplant
      2. May not occur if immunosuppression can be maintained at a stable and adequate level
   D. Site
      1. May occur throughout the graft
      2. Ileum is most commonly affected

E. Serum markers
    1. No specific serum markers are indicative of rejection of the intestine
    2. Plasma citrulline may be a possible indicator of rejection[19]
        a. A nonessential amino acid produced by the intestinal mucosa
        b. Currently under investigation
    3. Serum markers for nutritional adequacy are of limited value[20]
        a. Albumin
        b. Transferrin
        c. Retinoic acid
F. Symptoms of rejection
    1. No single symptom is a clear indicator
    2. Presents as a combination of clinical signs
        a. Fever
        b. Significant increase or decrease in stool output
        c. Abdominal distention
        d. Cramping
        e. Vomiting
        f. Abdominal pain and/or
        g. Change in the appearance of the stoma
G. Endoscopic findings
    1. Mild to moderate rejection
        a. Edema
        b. Granularity
        c. Erythema and/or duskiness
        d. Absent or decreased peristalsis
        e. Loss of normal velvety appearance
    2. Severe rejection
        a. Diffuse ulceration
        b. Aperistalsis
        c. Denuded mucosa with bleeding
    3. Definitive diagnosis through histology from intestinal biopsy[20]
        a. 4-6 sites biopsied throughout as much of graft as possible
        b. Histologic findings associated with rejection
            i.   Increased apoptotic bodies
            ii.   Presence of activated lymphocytes
            iii. Loss of goblet cells
            iv.   Blunted villae
            v.   Ulceration
        c. Histology of severe rejection[20]
            i.   Crypts between the villae are destroyed
            ii. Epithelium is sloughed
H. Chronic rejection
    1. May develop over a longer period of time
    2. May result from rejection that is partially treated or refractory to treatment
    3. Symptoms
        a. Chronic diarrhea
        b. Progressive weight loss
        c. Intermittent fevers
        d. High output
        e. Abdominal pain
        f. GI bleeding

4. Endoscopic findings
   a. Tubular appearance
   b. Thickened mucosal folds
   c. Pseudomembranes and/or
   d. Chronic ulcers
5. Histology[20]
   a. Limited cellular infiltrates
   b. Villous blunting
   c. Focal ulcerations
   d. Epithelia metaplasia
6. Full-thickness biopsies
   a. Completed on graft enterectomies
   b. Reveal thickening or obliteration of the intestinal arterioles causing compromised oxygenation of the intestinal mucosa

I. Treatment
1. Mild to moderate rejection
   a. Optimize tacrolimus levels (Table 12-8)
   b. Administer intravenous methylprednisolone as a bolus dose with decreasing cycled dosing over a short period of time, usually 5 days
   c. Adjunctive agents may be added to the baseline immunosuppressive regimen
   d. Repeat endoscopy with biopsy every 3-5 days to assess effect of treatment and determine further immunosuppressant management
2. Severe rejection (Table 12-9)
   a. Administration of muromonab-CD3 (Orthoclone®, OKT3) for maximum of 14 days
   b. Alternate treatment (1-4 doses) with rabbit antithymocyte globulin (Thymoglobulin®)
   c. Duration of therapy determined by subsequent histology
   d. Consider graft enterectomy if refractory to all available treatments and patient has increased complications related to infection from high levels of immunosuppression
   e. Retransplantation is possible, but survival rates are much lower than following the primary transplant

XVII. Post-endoscopy/biopsy monitoring
A. Surveillance endoscopies (Tables 12-10 and 12-11)
1. Obtained frequently within the first 3-6 months post-transplant
2. Also obtained whenever rejection is suspected
3. Ileostomy is created to facilitate frequent endoscopies and maintained up to 12 months post-transplant
4. Usually performed at patient's bedside in intensive care and in the GI suite when on the transplant/surgical unit
5. If sedation is not required:
   a. Resume preprocedure care
   b. Resume ordered diet
   c. Resume preprocedure activity
6. If patient is sedated:
   a. Monitor vital signs per hospital protocol
   b. Resume diet and activity when recovered
7. Hospitalized patients

TABLE 12-8

■ **Nursing Interventions: Effective Tacrolimus Administration and Monitoring**

Administer tacrolimus as ordered and on time, usually every 12 hours.

Administer doses within an hour of the prescribed time unless there is an order to hold a dose.

Achieve stable levels with consistency of administration.

Maintain NPO 1 hour before and after the oral dose or as per center protocol.

Administer whole capsules.

Use alternative administration strategies in pediatric patients as required, but identify and record a consistent method for that patient.

Obtain tacrolimus trough levels 10-12 hours after the previous dose.

Do not draw blood for the tacrolimus level through lines where tacrolimus has previously infused or is currently infusing if the patient has received tacrolimus intravenously.

Be aware of the desired tacrolimus level for the patient and alert the physician immediately to an inappropriate level.

Monitor patient for the most common side effects of tacrolimus:

- Neurotoxicities: insomnia, headache, burning or tingling of the hands and feet, tremors, photophobia, aphasia, confusion, seizures
- Nephrotoxicities: hyperkalemia, hypomagnesemia, hypertension, renal dysfunction
- GI distress: abdominal distress, nausea, vomiting, diarrhea
- Increased risk of infection: fever
- Hyperglycemia

Be aware of drug interactions that increase or decrease tacrolimus levels.

---

        a.   Monitored as above for possible complications
        b.   Frequent vital signs are not usually ordered
    8. Outpatient endoscopies
        a.   Usually intestinal recipients in the later postoperative period
        b.   Monitored in GI suite then discharged
    9. Patient education
        a.   Signs and symptoms of post-procedure complications
        b.   How to contact their transplant coordinator and/or physician in event of fever, discomfort, or bleeding
XVIII. Infection
    A. Consequence of high baseline levels of immunosuppression
    B. Incidence
        1. Leading cause of death in intestinal transplantation contributing to 46% of mortalities[18, 21]
        2. Must balance risk of infection from a highly immunosuppressed state and risk of rejection from decreased immunosuppression
        3. Factors contributing to the incidence of infection
            a.   Prolonged operative time

TABLE 12-9

■ **Nursing Interventions to Assess Rejection**

Administer immunosuppressive medications as ordered.

Assess the patient for the clinical signs of rejection:

- Fever
- Significantly increased or decreased stool output
- Change of consistency of stool to a more watery fluid
- Abdominal pain
- Distention
- Bleeding from the stoma or rectum
- Change in stoma color and/or
- Hypoactive bowel sounds

Notify the physician in the event of any of these symptoms.

Be aware of the desired tacrolimus level for the patient and any changes in that level. Notify the physician immediately for levels outside of the desired range.

Facilitate the endoscopy procedure as required in the GI suite or at bedside and provide post-procedure care per center protocol.

Administer immunosuppressive medications as ordered to treat rejection.

Monitor for drug toxicities secondary to increased levels.

Provide education for the family and patient in regard to the diagnosis of rejection, treatment, and potential side effects of treatment.

Provide emotional support for the patient/family in expressing anxiety and fear related to rejection.

Reassure the patient that rejection is a common complication of transplantation and can usually be treated.

      b. Preoperative status and the presence of liver disease
      c. Surgical complications
      d. Multiple surgeries
      e. Sepsis prior to transplant
      f. Inability to close the abdominal wall following implantation of organ(s)
      g. Presence of multiple invasive lines and catheters that compromise the skin barrier
   4. Cadaveric organ procurement
      a. Adds to risk of infection because adequate bowel preparation is not possible prior to the enterectomy
      b. Intestinal contents and gastrointestinal flora are transplanted with the graft
      c. Intestinal epithelium may be damaged if there is preservation injury to the graft resulting in bacterial translocation into the splanchnic venous system causing bacteremia[10]

TABLE 12-10
■ Nursing Interventions Prior to Endoscopy

Maintain NPO status as ordered: usually NPO for 4 hours prior to procedure if endoscopy is performed through the ileostomy and patient is sedated

Obtain labs within 3 days prior to the procedure or per center protocol: hemoglobin and hematocrit, platelet count, and PT/PTT

Notify the transplant physician or GI physician with any abnormalities.

Administer appropriate blood products or medications as ordered to correct abnormal levels.

Repeat labs after interventions are performed to assess correction.

Perform the ordered bowel preparation:

- Protocols vary by center
- Preparation for a lower endoscopy:
- Clears for 12 hours then NPO
- Administer GoLYTELY® on the evening prior to endoscopy
- Normal saline enemas as needed
- No bowel preparation for an upper endoscopy or ileoscopy

Administer intravenous bacterial prophylaxis if ordered.

Explain procedure and postprocedure care to patient/family.

Provide emotional support for fears or concerns they may have about the procedure, particularly if rejection is suspected.

C. Timing of infections
   1. Early (0-2 months)
      a. Usually due to surgical and technical complications, pneumonia and indwelling catheters[12]
      b. Bacterial infections
      c. Fungal infections
   2. Middle period (2-6 months)
      a. Cytomegalovirus (CMV)
      b. Epstein Barr virus (EBV)/post-transplant lymphoproliferative disease (PTLD)
      c. Adenovirus
   3. Long term
      a. EBV
      b. Community-acquired infections
         i. Influenza
         ii. Respiratory syncytial virus (RSV)
      c. Patients usually tolerate community-acquired infections well since their overall health is improved and immunosuppression is lower
   4. EBV/PTLD and CMV can occur any time there is a significant increase in the level of immunosuppression[12]

TABLE 12-11

■ Nursing Interventions Post-Endoscopy

Monitor vital signs frequently as ordered until awake. Notify the physician for fever, tachycardia, or hypotension.

Obtain postprocedure hemoglobin and hematocrit levels if ordered. Notify the physician with abnormal results.

Assess for postprocedure complications:

- Bleeding from the ileostomy due to intestinal perforation
- Abdominal discomfort or pain
- Hypoactive bowel sounds
- Firm abdomen secondary to an ileus

Assess for abdominal distention.

- Some distention is normal because air is inserted into the intestine to facilitate viewing and to obtain the biopsy
- Distention should decrease within hours as patient passes gas from the ileostomy or rectum and as physical activity is resumed
- Notify the physician of:
  - Prolonged or increased distention
  - Hypoactive or absent bowel sounds
  - Vomiting

Encourage the ordered diet and fluids when fully awake.

Resume preprocedure activity level when fully awake or as ordered.

Review the findings of the study with the patient/family, as explained by the transplant physician or gastroenterologist.

Assess understanding of the outcome and any required treatment.

5. Bacteremia related to severe rejection and central venous catheters can occur at any time
   a. Central venous catheters may be required for up to a year post-transplant
   b. Used to provide hydration, intravenous fluids/electrolytes, and medications
D. Bacterial infections
   1. Incidence
      a. Can occur at any time, but most commonly seen during the first three months post-transplant
      b. Incidence > 60%
   2. Common organisms[12, 22]
      a. *Enterobacter*
      b. *Klebsiella*
      c. *Pseudomonas* species
      d. Polymicrobial infections and antibiotic-resistant organisms, such as vancomycin-resistant enterococcus also occur[22]

3. Bacterial translocation
   a. Bacteria translocate from the transplanted intestine and travel to the peritoneal cavity through leakage from division of the lymphatics during procurement
   b. Peritonitis can occur in the immunocompromised patient
   c. Bacteria can also move into the portal circulation and progress to other sites
4. Bacterial overgrowth
   a. Defined as $> 10^9$ colony-forming units per milliliter of stool
   b. High correlation between bacteria identified in stool and those in the blood
   c. Overgrowth can lead to translocation when the intestinal mucosa is damaged through ischemia, reperfusion injury, or rejection[17]
5. Signs and symptoms of bacterial infection may include:
   a. Fever, usually $\geq 101°$ F or $38.5°$ C
   b. Flu-like symptoms: malaise, lethargy, decreased appetite, irritability/change in behavior (pediatrics)
   c. Catheter or tube insertion sites that are erythematous, swollen, tender
   d. Wound site abnormalities: erythema, purulent drainage, tenderness, swelling
   e. Wound dehiscence
   f. Changes in respiratory status: tachypnea, decreased breath sounds, cough
   g. Changes in drainage: purulence, cloudy urine, stool consistency and odor
6. Diagnosis
   a. Central and peripheral blood cultures
   b. Cultures of the wound, throat, urine, sputum, JP drainage, and/or stool should be obtained as ordered
   c. Chest x-ray particularly in the setting of respiratory symptoms
   d. Abdominal CT scan to assess the source of infection
7. Treatment
   a. Broad-spectrum antibiotics administered after cultures are obtained based on the apparent etiology of fever
   b. Antimicrobial treatment adjusted based on the sensitivity of the identified organism
   c. Immunosuppression may be decreased with caution, particularly in the setting of severe polymicrobial infections
      i. Closely monitor immunosuppressant levels and report any levels that are not within the desired therapeutic range
      ii. Observe patient for signs and symptoms of rejection
   d. Infected wounds
      i. Wet to dry dressing changes with daily assessment
      ii. Dressing changes completed two to four times daily depending on the extent of the wound, amount of drainage, and amount of granulation tissue
   e. Bacterial pneumonia
      i. Nursing interventions vary depending on the severity of respiratory compromise
      ii. Complete routine respiratory assessments
      iii. Administer IV antibiotics as ordered

   iv. Monitor supplemental oxygen flow, oxygen saturation, and/or blood gases

   v. Monitor the patient on mechanical ventilation for severe respiratory compromise

   vi. Perform endotracheal suction per hospital protocol if ventilated

   vii. Encourage coughing and deep breathing

   viii. Reposition the patient every 2 hours or as ordered

   ix. Administer aerosols if not given by Respiratory Therapy

  f. Central line infections

   i. Treated with intravenous antibiotics

   ii. Blood cultures are drawn daily until negative

   iii. Treatment usually continues for 14 days from the first negative blood culture for that organism

   iv. Central line may be removed in some cases[23]

    a) May be changed over a guide wire and a temporary line inserted in patients with limited access

    b) After treatment is complete, another permanent line will be placed

  g. Selective intestinal decontamination

   i. Administered in patients with persistent bacteremias with enteric organisms

   ii. Treatment protocols vary by center

   iii. Common practice is to administer colistimethate, tobramycin, and amphotericin by an enteral route two to three times daily for two weeks every month[17]

 E. Fungal infections

  1. Less common than bacterial infections

  2. Usually occur in the early postoperative period

  3. Risk factors

   a. Deteriorating health status prior to transplant

   b. Surgical complications (particularly intestinal leaks)

   c. Surgical re-explorations

   d. Polymicrobial therapy

   e. High levels of immunosuppression

   f. Disruption of the mucosal barrier leading to translocation

   g. Indwelling catheters

  4. *Candida albicans* (noninvasive infection)

   a. Most common fungal infection following intestinal transplantation

   b. Site

    i. Oropharynx, esophagus, or genitalia

    ii. Prophylaxis with oral nystatin during the first 3 months post-transplant and when immunosuppression is maximized to treat rejection

   c. Signs and symptoms

    i. White plaques on oral mucosa or tongue

    ii. Red pinpoint rash of the buttocks or genitalia (pediatrics)

    iii. Vaginal discharge and itching

   d. Treatment

    i. If receiving prophylaxis, dosage frequency may be increased and/or a second agent added

   ii.   Nystatin or clotrimazole are commonly prescribed
   iii. Fluconazole prescribed if infection is refractory to nystatin
         a) Fluconazole is known to increase tacrolimus levels
         b) Dose of tacrolimus must be adjusted to prevent toxicity
         c) Tacrolimus levels during treatment with oral or intravenous fluconazole must be monitored carefully
         d) Tacrolimus dosing changes made when therapy is initiated and discontinued to maintain appropriate levels
   5. *Candida albicans* (systemic infection)
      a. Treated with intravenous fluconazole or amphotericin B
      b. Monitor renal function closely in patients receiving tacrolimus and intravenous amphotericin due to nephrotoxicity of each
      c. Renal-adjusted doses of amphotericin or a liposomal amphotericin product (Abelcet® or AmBisome®) should be used in patients with nephrotoxicity
      d. Assess for fungal abscess by CT scan
      e. Assess for cardiac vegetations by an echocardiogram if a central venous line is present[17]
   6. Aspergillus
      a. Rare fungal infection
      b. Carries a high mortality
      c. Site
          i.   Lungs are the most common site of a primary infection
          ii. Sinuses
          iii. Metastatic disease seen in central nervous system (CNS), liver, and/or kidneys
      d. Symptoms
          i.   Isolated fever without symptoms of rejection
          ii. Dyspnea
          iii. Hypoxia
          iv. Sinusitis: headache, facial pain, and facial edema
          v.   CNS symptoms: headache, lethargy, hemiparesis, seizure
      e. Diagnosis
          i.   CXR and CT scan to observe for nodular pneumonias with indistinct margins
          ii. CT scans of the sinuses or brain
      f. Treatment
          i.   Prolonged treatment, usually longer than 1 month
          ii. Intravenous amphotericin, a liposomal amphotericin product, or combination therapy with 5-Flucytosine
F.   Viral infections
   1. Cytomegalovirus (CMV) (Table 12-12)
      a. Common community-acquired infection of the herpes virus family
      b. Usually does not cause significant morbidity in the immunocompetent person
      c. More serious in intestine transplant recipients, but outcomes are generally favorable when diagnosed and treated early
      d. Risk factors
          i.   Donor-recipient CMV serology mismatch
               a) CMV-negative recipient receiving a CMV-positive intestine is at risk for primary CMV disease

TABLE 12-12

■ Nursing Interventions: Monitoring for CMV Infection

Monitor for fever and report temperatures > 101° F/38.5° C.

Monitor for increased stool output and GI symptoms.

Obtain serial CMV-PCRs, CBC, and other laboratory tests as ordered.

Monitor serial CMV-PCRs for response to treatment.

Monitor CBC results for leukopenia and thrombocytopenia.

Provide post-endoscopy care per protocol.

Administer intravenous antiviral therapy as ordered.

Monitor for signs and symptoms of nephrotoxicity.

Be aware that changes may be made in the level of immunosuppression during treatment for CMV. Notify the physician of any tacrolimus levels that are not within the desired range.

Provide patient/family with information about CMV disease, lab tests, endoscopy findings, and treatment. Reinforce teaching as necessary.

        b) Mismatch may be avoided in isolated intestine transplantation in some centers
     ii. High levels of immunosuppression
        a) Interferes with the body's normal immunologic response to the virus
   e. Prophylaxis
     i. Protocols vary by center
     ii. CMV-negative recipient receiving a CMV positive intestine receives 14 days of intravenous ganciclovir
     iii. Oral valganciclovir may be ordered to complete three months of therapy
     iv. Some protocols include CMV immunoglobulin (Cyto-Gam®) every other week for 2 months, then monthly for 2 months[17]
     v. Patients receiving intensified immunosuppression during treatment for rejection may also receive ganciclovir daily until baseline immunosuppressive therapy is resumed
   f. Symptoms[12]
     i. Patient may be asymptomatic
     ii. Most commonly affects the gastrointestinal tract
     iii. Fever
     iv. Flu-like symptoms
     v. Diarrhea
     vi. Varying degrees of gastroenteritis
     vii. Leucopenia
     viii. Atypical lymphocytosis
     ix. Thrombocytopenia
     x. Myalgias
     xi. Arthralgia
     xii. Malaise

        xiii. Anorexia

  g. Diagnosis

      i. CMV-PCR: measurement of CMV viral load in peripheral blood with polymerase chain reaction (PCR)

      ii. Patients are considered CMV-PCR negative if no CMV is detected.[17]

      iii. An endoscopy with biopsy performed to assess the degree of CMV enteritis

        a) Ulcerations within normal intestinal mucosa seen on endoscopy

        b) Histology reveals CMV inclusion bodies with inflammatory changes[24]

      iv. Invasive disease most commonly found in the gastrointestinal tract and liver

      v. Can also occur, although rarely, as CMV pneumonitis, retinitis, or as central nervous system disease

  h. Treatment

      i. Intravenous ganciclovir for 14-21 days or until the CMV-PCR is nondetectable

      ii. Baseline immunosuppression usually maintained, but may be decreased if the patient is deteriorating

      iii. Serial CMV-PCRs are followed as a response to therapy

      iv. Improved symptoms usually seen within 5-7 days

      v. Foscarnet used if resistant to ganciclovir[12]

      vi. Cidofovir is used in cases of foscarnet-resistant CMV[12]

      vii. Monitor renal function closely due to the nephrotoxicity of these agents and concomitant use of tacrolimus

  i. Nursing considerations

      i. Bear in mind that some symptoms of CMV enteritis appear similar to those of rejection

      ii. Be aware of the patients' risk factors for developing CMV

        a) Donor/recipient CMV status

        b) History of immunosuppression.

2. Epstein-Barr virus (EBV) and EBV-associated lymphoproliferative disease (PTLD) (Table 12-13)

  a. Includes a range of illnesses from a nonspecific viremia to polyclonal or monoclonal disease, and ultimately, lymphoma

  b. Significant cause of morbidity and mortality following intestine transplantation

  c. Risk

      i. Risk is highest in first year post-transplant, but PTLD can occur at any time

      ii. Intestine recipients have the highest risk of developing PTLD of all solid organ transplants due to the need for prolonged elevated levels of immunosuppression

      iii. Use of muromonab-CD3 (OKT3)[12]

      iv. EBV seropositive donor into an EBV seronegative recipient

        a) Pediatric recipients at greater risk because they are usually seronegative

      v. Recipient splenectomy is associated with a higher incidence of PTLD[12]

  d. Incidence

TABLE 12-13

■ **Nursing Interventions: Monitoring for EBV/PTLD**

Be aware of the patient's unique risk factors for EBV/PTLD.

Monitor for fever and report temperatures $\geq$40° C.

Monitor for clinical symptoms of EBV:

- Diarrhea

- Bloody stools

- Tonsilar enlargement (often with exudate)

- Peripheral lymphadenopathy

- Fatigue

- Malaise

- Decreased appetite

Obtain an EBV-PCR, CBC, and other laboratory tests as ordered.

Monitor serial EBV-PCRs for response to treatment.

Monitor CBC results for pancytopenia, leukopenia, and atypical lymphocytosis.

Facilitate procedures such as CT scan and endoscopy.

Provide post-endoscopy care per protocol.

Administer intravenous antiviral therapy as ordered.

Be aware that changes may be made in the level of immunosuppression during treatment for EBV/PTLD. Notify the physician of any tacrolimus levels that are not within the desired range.

Provide the patient/family with information about EBV/PTLD, lab tests, endoscopy findings, and treatment. Reinforce teaching as necessary.

Provide supportive care to the patient and family during diagnosis and treatment.

      i. Adults: 3.4% for intestine grafts, 2.9% for combined liver and intestine grafts, 6% for multivisceral transplants18
     ii. Pediatrics: 11.1% for intestine grafts, 10.4% for combined liver and intestine grafts, and 18.6% for multivisceral transplants[18]
  e. Evaluating EBV disease
      i. Measurement of EBV viral load in peripheral blood with polymerase chain reaction (PCR)
     ii. Serial EBV-PCRs are monitored frequently during the first year post-transplant in patients who are at greater risk
    iii. There is an association of elevated EBV viral loads and PTLD[25]
  f. Signs and symptoms of EBV[17]
      i. High fever (40° C) for at least 3 days
     ii. Diarrhea
    iii. Bloody stools

        iv. Tonsilar enlargement (often with exudate)

        v. Peripheral lymphadenopathy

        vi. Fatigue

        vii. Malaise

        viii. Decreased appetite

        ix. Pancytopenia

        x. Leukopenia

        xi. Atypical lymphocytosis

    g. Diagnosis

        i. EBV-PCR level

        ii. Endoscopy with tissue biopsy

        iii. CT scan of the neck, chest, abdomen, and pelvis

        iv. Lymph node biopsy may be completed

        v. Diagnosis confirmed through tissue histology

    h. Treatment

        i. Varies by center

        ii. The essential component of care lies in decreasing the level of immunosuppression and vigilant surveillance[26, 27]

        iii. Tacrolimus levels may be decreased by 25% to 50% to maintain levels of 5-7 ng/ml

        iv. Steroid dosage may be decreased to a lower baseline level if receiving steroids

        v. Antiviral therapy administered per transplant center protocol

           a) Intravenous ganciclovir

           b) Cytomegalovirus immune globulin (CytoGam®) or intravenous immune globulin (IVIG)

        vi. Close follow-up through weekly endoscopies with biopsy and serial EBV-PCRs

        vii. Treatment continued until there is clinical and virological evidence that EBV or PTLD has resolved

        viii. Other therapies with varying success for PTLD that is refractory to standard management[25, 27, 28]

           a) Anti-CD20 antibody (rituxumab)

           b) Interferon-alpha

           c) Cytotoxic chemotherapy

           d) Radiation

           e) Surgical resection

        ix. Prognosis is poor in patients who have disease involving more than one site, CNS involvement, monoclonal disease, EBV-negative PTLD, T or NK cell PTLD, or the presence of tumor suppressor genes[25]

XXI. Nutrition (Table 12-14)

    A. Goal of intestinal transplantation is to provide the patient's nutritional requirements enterally without TPN support

    B. Total parental nutrition

        1. Required by most patients for the first several weeks post-transplant

        2. ITR reports that 75% of patients are completely free of TPN within 6 months post-transplant[4]

        3. Intravenous nutritional support may be needed during episodes of severe rejection or prolonged infection

TABLE 12-14

■ **Nursing Interventions Related to Nutritional Needs**

Provide enteral and/or oral feedings as ordered.

Encourage oral intake.

Maintain an accurate calorie count if ordered.

Assess tolerance to feeds by observing the patient for:

- Change in stool consistency and output
- Weight gain or loss
- Abdominal distention
- Cramping
- Nausea
- Emesis

Maintain strict intake and output records.

Report changes in stool output.

Administer motility agents as ordered.

Monitor albumin levels.

Encourage oral intake.

Obtain the patient's weight at the same time every day.

Facilitate testing as ordered and per hospital protocols for:

- Fecal fat collection
- D-xylose testing
- Calorie counts

Facilitate team consultations related to nutritional needs:

- Dietary
- Physical Therapy
- Speech Therapy
- Occupational Therapy

4. Pediatric patients may require intermittent periods of partial TPN to support growth and development

C. Enteral feeds
   1. Upper gastrointestinal contrast study is completed to evaluate the integrity of the intestinal anastomoses before starting feeds
   2. Enteral feedings are begun if there are no confirmed intestinal leaks and peristalsis has resumed
   3. Feeding routines vary by center, the type of transplant, and post-operative complications

4. Enteral feeds usually begun within the first postoperative week through the jejunostomy tube then transitioned to gastrostomy tube feedings
5. Formulas
   a. Ideal formula is one that provides maximal calories with a minimal volume without being hyperosmolar[10]
   b. Should contain medium chain triglycerides as fat content and be supplemented with glutamine and/or arginine which are believed to aid in bowel adaptation[10]
   c. A low osmolality isotonic dipeptide formula containing medium chain triglycerides and glutamine is preferred for children[17]
6. Feedings usually begun with half-strength formula at a low rate, usually 5 cc/hr in children and 10 cc/hr in adults, then slowly increased by 5 cc/hr every 12-24 hours as tolerated
7. Formula strength is increased to ¾ strength, then to full strength after the goal rate has been achieved
8. Since fat malabsorption is common, Vitamin ADEK is often used to provide water soluble forms of fat soluble vitamins, water-soluble vitamins, and zinc[29]
9. Additional zinc may be required in patients with high outputs at 1 to 1.5 times the recommended dietary allowance (RDA)[29]
10. Nutrition consults and continued follow-up by a dietician dedicated to the patients nutritional needs are essential
11. Common complaints as enteral feedings are optimized include abdominal pain, nausea, vomiting, or increased output
    a. Discontinue or reduce rate of feeding until the etiology of the symptoms is identified
    b. Patients who received all nutrition parentally prior to transplant with minimal oral intake may be uncomfortable with GT feedings because they are not accustomed to a large gastric volume
    c. Decreased gastric motility may occur related to:
       i. Original disease
       ii. Disuse of the stomach prior to transplant
       iii. Dysmotility of transplanted stomach as part of a multivisceral graft
    d. Nursing interventions for abdominal discomfort in the absence of rejection
       i. Administer enteral feeds at a slower rate over a longer period of time
       ii. Administer metoclopramide intravenously or orally to increase gastric motility and/or
       iii. Change the enteral formula
12. Stool output
    a. Considered excessive if greater than 1-2 L/day for adults or 40-60 ml/kg/day for children in the absence of rejection or other pathology
    b. Treatment
       i. Treatment begun with a single motility agent then combination therapy until an acceptable output is achieved
       ii. Motility agents
          a) Loperamide
          b) Paregoric

        c) Diphenoxylate hydrochloride and atropine (Lomotil®)

        d) Cyproheptadine hydrochloride (Levsin®) cholestyramine

        e) Clonidine

        f) Tincture of opium and/or

        g) Fiber supplements

           1) Pectin

           2) Benefiber®

    iii. Intravenous or subcutaneous somatostatin used when output is extremely high

    iv. Intravenous hydration required to stabilize electrolyte levels until output decreases

13. Oral diet
    a. Offered when tube feedings are begun
    b. Begin oral feeds with clear liquids then advance as tolerated

14. Oral aversion
    a. Common, particularly in pediatric intestinal recipients
    b. Factors contributing to oral aversion[30]
       i. Early age of onset of short gut syndrome with initiation of TPN and limited/no oral feedings
       ii. Intermittent and/or extended periods of having nothing by mouth
       iii. Development of a hypergag reflex
       iv. Hospital environment
       v. Behavioral issues
       vi. Parenting behaviors
       vii. Limited experiences with food textures, tastes, and aromas
    c. Interventions/treatment
       i. Early consultation prior to transplant with occupational and speech therapy
       ii. Inpatient feeding rehabilitation programs
       iii. Psychological counseling and intervention through child development programs

15. Food allergies
    a. Symptoms
       i. Increased stool output
       ii. Changes in stool consistency
       iii. Abdominal distention/pain
       iv. Cramping
       v. Eosinophilia
       vi. Weight loss
       vii. Failure to thrive
    b. Diagnosis
       i. Serum IgE levels
       ii. Intestinal tissue biopsy showing eosinophilia
       iii. Serum radioallergosorbent testing (RAST®)
          a) Reported as Class 0 (no allergy) to Class 4 (high allergy)
          b) Class 3 and 4 foods are restricted from diet
       iv. Most common food allergies are to milk protein, lactose, wheat, peanuts, and eggs[31]
    c. Treatment

           i.   Dietary restrictions

          ii. Low dose prednisone may be prescribed

16. Outcome
    a. Long-term nutritional goal is ability to tolerate a regular oral diet that maintains appropriate growth/weight without intravenous fluids, enteral nutrition or parenteral supplementation
    b. Weight gain and growth may be effected by repeated or prolonged episodes of rejection and infection
    c. Many adults achieve nutritional goal within a year
    d. May take pediatric recipients longer to achieve goal
       i. Improvements are seen but attaining linear growth is challenging in the majority of patients[32]
       ii. Routinely monitor height and weight
       iii. Adjust and maintain calorie requirements based on the absorptive ability of the graft
       iv. Decrease steroid use when possible

XX. Impaired wound healing (Table 12-15)
    A. Impaired or delayed wound healing common in the early post-operative period
    B. Contributing factors
       1. Patient's pretransplant nutritional status
       2. Concomitant liver disease
       3. Post-transplant complications
       4. Surgical reexplorations
       5. Staged closing of the abdominal wound secondary to surgical complications
       6. Inadequate nutritional intake post-transplant
       7. Prolonged use of steroids

TABLE 12-15

■ **Nursing Interventions: Compromised Skin Integrity[33]**

Monitor abdominal wound routinely for bleeding, infection, dehiscence, and evisceration.

Instruct patient on abdominal splinting techniques when coughing, sneezing or vomiting to decrease pressure on the site.

Assess wound site when cleaning and changing the dressing.

Pack wounds with wet to dry dressings and change twice daily or as ordered.

Monitor wound site for signs of infection including erythema, edema, wound separation, localized pain, and purulent drainage.

Obtain cultures of wound drainage as ordered.

Report abnormalities to the surgeon.

Monitor nutritional intake.

Administer antibiotics as ordered for positive wound cultures.

Consult enterostomal nursing specialist as needed for skin care concerns.

      C. Compromised skin integrity
          1. Extensive abdominal incision
          2. Ileostomy
          3. Puncture wounds
              a. Jackson-Pratt drain sites
              b. Enteral feeding tube insertion sites
              c. Central lines
              d. Venous catheters
          4. Other wound sites related to complications
              a. Chest tubes to drain pleural effusions
              b. Percutaneous transhepatic cathether for biliary duct complications
              c. Abdominal fistulas
              d. Skin ulcerations/pressure ulcers
      D. Wound healing
          1. Achieved through optimizing nutrition
              a. Maximize calories
                  i. May require short-term TPN in cases of serious wound complications
              b. Increased protein
          2. Meticulous wound care
          3. Minimizing/eliminating steroids when possible
XXI. Ileostomy care (Table 12-16)
      A. Pretransplant education regarding ileostomy care is essential
          1. Rationale for ileostomy
          2. Basic ileostomy care

TABLE 12-16

■ Nursing Interventions Related to Output and Ileostomy Care

Monitor the patient for any subjective complaints of cramping, abdominal pain, or nausea.

Examine the patient for abdominal distension and auscultate for bowel sounds.

Maintain accurate intake and output records.

Administer intravenous fluids as ordered to maintain electrolyte and fluid balance secondary to an increased output.

Administer antidiarrheal medications as ordered.

Examine ileostomy output for color and consistency.

Monitor stoma tissue for changes in color, texture, and size.

Report bleeding or changes in output to the physician.

Provide the appropriate ileostomy appliance and meticulous skin care.

Facilitate consultation with the enterostomal therapy nurse.

Provide teaching sessions on ileostomy care.

Facilitate ordering and delivery of ostomy supplies prior to discharge with the ET nurse or discharge planner.

3. View stoma appliances or pictures of appliances
4. Provide emotional support through partnering the patient with another recipient who has an ileostomy
5. Discuss the plan for ileostomy closure with the patient if he/she is a candidate for closure

B. Reinforce teaching post-transplant through collaborative effort by the enterostomal therapy (ET) nurse and staff nurse to design an individualized nursing care plan to meet patient's needs

C. Adults and older children should be able to provide self-care of the ileostomy prior to discharge from the hospital
   1. A support person, parent, or spouse should also be taught ileostomy care

D. Stoma surveillance[34]
   1. Routine surveillance may lead to early detection of complications
   2. Normal stoma is comparable in color and moistness to oral mucosa
   3. Monitor stoma site for changes in tissue color, texture, or size
      a. Change in color, particularly a deeper red or dusky appearance, may indicate rejection, an internal obstruction, or a prolapse
      b. Texture change may indicate rejection or infection
      c. Size changes may be due to inflammation from rejection or obstruction/prolapse
   4. Other abnormal findings
      a. Ulcerations
      b. Stomal prolapse
      c. Bleeding
   5. Monitoring color, amount, and consistency of output to further assess complications
      a. Stool color
         i. Ranges from deep brown to light yellow depending on the patient's diet and medical status
      b. Amount varies depending on:
         i. Presence of rejection or infection
         ii. Oral/enteral intake
         iii. Diet
         iv. Absorption/motility issues
         v. Intestinal obstruction or ileus
         vi. Output changes should be correlated to formula or diet changes, infusion rate, or route
         vii. Standard output for adults is 1-2 L per day
         viii. Standard output for children is 40-60 cc/kg/day
         ix. Maintain accurate intake and output records
         x. Be aware of the patient's normal output range
         xi. Administer intravenous replacement fluids as ordered to prevent fluid and electrolyte imbalance in cases of high output
      c. Stool consistency variable based on:
         i. Diet
         ii. Amount of oral/enteral intake
         iii. Presence of rejection or infection
         iv. Consistency ranges from a very thick fluid to a watery effluent
            a) Watery diarrhea may be associated with rejection, infection, or food allergies

b) Hypermotility and decreased absorption results in a more watery stool
  v. Improving consistency
   a) Antidiarrheal medications administered to slow transit time and increase absorption
   b) Fiber added to enteral feedings to decrease transit time and improve absorption
  vi. Monitor for bleeding from the ostomy site
   a) Bleeding is of concern and may be a sign of rejection or infection
   b) Can occur following an intestinal biopsy and is usually self-limiting
   c) Superficial bleeding of the stoma tissue may occur from localized trauma when cleaning the site or when changing the ostomy appliance
   d) Any bleeding should be reported to a physician immediately
   e) An ET nurse is an invaluable resource in choosing appliances for an optimal and comfortable fit

XXII. Self-care deficit
 A. Learn self-care routines
  1. Patient should participate in formal and informal teaching sessions with the transplant nurse to reinforce previous education
   a. Importance of immunosuppression and stable levels
   b. Transplant medications
   c. Signs and symptoms of infection
   d. Signs and symptoms of rejection
   e. Ileostomy care
   f. Care of feeding tubes
   g. Central line care
   h. Maintaining records of intake and output, vital signs, weight
   i. Importance of routine medical follow-up
   j. Long-term care issues
  2. Design, review and implement a medication schedule with the patient and family to evaluate the patient's ability to adhere to that routine
  3. Implement changes to facilitate adherence
  4. Adherence can be affected by:
   a. Perceived or actual side effects
   b. Inability to obtain medications due to physical limitations
   c. Distance from the pharmacy
   d. Availability of medications
   e. Insurance coverage
  5. Encourage and facilitate discussions with the patient and family to assess any mitigating psychosocial issues, depression, family support, and/or financial concerns that effect adherence
  6. Facilitate consultations with the social worker, psychologist/psychiatrist, financial counselor, child life specialist, and or pastoral care as needed
 B. Activity
  1. Recuperation can be challenging for many patients, particularly when critically ill and debilitated prior to transplant

2. Activity is increased as tolerated by the patient postoperatively
3. Physical therapy should be consulted early in the postoperative period to work on strengthening and endurance as the patient recovers
4. Patients with an extended postoperative course and multiple complications may benefit from more extensive rehabilitation

REFERENCES

1. Pritchard TJ, Kirkman RL. Small bowel transplantation. *World J Surgery,* 1985; 9: 860-886.
2. Asfar S, Atkinson P, Ghent C, et al. Small bowel transplantation. *Transplant Proc,* 1966; 28: 2751.
3. Goulet O, Frederique S, Dominique C, et al. Intestinal transplantation in children: Paris report. Abstract 0-96. IXth International Small Bowel Transplantation Symposium. Brussels, July 2, 2005.
4. Grant D. Update from the Intestinal Transplant Registry. Abstract O-105. IXth International Small Bowel Transplantation Symposium. Brussels, July 2, 2005. Web access: http://www.lhsc.on.ca/itr/. Accessed 3/7/07.
5. Goulet O, Ruemmele F, Lacaille F, et al. Irreversible intestinal failure. *J Ped Gastroenterol Nutr,* 2004; 38: 250-269.
6. Andersen D, DeVoll-Zabrocki A, Brown C, et al. Intestinal transplantation in pediatric patients: A nursing challenge: Part one: Evaluation for intestinal transplantation. *Gastroenterol Nurs,* 1999; 23(1): 3-9.
7. Reyes J, Mazariegos G, Bond G, et al. Pediatric intestinal transplantation: Historical notes, principles and controversies. *Ped Transplant,* 2002; 6: 193-207.
8. Pirenne J. Advances in Intestinal Transplantation: Report from the VII International Small Bowel Transplant Symposium. Medscape Transplantation, 2002. www.medscape.com/Medsapre/transplantation/journal/2002/v03.n01/. Accessed 3/7/07.
9. Horslen SP, Kaufman SS, Sudan DL, et al. Isolated liver transplantation in infants with total parenteral nutrition-associated end-stage liver disease. *Transplant Proc,* 2000; 32: 1241.
10. Fryer J. Intestine transplantation. In Stuart F, Abecassis M, Kaufman D, (Eds.). *Organ Transplantation,* 2nd ed. Georgetown, TX: Landes Bioscience; 2003. 244-460.
11. Spada M, Allessiani M, Fabbi M, et al. Bacterial translocation is enhanced in pig intestinal transplantation when the colon is included in the graft. *Transplant Proc,* 1996; 28(5): 2658.
12. Reyes J, Green M. Risks and epidemiology of infection. In Bowden R, Ljungman P, Paya C, (Eds.). *Transplant Infections,* 2nd ed. New York: Lippincott Williams & Wilkins, 2004. 132-139.
13. Reyes J, Bueno J, Kocochis S, et al. Current status of intestinal transplantation in children. *J Ped Surg,* 1998; 33: 243-254.
14. Reyes J, Abu-Elmagd K. Small bowel and liver transplantation in children. In: Kelly DA, (Ed.). *Diseases of the Biliary System in Children.* Oxford: Blackwell Science, Ltd.; 1999. 313-331.
15. Kim J, Fryer J, Craig RM. Absorptive function following intestinal transplantation. *Dig Dis Sci,* 1998; 43(9): 1925-1930.
16. Siniscalchi A, Begliomini B, DePietri L, et al. Pain management after small bowel transplant. *Transplant Proc,* 2002; 34(3): 969-970.
17. Peter A, Telkes C, Varga M. Endoscopic diagnosis of cytomegalovirus infection of upper gastrointestinal tract in solid organ transplant recipients: Hungarian single-center experience. *Clin Transplant,* 2004 Oct; 18(5): 580-584.
18. Grant D, Abu-Elmadg K, Reyes J, et al. 2003 report of the intestine transplant registry: A new era has dawned. *Ann Surg,* 2005; 241(4): 607-613.
19. Pappas P, Tzakis A, Gaynor J, et al. An analysis of the association between serum citrulline and acute rejection among 26 recipients of intestinal transplant. *Am J Transplant,* 2004; 4: 1124-1132.

20. Mazariegos G, Reyes J, Abu-Elmagd K, Starzl T. Intestinal and Multiple Organ Transplantation. In Shoemaker, Ayers, et al. *Critical Care Medicine*. 2004.

21. Roberts CA, Radio S, Markin R, et al. Histopathologic evaluation of primary intestinal transplant recipients at autopsy: A single center experience. *Transplant Proc,* 2000; 32: 1202-1204.

22. Sigurdsson L, Reyes J, Kocoshis S, et al. Bacteremia after intestinal transplantation in children correlates temporarily with rejection or gastrointestinal lymphoproliferative disease. *Transplantation,* 2002; 70: 302-305.

23. Andersen D, DeVoll-Zabrocki A, Brown D, et al. Intestinal transplantation in pediatric patients: A nursing challenge. Part 2: Intestinal transplantation and the immediate post-operative period. *Gastroenterol Nurs,* 2000; 23(5): 201-09.

24. Bueno J, Green M, Kocoshis S, et al. Cytomegalovirus infection after intestinal transplantation in children. *Clin Infect Dis,* 1997; 25: 1078-1083.

25. Green M, Webber S. Post-transplantation lymphoproliferative disorders. *Ped Clin North Am,* 2003; 50: 1471-1491.

26. Shroff R, Rees L. The post-transplant lymphoproliferative disorder – a literature review. *Ped Nephrol,* 2004; 19: 369-377.

27. Green M. Management of Epstein-Barr virus-induced post-transplant lymphoproliferative disease in recipients of solid organ transplantation. *Am J Transplant,* 2001; 1(2): 103-108.

28. Berney T, Delis S, Kato T, et al. Successful treatment of post-transplant lymphoproliferative disease with prolonged rituximab treatment in intestinal transplant recipients. *Transplantation,* 2002; 74(7): 1000-1006.

29. Kowalski L, Nucci A, Reyes J. Intestinal transplantation. In Rolandelli RH, Boullata J, Compher C (Eds.). *Clinical Nutrition: Enteral and Tube Feeding*, 4th ed. Philadelphia: Elsevier, 2005. 523-529.

30. Kosmach-Park B. Intestinal transplantation in pediatric patients. *Prog Transplant,* 2002; 12(2): 97-113.

31. Koehler A, Yaworski J, Gardner M, et al. Coordinated interdisciplinary management of pediatric intestinal failure: A 2-year review. *J Ped Surg,* 2000; 35(2): 380-385.

32. Nucci A, Barksdale E, Beserock N, et al. Long-term nutritional outcome after pediatric intestinal transplantation. *J Ped Surg,* 2002; 37(3): 460-463.

33. Killman, K. Generic care plan for the surgical client. In Carpenito-Moyet L, Juall L, (Eds.). *Nursing Care Plans and Documentation: Nursing Diagnoses and Collaborative Practice*, 4th ed. Philadelphia: Lippincott, Williams & Wilkins, 2004.

34. Carpenito-Moyet L, Juall L. Ileosotomy. In Carpenito-Moyet L and Juall L, (Eds.). *Nursing Care Plans and Documentation: Nursing Diagnoses and Collaborative Practice*, 4th ed. Philadelphia: Lippincott, Williams & Wilkins, 2004.

REVIEW QUESTIONS

1. Which of the following is *not* descriptive of short gut syndrome?
   a. Inadequate gut mass to maintain fluid and nutritional requirements
   b. Always includes liver disease
   c. Can be due to motility or absorptive disorders
   d. Nutrition supplied primarily by TPN

2. In the small intestine, most absorption occurs in the:
   a. Jejunum
   b. Ileum
   c. Duodenum and jejunum
   d. Ileum and jejunum

3. You are caring for a 23-year-old female who is listed for a multivisceral transplant. She is ill but stable and is hospitalized for supportive care as she waits for an organ. Which of the following would preclude transplant when an organ is offered?
   a. Positive blood cultures with *Klebsiella*
   b. History of adherence issues
   c. Ammonia level of 200 µmol/L
   d. Seizure disorder controlled with phenytoin

4. You are caring for a 10-year-old boy following isolated intestine transplant on postoperative day 2. He has become increasingly tachycardic and his blood pressure is 80/55. JP drainage has increased serosanguineous fluid. The abdomen is mildly distended. His hemoglobin is 9.2 g%. The ileostomy drainage is 40cc/kg/d and watery brown. What do you suspect?
   a. Vascular thrombosis
   b. Postoperative hemorrhage
   c. Acute rejection
   d. Leak at the anastomoses of the jejunum and duodenum

5. During the early postoperative period (weeks 1-6), surveillance endoscopies are performed:
   a. If the stool output is 1-2 L/day in an adult
   b. If tacrolimus levels are < 10 ng/ml
   c. Twice weekly
   d. Only if febrile

6. Your patient is a 35-year-old female at 2 weeks post intestine transplant. Enteral feedings via a GT are ordered at 40 cc/hr continuously. Her complaints of nausea are increasing and she has vomited a large amount of formula. She is afebrile. What is your first nursing intervention prior to informing the physician?
   a. Stop the infusion of formula
   b. Decrease the rate to 20 cc/hr
   c. Increase the IV fluid rate
   d. Assess the ileostomy drainage

7. In this patient (#6), what other issue might be considered in regard to nausea and vomiting?
   a. Rejection
   b. Decreased gastric motility
   c. Food allergies
   d. Oral aversion

Correct answers:

1. b	5. c
2. c	6. a
3. a	7. b
4. b	

13
Kidney Transplantation

MARY JO HOLECHEK

GREG ARMSTRONG

INTRODUCTION

I. Transplantation provides an opportunity to leave the rigors of dialysis behind and improve the quality of life for chronic kidney disease patients.
- A. Thousands of patients are awaiting a new kidney through registries in countries worldwide.
- B. Table 13-1 provides data on patients awaiting renal transplantation in the United States, Australia, Eurotransplant, and the United Kingdom[1-4]
- C. In the U.S. there are also 2,579 individuals awaiting simultaneous kidney-pancreas transplantation.[1]
- D. There are also thousands of others throughout the world in the process of being evaluated or scheduled for living donor transplantation.
- E. Economically, it is the most cost-effective treatment for chronic kidney disease.[5, 6]

II. This chapter provides information on the evaluation and preparation for kidney transplantation and the complex postoperative nursing care required.
- A. To have a clear understanding of both the pre- and the postrenal transplant process, it is necessary to have knowledge of renal functions, causes of chronic kidney disease (CKD), and the manifestations of abnormal renal function.

TABLE 13-1

■ **Patients Awaiting Renal Transplant (March 2006)**

Country	Number of patients
United States[1]	68,983
Australia[2]	1,600
Eurotransplant[3] Austria, Belgium, Germany, Luxembourg, the Netherlands	11,950
United Kingdom[4]	5,074

B. In most cases, early kidney disease is a silent and insidious process.
1. Patients accommodate to their worsening physiological condition without realizing they are doing so and often without being aware they have a health problem.
2. Renal failure often is not recognized until the patients have irreversibly lost a significant percentage of their kidney function and have multiple manifestations of renal disease.
3. The state where all or most kidney function has been lost and dialysis is indicated has traditionally been referred to as end-stage renal disease (ESRD).
4. A newer term to describe this state is chronic kidney disease (CKD) and this term will be used throughout this chapter.

III. Renal function: The kidneys:
A. Are paired organs
B. Sit behind the peritoneum at approximately the level of the first lumbar vertebra
C. Receive their blood supply via the renal arteries and are drained via the renal veins.
1. It is not uncommon to have two to three renal arteries supplying each kidney.
2. It is less common to have multiple renal veins
D. Perform numerous functions (see Table 13-2).[7]
1. Primary product, urine, is drained via the ureters into the urinary bladder.
   a. On occasion, there may be two ureters from a single kidney.
   b. The bladder is a hollow muscular organ that is readily distensible and has a capacity of 500 cc.
2. The urine produced contains waste products, electrolytes, and other substances outlined in Table 13-3.[7]
3. Abnormalities in the urine composition such as the presence of protein, blood cells, glucose, or other substances can indicate renal or systemic disease.
4. The basic functional unit of the kidney is the nephron, with each kidney having approximately 1 million nephrons.[8]
   a. Each nephron is capable of carrying out all of the functions of the kidney.
   b. About 50% of the nephrons must be impaired before the creatinine will rise.
5. When the kidneys fail, dialysis or transplantation is required to sustain life.

IV. Causes of chronic kidney disease
A. The causes of CKD are many (Table 13-4), but diabetes mellitus, hypertension, and glomerulonephritis account for the majority of patients with CKD.
1. These three diseases account for almost 80% of all patients on dialysis.[9]
2. Diabetes is the most common cause of chronic kidney disease.
B. Although all forms of glomerulonephritis may recur, focal segmental glomerulosclerosis has the highest rate of recurrence.
C. Other causes of CKD that may recur include Henoch-Schönlein purpura, amyloidosis, hemolytic-uremic syndrome, and oxalosis.[11]

TABLE 13-2

■ Major Kidney Functions[7]

- Excretion of most metabolic end-products of the body

- Control of fluid and electrolyte balance

- Maintenance of acid/base balance

- Production of erythropoietin for stimulation of red blood cell production

- Activation of vitamin D to facilitate calcium absorption

- Production of renin as part of the renin/angiotensin system for blood pressure control

TABLE 13-3

■ Urine Composition[7]

Common Substances Found in Urine

Water

Nitrogenous waste products: creatinine, urea, uric acid, ammonia

Electrolytes: sodium, potassium, ammonia, chloride, bicarbonate, phosphate, sulfate, minerals

Hormones

Other: drug metabolites, bacterial toxins, pigments

Abnormal substances: glucose, albumin, protein, red blood cells, white blood cells, casts, calculi

      D. Patients with polycystic kidney disease may require bilateral nephrectomy before transplant if the cysts are large, cause frequent infection or bleeding, or impinge on surrounding structures.

  V. Chronic kidney disease stages

      A. In most cases, CKD occurs over months to years, although some diseases such as rapidly progressive glomerulonephritis can cause permanent damage within weeks or months.

      B. Chronic kidney disease is differentiated from acute disease in that the damage to the kidney lasts for more than 3 months in CKD.

      C. Gradual loss of kidney function is described in five stages (Table 13-5) that have been clearly defined in the Clinical Practice Guidelines by the Kidney Disease Outcomes Quality Initiative (K/DOQI).[12]

         1. The staging of CKD enables clinical practice guidelines and performance measures to be used as tools for improving the evaluation and management of CKD.

         2. The two primary markers used to define the stages of disease are:

            a. Damage to the kidneys as manifested by abnormalities in blood and/or urine (BUN, creatinine, etc.)

            b. Level of kidney function as measured by the glomerular filtration rate (GFR)

TABLE 13-4

■ **Major Causes of Chronic Kidney Disease[2, 10]**

Most common causes of CKD:
- Diabetes mellitus
- Hypertension
- Glomerulonephritis

Cystic disorders:
- Polycystic kidney disease
- Medullary cystic disease
- Acquired cystic diseases

Urinary tract abnormalities:
- Reflux nephropathy
- Posterior ureteral valves
- Neurogenic bladder

Tubular disorders:
- Renal tubular acidosis
- Fanconi's syndrome

Obstructive disorders:
- Renal calculi
- Retroperitoneal fibrosis
- Prostatic hypertrophy

Auto-immune disorders:
- Goodpasture's disease
- Wegener's disease
- Systemic lupus erythematosis
- IgA nephropathy

Hemolytic disorders:
- Hemolytic-uremic syndrome
- Thrombotic thrombocytopenic purpura

Nephrotoxic agents:
- Cyclosporine
- Gentamicin
- Nonsteroidal anti-inflammatory drugs
- Analgesics
- Intravenous contrast dyes

Cancers:
- Multiple myeloma
- Renal cell cancer

Congenital disorders:
- Renal agenesis
- Renal aplasia

Other:
- Amyloidosis
- Oxalosis
- Henoch-Schönlein purpura
- Interstitial nephritis
- Nephrotic syndrome
- Focal segmental glomerulosclerosis (FSGS)
- HIV nephropathy
- Pyelonephritis

TABLE 13-5

■ **Stages of Chronic Kidney Disease**

Stage	Description	GFR (ml/minute)
1	Kidney damage with normal or increased GFR	Equal to or greater than 90
2	Kidney damage with mild decrease in GFR	60–89
3	Moderate decrease in GFR	30–59
4	Severe decrease in GFR	15–29
5	Kidney failure	Less than 15 (or dialysis)

Data from K/DOQI Clinical Guidelines for Chronic Kidney Disease: Evaluation, Classification, and Stratification[12]

3. The stages also indicate how soon renal replacement therapy may be required.
4. Those in stage 4 should be preparing for dialysis by having access placed or seeking a living donor for pre-emptive transplant.
5. Those who have reached stage 5 are in need of immediate renal replacement therapy.

VI. Manifestations of chronic kidney disease (CKD)
   A. Chronic kidney disease as it progresses leads to a syndrome known as uremia, which literally means urine in the blood and refers to the build-up of waste products, excess electrolytes, and toxins in the blood.
   B. Physical signs and symptoms develop due to the presence of unfiltered waste products and the loss of kidney function.
      1. Chronic kidney disease can affect the most elemental of patient parameters, the vital signs.
         a. Despite an increased susceptibility to infection, CKD patients may have a subnormal temperature as blood urea nitrogen acts as a hypothermic agent.
         b. Tachycardia is often present in response to cardiac and volume changes.
         c. Tachypnea can be present as a compensatory response to metabolic acidosis.
         d. Blood pressure can be normal, but is often elevated due to the cardiovascular changes that occur in many diseases that cause kidney disease.
      2. Chronic kidney disease evolves into a multi-system disease affecting many aspects of bodily function.
      3. Table 13-6 describes clinical symptoms that may develop with a diagnosis of CKD.
   C. Although dialysis can improve fluid and electrolyte balance and remove waste products, other measures are necessary to prevent and treat the many symptoms and complications of CKD:
      1. Dietary restrictions
      2. Antihypertensive therapy

TABLE 13-6

■ **Systemic Effects of Chronic Kidney Disease**[7, 13, 14, 15]

System	Effect of Disturbance
Cardiovascular disturbances	Hypertension Left ventricular hypertrophy Congestive heart failure Pericarditis Pericardial effusion Pericardial tamponade Edema of extremities
Gastrointestinal disturbances	Uremic fetor Nausea Vomiting Gastritis Diarrhea Anorexia Gastrointestinal bleeding Stomatitis Gastritis Peptic ulcer disease
Musculoskeletal disturbances	Renal osteodystrophy Osteitis fibrosa/osteomalacia Muscle wasting Muscle irritability Bone pain Bone fractures
Pulmonary disturbances	Pulmonary edema Pleuritis Dyspnea Pneumonia Tachypnea
Hematologic disturbances	Anemia Impaired platelet function Infection
Neurologic disturbances	Drowsiness, fatigue Muscle twitching Headache Confusion Delirium Tremors Seizures Coma Peripheral neuropathy Sleep disturbances Paresthesias Restless legs syndrome Motor weakness

System	Effect of Disturbance
Genitourinary disturbances	Oliguria Anuria Urinary tract infections Proteinuria
Metabolic/electrolyte/acid-base disturbances	Hyperkalemia Hyperlipidemia Acidosis Hypo/hypercalcemia Hypoalbuminemia Hyperphosphatemia Carbohydrate intolerance Waste product accumulation
Endocrine disturbances	Altered insulin metabolism Reduced insulin requirements Peripheral insulin resistance Thyroid abnormalities Hyperparathyroidism
Reproductive disturbances	Amenorrhea Impotence Infertility
Integumentary disturbances	Uremic frost Pallor, pigmentation changes Pruritus, dry/scaly skin Ecchymosis Excoriations Calcium-phosphate deposits
Psychologic disturbances	Anxiety Depression Noncompliance Denial Psychosis

      3. Iron replacement
      4. Stimulation of red blood cell production
      5. Control of calcium and phosphate levels
  VII. Radiologic and invasive testing for chronic kidney disease
     A. As described earlier, CKD is defined by stages that enable the application of guidelines for treatment and management.
       1. In order to determine the stage of CKD and the underlying cause of the CKD, it is usually necessary to undertake both radiologic and invasive tests in addition to routine lab work.
       2. Imaging of the kidneys provides information on the size and any structural abnormalities of the kidneys:
         a. Renal or abdominal ultrasound
         b. Computed tomography (CT)
         c. Magnetic resonance imaging (MRI)
       3. A renal biopsy provides tissue for histological classification of the disease.

      4. A 24-hour urine for creatinine and protein may be collected and provides information regarding the severity of the kidney disease.

      5. An excellent test to determine the degree of renal dysfunction is a nuclear medicine glomerular filtration rate.

      6. These diagnostic studies provide information regarding the potential causes and reversibility of the kidney disease and help guide treatment and prevention of further loss of function.

VIII. Evaluation of kidney transplant candidates

    A. The assessment process and acceptance criteria for renal transplant candidates differ from program to program and from country to country.

      1. Patients who may be considered acceptable candidates by one program may be deemed unacceptable by another.

      2. There is no one set of definitive acceptance or rejection criteria or methodology for assessment.

    B. Physical assessment

      1. Physiologically, the potential candidate needs to be able to undergo and withstand the transplant procedure itself and have a low risk of long-term morbidity and mortality.

      2. Cardiovascular function, respiratory status, body mass index, and the absence of defined contraindications form the basis of the assessment.

      3. Generally accepted contraindications are given in Table 13-7.

      4. Although some of these criteria and/or contraindications will exclude a patient at the time of initial assessment, if they can be resolved, the patient can be reassessed.

      5. Examples of this would be obese patients who complete a weight reduction program or patients with symptomatic coronary artery disease who undergo coronary artery bypass graft.

      6. Older age, in itself, is not a definitive contraindication since physiologic age is more important than chronologic age.

TABLE 13-7

■ Contraindications to Kidney Transplantation[9, 11, 16]

- Active or current malignancy
- Active infection
- Obesity
- Significant peripheral vascular disease (that would interfere with surgical anastomoses)
- Untreatable end-stage diseases of other organs: e.g., inoperable coronary artery or valvular disease, severe cardiomyopathy, end-stage emphysema
- Active inflammatory disease (systemic)
- Noncompliance
- Active substance abuse
- Untreated psychiatric illness or mental incapacity without an adequate support system
- Active peptic ulcer disease
- Limited life expectancy: transplant program dependent

7. Physical assessment is aimed at determining patients' potential morbidity and mortality both in the short and long term.

8. A battery of laboratory, tissue and blood typing, radiologic and diagnostic tests are required to determine the state of a potential candidate's health. See Table 13-8.

9. Certain patients may require additional tests and procedures depending on their medical history.

10. Based on the evaluation results, the program staff will determine if candidates fall within the range of acceptable risk.

11. It needs to be understood that if a patient is rejected on one occasion, periodic reevaluation may be considered for changed circumstances.

IX. Psychosocial assessment

   A. The psychosocial assessment of patients is of particular importance to the long-term success of kidney transplantation.

      1. Major components of the psychosocial evaluation include:

         a. Psychiatric history

         b. Compliance history

         c. Substance abuse history

         d. Mental status

         e. Social history

         f. Availability of social support

         g. Family social and mental health history

         h. Perceived health, coping style, and quality of life[17]

         i. Any cultural or religious concerns

            i. Are there any objections to receiving blood or blood products?

            ii. Certain religious faiths such as Jehovah's Witnesses do not accept blood products under any circumstances.

            iii. The risks of this belief must be carefully discussed before proceeding to the operating room.

            iv. Consideration must be given, as well, to cultural rules such as Muslim women needing to keep their heads covered.

         j. When the nursing assessment indicates that cultural or religious norms could be an issue, they should be fully investigated, seeking experts as needed, to ensure that no cultural rules are violated.

            i. Are there dietary restrictions?

            ii. Use of herbal or alternative therapies

         k. (See Chapter 1: Transplant Evaluation and Chapter 16: Psychosocial Issues in Transplantation for additional information.)

         l. Patients need to either be able to care for themselves post-transplant or have a support network in place that is capable of assisting them in doing so.

         m. Post-transplant self care is critical to graft and, at times, patient survival.

         n. Regular attendance at post-transplant clinics, compliance with medication regimens, and awareness of the signs and symptoms of rejection and infection are all the responsibility of the patients or their support network.

TABLE 13-8

■ **Pretransplant Tests and Investigations for Potential Kidney Transplant Recipients**[9, 11]

Laboratory Tests: Blood and Urine	*Hematology*: • Complete blood count (CBC) with differential • PT, INR, PTT *Chemistry panel*: • Sodium, potassium, carbon dioxide, chloride, creatinine, blood urea nitrogen, blood glucose *Liver Function Tests* *Urine*: • (If patient is able to produce urine) • Culture, urinalysis, 24-hour urine for protein and creatinine *Serology*: • Hepatitis B surface antigen and antibodies • Hepatitis C PCR • CMV, EBV, HSV, VZV • HIV • VDRL *Other*: • Papanicolaou (PAP) smear • Prostate specific antigen (men 50 or older) • PPD • Hemoglobin A1C (diabetics) • Pregnancy test (females)
Tissue and Blood Typing Tests	• ABO blood typing • Tissue typing • Panel reactive antibodies (PRA) • Cross-match
Radiologic/Diagnostic Tests	• Chest X-ray • Electrocardiogram • Pulmonary function tests* • Mammogram (women 40 or older) • Cardiac echocardiogram* • Stress test* • Cardiac catheterization* • Abdominal computed tomography* • Magnetic resonance imaging* • Noninvasive vascular studies* • Voiding cystourethrogram (VCUG)
Physical Exams	• Full history and physical • Gynecologic exam (females) • Prostate exam (males)

*If indicated by exam or other studies.

aPTT=activated partial thromboplastin time, CMV=cytomegalovirus, EBV=Epstein-Barr virus, HIV=human immunodeficiency virus, HSV=herpes simplex virus, INR=international normalized ratio, PCR=polymerase chain reaction, PPD=purified protein derivative, PT=prothrombin time, VDRL=venereal disease research laboratories, VZV=varicella-zoster virus.

2. As well as assessing patients' and support networks' ability to cope with the rigors of post-transplant life, an assessment of patients' history of adherence to medical management must be done.
   a. Patients should demonstrate reliability in this regard before being allowed to proceed.
   b. For patients who have not been able to demonstrate consistent compliance, contracts of varying lengths can be set up detailing criteria the patients must meet to be accepted for transplantation in the future.
      i. This is not an accepted practice in all countries (i.e., Australia)
3. Patients who are actively abusing illegal or legal substances or have an untreated psychiatric disorders are not good candidates for transplantation.[18]
4. For all patients, ensuring that they have a current and long-term source of income to cover hospitalization, their medications, and post-transplantation costs is essential.
   a. In a large number of Western countries, organ transplant services and medications are provided to patients either free of charge or with minimal charge through national health services or national social insurance schemes.
   b. In the United States, the coverage for transplantation and medications required post-transplantation can be covered by a wide variety of private and governmental insurance programs.
      i. For those with adequate insurance, the appropriate approvals and authorizations are obtained.
      ii. Those who are uninsured or underinsured are assisted in completing the paperwork necessary to obtain adequate coverage.
      iii. No kidney patients are ever refused transplantation on the basis of inability to pay.
B. Psychosocial evaluations should be completed by a trained professional such as a social worker.
C. Additional assessment by a psychologist or psychiatrist familiar with transplantation may be necessary in cases where the initial assessment is equivocal or for individuals with significant psychiatric or compliance issues.

X. Pretransplant patient education and the evaluation process
   A. Not only is the patient assessment process a time when the program staff evaluates patients, but it is also a time to educate patients and their supporters.
   B. Clear, concise, understandable, and structured education sessions should be provided to all potential transplant patients and their supporters.
   C. Topics should include:
      1. The transplant evaluation process
      2. Responsibilities while awaiting transplant
      3. Transplant surgery
      4. Post-transplantation management and responsibilities
      5. Importance of medication compliance
      6. Outcome data
      7. Potential complications
      8. Options of living versus deceased donor transplantation

D. These sessions ideally should occur at the first stage of the patient evaluation process.
1. Early education provides benefits to both the patients and the transplant team.

E. Introducing patients and families to other patients who have been transplanted is often helpful.

F. Provide patients with time to ask questions.

G. Provide patients and families with information on support groups and continuing education on transplantation.

H. Table 13-9 describes benefits of early patient education.

XI. Living versus deceased donor transplantation

A. For those patients who are accepted as a transplant candidate and have potential live donors, efforts should be directed towards early live donor transplantation.
1. Living donor assessment may entail the evaluation of a number of potential donors.
2. The general assessment requirements for living donor transplantation are provided in Table 13-10. It should be noted that these criteria can vary from program to program.

XII. Deceased donor waiting list patient maintenance

A. If a living donor transplant is not an option, patients will be placed on the deceased donor transplant waiting list.

B. Waiting times can vary widely depending on patient location, blood type, age, severity of disease, panel reactive antibodies (PRA), and other factors.

C. In the United States, median waiting times range from 2 to 4.8 years.[19]

D. It is necessary to have a process whereby the physical and psychosocial status of listed patients is reviewed on a regular basis to ensure their ongoing suitability.

E. Close liaison with dialysis programs is important to ensure timely communication of changes in patients' condition.

F. Additionally, regular blood work results must be supplied to the tissue typing laboratories for assessment of the PRA and, depending on local protocols, pretransplant donor/recipient cross-match.

XIII. Transplant surgery preparation

A. Kidney transplantation can be either an elective procedure as is the case with live donor transplant or an emergency procedure when the kidney is donated by a deceased donor.

TABLE 13-9

■ **Benefits of Early Patient Education**

- Ensures patients have a solid understanding of what may be in front of them

- Allows patients and their support system to make informed decisions regarding their willingness to proceed to transplant before they and the program commit resources to their evaluation

- Lets patients know what is required of them

- Introduces the concept of living donor transplant early in the process, thereby enabling early identification of potential live donors and possible early transplant

- Allows the program to assess the cognitive ability of the patients and their supporters

TABLE 13-10

■ Required Testing for Living Donors

- History and physical
- Routine blood tests: complete blood count (CBC), chemistry panel, liver function tests, lipid panel, glucose tolerance test (GTT)
- Serology: hepatitis B and C screening, HIV, CMV, EBV
- Urine tests: urinalysis, urine culture, 24-hour urine for protein and creatinine clearance, pregnancy testing (females)
- ABO typing, tissue typing and cross-match
- Nephrology/urologic evaluation
- Chest X-ray
- Electrocardiogram
- Cardiac stress test (if >50 years old)
- Magnetic resonance imaging (MRI), angiography, or 3D computed tomography
- Psychosocial assessment

CMV=cytomegalovirus, EBV=Epstein-Barr virus, HIV=human immunodeficiency virus

B. Live donor transplantation has a number of advantages over deceased donor transplant.
   1. Condition of the recipient can be maximized.
   2. Organ storage time is minimized prior to the transplant.
   3. Incidence of delayed graft function is decreased.
   4. Short- and long-term outcomes are better.
   5. The organ is not subjected to the physiological insults that accompany brain death.[20]
   6. Patient can be dialyzed prior to final preparation for surgery.
   7. All relevant tests and investigations can be completed.[9, 11]
C. Deceased donor transplant in comparison provides a much shorter time for patient preparation.
   1. When an organ becomes available the patient is contacted and detailed information is sought regarding recent medical history, date of last dialysis, and whether they have received any recent blood transfusions.
   2. Questions are directed at ascertaining if there are any impediments to transplant:
      a. Any cardiovascular events (myocardial infarction, stroke)
      b. Recent infections or fevers
      c. New diagnoses of cancer or any other major medical or surgical events
D. If no contraindications are identified, the patient is asked to proceed immediately to the hospital.
E. Upon admission:
   1. Vital signs are checked.
   2. Blood samples are taken.
   3. If not anuric, a urine sample is sent for analysis and culture.

4. A throat culture may be ordered.
5. Full history and physical
6. CXR
7. EKG
8. Patient is dialyzed, if necessary.
9. Table 13-11 provides a list of preoperative tests for kidney transplantation.

F. Careful attention should be paid to the results that are critical to patient survival and transplant outcome.

1. If the patient is febrile or has an elevated white blood cell count, infection must be ruled out before proceeding to transplantation.
2. If the potassium is elevated, dialysis will be required to prevent intra-operative arrhythmias.
3. Coagulation study results such as the partial thromboplastin time (PT), international normalized ratio (INR), and activated partial thromboplastin time (aPTT) must be reviewed given that clotting dysfunction may be present.
   a. A prolonged PT, INR, or PTT may necessitate the use of vitamin K or fresh frozen plasma to minimize intra-operative bleeding.
   b. Anticoagulants and antiplatelet agents such as warfarin, aspirin, and clopidogrel must be discontinued and reversed when possible.
4. Although a low hemoglobin level is common in renal failure patients, a hemoglobin level of 8 to 8.5 gm/dL may predispose patients to cardiac ischemic events and necessitate preoperative transfusion.
5. Untreated pneumonias or suspicious lesions on the CXR or serious EKG abnormalities may result in cancellation of the case.
6. The cytomegalovirus (CMV) status should also be determined as more aggressive antiviral therapy may be needed postoperatively for CMV-negative recipients who receive CMV-positive kidneys.
7. Confirmation of tissue typing, compatibility of ABO blood group between donors and recipients, and a negative donor/recipient cross-match result is of utmost importance to a successful outcome.

TABLE 13-11

■ Preoperative Tests for Kidney Transplantation

- History and physical including vital signs, weight, height, and oxygen saturation
- Routine blood tests: CBC, chemistry panel, calcium, phosphate, magnesium, liver function tests, PT, INR, aPTT
- Routine urine tests: urinalysis, pregnancy test (females)
- Type and cross-match for blood (2-4 units)
- ABO typing
- Tissue typing and final cross-match with donor
- Chest X-ray
- Electrocardiogram

aPTT=activated partial thromboplastin time, CBC=complete blood count, INR=international normalized ratio, PTT=partial thromboplastin time

8. Incompatibility of ABO blood groups and/or a positive cross-match can lead to an immediate hyperacute rejection of the organ.
   a. These results must be ascertained prior to going to surgery.
9. If the final assessment indicates the patient is in good health and the cross-match with the donor is negative, the final preparation for surgery is initiated.
10. As with any surgical procedure, the patients are not to have any oral intake from the moment they are called in for transplant.
    a. Critical medications can be given by mouth with sips of water.
    b. Several units of blood should be typed and crossed for the unlikely event of intra-operative bleeding
    c. Generally patients are given a third or fourth generation cephalosporin on call to the operating room.
    d. Mycophenolate mofetil or a similar immunosuppressant drug may be given prior to surgery.
    e. An intravenous corticosteroid such as dexamethasone or methylprednisolone may be given just prior to or early in the transplant surgery.
    f. Both of these drugs initiate suppression of the immune system to prevent rejection.
    g. If a graft or native fistula is present, the affected extremity should be labeled "no procedures."
    h. Abdominal scrubs may be done to decrease the infection risk.
    i. For peritoneal dialysis patients, the abdomen should be drained just prior to going to surgery and the peritoneal catheter capped.
11. Throughout the preparation for surgery, close attention should be given to the emotional state of the patient, family, and supporters as it is a time of great anxiety and uncertainty.

XIV. Transplant surgery
   A. Upon arrival in the operating room (OR), the patient is placed in a supine position on the OR table and is prepared for surgery by the anesthesia team.
      1. A central venous catheter is inserted and an arterial line may be placed.
      2. The patient is then anesthetized.
      3. Prophylactic antibiotics are usually given at this time if they were not given on call.
      4. Once the patient is asleep a bladder catheter is placed and several hundred milliliters of normal saline or antibiotic solution is instilled into the bladder.
         a. Antibiotic solutions help decontaminate the bladder.
         b. The fluid instilled also distends the bladder facilitating locating the bladder and completing the ureteric anastomosis.
      5. The operative site is shaved and prepared with a topical anti-infective cleansing agent such as povodine iodine and the patient is draped.
   B. The usual placement of the kidney is extraperitoneal in the iliac fossa.
      1. Allows easy access to the iliac vessels and the urinary bladder
      2. Provides easy access if a biopsy is required.
      3. Alternative placements may be used and are indicated by the recipient size or if both donor kidneys are to be used in the recipient.

a. If the donor kidneys are from a small child, then both kidneys may be implanted en bloc in the abdomen.

b. Intra-abdominal placement may also be used if the patient has had previous transplants, multiple abdominal surgeries, or the iliac vessels are unsuitable for anastomosis due to vessel disease.

4. A curved incision is made beginning near the iliac crest and ending above the symphysis pubis in the left or right lower abdomen.

a. The side chosen depends on:
    i.   The donor kidney
    ii. Surgeon's assessment
    iii. Future plans for pancreas transplant: use left side if pancreas transplant is anticipated
    iv. Previous surgery

b. Muscle layers are divided and the peritoneum is retracted superiorly

c. Iliac vessels (external, internal common) are identified.

d. Selected vessels are dissected out, slung with vascular slings, and clamped proximal and distal to the chosen anastomosis site.

e. The anastomoses may be end to end or end to side.

f. Anatomy of the kidney and the quality of both the donor and recipient vessels determines the method of anastomosis.

g. When venous and arterial anastomoses are completed, the clamps are released.
    i.   The kidney should turn pink and produce urine.
    ii. Furosemide or mannitol may be given at this time to stimulate urine production.
    iii. Each vascular anastomosis is checked carefully for leaks.
    iv. If none are noted, the surgeon will proceed to the bladder anastomosis.

h. In most cases, the bladder dome is exposed and the muscle is divided along a length of about 4 to 5 cm.
    i.   A small incision at the distal end of the muscle incision is used to open the bladder mucosa.
    ii. A small cut is made in the end of the donor ureter to open it out or splay it and it is anastomosed to the mucosa.
    iii. At many institutions, the anastomosis is over a ureteric stent to ensure patency and facilitate healing of the vesicoureteral anastomosis.
    iv. The muscle is then closed over the ureter forming a tunnel that acts as an antireflux valve compressing the ureter as the bladder fills.

i. A final check for hemostasis and the positioning of the vessels is done before closure.

j. One or two low-pressure drains may be placed in the surgical bed.

k. A standard wound closure is performed using staples or sutures and the anesthetic is reversed.[11]

XV. Post-transplant care: Monitoring and maintenance

A. Once the surgical transplantation procedure is completed, transplant recipients will be transferred to the intensive care unit (ICU) or transplant unit for close monitoring and care.

B. Recipients transferred to the ICU can expect to be there for approximately 24 hours and then transfer to the inpatient transplant unit. Recipients will arrive with:
1. Urinary catheter
2. Central line
3. Possibly one or more wound drains
4. An arterial line
5. Endotracheal tube is usually removed in the OR or recovery room
C. Nursing care will include postoperative management that includes assessing:
1. Vital signs: parameters should be followed at least hourly and then every 4 hours after transfer to the general transplant floor.
    a. Temperature
        i.   If elevated, may indicate postoperative atelectasis, dehydration, infection, and/or rejection.
        ii. Transplant recipients may not be able to mount a normal fever response due to the effects of immunosuppressant drugs.[21]
        iii. Nurses must assess for other indicators of infections as well.
        iv. Suspected atelectasis should be addressed with aggressive pulmonary toilet and dehydration with increased fluid infusion.
        v.   Possible infections should be evaluated by obtaining blood and urine cultures and a chest x-ray.
        vi. Suspected rejection will require a biopsy for confirmation.
    b. Heart rate
        i.   Bradycardia may indicate a cardiac problem such as heart block or excessive beta blockade (e.g., metoprolol) being used for rate or blood pressure control or hypomagnesemia.
        ii. Tachycardia can be a sign of febrile illness, rebound tachycardia due to the rapid discontinuation of alpha-adrenergic stimulators (e.g., clonidine), or volume status changes such as hypovolemia related to bleeding or dehydration.
    c. Respiratory rate
        i.   Decreased respirations may be a sign of oversedation or cardiopulmonary problems.
        ii. Rapid respirations may be a response to acidosis or fluid overload.
        iii. Abnormal respiratory patterns should be further investigated by monitoring oxygen saturation levels and, if indicated, arterial blood gases.
    d. Blood pressure (BP)
        i.   Both hypotension and hypertension are detrimental to renal function.
        ii. Causes of hypotension include:
             a) Bleeding
             b) Dehydration
             c) Sepsis
             d) Medications
             e) Adrenal insufficiency
             f) Neuropathy

g) Can lead to poor perfusion of the renal transplant resulting in:
1) Acute tubular necrosis (ATN)
2) Delayed graft function (DGF)
3) Vascular thrombosis[22]
iii. Causes of hypertension are:
a) Persistent chronic hypertension
b) Rebound hypertension due to cessation of an adrenergic agent
c) Volume overload
iv. Hypertension can be worsened postoperatively due to:
a) Steroids
b) Calcineurin inhibitors such as tacrolimus
c) Development of renal artery stenosis[23]
d) Pain and hypoxia[24]
v. Persistent hypertension can damage the new kidney, increase the risk of vascular leaks, and increase the chance of cerebrovascular events.[22, 24]
vi. Systolic BP that exceeds 180 mm Hg should receive immediate treatment.[24]
vii. Systolic BP should be kept above 110 mm Hg to avoid complications associated with poor perfusion.[25]
viii. The etiology, associated symptoms, and treatments for hypotension and hypertension are varied. See Tables 13-12 and 13-13 for more information.
2. Lab/blood work:
a. Basic laboratory values provide excellent information regarding kidney function, electrolyte balance, metabolic function, and the presence of postoperative bleeding or infection.
b. The surgical transplant procedure can cause some electrolyte imbalances such as hyponatremia related to IV infusion of ½ normal saline as a replacement fluid.
c. CKD patients have significant lab value abnormalities pretransplantation such as hypocalcemia and anemia, many of which can persist for a time postoperatively especially if the kidney does not function immediately.
d. Careful attention to lab values can prevent or allow for the early treatment of complications.
e. Laboratory indicators of ATN or early nonfunction of the kidney include:
i. Hyponatremia related to the dilutional effect of fluid retention when the kidney is unable to excrete body water
ii. Indicators that the kidney is unable to excrete waste products include:
a) Hyperkalemia
b) Increased blood urea nitrogen (BUN)
c) Increased serum creatinine
d) Hypermagesemia
e) Hyperphosphatemia
f) Decreased carbon dioxide level
1) Carbon dioxide is an indirect measure of bicarbonate

TABLE 13-12

■ **Hypotension: Monitoring and Maintenance**[22, 23, 24]

Etiology	Associated Signs & Symptoms	Treatment
Postoperative bleeding	Dizziness	*Bleeding:*
	Decreased level of consciousness	Surgical exploration to identify and ligate source
	Tachycardia	Red blood cell transfusions
		Fluid boluses
		Administration of vasoconstrictive agents (e.g., Neo-Synephrine)
Dehydration related to postoperative osmotic diuresis		*Dehydration:*
		Fluid boluses
		Maintenance intravenous fluids (IV)
		Replacement of urine output cc for cc with ½ normal saline or 0.9% normal saline
Sepsis	Increased temperature (in sepsis)	*Sepsis:*
		Fluid boluses
	Tachycardia	Cultures
		Antibiotics
		Administration of vasoconstrictive agents, if indicated
Antihypertensive medications		*Antihypertensive-Induced:*
		Withhold antihypertensives
		Adrenal insufficiency/ autonomic neuropathy
		Midodrine or florinef administration
Adrenal insufficiency		*General Treatment for All Etiologies:*
Autonomic neuropathy		Limit activity
		Frequent vital signs
		Renal ultrasound to assess blood flow to kidney
		Evaluate response
		Consultation with physician

TABLE 13-13

■ **Hypertension: Monitoring and Maintenance**

Etiology	Associated Signs and Symptoms	Treatment
Persistent chronic hypertension	Can be asymptomatic Headache	Resume preoperative antihypertensives as ordered by physician/nurse practitioner
Rebound hypertension due to stopping alpha adrenergic receptor stimulator		If patient was on alpha-adrenergic agent, resume to prevent rebound hypertension
		Add additional agents (IV and oral) as ordered by physician/nurse practitioner
Volume overload		If volume related, reduce IV infusion rates and/or replacement fluids
Pain		Pain control
Hypoxia		Oxygenation to maintain oxygen saturation > 92%
		Frequent vital signs and consultation with health care provider as status changes

        2) Levels falls when acid accumulates in renal failure

e. If the new kidney works immediately, it is expected that the BUN and creatinine will begin to fall.

    i. Hyponatremia may occur related to aggressive fluid replacement and can usually be corrected by:

        a) Decreasing the amount of fluid infused

        b) Increasing the sodium content

    ii. Hypokalemia, hypophosphatemia, and hypomagenesemia may develop as the kidney begins to function and significant diuresis occurs.

    iii. A decreased carbon dioxide level may persist.

f. All of these values require assessment to determine if the recipient is in ATN or experiencing rejection so the appropriate treatment can be initiated.

g. See Table 13-14 for normal values for common electrolytes/metabolites.

h. See Table 13-15 for electrolyte/metabolic disorders in kidney transplant recipients.[15, 25, 26, 27, 28]

i. Lab work can also provide indications of postoperative bleeding.

j. CKD patients have a chronic anemia related to their kidney failure.

    i. Many patients at the time of transplant can have a hematocrit of 25% or less.

TABLE 13-14

■ **Normal Values for Common Electrolytes/Metabolites**

Electrolyte	Normal Range
Sodium	135-148 mEq/L
Potassium	3.5-5.0 mEq/L
Chloride	96-109 mEq/L
Creatinine	0.5-1.2 mg/dL
Blood urea nitrogen	7-22 mg/dL
Glucose	60-109 mg/dL
Phosphate	2.7-4.5 mg/dL
Calcium	8.4-10.5 mg/dL
Magnesium	1.3-2.0 mEq/L
Carbon dioxide	21-30 mEq/L

Values are based on the Johns Hopkins Hospital, Baltimore, MD, reference laboratory normal values. See Appendix B for comparable SI units.

      ii. Post-transplant, it is essential to assess the trend of the hematocrit (Hct) and hemoglobin (Hgb) in reference to the preoperative levels.

      iii. If there is a significant decrease in the Hct/Hgb then a full work-up to assess for bleeding should be initiated including serial Hct/Hgb testing, renal ultrasound, and CT scan.

      iv. Attention should also be given to the platelet (PLT) count to ensure that it is in the normal range and is not contributing to a bleeding episode.

      v. The prothrombin (PT) and activated partial thromboplastin (aPTT) times should also be reviewed to determine if they are abnormal.

   k. Blood work can also provide an early warning of infection in transplant recipients.

      i. An elevated white blood cell count (WBC), erythrocyte sedimentation rate (ESR), and C-reactive protein can indicate the presence of an infection.

      ii. An elevated WBC may develop in response to high doses of steroids.

      iii. An elevation of any of these parameters warrants further investigation.

3. Hemodynamic status:

   a. Hemodynamic monitoring is of paramount importance for kidney transplant recipients as the success of the transplant and prevention of complications revolves around tight control of fluid balance and the BP.

   b. The nursing assessment should include[29]:

      i. Vital signs as discussed above

      ii. Genitourinary assessment (see below)

TABLE 13-15

■ **Electrolyte/Metabolic Disorders in Kidney Transplant Recipients**[15, 25, 26, 27, 28]

Abnormality	Etiology	Clinical Presentation	Treatment
Hypernatremia	Dehydration Osmotic diuresis post-transplantation Large volume NS infusions IV sodium bicarbonate	Fever, thirst Dry mucous membranes, flushing Restlessness, agitation, confusion Weakness, twitching, seizures, coma Decreased urine output If due to water loss: decreased weight, BP, CVP and increased pulse If due to Na+ excess: Increased weight, BP, CVP, edema, weak pulse	If due to water losses: Rehydration with D_5W or hypotonic saline If due to Na+ excess: Restrict Na+, administer D_5W and diuretics Gradual correction of hypernatremia essential to prevent cerebral and pulmonary edema
Hyponatremia	Fluid overload Osmotic diuresis with impaired concentrating ability post-transplantation Large volume hypotonic saline infusions (e.g., ¼ or ½ NS) Diuretics Gastrointestinal losses: vomiting, NG suction, diarrhea	If due to water excess: Headache, weakness, confusion Muscle weakness, seizures, coma Nausea, vomiting Increased weight, BP, CVP, P, and edema If due to Na+ losses: Irritability, confusion, anxiety Thirst, dry mucous membranes Muscle weakness, tremors, seizures Decreased weight, BP, CVP, and increased P	If due to water excess: Fluid restriction Careful use of diuretics Dialysis If due to Na+ losses: Stop hypotonic infusions NS infusion Stop diuretics, if indicated In life-threatening situations: 3-5% hypertonic NS with great caution Rapid over correction of hyponatremia can cause central pontine myelinolysis
Hyperkalemia	Renal insufficiency/failure Acute Tubular Necrosis (ATN) Calcineurin inhibitors Beta blockers Angiotensin-converting enzyme inhibitors (ACEI) Oral PO_4 supplements Potassium-sparing diuretics (e.g., spironolactone) Bleeding/cell damage Metabolic acidosis	Lethargy, confusion Muscle irritability, muscle cramps, muscle weakness, flaccid paralysis, paresthesias, hyperactive reflexes Abdominal cramps, nausea, diarrhea EKG changes: Tall peaked T waves, prolonged PR interval, ST segment depression, widened QRS Tachycardia that can proceed to bradycardia, ventricular fibrillation, cardiac arrest.	Eliminate IV/drug sources of K+ (e.g., beta-blockers, ACEI, oral PO_4 supplements, spironolactone) Restrict dietary intake of K+ Diuretics Sodium polystyrene sulfonate (Kayexalate®) if no ileus Dextrose 50% and insulin Keep calcineurin inhibitor levels within therapeutic range Calcium gluconate or chloride to increase threshold for arrhythmias Sodium bicarbonate if metabolic acidosis present Dialysis

Abnormality	Etiology	Clinical Presentation	Treatment
Hypokalemia	Osmotic diuresis post-transplantation Diuretics Gastrointestinal losses Magnesium depletion Alkalosis Renal tubular acidosis Steroid therapy	Fatigue, confusion, dizziness Muscle weakness, leg cramps, paresthesias, decreased reflexes Respiratory paralysis Nausea, vomiting, ileus, constipation EKG changes: ST depression, flattened or inverted T waves, U wave present. Cardiac arrest	IV or oral K+ supplements Increase dietary intake of K+ Stop diuretics, if possible Magnesium supplementation, if indicated Correct alkalosis
Hypermagnesemia	Renal insufficiency/failure Excessive supplementation Mg-containing laxatives or antacids	Lethargy, fatigue, drowsiness, confusion Muscle weakness, decreased/absent reflexes, flaccid paralysis, seizures Depressed R, respiratory muscle paralysis Bradycardia, weak pulse, hypotension, heart block, cardiac arrest	Restrict dietary Mg Avoid Mg-containing products Dialysis Hydration and diuretics IV Ca gluconate to oppose cardiotoxic effects of Mg
Hypomagnesemia	Calcineurin inhibitor-induced Excessive urine output Diuretics Gastrointestinal losses: diarrhea/vomiting/NG suction Malnutrition	Dizziness, lethargy, confusion Twitching, tremors, seizures, coma Muscle weakness, leg/foot cramps EKG: flat or inverted T waves, ST segment depression, prolonged QT interval	Increase dietary intake of Mg (fish, green vegetables) Oral Mg supplements IV Mg supplements
Hyperphosphatemia	Renal insufficiency/failure Secondary hyperparathyroidism with hypocalcemia PO_4–containing enemas	Muscle weakness and cramping, tetany, seizures Hypocalcemia Ca-PO_4 deposits in the soft tissues, blood vessels, skin, and organs (heart, brain, eyes) Joint pain related to deposits	Restrict dietary PO_4 (dairy products) Phosphate binders (e.g., calcium acetate, sevelamer) Activated vitamin D (IV and oral) Ca supplements Dialysis
Hypophosphatemia	Increased post-transplant urinary excretion Phosphaturia due to glucocorticoid-induced gluconeogenesis PO_4 binders Hypercalcemia Poor oral intake	Fatigue, confusion Muscle weakness, tremor, paresthesias Diaphragmatic weakness Cardiac arrhythmias Osteomalacia	Increase dietary intake of PO_4 Oral PO_4 supplements (e.g., K phos neutral) IV PO_4 supplementation (sodium phosphate)

(Continued next page.)

Abnormality	Etiology	Clinical Presentation	Treatment
Hypocalcemia	Chronic kidney disease Hyperphosphatemia Vitamin D deficiency Inadequate oral intake of Ca and vitamin D Loop diuretics Citrate in blood products	Depression, lethargy, confusion, irritability, fatigue Perioral and extremity numbness and tingling, hyperactive reflexes, muscle cramps, + Chvostek's and + Trousseau's signs, tetany, seizures Bone pain Abdominal cramps, constipation, nausea, vomiting EKG changes: prolonged ST and QT, ventricular tachycardia	Increase dietary intake of Ca and vitamin D Oral calcium supplements IV calcium supplements (Ca gluconate or chloride) Vitamin D supplements (IV and oral) High Ca dialysate
Decreased carbon dioxide	Renal insufficiency/failure Diabetic ketoacidosis Diarrhea Malnutrition	Drowsiness, confusion, headache, coma Deep, rapid R (Kussmaul) Arrhythmias, if K+ elevated Nausea, vomiting, diarrhea	Sodium bicarbonate (IV or oral) Correct hyperkalemia Dialysis

BP=blood pressure, Ca=calcium, CVP=central venous pressure, EKG=electrocardiogram, IV=intravenous, K+=potassium, Mg=magnesium, Na+=sodium, NG=nasogastric, NS=Normal saline, PO_4=phosphate, P=pulse, R=respirations

    iii. Pulmonary assessments (see below)

    iv. Cardiovascular assessments

        a) It is crucial that the heart be functioning properly to ensure adequate fluid management.

        b) Many programs require cardiac monitoring of transplant recipients for 24 hours to assess effects of fluid alterations, observe for electrocardiogram (EKG) indications of electrolyte abnormalities such as hyperkalemia, and to identify life-threatening arrhythmias such as atrial fibrillation.

        c) Although cardiac monitoring is the standard of care in the United States, it is not considered necessary, in most cases, in countries such as Australia and the United Kingdom.

        d) A CVP of 6 to 12 cm H_2O should be adequate to prevent hypotension and hypoperfusion of the kidney or hypertension and fluid overload.[25]

        e) Absence of lower extremity pulses particularly on the side of the transplant could herald a serious vascular complication and requires immediate attention.

    v. Fluid balance

        a) Strict intake and output

        b) Daily weights

        c) Peripheral edema screening

4. Genitourinary system
   a. Recipients who have received a living donor transplant or a deceased donor organ with a short cold ischemia time (CIT, cold storage time) may anticipate immediate graft function.
   b. Delayed graft function may be expected for a deceased donor recipient with a prolonged CIT or technical problems. The nursing care can be very different in each situation.
   c. Strict intake and output (I&O) is essential.
      i. An estimate of an acceptable hourly output should be determined considering donor characteristics, operative history, and patient's preoperative output.
      ii. If patients do not achieve this goal then the health care provider (physician and/or nurse practitioner) should be notified to discuss strategies to increase the output.[24]
   d. Daily weights and central venous pressures (CVP) in conjunction with clinical assessment of the patient will help determine if the patient is maintaining fluid balance.
   e. The presence of truncal and lower extremity edema provides clues as to the fluid status of a patient.
      i. Peripheral edema and pulses in the lower extremities should be assessed at least once every 8 hours.
      ii. Edema that is greater in the extremity on the side of the transplant could simply be related to the surgery or could indicate a deep vein thrombosis or lymphocele.
      iii. Nurse must consider what the patient is receiving orally and particularly through IV infusions.
   f. Most transplant patients will receive maintenance IV fluids, a carrier for patient controlled analgesia, and hourly urine replacements.
      i. Fluid boluses may be ordered for patients whose urine outputs are inadequate.
      ii. There must be constant adjustment to IV infusion rates factoring in the patients' hemodynamic state.
      iii. If balance is not maintained volume related complications can develop rapidly with serious consequences.
   g. Hypervolemia is quite common both in patients with immediate and delayed function. Causes include:
      i. Intra-operative overhydration
      ii. Cardiac dysfunction
      iii. Primary nonfunction of the kidney
      iv. Simple obstruction of the urinary catheter.
      v. Assessment of hypervolemia may reveal the following symptoms:
         a) Shortness of breath
         b) Decreased oxygenation
         c) Rales, rhonchi, wheezing
         d) Dyspnea
         e) Pulmonary and/or peripheral edema
         f) Increased weight
         g) Hypertension
         h) Elevated CVP
         i) Distended neck veins

    j)   Presence of an S_3 on cardiac auscultation[23, 24]

    k)   Pleural effusions

    l)   Decreased oxygen saturation

vi.   When a patient demonstrates hypervolemia with a decreased urine output, one of the first assessments should be of the urinary catheter to ensure it is patent.

    a)   The patient's abdomen should be examined for distention and pain over the bladder.

    b)   The catheter should be observed for the presence of clots or hematuria.

       1)   Particularly if the urine output has dropped off suddenly, the suspicion that clots may be occluding the catheter should be evaluated.

    c)   The primary care provider should be notified and, if directed, the nurse may gently flush the catheter with 30 cc of normal saline.[24]

    d)   If there are no noticeable clots flushed through and the urine output remains low treatment for hypervolemia should be initiated.

vii.   Treatment of hypervolemia includes diuretics, decreasing IV infusion rates, and dialysis.[23, 24]

m. Hypovolemia can lead to hypotension, hypoperfusion, and ATN.

   i.   Common etiologies of hypovolemia are:

    a)   Inadequate IV or oral intake of fluids

    b)   Osmotic diuresis

    c)   Bleeding

   ii.   BP and CVP can provide vital information regarding intravascular fluid status. Central venous pressures below 6 and systolic BP readings of <110 mm Hg warrant immediate attention.

   iii.   Clinical signs of hypovolemia include:

    a)   Decreased urine output

    b)   Decreased BP

    c)   Decreased weight

    d)   Tachycardia

    e)   Increased bleeding from the wound and the drain

    f)   Pallor

    g)   Hypoxia

    h)   Poor skin turgor

    i)   Dry mucous membranes

    j)   Weakness

    k)   Mental status changes

   iii.   A renal ultrasound may be ordered to assess the blood flow to the kidney.

   iv.   Identifying the etiology of the hypovolemia guides the treatment plan.

   v.   If a patient is simply fluid depleted, fluid boluses are a quick, effective means of rehydration.

   vi.   If diuretics are in use, they should be discontinued.

   vii.   Antihypertensive drugs should be withheld until the BP stabilizes.

viii. If bleeding is suspected and confirmed by a precipitous fall in the Hct/Hgb then red blood cells transfusions (RBC) are indicated.

ix. Active bleeding will require returning to the OR for exploration.

x. Hypovolemia regardless of cause should be reported to the primary health care provider immediately.

5. Pulmonary assessment and management

   a. Respiratory assessment also provides information regarding the hemodynamic status.

   b. The patient should be assessed for rales, rhonchi, wheezing, and any other indicators of difficult air passage due to the presence of fluid.

   c. Through auscultation and radiologic studies the potential presence of effusions should be assessed.

   d. The oxygen saturation level should be monitored

   e. Most patients receive oxygen for the first 24 hours postoperatively and should be able to maintain oxygen levels in excess of 92% or better.

   f. Oxygen can be weaned when the patient is able to maintain this level on room air.

   g. To prevent infection turning, coughing, and deep breathing are essential components of care along with the use of assist devices such as the incentive spirometer and flutter valve.

   h. Patients should be out of bed by the first postoperative day and spend as much time as possible ambulating or sitting in the chair to prevent respiratory infections related to atelectasis and inactivity.[30]

6. Neurologic status

   a. Renal transplant recipients should be neurologically intact postoperatively, but the effects of anesthesia, narcotics, and immunosuppressants can have a negative impact.

   b. All patients should be examined for level of consciousness, orientation, and motor and cognitive function.

   c. Disorientation, agitation, and inability to follow commands or move the extremities should be reported immediately.

   d. Special attention should be paid to the presence of tremors particularly of the hands associated with tacrolimus toxicity.[30]

   e. Leukoencephalopathy is a rare toxicity associated with tacrolimus and can cause significant mental status changes and usually requires cessation or reduction of the dose of the drug.[31]

   f. Delirium is not uncommon post-transplant and has been associated with immunosuppressant agents and can be worsened by advanced age and concomitant medical conditions.[32]

     i. When possible, the offending agent should be discontinued or used at the lowest possible dose.

     ii. When acute delirium occurs haloperidol is usually effective.

     iii. Narcotics should be discontinued as early as possible.

   g. It is important to make sure the patient is neurologically intact before initiating patient education.

   h. Seizures have been reported with calcineurin inhibitor toxicity as well as hyponatremia.

7. Gastrointestinal tract
   a. The nurse should assess the patient every 8 hours for:
      i. Bowel sounds
      ii. Abdominal distention
      iii. Eructation, flatus
      iv. Bowel movement (including consistency of stool)
      v. Ability to tolerate fluids
   b. If the patient has an ostomy, the stoma should be examined and the quantity of stool should be recorded.
   c. Common gastrointestinal (GI) problems reported postoperatively include nausea and vomiting, constipation, diarrhea, and anorexia.
      i. Nausea, vomiting, and constipation are generally due to the effects of residual renal disease, anesthesia, and narcotic usage.
         a) Nausea and vomiting generally abate after several days, but can be treated acutely with antiemetics such as dolasetron or promethazine or motility agents such as metoclopramide.
         b) Constipation can be treated by eliminating narcotics as early as possible, increasing fluid intake, ambulation, a high-fiber diet, stool softeners, laxatives, and enemas.
         c) The dietitian can be consulted to assist with providing a high-fiber diet.
      ii. Diarrhea is usually medication-related, but cultures should always be sent to confirm the absence of infection.
         a) Mycophenolate mofetil (CellCept®), phosphate supplements, and magnesium oxide can cause diarrhea.
         b) Mycophenolate mofetil cannot be stopped, but the dose can be decreased at the direction of the health care provider for persistent diarrhea.
         c) Oral magnesium oxide and phosphate supplements can be discontinued and IV magnesium and phosphate substituted.
         d) If stool cultures are positive, the appropriate antibiotics should be initiated.
         e) If the stool cultures are negative and the diarrhea persists then antimotility agents such as loperamide may be administered.
         f) Until the diarrhea is controlled, adequate hydration is essential to maintain the BP and prevent hypoperfusion of the new kidney.
      iii. Some patients complain of stomach discomfort and anorexia.
         a) Both mycophenolate mofetil and steroids can irritate the GI tract.
         b) Generally, this can be managed with the prescription of an H_2 blocker such as omeprazole or pantoprazole.
8. Hematologic system: There are two major hematologic concerns post-transplantation, infection and anemia.
   a. Infection: elevated WBC

    i. As has been previously discussed transplant recipients are at great risk for infection related to the immunosuppression, surgical procedure, and comorbid illnesses.[33]

    ii. Potential post-transplant infections and their treatments are discussed in Chapter 5, Transplant Complications: Infections.

    iii. Of note, transplant recipients have a urinary catheter in place for 3 to 4 days after surgery to allow the bladder anastomosis to heal.

       a) A urinalysis and urine culture should be sent if a UTI is suspected.

       b) Urinary tract infections should also be assessed after the catheter is removed.

       c) The nurse should observe patients closely for signs and symptoms of urinary tract infection (UTI) including:

          1) Urethral burning

          2) Cloudy, foul-smelling urine

          3) Frequency

          4) Pain on urination

          5) Dribbling

          6) Difficulty initiating a stream

  b. Anemia

    i. Chronic kidney disease causes anemia as the failed kidneys are no longer able to produce the erythropoietin necessary to stimulate the bone marrow to produce new RBCs.

    ii. This anemia persists post-transplant and can be worsened by operative blood losses.

    iii. The Hct/Hgb, ferritin, transferrin percent saturation (TSAT), and reticulocyte count should be assessed.

    iv. The Kidney Disease Outcomes Quality Initiative (K-DOQI) recommends that the Hct be 33-36% and the Hgb be 11-12%.[34]

    v. Both darbopoietin alfa and epoietin alfa that stimulate RBC production can be used to increase the Hct/Hgb.

    vi. It is essential that iron stores be adequate for erythropoiesis to take place.

       a) Iron, if required, can be supplemented orally or by the IV route (iron dextran, iron gluconate, iron sucrose).

       b) TSAT should be > or equal to 20%.

       c) Ferritin > or equal to 100 ng/ml.[34]

    vii. Correction of anemia is essential to prevent fatigue, improve the quality of life, and reduce morbidity and mortality.

9. Wound and drainage

  a. All transplant recipients are as risk for impaired wound healing related to the steroids they receive which can interfere with tissue healing and increased risk of infection due to immunosuppressant effects.

  b. Wounds should be watched for abnormal wound drainage, evidence of infection, or dehiscence.

  c. If a drain is present, volume, consistency, and color of the effluent should be noted.

      i.   The drain should be emptied and the bulb recompressed every 8 hours and as needed.

      ii. If there is excessive serosanguineous or bloody drainage from the wound or the wound drain, the Hct/Hgb and vital signs should be checked.

d. If a significant Hct/Hgb drop is noted and the vitals signs are consistent with bleeding (decreased BP, tachycardia), the health care provider should be notified and the appropriate radiologic testing performed.

      i.   A renal ultrasound or CT may be ordered.

      ii. To alleviate their anxiety, patients should be kept informed of what is happening and reassured that all the appropriate measures are being taken.

e. If active bleeding is occurring, the patient will likely return to the OR for exploration.

      i.   While the patient waits for transfer to the OR, fluid boluses and RBC transfusions may be required to stabilize the patient.

f. Excessive clear or yellow fluid drainage from the wound can indicate a urine leak, lymphocele, or seroma.

      i.   One of the first actions to take in this situation is to send the fluid for analysis including creatinine and a cell count.

      ii. If the creatinine of the fluid is well in excess of the serum creatinine, then a urine leak is likely.

      iii. Lymphocytes present in the fluid can be due to a lymphocele.

      iv. Fluid with a normal creatinine and no cells may represent a seroma.

      v. The health care provider should be advised of any abnormal findings.

      vi. Suspicion of a urine leak will require a renal scan for confirmation and urinary catheter placement to decompress the bladder.

      vii. If the fluid drainage is not deemed to be abnormal, frequent dressing changes with careful skin care may be the only care require until the excessive drainage abates.

g. The primary wound and drain site should be assessed at least twice a day for infection.

      i.   Purulent drainage, erythema, pain, and tenderness are all indicators of infection.

      ii. The wounds should also be observed for any necrosis.

      iii. Most transplant recipients receive IV antibiotics for 24 hours perioperatively to minimize the risk of wound infections.

h. If infection develops, the primary health care provider should be informed.

      i.   The nurse can expect to send wound cultures, initiate antibiotics, and provide local wound care.

      ii. Simple wounds may require cleaning with NS and the application of a dry sterile dressing.

      iii. The wound can be left open to air when drainage ceases.

      iv. The wound drain should have a dry drain dressing around it until it is removed.

v.   Infected wounds may be opened and packed with NS gauze or an agent designed to disinfect the wound such as chlorpactin or debride the wound such as an enzymatic ointment (e.g., Accuzyme®).

vi. Complex wounds will require consultation with a wound care specialist who has knowledge of state of the art treatments.

vii. Pulse lavage where a small stream of fluid is used to debride the wound may be needed for wounds with a large amount of nonviable tissue.

viii. The dietitian should also be consulted to provide a diet that will promote wound healing.

ix. At the time of discharge, if complex wound care is still required, a home nursing referral should be made.

x.   A final assessment parameter for wounds is the intactness of the sutures both external and fascial.

a)   The wound edges should be observed for any separation or evidence of fascial dehiscence.

b)   If the wound edges separate, it should be reported to the primary health care provider.

c)   If the separation is due to infection, wound care can be initiated as described above.

d)   If bowel is noted through the wound opening appearing as a moist, shiny, tubular structure, the surgeon should be notified immediately as this is a medical emergency that could result in herniation or obstruction of the bowel.

e)   Dehiscence occurs when the fascial sutures break.

1)   The exposed bowel should be covered with a nonadherent dressing, an abdominal binder applied, and the patient placed on strict bed rest.

2)   As soon as possible the patient should return to the OR for exploration and fascial closure.

10. Pain management

a.   Pain is expected after any major surgical procedure.

b.   The nursing assessment for pain should include a subjective pain scale rating, visual inspection, and physical examination.

c.   Severe and rapidly escalating pain is unusual and may warn of a serious complication such as bleeding or fascial dehiscence.

d.   Typical pain manifests as discomfort directly over the transplant surgical site that worsens with movement.

e.   Most patients will receive patient controlled anesthesia (PCA) where the patient can deliver IV pain medication independently with the push of a button.

i.   Usually morphine or fentanyl is used.

ii. Both of these drugs are metabolized by the liver.[24]

iii. Meperidine, also metabolized by the liver, but dependent on the kidneys for excretion of the metabolites, is contraindicated in renal disease as the retained metabolites can cause seizures.[35]

iv. Ketorolac[35] and other nonsteroidal anti-inflammatory drugs should be avoided as they can block vasodilatory prostaglandins impairing renal perfusion.

v. Within 24 to 48 hours, most patients are ready to transition to oral pain medication such as oxycodone or propoxyphene.

vi. Because of the constipating effects of narcotics, a bowel regimen should be initiated that includes docusate sodium to soften the stool, ambulation, fluids, and a high-fiber diet.

vii. Laxatives and enemas can be administered as required.

viii. It is important to remember that if the new kidney has limited function, phosphate and magnesium-containing laxatives and enemas should be avoided.

11. Administering immunosuppression agents and monitoring for side effects

a. Management of antirejection medications requires a significant amount of nursing time.

b. Most renal transplant recipients are on a triple drug regimen including tacrolimus or cyclosporine, prednisone, and mycophenolate mofetil.

c. Sirolimus is at times substituted for one of these drugs if a patient is intolerant.

d. Drug levels can be followed for tacrolimus, cyclosporine, and sirolimus.

e. Nurses play an important role in monitoring these levels, assessing for toxicities, and collaborating with the doctors to make dose adjustments.

f. Some patients will receive induction therapy starting just before or immediately after the transplant with thymoglobulin or muromonab CD3, if delayed graft function is anticipated.

i. Induction therapy can continue daily for days to a week.

ii. Both of thymoglobulin and muromonab CD3 can also be used if T-cell rejection develops.

iii. See Chapter 4, Transplant Pharmacology, for information regarding dosing, indications, side effects, drug interactions, and nursing implications of these and other transplant-related drugs.

12. Mobility and self-care capability

a. One of the goals of transplantation is to allow transplant recipients to resume as normal a life as possible.

b. Post-transplant it is vital to assess patients' mobility and ambulation skills, ability to carry out activities of daily living independently, and motivation to participate actively in care.

c. Activity should be encouraged to the level that is ordered by the physician and, in most cases, this will be ambulation early on postoperative day 1.

d. The patients should remain out of bed for as much of the day as possible.

e. The incentive spirometer and flutter valve should be used every hour while awake.

f. Activity and respiratory devices will help prevent postoperative atelectasis and respiratory infections.

g. If a patient is debilitated or has other physical impairments, physical, occupational, and speech therapy consults should be obtained as needed.

h. Family members and friends should be encouraged to participate in the care and the primary caregiver at home should be identified.

i. Deep vein thrombosis (DVT) is a postoperative risk and it can be ameliorated by early activity as described above.

j. The use of support stockings, automatic compression devices, and subcutaneous heparin can also help prevent DVT.

13. Nutrition

a. As noted in the GI section, transplant patients may experience anorexia and other complications that reduce their caloric intake.

b. As the GI tract is minimally disturbed during transplant surgery, patients can begin a clear liquid diet on postsurgical day 1 and then advance as tolerated.

c. The nurse should assess daily caloric intake, daily weights factoring in fluid shifts, prealbumin, transferrin percent saturation, total protein, and albumin.

   i. If any of these values are subtherapeutic or a patient has a special need such as diabetes mellitus or weight or lipid reduction, the doctor and dietitian should be notified so that a dietary plan can be developed.

d. Medications that may facilitate eating should be administered including antiemetics, motility agents, and H_2 blockers.

e. Calorie counts should be obtained if inadequate oral intake is suspected.

f. For the rare transplant patient who cannot consume sufficient calories orally, calories should be provided enterally or parenterally.

g. Adequate nutrition is essential for carrying out activities of daily living and wound healing.

14. Psychosocial

a. The psychosocial status of new transplant recipients must be watched closely as well, as patients adjust to this life-changing event and the effects of anesthesia, narcotics, and the new immunosuppressant medications.

XVI. Renal transplant potential complications: Monitoring, maintenance

A. Post-transplant nursing care is complex. Despite vigilant medical and nursing care, complications can develop.

B. Some of the most common complications include:

1. Acute tubular necrosis (ATN)

a. Refers to the condition where the newly transplanted kidney does not function in the absence of rejection or obstruction.

b. Can occur due to a prolonged CIT, prolonged warm ischemia time, hypoperfusion, and hypotension.[24, 30]

c. Premortem donor incidents such as hypotension or cardiac or respiratory arrest are contributing factors to ATN.[36]

    d. ATN presents as renal failure with an elevated BUN, creatinine, potassium, phosphate, and magnesium; anuria or oliguria; increased weight; shortness of breath; pulmonary edema; lower extremity edema; and decreased oxygenation.

    e. Severity of the signs and symptoms depends on the severity of the ATN.

    f. If there are no life-threatening lab abnormalities such as hyperkalemia or fluid overload causing pulmonary edema, then watchful waiting will be the treatment strategy.

    g. There is no direct treatment for ATN, but if it is expected at the time of transplant, induction therapy may be initiated.

        i. An induction agent such as thymoglobulin may be used so calcineurin inhibitors can be withheld thus avoiding the introduction of a nephrotoxin that could further impair function in the immediate postoperative period.

    h. Renal ultrasounds and renal scans should be done periodically to ensure adequate flow, absence of collections or hydronephrosis, or absence of a urine leak.[22]

    i. The patient will be observed closely waiting for the kidney function to improve or the need for dialysis to become apparent.

    j. This is a very frustrating time for the patient as the expectation is that the new kidney will function immediately.

    k. Throughout this period the patient will remain on a renal diet and phosphate binders.

    l. If ATN persists for greater than 5 to 7 days then a kidney biopsy should be done to ensure there is not a concurrent episode of rejection.[22]

    m. Recovery from ATN can take days to weeks.

2. Transplant rejection

    a. Despite advances in immunology, tissue-typing, cross-matching techniques, surgical strategies, and immunosuppressive agents, rejection remains a key cause of graft dysfunction and loss.

    b. Rejection is categorized into four types based on the etiology and time of onset (Table 13-16):

        i. Hyperacute

        ii. Accelerated

        iii. Acute

        iv. Chronic[22, 25, 30]

    c. The two primary causes of rejection are T-cell (cell-mediated, cellular) rejection and B-cell (antibody-mediated, humoral) rejection.

    d. Rejection is diagnosed based on the clinical presentation of the patient and biopsy findings.

    e. A renal scan may show decreased flow to further confirm the diagnosis.

    f. Treatment varies based on the primary cause and severity of the rejection episode.

    g. Acute rejection due to T-cell activation is the most common type of rejection, accounting for about 90% of all rejection episodes.

        i. Most episodes occur within the first 3 months after transplantation.[37]

TABLE 13-16

■ Types of Kidney Transplant Rejection and Their Treatment[25, 30, 37, 38, 39]

Type	Onset	Etiology	Clinical Presentation	Treatment
Hyperacute Rejection	Occurs within minutes or hours of transplantation	B-cell, Ab-mediated, Humoral Preformed cytotoxic B-cells attack the new kidney	Graft becomes cyanotic, can rupture Irreversible condition Anuria *Bx findings:* Fibrinoid necrosis, fibrin thrombi, marginating neutrophils, ischemic necrosis. marked interstitial hemorrhage	None Transplant nephrectomy Wound is usually not even closed before damage occurs
Accelerated Rejection	Occurs 24 hours to 5 days post transplantation	B-cell Ab-mediated Humoral Due to pre-sensitization from prior exposure to one or more of the donor's antigens May have a cellular component	Fever Edema Abdominal pain or tenderness over graft site Increased BUN, Cr Increased weight and BP Decreased UOP + XM or antibody screen + for DSA *Bx findings:* +C4D, marginating neutrophils	Plasmapheresis: Removes all Ab IVIG: replenishes good Ab and modulates immune system over time so that Ab is no longer made or responded to
Acute Rejection	Occurs days to weeks after transplantation	T-cell Cell-mediated Cellular Inflammatory response	Fever Myalgias/arthralgias Edema Gross hematuria Abdominal pain or tenderness over graft site Increased BUN, Cr Increased weight and BP Decreased UOP *Bx findings:* Interstitial edema, tubulitis, mononuclear infiltration, arteritis, fibrinoid necrosis, Banff Grade 1-3.	*Mild-Moderate*: Banff Grade 1-2: IV steroids *Moderate to Severe*: Banff Grade 2-3: Thymoglobulin Muromonab CD3
Chronic Rejection	Months to years after transplantation, insidious	Not well defined Immune and nonimmune mechanisms involved	Chronic renal failure Elevated BUN, Cr Electrolyte abnormalities Edema Increased BP and weight Decreased UOP *Bx findings:* Tubular atrophy, glomerulosclerosis, interstitial fibrosis	None Progression may be slowed by discontinuing calcineurin inhibitors Retransplant

Ab=antibody, BUN=blood urea nitrogen, Bx=biopsy, Cr=creatinine, XM=cross-match, DSA=donor specific antibody, IVIG=intravenous immune globulin, +=positive, UOP=urine output

      ii. The severity of T-cell rejection is rated using the Banff 97 Grading System.[40]

      iii. The severity is determined by looking at the degree of tubulitis and arteritis.

         a) The grades are borderline, 1A, 1B, 2A, 2B, and 3.

         b) Borderline is the mildest form and easiest to reverse; whereas Grade 3 is the most severe and most difficult to reverse.

         c) The grade guides what the treatment plan will be.

  h. B-cell rejection is characterized on biopsy by marginating neutrophils and a positive C4D that is an end product of complement degradation.

  i. The kidney biopsy is an integral part of diagnosing rejection.

      i. It is important to establish that coagulation studies and the platelet count are within normal limits before attempting a kidney biopsy.

      ii. Prior to the biopsy being done the patients need to be educated about its purpose, how the results will guide treatment, and postbiopsy care.

      iii. Patients can expect to have some pain over the biopsy site and to be on bed rest for several hours lying on the biopsy site with a pressure roll to facilitate hemostasis and prevent postbiopsy bleeding.

      iv. They should be aware that frequent vital signs will be done along with a postbiopsy Hct/Hgb to assess for significant bleeding.

      v. Any new onset hematuria or the presence of clots in the urine will be observed for and will be reported immediately to the health care provider.

      vi. If postbiopsy bleeding is suspected, a repeat ultrasound will be done to check for evidence of bleeding.

  j. During treatment for rejection, it is essential to reassure patients that rejection is usually reversible.

      i. This is an anxiety-producing time due to the uncertainty.

      ii. Providing information to patients will help to ease the concerns of the patients and their families.

3. Surgical complications: Assessment and management

  a. Despite care and caution during the surgical procedure to place a kidney transplant, complications can occur (Table 13-17).

  b. The nurse must be vigilant in monitoring for the occurrence of complications.

  c. Attention to subtle changes can help clarify the diagnosis as the clinical presentation of many of the complications is similar.

  d. The most common early complications are:

      i. Urine leaks

      ii. Lymphoceles

      iii. Renal vein thrombosis

      iv. Ureteral obstruction

      v. Wound infections and bleeding are also complications, but have been previously discussed

      vi. Infectious complications (see Chapter 5)

TABLE 13-17

■ Surgical Complications of Kidney Transplantation[20, 25, 30, 38]

Complication	Etiology	Clinical Presentation	Diagnostic Studies	Treatment
Urine leak	Uretero-neocystostomy (anastomotic) leak Necrosis of ureter due to interrupted blood supply Tight ureteral stenosis	Sudden loss of kidney function Decreased UOP Increased BUN/Cr Pain over transplant site Drainage of yellow fluid from wound in large quantities	Cr on drain fluid; Cr of fluid is higher than serum Cr Renal scan: shows extravasation of dye outside urinary tract Renal US: shows fluid collection or mass CT cystogram: shows extravasation of dye	*Conservative for small leak*: Insertion of urinary catheter to decompress bladder Nephrostomy tube placement *Larger leaks or Necrotic Ureter*: Surgical repair
Lymphocele	Severed lymphatics in iliac region without ligation resulting in fluid collecting around transplanted kidney	Decreased kidney function Decreased UOP Increased BUN/Cr Pain over transplant site Leg swelling on the side of the transplant due compression of iliac vessels Incontinence, frequency due to pressure on the bladder	Renal US: round, septated collection CT scan: collection Needle aspiration of collection: a high protein content is consistent with lymphocele	Watchful waiting for small noncompressive collections Percutaneous drainage for large collections Instillation of sclerosing agent via drain (e.g., Betadine or tetracycline) Surgical drainage with marsupialization into the peritoneum for persistent recurrent collections
Graft thrombosis	Can be arterial or venous Due to clots, anastomotic problems, and rarely, due to cytokine release seen with muromonab CD3 infusion	Sudden cessation in urine production Graft tenderness and swelling Elevated BUN/Cr Hematuria with venous thrombosis	Renal US with high impedence through artery with reversed diastolic flow Renal scan: No flow	Immediate return to the operating room for surgical exploration Nephrectomy if kidney is thrombosed
Ureteral obstruction	Blood clots Anastomotic complications Ureteral sloughing Ureteral fibrosis due to infection or ischemia Lymphocele Hematoma	Impaired renal function Hydronephrosis Decreased UOP Pain over transplant site Elevated BUN/Cr	Renal US Intravenous pyelogram Retrograde pyelogram Percutaneous antegrade pyelogram Renal scan	Percutaneous balloon dilatation, if stricture present Nephrostomy tube placement Surgical repair Correction of lymphocele, if present (as described above) Percutaneous or surgical drainage, if hematoma present
Renal artery stenosis	Technical complications at anastomosis Occurs months to years after transplantation	Uncontrolled hypertension Impaired renal function Bruit over anastomosis	Arteriogram with minimal dye	Angioplasty to dilate stenotic area Surgical repair if not amenable to angioplasty

BUN = blood urea nitrogen, Cr = creatinine, UOP = urine output, US = ultrasound.

e.   Renal artery stenosis is a late complication.

4. Endocrine and metabolic dysfunction post transplantation

   a.   Bone disease related to hyperparathyroidism and medications. Bone disease is discussed in Chapter 6, Transplant Complications: Non-Infectious.

   b.   Diabetes mellitus

   i.   Diabetes mellitus is the number-one cause of end-stage renal disease in the United States, so many patients who are transplanted have this illness.[41]

   ii.   Others may develop type 2 diabetes mellitus post-transplant.

   iii.   Medications required to prevent rejection are directly responsible for making diabetes mellitus more difficult to manage in those with pre-existing disease and causing *de novo* disease.

   a)   Steroids increase peripheral insulin resistance and alter pancreatic beta cell secretion.

   b)   Calcineurin inhibitors alter peripheral insulin sensitivity and decrease islet cell function.[26]

   iv.   For those with pre-existing diabetes mellitus, insulin requirements may likely increase.

   v.   For those with *de novo* disease, they now have the added burden to learn about diabetes mellitus and how to manage the disease in addition to their transplant.

   vi.   The signs and symptoms that should be monitored for include:

   a)   Blood glucose levels consistently greater than 110

   b)   Polydipsia, polyuria, polyphagia

   c)   Possibly blurred vision

   vii.   Blood glucose readings should be checked before each meal and at bedtime and a regimen designed to keep blood glucoses in the normal range using a combination of diet, oral antihypoglycemic agents, insulin, and exercise.

   viii.   When possible, doses of steroids and calcineurin inhibitors should be reduced to the lowest possible dose to prevent rejection, but not worsen the diabetes mellitus.

   ix.   Both the diabetes educator and dietitian should be consulted for patients who are new to diabetes mellitus.

   x.   Any patient with diabetes mellitus who is overweight should be instructed regarding weight loss.

   xi.   A home care referral will be crucial to continued success with the management of diabetes mellitus and the new transplant after the patient returns home.

   xii.   The hemoglobin A1C should be followed to assess long-term compliance and efficacy with the prescribed regimen.

   xiii.   In addition to assessing and treating hyperglycemia, the nurse must observe closely for and teach the patients about hypoglycemia.

   xiv.   Hypoglycemic symptoms usually present when the blood glucose falls below 60 to 70 mg/dL and include:

   a)   Cool, clammy skin

   b)   Diaphoresis

   c)   Nausea and vomiting

        d) Decreased mental status

        e) Agitation

        f) Feeling of impending doom

    xv. If hypoglycemia occurs, carbohydrates should be administered immediately in the form of sweetened juices or hard candy if the patient is alert, or IV dextrose 50% if the patient is unconscious or unable to swallow.

    xvi. Patients should be taught how to manage these episodes at home. For additional information, see Chapter 5, Transplant Complications: Non-Infectious.

XVII. Discharge planning and education

    A. Preparing transplant patients and their families for discharge is a major undertaking.

    B. They are not just learning about their new organ(s), but to manage numerous medications as well.

    C. They must also be taught to observe for symptoms of complications such as infection and rejection.

    D. Discharge planning and education is discussed in Chapter 3, Patient Education and Discharge Planning.

XVIII. Summary

    A. Kidney transplantation is a multi-faceted and ever-changing process. It begins with careful evaluation of the patient and continues for as long as the patient has a viable transplant.

    B. The success of transplantation depends on the quality of the organ provided, the patient's ability to actively participate in care, presence of complications and comorbid conditions, and close follow-up care.

    C. Transplantation presents significant challenges for kidney disease patients, their families, and the transplant team, but it also provides these patients the opportunity to transform their lives and escape many of the complications of CKD and dialysis.

REFERENCES

1. United Network for Organ Sharing (UNOS). Kidney and kidney-pancreas waiting list statistics. Available at: http://www.unos.org/data/default. asp?displayType=usData. Accessed 3/7/06.

2. McDonald SP, Russ GR. ANZDATA Registry Report 2004. Adelaide, South Australia, 2005.

3. Eurotransplant Website. Waiting list statistics. Available at: http://www. eurotransplant.nl/files/statistics/ active_waitinglist.html. Accessed 3/6/06.

4. Ansell D, Feest T, Ahmad A, Rao R (Eds.). The Seventh Annual Report of the United Kingdom Renal Registry 2004. Available at: http://www.renal-reg.com/report%202004/cover_Frame. htm. Accessed 6/26/05.

5. Arredondo A, Rangel R, de Icaza E. Cost effectiveness of interventions for end-stage renal disease. *Revistta Saude Publica*, 1998; 32(6): 556-565.

6. Wilfe RA, Ashby VB, Milford EL, et al. Comparison of mortality in all patients in dialysis, patients on dialysis awaiting transplantation, and recipients of first cadaveric transplant. *N Engl J Med*, 1999; 341: 1725-1730.

7. Guyton AC. *Human Physiology and Mechanisms of Disease*. Philadelphia: WB Saunders; 1982.

8. Preisig P, Chmielewski C, Keen M, Holechek MJ, et al. Renal physiology. In Parker J, (Ed.). *Contemporary Nephrology Nursing*. Pitman, NJ: Anthony J. Janetti, Inc.; 1998. 129-176.

9. Holechek MJ. Kidney transplantation. In Cupples SA, Ohler L (Eds.). *Solid Organ Transplantation*. New York: Springer; 2003.

10. Richard C. Assessment of renal structure and function. In Lancaster L (Ed.). *Core Curriculum for Nephrology Nursing*. Pitman, NJ: Anthony J. Janetti, Inc.; 2001. 57-82.

11. Majid A, Kingsnorth AN (Eds.). *Advanced Surgical Practice*. London: Greenwich Medical Media; 2003.

12. National Kidney Foundation (NKF). K/DOQI Clinical Practice Guidelines for chronic kidney disease: Evaluation, classification, and stratification. Available at: http://www.kidney.org/professionals/kdoqi/guidelines_ckd/toc.htm. Accessed 6/22/05.

13. Anthony CP, Thibodeau GA. *Anatomy and Physiology*. St. Louis: CV Mosby; 1975.

14. Holechek MJ. Acute renal failure and chronic kidney disease. In Lewis SL, Heitkemper MM, Dirksen SR (Eds.). *Medical Surgical Nursing: Assessment and Management of Clinical Problems*. St. Louis: Mosby; 2004. 1210-1246.

15. Lancaster LE. Systemic manifestations of renal failure. In Lancaster LE (Ed.). *Core Curriculum for Nephrology Nursing*, 4th ed. Pitman, NJ: Anthony J. Janetti, Inc.; 2001. 117-158.

16. Corsini JM, White-Williams C, Cupples SA. Evaluation of patients for solid organ transplantation. In Cupples SA, Ohler L (Eds.). *Transplantation Nursing Secrets*. Phildelphia: Hanley & Belfus; 2003. 27-44.

17. Dew MA, Switzer GE, DiMartini AF, et al. Psychosocial assessments and outcomes in organ transplantation. *Prog Transplant*, 2000; 10: 239-259.

18. Harrison JD, Cupples SA. Psychosocial issue in transplantation. In Cupples SA, Ohler L (Eds.). *Transplantation Nursing Secrets*. Phildelphia: Hanley & Belfus; 2003. 45-60.

19. Organ Procurement and Transplantation Network. Kaplan-Meier median waiting times for resitrations listed: 1996-2001. Available at: http://www.optn.org/latestData/rptStrat.asp. Accessed 2/15/05.

20. Gritsch HA, Rosenthal JT. The transplant operation and its surgical complications. In Danovitch RM (Ed.). *Handbook of Kidney Transplantation*, 3rd ed. Philadelphia: Lippincott, Williams & Wilkins; 2001. 146-162.

21. Kubak BM, Pegues DA, Holt CD. Infectious complications of kidney transplantation and their management. In Danovitch RM (Ed.). *Handbook of Kidney Transplantation*, 3rd ed. Philadelphia: Lippincott, Williams & Wilkins; 2001. 221-262.

22. Amend WJ, Flavio V, Tomlanovich SJ. The first two transplanatation months. In Danovitch RM (Ed.). *Handbook of Kidney Transplantation*, 3rd ed. Philadelphia: Lippincott, Williams & Wilkins; 2001. 163-181.

23. Bartucci MR. Kidney transplantation: State of the art. *AACN Clinical Issues*, 1999; 10: 153-163.

24. Barone CP, Martin-Watson, AL, Barone, GW. The post-operative care of the adult renal transplant recipient. *MedSurg Nurs*, 2004; 13: 296-303.

25. Mudge C, Carlson L, Brennan P. Transplantation. In Parker J (Ed.). *Contemporary Nephrology Nursing*. Pitman, NJ: Anthony J. Janetti, Inc.; 1998. 695-776.

26. Guichard SW. Nutrition in the kidney transplant recipient. In Danovitch RM (Ed.). *Handbook of Kidney Transplantation*, 3rd ed. Philadelphia: Lippincott, Williams & Wilkins; 2001. 394-410.

27. Malick LB. Fluid, electrolyte, and acid-base imbalances. In Lewis SL, Heitkemper MM, Dirksen SR (Eds.). *Medical Surgical Nursing: Assessment and Management of Clinical Problems*. St. Louis: Mosby; 2004. 316-358.

28. Stark, JL. The renal system. In Alspach JG (Ed.). *Core Curriculum for Critical Care Nursing*, 4th ed. Philadelphia: WB Saunders; 1991. 472-608.

29. Gharbieh PA. Renal transplant: Surgical and psychologic hazards. *Crit Care Nurse*, 1988; 8: 58-71.

30. Bartucci MR, Schanbacher B. Renal transplantation. In Lancaster LE (Ed.). *Core Curriculum for Nephrology Nursing*, 4th ed. Pitman, NJ: Anthony J. Janetti, Inc.; 2001. 501-522.

31. Crowder CD, Guyure KA, Drachenberg CB, Werner J, et al. Successful outcome of a progressive multi-focal leukoencephalopathy in a renal transplant recipient. *Am J Transplant*, 2005; 5: 1151-1158.

32. Dyrud JE. Post-transplantation delirium: A review. *Curr Op Organ Transplant*, 2004; 9: 428-431.

33. Varon NF, Alangaden GJ. Emerging trends in infections among renal transplant recipients. *Exp Rev Anti-infective Ther,* 2004; 2: 95-109.

34. National Kidney Foundation. K/DOQI Clinical Practice Guidelines for anemia of chronic kidney disease, 2000. *Am J Kid Dis,* 2001; 37:S182-S238.

35. Barone CP, Lightfoot ML, Barone GW. The post-anesthesia care of an adult renal transplant recipient. *J PeriAnesthesia Nurs,* 2003; 18: 32-41.

36. Jacobsson PK, Cohan JL. Kidney transplantation. In Williams BA, et al., (Eds.). *Organ Transplantation: A Manual for Nurses.* New York: Springer; 1991.

37. Helderman JH, Goral S. Transplant immunobiology. In Danovitch RM (Ed.). *Handbook of Kidney Transplantation,* 3rd ed. Philadelphia: Lippincott, Williams & Wilkins; 2001. 17-38.

38. Holechek MJ, Paredes M. Kidney transplantation. In Cupples SA, Ohler L (Eds.). *Transplantation Nursing Secrets.* Phildelphia: Hanley & Belfus; 2003. 127-142.

39. Nast CN, Cohen AH. Pathology of kidney transplantation. In Danovitch RM (Ed.). *Handbook of Kidney Transplantation,* 3rd ed. Philadelphia: Lippincott, Williams & Wilkins; 2001. 290-312.

40. Racusen L, Solez K, Colvin R. The Banff 97 working classification of renal allograft pathology. *Kid Internat,* 1999; 55: 713-723.

41. Levey AS, Coresh J, Balk E, Kausz AT, et al. National Kidney Foundation guidelines for chronic kidney disease: Evaluation, classification, and stratification. *Ann Intern Med,* 2003; 139: 137-147.

REVIEW QUESTIONS

1. The most common causes of chronic kidney disease (CKD) include which of the following disorders?
   1. Hypertension
   2. Congestive heart failure
   3. Diabetes
   4. Glomerulonephritis

   a. 1, 2, 3
   b. 2, 3, 4
   c. All of the above
   d. 1, 3, 4

2. Clinical systemic symptoms that may develop with CKD include which of the following?
   1. Amenorrhea, impotence
   2. Pallor, pruritus
   3. Hyperkalemia, acidosis
   4. Muscle twitching, seizures

   a. 1, 3, 4
   b. 1, 2, 3
   c. All of the above
   d. 1 and 3 only

3. The severity of T-cell rejection is rated using the Banff 97 Grading System. The severity of T cell rejection is determined by the degree of:
   a. Proliferating B cells
   b. Circulating donor antibodies
   c. Tubulitis and arteritis
   d. Tubular atrophy

4. Acute tubular necrosis (ATN) may occur in kidney recipients during the immediate postoperative phase. Donor factors that may affect the development of ATN in the newly transplanted kidney include which of the following?
   1. Hypotension during the donor management phase
   2. Cardiac or respiratory arrest
   3. Ventilator-associated pneumonia
   4. Fluid overload during donor management

   a. 1 and 3
   b. 1 and 2
   c. 2 and 3
   d. 3 and 4

5. ATN presents as renal failure in the absence of rejection or obstruction. Signs of ATN include which of the following?
   1. Increased BUN and creatinine
   2. Anuria or oliguria
   3. Pulmonary edema
   4. Elevated potassium and magnesium levels

   a. 1, 2, 3
   b. 1, 2, 4
   c. All of the above
   d. 1 and 2 only

6. Potential complications following renal transplantation during the immediate postoperative phase include which of the following?
   1. Urine leaks, ATN
   2. Ureteral obstruction
   3. Infections
   4. Lymphoceles

   a. All of the above
   b. 1, 2, 3
   c. 1 and 3
   d. 1 and 4

7. To prevent hypoperfusion of the kidney during the immediate postoperative phase, the central venous pressure (CVP) should be maintained:
   a. between 4-6 mm H_2O
   b. between 6-8 mm H_2O
   c. between 8-12 mm H_2O
   d. > 12 mm H_2O

8. Edema in the lower extremity on the same side of the renal transplant could indicate which of the following problems?
   a. Acute rejection
   b. Deep vein thrombosis (DVT)
   c. Lymphocele
   d. All the above
   e. b and c

9. Prior to a renal biopsy, which of the following tests should be evaluated?
   a. Platelet count
   b. Coagulation studies
   c. Hematocrit
   d. a and b
   e. b and c

10. Following a renal biopsy the most important nursing intervention(s) are:
    a. Ensuring that the patient is lying on the opposite side of the biopsy site
    b. Applying pressure to the biopsy site by having the patient lie on that side
    c. Checking urine for clots
    d. a and c
    e. b and c

14 Pancreas and Kidney-Pancreas Transplantation

MICHELE D. BLAKELY

DIANE LEPLEY

TERRI ACHANZAR

INTRODUCTION

I. Overview
   A. Worldwide, approximately 194 million people have been diagnosed with diabetes, giving it the distinction of being one of the most common non-communicable diseases.[1]
   B. In the United States, there are 18.2 million people, or 6.3% of the population, who have diabetes.[2]
   C. Diabetes is classified into two main types: type 1 and type 2.
      1. Type 1 diabetes results from cellular-mediated autoimmune destruction of pancreatic islet beta-cells causing the loss of insulin production.
         a. Type 1 diabetes (insulin-dependent), affects 5%-10% of those with diabetes and most often occurs during childhood or adolescence.[3]
         b. Approximately 34% of individuals with type 1 diabetes develop end-stage renal disease (ESRD) as a secondary complication within 15 years of disease onset.[4]
      2. Type 2 diabetes (noninsulin-dependent) is the more common type, affecting 90%-95% of those with diabetes.[3]
         a. Type 2 diabetes usually occurs after age 40 and is characterized by insulin resistance and relative insulin deficiency.
         b. In recent years, there has been an increase in type 2 diabetes diagnosed in children and adolescents.
         c. Obesity and diet are associated with development of type 2 diabetes.
   D. Pancreas transplantation has been performed since 1967.[5]
   E. Goals of pancreas transplantation are:
      1. To improve the health of patients who have insulin-dependent diabetes.
      2. To replace exogenous insulin therapy with a suitable pancreas from a deceased donor.
   F. The International Pancreas Transplant Registry (IPTR) reports:[5]
      1. 21,208 pancreas transplants were performed between 1967 and 2003.

2.   15,953 transplants were performed in the United States during the same period.
3.   5,555 pancreas transplants were performed outside the U.S.
4.   Types of pancreas transplant and outcomes are reported in Table 14-1.
5.   Distribution of pancreas transplant volume by type of transplant is reported in Figure 14-1.

G.   Patients with severe or "brittle" diabetes are very limited in their ability to pursue normal activities of daily living due to:
1.   Frequent problems with high and/or low blood sugar
2.   The possibility of vascular complications such as:
   a.   Gastroparesis
   b.   Diabetic retinopathy
   c.   Peripheral neuropathy
   d.   Accelerated cardiovascular disease.

H.   Most patients tend to do very well with a pancreas transplant.
1.   Quality of life may be dramatically enhanced.
2.   Progression of complications of diabetes may be arrested.

II.   Indications
A.   Most candidates for pancreas transplant have had type I diabetes manifested by poor metabolic control for many years.
B.   Individuals requiring total pancreatectomy.
C.   Patients with type 2 diabetes are seldom evaluated for pancreas transplantation.

III.   Candidate selection criteria
A.   Objective measures of end organ failure include:
1.   Mean duration of diabetes (23-27 years)
2.   C-peptide < 0.8 ng/ml
3.   Frequent or severe metabolic complications:
   a.   Hypo-/hyperglycemia
   b.   Ketoacidosis
   c.   Hypoglycemic unawareness despite optimized medical management

TABLE 14-1

■ Pancreas Transplants and Outcomes

Procedure	1 Yr. Patient Survival*	1 Yr. Graft Survival*	5 Yr. Graft Survival*
Pancreas transplant alone (PTA)	98%	78%	81%
Simultaneous pancreas-kidney transplant (SPK)	95%	pancreas 85%	70%
		kidney 92%	70%
Pancreas after kidney transplant (PAK)	95%	94%	78%

*According to 2003 IPTR data

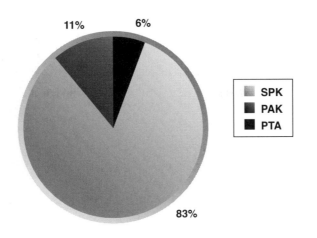

11%   6%

83%

SPK
PAK
PTA

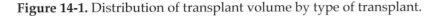

Figure 14-1. Distribution of transplant volume by type of transplant.

4. Minimal evidence of secondary complications such as:
   a. Peripheral neuropathy
   b. Retinopathy
   c. Gastroparesis
   d. Nephropathy
   e. Coronary artery disease
  B. Subjective measures of end organ failure
   1. Numbness in extremities
   2. Lethargy
   3. Nausea
   4. Dizziness
   5. Blurred or low vision
IV. Surgical approach
  A. Native kidneys or pancreas are not removed during the transplant operative procedure.
   1. Allows the exocrine function of the native pancreas to be preserved
  B. There are two surgical approaches to handle exocrine secretions produced by the transplanted pancreas.
   1. Exocrine secretions are generally drained into:
    a. Bowel (enteric drainage [ED])
     i. When the pancreas is drained enterically, much of the approximate two liters of fluid is reabsorbed in the bowel.
     ii. The donor portal vein is anastomosed to the side of the recipient's superior mesenteric vein.
     iii. The transplanted duodenal segment is attached to the recipient's jejunum to establish exocrine drainage.
     iv. The enteric drainage technique is shown in Figure 14-2.
    b. Bladder drainage (BD)
     i. The systemic-bladder drainage technique directs venous outflow and insulin drainage into the iliac vein
     ii. Exocrine drainage is via anastomosis of a donor duodenal segment to the recipient's urinary bladder.[8]
     iii. The bladder drainage technique is shown in Figure 14-3.

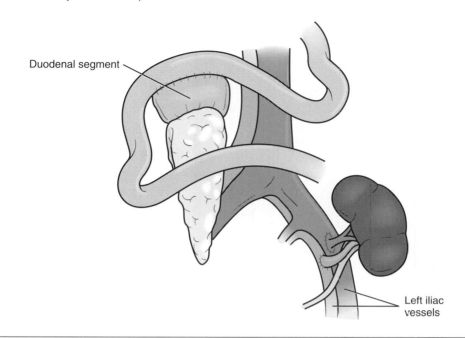

Figure 14-2. Enteric drainage technique.

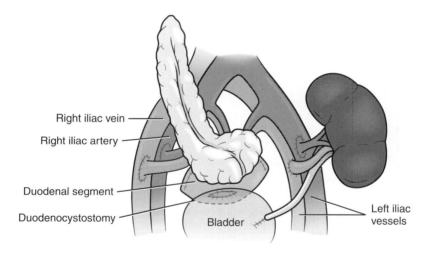

Figure 14-3. Technique of a combined pancreas-kidney transplantation through a lower midline approach.

      iv. The benefit of bladder drainage is that rejection episodes in the pancreas can be detected more readily by measuring the exocrine enzyme (amylase) in the urine.

      v. Bladder drainage may predispose the patient to:

         a) Dehydration

         b) Cystitis

         c) Metabolic acidosis

            1) Large amounts of sodium bicarbonate are emptied into the bladder.

2. According to IPTR, there was no significant difference in the success rates between ED and BD pancrease transplant surgical technique in simultaneous pancreas-kidney recipients.[5]
    a. Most centers use the enteric drainage technique.
    b. Approximately 15%-20% of BD recipients undergo a surgical procedure called "enteric conversion."
        i. Moves the duodenal segment from the bladder to the bowel in the first 3 years following transplant.
3. When the pancreas is transplanted simultaneously with a kidney from the same donor, the kidney can serve as the early rejection detection mechanism.

V. Candidate evaluation testing
  A. Protocols to evaluate candidates may vary by institution and are individualized according to candidate's medical history and physical examination.
    1. Table 14-2 lists typical evaluation tests.

VI. Preoperative principles of patient education
  A. Before providing education, assess the patient for:
    1. Readiness to learn
    2. Barriers to learning
  B. Inquire about patient's expected outcomes and preferred learning style.
  C. Common topics for preoperative patient education include:
    1. Preoperative testing:
      a. Laboratory testing
      b. Chest x-ray
      c. EKG
    2. Preoperative medication:
      a. Bowel preparation.
        i. Pancreas transplant is an intra-abdominal procedure and requires sterilization of the bowel to minimize risk of post-transplant infections.
      b. Immunosuppression may be administered preoperatively.
        i. The standard immunosuppression for pancreas transplants today is:
          a) Tacrolimus (TAC, Prograf, FK506)
          b) MMF (mycophenolate mofeteil, CellCept)
          c) Prednisone (steroids)

VII. Post-transplant course (Table 14-3)
  A. Average length of stay: 7-14 days
  B. Average length of surgical procedure: 4-8 hours
  C. May require 24-48 hour stay in intensive care unit for cardiac monitoring
  D. Postoperative tubes, drains, and devices:
    1. Nasogastric (NG) tube in place for approximately 1-2 days until bowel function returns
    2. Foley catheter in place for 3-8 days
    3. Compression stockings or device to prevent deep vein thrombosis
    4. Incentive spirometer—cough and deep breathe 10 times an hour while awake
    5. Central venous catheter for parenteral medications and fluid management until diet is advanced

TABLE 14-2

■ **Typical Evaluation Tests**

Laboratory	Cardiovascular
• Electrolyte panel	• 12-lead EKG
• Phosphate, magnesium	• Chest X-ray
• Uric acid	• Echocardiogram
• Liver function tests	• Ultrasound of carotid arteries
• Hgb A-1C	• Nuclear stress test/or cardiac catheterization
• C-peptide	• Doppler ultrasound of peripheral vessels to detect vascular disease
• Fasting lipid panel	
• Amylase, lipase	• Letter of clearance from cardiologist
• CBC with differential	
• Coagulation profile	
• Serologies (CMV, HIV, EBV, HBV surface antigen, antibody and core antibody, HCV antibody, HAV IgG)	
• Urinalysis	
• 24-hour protein/creatinine clearance	
• Glomerular filtration rate	
• Thyroid function studies (T_3,T_4,TSH) FANA, ANA	
• Blood type (ABO/Rh)	
• Prostate specific antigen	
• PAP smear	

Immunogenetics	Radiology
• PRA	• Bone density scan
• HLA typing /tissue typing	• Mammogram
	• Sigmoidoscopy/barium enema or colonoscopy

Dental exam	Psychosocial and financial consultation

CBC = complete blood count; Hgb A-1C = glycosylated hemoglobin; CMV = cytomegalovirus; EBV = Epstein Barr virus; HCV = hepatitis C; HBV = hepatitis B; T_3 = triiodothyronine; T_4 = thyroxine; TSH = thyroid-stimulating hormone; FANA = immunofluorescent antinuclear antibody; ANA = antinuclear antibody; PRA = preformed reactive antibody; HLA = human lymphocyte antibody; EKG = electrocardiogram

TABLE 14-3

■ **Potential Complications and Appropriate Interventions**[22]

Potential complication	Report signs and symptoms	Intervene as ordered by physician	Collaborate with multidisciplinary team
Impaired wound healing	Wound leakage Purulent drainage Edge separation Redness Necrosis Dehiscence	Wound care Enzymatic debridement Antibiotics Hyperbaric oxygen treatments	Physician Wound-care nurse Nutritionist
Fluid and electrolyte imbalance	Poor skin turgor Changes in daily weight EKG rhythm disturbance Dry mucous membranes Decreased urine output Mental status changes Dyspnea Rales Edema Distended neck veins	Daily weights Replace urine output and nasogastric drainage with IV fluids Replace electrolytes	Nutritionist Physician
Hypoglycemia	Cool and clammy skin Diaphoresis Mental status changes Palpitations	Perform capillary blood glucose measurements Administer glucose Offer carbohydrates	Diabetes educator Nutritionist
Hyperglycemia	Polyuria, polydipsia Fatigue, blurred vision	Perform capillary blood glucose measurements Administer insulin as prescribed	Physician Pharmacist Diabetes educator Nutritionist
Hypotension	Vital sign changes Orthostatic hypotension Dizziness	Fluid boluses Monitor I & O	Limit activities Evaluate response to interventions; e.g., increased frequency of vital sign monitoring
Hypertension	Headaches	Administer vasoactive drugs as prescribed Monitor I & O	Physician Pharmacist

(Continued next page.)

Potential complication	Report signs and symptoms	Intervene as ordered by physician	Collaborate with multidisciplinary team
Altered bowel function	Abdominal pain Constipation Abdominal distention	GI stimulants Stool softeners, laxatives Suppositories, enemas Increase activity Encourage adequate fluid and fiber intake Ensure patient has a bowel movement at least every other day	Physician
Diarrhea	Diarrhea Amount and consistency of stools Stoma condition if applicable	Evaluate response to prescribed medications Reinforce patient's knowledge on decreased GI motility and adverse effect of constipation to pancreas graft	
Altered nutrition	Low serum albumin Changes in appetite Weight changes	Calorie counts Enteral and parenteral nutritional supplements	Nutritionist Ancillary nursing staff
Altered mobility/ self-care deficit	Level of independence with activities of daily living and ambulation	Incentive spirometer volumes Encourage/assist with mobility Involve family or other caregiver	Physical therapist Respiratory therapist

    E. Pain management:
      1. It is important to continually assess the patient's level of pain and response to analgesia throughout hospitalization.
      2. Strategies to manage pain are guided by institutional protocols.
    F. Anti-rejection medication (Tables 14-4 and 14-5):
      1. Most patients receiving pancreas transplants will receive triple therapy immunosuppression.
      2. Some centers try to avoid steroids owing to their impact on blood glucose levels.
      3. Antilymphocyte induction therapy is being used by some pancreas transplant centers.
    G. Blood transfusion:
      1. Although a rare occurrence post-transplant, it is important to instruct patients that any surgical procedure may result in blood loss that necessitates replacement with blood products.

a. Assessment and documentation of the patient's willingness to accept blood products during preoperative nursing should be performed.

b. If transfusion is indicated, most institutions recommend utilizing CMV-negative blood products to minimize transmission or reactivation of CMV virus post-transplant.

H. Activity:

1. Patients should be out of bed postoperative day 1 and advance activity as tolerated.

I. Incisional care:

TABLE 14-4
■ Common Pharmacologic Therapeutics

Immunosuppressive drugs	Common side effects and drug interactions[23,24,25]	Nursing considerations
Corticosteroids Methylprednisolone Prednisone	Sodium and fluid retention, potassium loss, hypertension, circulatory collapse, tachycardia, muscle weakness, severe arthralgia, pathologic fracture of long bones, osteoporosis, impaired wound healing, petechiae and ecchymoses, facial erythema, acne, hyperglycemia, flushing, sweating, mood and behavioral changes, aggression, thrombophlebitis, embolism, fungal infections, increased intraocular pressure, blurred vision, peptic ulcer, GI hemorrhage, increased appetite, pancreatitis, thrombocytopenia *Interacts with*: barbiturates, salicylates, phenytoin, rifampin, vaccines, toxoids	May be divided into morning and afternoon dose to help control post prednisone hyperglycemia[11] Rapid infusion may cause circulatory collapse[23] Give prednisone with food or milk to decrease GI symptoms Psychological derangements may occur while on therapy[23] Monitor serum potassium, serum and urine glucose levels, blood pressure, urine output, and edema
Calcineurin inhibitors Cyclosporine (Sandimmune, Neoral, Gengraf)	Renal dysfunction, hepatotoxicity, pancreatitis, gum hyperplasia, oral Candida, rash, acne, hirsutism, tremors, seizures, albuminuria, hyperglycemia, proteinuria, hyperkalemia, hypomagnesemia, hyperlipidemia, hyperuricemia *Increase drug levels*: calcium channel blockers, cimetidine, corticosteroids, foscarnet, ketoconazole, fluconazole, metoclopramide, oral contraceptives, NSAIDs,[24] erythromycin, allopurinol, colchicin[23] *Decrease drug levels*: phenytoin, phenobarbitol	Monitor drug levels Grapefruit juice increases serum concentrations Avoid live vaccinations

(Continued next page.)

Immunosuppressive drugs	Common side effects and drug interactions[23,24,25]	Nursing considerations
Tacrolimus (Prograf)	Hypertension, hyperkalemia, hyperglycemia, renal dysfunction, tremors, insomnia, paresthesia, hypomagnesemia, anemia, leukocytosis, thrombocytopenia, nausea, diarrhea, GI bleeding, paresthesia, chills, seizures, UTI, albuminuria, hematuria, proteinuria, hirsutism, hyperuricemia, pleural effusion, dyspnea, rash, flushing, itching alopecia, blurred vision, photophobia, anaphylaxis *Increase drug levels*: antifungals, calcium channel blockers, cimetidine, erythromycin, mycophenolate mofetil, ketoconazole, fluconazole, erythromycin, metoclopramide, cyclosporine, clotrimazole *Decreased blood levels:* phenobarbital, phenytoin[24]	Monitor hemoglobin, WBC, platelets, hepatic panel Give with meals to reduce GI upset Monitor drug levels Grapefruit juice increases serum concentrations Avoid live vaccinations
Antimetabolites		
Mycophenolate mofetil (CellCept, Myfortic)	Diarrhea, vomiting, stomatitis, GI bleed, leukopenia, anemia, thrombocytopenia, pancytopenia, rash, respiratory infection, tremors, dizziness, insomnia, headaches, fever, peripheral edema, hypercholesterolemia, hypophosphatemia, hyperkalemia, hypokalemia, hyperglycemia, UTI, hematuria, renal tubular necrosis, hypertension, chest pain, lymphoma, nonmelanoma skin carcinoma *Interacts with:* magnesium and aluminum hydroxides *Increases concentration:* of acyclovir and ganciclovir	Monitor drug levels Monitor CBC and hepatic panel Give alone for better absorption Avoid taking within 2 hours of magnesium oxide
Azathioprine (Imuran)	Leukopenia, infection, nausea, vomiting, neoplasia *Interacts with:* ACE inhibitors If given with allopurinol, may cause severe pancytopenia[23]	Monitor WBC

Immunosuppressive drugs	Common side effects and drug interactions[23,24,25]	Nursing considerations
Monoclonal and polyclonal antibody products		
Muromonab CD3	**Possible anaphylactoid reactions:** cytokine release syndrome: from mild flu-like syndrome to severe life-threatening shock-like reaction with first few doses, neuropsychiatric events: seizures, encephalopathy, cerebral edema, aseptic meningitis, headache, risk of infection and neoplasia[23]	A clear chest x-ray pre injection Administer prophylactic methylprednisolone 1 to 4 hours prior to injection[23] and antipyretic if temperature is 37.8° C prior to injection. Monitor antimurine antibody titers after therapy Have emergency drugs and equipment on hand
Antithymocyte globulin	*(Equine)* **Possible anaphylactoid reactions:** fever, chills, leukopenia, dermatologic reactions, thrombocytopenia, arthralgia, night sweats, peripheral thrombophlebitis, chest and/or back pain, nausea, vomiting, pain at infusion site, stomatitis *Interacts with:* dextrose injection, USP *(Rabbit)* Abdominal pain, headache, malaise, dyspnea, fever, chills, leukopenia, dermatologic reactions, thrombocytopenia	Discontinue infusion if signs and symptoms of anaphylaxis are observed[23] Have emergency drugs and equipment on hand Monitor CBC for leukopenia and thrombocytopenia
Daclizumab (Zenapax)	**Possible anaphylactoid reactions:** increased risk for lymphoproliferative disorders and opportunistic infections[23] Chest pain, edema, tachycardia, thrombosis, dizziness, tremor, cellulites, impaired wound healing, renal tubular necrosis, musculoskeletal pain, pulmonary edema[25]	Monitor cardiorespiratory and renal functions Watch for hypersensitivity reactions

(Continued next page.)

Immunosuppressive drugs	Common side effects and drug interactions[23,24,25]	Nursing considerations
Basiliximab (Simulect)	**Possible anaphylactoid reactions:** increased risk for lymphoproliferative disorders and opportunistic infections[23] Peripheral edema, hypertension, atrial fibrillation, dyspnea, anemia, tremor, constipation[25]	Monitor cardiovascular, respiratory and renal functions
Other		
Sirolimus (Rapamune)	Hyperlipidemia, hypertension, abnormal liver function tests, anemia, leukopenia, thrombocytopenia, GI disturbances, atrial fibrillation, CHF, hypotension, palpitation, tremors, insomnia, paresthesia, chills, hematuria, proteinuria, hyperglycemia, edema, hypophosphatemia, hyperkalemia, hyperuricemia, hypokalemia, hypomagnesemia, rash, acne, blurred vision, photophobia,[24] delayed wound healing, development of lymphocele, impaired renal function in combination with cyclosporine[23] *Increase drug levels*: cyclosporine, diltiazem, rifampin, ketoconazole, calcium channel blockers, antifungal agents, erythromycin *Decrease drug levels*: phenobarbital, phenytoin, rifabutin, rifapentin, St. John's wort	Use consistently with or without food; alters bioavailability Do not use with grapefruit juice Monitor drug levels Monitor hepatic panel Monitor lipid profile; lipid-lowering agents if needed Reduce or discontinue dose if leukocytes <3000/mm^3; platelets < 1000,000/ mm^3 [24]

     1. Midline abdominal incision dressing should be changed daily or as needed.
     2. Staples or sutures will remain for approximately 3 weeks after surgery.
   J. Emotional considerations
     1. Transplantation is emotionally stressful and demanding.
     2. Most patients cope better when they know what to expect from pancreas transplant.
     3. Patients, as well as family members, are likely to need special support.
     4. Patients and families may feel excited and hopeful to be starting the transplant procedure and, at the same time, feel anxiety about what is ahead.
     5. Reassure the patient and family that these feelings are natural and encourage the sharing of feelings.

TABLE 14-5
■ Commonly Prescribed Non-Immunosuppressive Drugs

Antimicrobials	
antibiotics	Trimethoprim-sulfamethoxazole against *Pneumocystis carinii* pneumonia and UTI; penicillins with beta lactamase inhibitor, quinolones, cephalosporins, aminoglycosides, linezolid
antifungals	Anti *Candida albicans*: nystatin, clotrimazole; Broad spectrum: fluconazole, ketoconazole; Anti Streptomyces: amphotericin B
antivirals	Anti herpes: acyclovir, valacyclovir, famciclovir
	Anti cytomegalovirus: ganciclovir, valgancyclovir, immunoglobulin, cytogam, foscarnet
Supplements	Sodium bicarbonate, magnesium oxide, potassium phosphate
Analgesics	Narcotics, non-narcotics, muscle relaxants
Cardiovascular	Beta blockers, ACE inhibitors, calcium channel blockers cholesterol-lowering agents, diuretics
Anti-ulcers	Hydrogen ion (H_2) blockers, proton pump inhibitors (PPI), antacids
Insulin and anti-hyperglycemics	Long-acting, regular insulin sliding scale, oral hypoglycemic agents

6. The availability of services such as support groups, counseling, and social workers is an important consideration to ensure optimal emotional adjustment.
7. It is important to reinforce the fact that transplantation is not a cure for either diabetes or renal failure.
   a. It is another treatment option.
   b. With improved surgical techniques and new drug therapies, it has become a more desirable approach to treating diabetes while enhancing a person's quality of life.
K. Driving restrictions and weight lifting restrictions will apply during the first 1-2 months post-transplant.
VIII. Post pancreas transplant care
   A. The initial postoperative period necessitates close monitoring of:
      1. Cardiac stability
      2. Fluid and electrolyte balance
      3. Metabolic function
   B. A well-documented nursing assessment is essential in providing immediate and accurate intervention during this critical phase of recovery.
   C. Vital signs
      1. Temperature accepted values: 36.8°–37.5° C
         a. Report if below 36° C or greater than 38° C
         b. In SPK, elevations may indicate:
            i. Infection
            ii. Pancreatitis
            iii. Acute rejection
      2. Pulse accepted values: 60–80 bpm

> a. Report if below 60 or above 84 bpm
3. Blood pressure accepted values: 120/80 mm Hg, systolic below 130 mm Hg
   a. Parameters usually individualized
   b. Report if readings beyond prescribed parameters
   c. Record supine and upright
      i. Orthostatic hypotension is common secondary to volume depletion.
   d. Diastolic greater than 100 mm Hg should be controlled with antihypertensives.
D. Central venous pressure (CVP) acceptable readings: 10–15 cm H_2O[9]
E. Weight
   1. Obtain baseline weight on admission.
   2. Record immediate postoperative weight.
   3. Record daily weight preferably at the same hour using the same scale.
   4. Report significant weight gain or loss.
F. Fluid and electrolyte imbalance
   1. Postoperative ileus, nausea, and vomiting are commonly seen due to prevalence of gastroparesis in diabetic patients.
      a. May contribute to fluid and electrolyte imbalance.
   2. NG tube is commonly placed until bowel function improves to avoid problems associated with decreased motility.
      a. Strict hourly measurement of fluid intake and output detects rapid dehydration.
   3. Imbalance is most common in bladder drained pancreas recipients due to the large amount of fluid loss
      a. Each day, the transplanted pancreas excretes into the bladder approximately 500 ml of fluid rich in bicarbonate and pancreatic enzymes.[17]
   4. Drainage from NG tube, surgical drains, pancreatic drains, and incision dressings must be carefully measured.
   5. Signs of dehydration such as poor skin turgor, a decrease in daily weight, dry mucous membranes, changes in vital signs, and decreased urine output should be reported.
      a. Laboratory values of dehydrated patients would show increased levels of blood urea nitrogen and creatinine, and decreased carbon dioxide.[9]
   6. The physician should be notified if:
      a. Urine output <50 ml and >200 ml per hour[9] in the first 24 hours post-transplant
   7. Interventions to correct fluid and electrolyte imbalance should include:
      a. Administer intravenous fluids to replace urine and NG tube output milliliter per milliliter in the first 24 hours following transplantation.
      b. Maintain CVP greater than 10 cm H_2O.
      c. Intravenous fluids initially do not contain glucose until the blood sugar is below 120 mg/dl.[9]
      d. Albumin is administered to restore plasma volume.
      e. IV fluids containing bicarbonate may be administered to prevent dehydration and correct metabolic acidosis.[8]

      f.   Dehydration and metabolic acidosis will remain a threat as long as the pancreas drains into the bladder.

      g.   Patients must be reminded to maintain adequate hydration.

    8.   Electrolytes are replaced either intravenously or orally.

IX. Pancreatic graft function

    A. Monitored by:

        1.   Serum glucose levels

        2.   Serum amylase concentrations

        3.   Glycosylated hemoglobin

        4.   C-peptide

    B. Serum glucose

        1.   Hyperglycemia often occurs related to the diabetogenic effect of high dose corticosteroids and cyclosporine or tacrolimus.

        2.   Glucose testing can be as frequent as 1 to 2 hours routinely.[9]

        3.   Insulin drip may be ordered for the first 24 to 48 hours post-transplantation.[11]

        4.   As pancreas function improves, the need for insulin decreases.

    C. Patient education includes:

        1.   Blood glucose self-monitoring

        2.   Use of regular insulin in a sliding scale for periods of hyperglycemia.

        3.   Consideration of the patient's degree of visual impairment.

    D. Serum amylase and lipase

        1.   May be elevated during the following events:

            a.   Pancreatitis–may occur in 48-96 hours

            b.   Venous thrombosis

            c.   Anastomotic leak

            d.   After a pancreas biopsy

        2.   Not useful in diagnosing pancreas graft rejection.

            a.   May be elevated for a short period prior to a decrease in urine amylase[12]

            b.   May be transiently elevated 48 to 96 hours post-transplant [10.]

               i.   Secondary to a degree of pancreatitis resulting from:

                   a)   Damage to the organ during cold ischemia preservation

                   b)   Handling of the organ during surgery[8]

              ii.   May also be elevated after a transplant pancreas biopsy

             iii. Serum lipase rises later than amylase and stays elevated up to 14 days [13]

    E. Urine amylase

        1.   An 8-hour urine collection is a way of monitoring for organ rejection in bladder-drained pancreas transplants.

        2.   Frequent testing is done, preferably from urine samples collected at the same hours of the day for better comparison of results.

        3.   Amylase levels are also monitored in pancreatic drain if there is one.[8]

        4.   Times of urine collection and the volume of urine collected must be carefully documented.

        5.   A convenient collecting time period would be for 8 hours through the night.

      a. Specimens should be refrigerated or maintained on ice and sent to the laboratory as soon as collection is completed[14] the next morning.

    6. Two-, six-, or twelve-hour urine collections may also be ordered.

    7. Baseline values for a patient with good initial graft function may be between 1500 to 7000 IU/hour within a few days following transplantation.[12]

    8. Less frequent monitoring is required in later weeks after transplant surgery.

F. Glycosylated hemoglobin
    1. HbA$_1$C should normalize with a well-functioning pancreas graft.
    2. Normal levels of 2.5% to 5.9% indicate good diabetic control and are maintained as long as the allograft functions.[15]

G. C-peptide level
    1. Determines function of the insulin-producing beta cells of the islet of Langerhans
    2. The absence of C-peptide indicates no beta cell function or insulin production.
       a. Its presence indicates residual beta cell function.[13]
          i. Normal values are 0.9–4.2 ng/ml[14] (SI units = 0.17–0.66 μmol/l)
          ii. Usually tested several hours after transplant

H. Serum bicarbonate
    1. Levels should be watched closely in a bladder-drained pancreas.
       a. The transplanted organ excretes large amounts of bicarbonate-rich pancreatic secretions into the bladder for weeks following transplantation.
       b. May lead to dehydration, orthostatic hypotension, and acidosis
       c. Supplemental sodium bicarbonate with doses as high as 100 to 150 mEq/day is administered to minimize the degree of metabolic acidosis.[16]
    2. In enteric-drained transplants, the excreted pancreatic enzymes and bicarbonate drain into the intestine for reabsorption.
       a. Problems of acidosis and dehydration are not as pronounced.

I. Immunosuppressant drug levels
    1. Measured daily while the patient is in hospital
    2. Measures a trough level of the previous dose
    3. Medications monitored with trough levels include:
       a. Tacrolimus
       b. Cyclosporine
       c. Sirolimus
       d. Mycophenolic acid
    4. Dosing is adjusted according to institutional guidelines.
       a. Therapeutic target levels are determined for individual patients based on the length of time since transplantation.
       b. In managing their care after discharge, patients will be expected to develop the understanding and skill of changing dosages when the physician or transplant coordinator informs them of such adjustments.
          i. Patients are instructed to withhold their morning dose until blood is drawn to test drug levels.

        ii.   Patients should be made aware of their target levels and dose changes.

   c. Dose changes when self-medicating with nurse supervision provides the patient a rehearsal of self-care after discharge.

        i.   The challenge for the transplant patient after discharge from the hospital is maintaining a schedule of medications.

        ii.   The challenge for the nurse is assisting the patient in establishing a regimen he/she can adhere to at home.

        iii.   Discharge instructions on medications should not be considered redundant.

           a)   Repetition is necessary because:

              1)   The degree of stress diminishes retention of new information.

              2)   The medication regimen is often complex.

   d. In the outpatient setting, a continuous assessment for side effects and unfavorable drug interactions must be made.

        i.   Patients must be encouraged to report any adverse effects experienced.

        ii.   Patients must be taught to inform the transplant nurse, nurse coordinator, or physician of additional medications prescribed by other care providers.

J.   Postoperative complications

   1.   These complications were the major causes of graft loss (>60%) in the first 6 months post-transplant in all categories of U.S. transplant recipients.[5]

      a. Vascular thrombosis

        i.   Vascular thrombosis is one of several early complications following pancreas transplant.

        ii.   Many transplant centers use various anticoagulation therapies either alone or in conjunction with antiplatelet options to decrease graft thrombosis such as:

           a)   Intravenous heparin

           b)   Enoxaparin

           c)   Aspirin

        iii.   Thrombosis generally occurs within 24-48 hours after transplant and can be venous or arterial in origin, although venous is more common.[10-18]

        iv.   A patient experiencing a vascular thrombosis may present with:

           a)   Acute abdominal pain

           b)   Elevated serum amylase levels

           c)   Elevated blood glucose levels

        v.   Arterial thrombosis presents with:

           a)   An abrupt rise in glucose levels

           b)   Serum amylase levels remaining stable

           c)   Abdominal examination usually unremarkable

           d)   Exploratory surgery usually necessary

        vi.   One strategy to prevent vascular thrombosis is cautious handling of the organ during procurement.[18-26]

        vii.   In many cases, graft pancreatectomy follows if the graft is not salvageable.[26]

      b. Pancreatitis

    i.   Allograft pancreatitis is a relatively common postoperative occurrence.[10-26]

    ii.   Serum amylase levels may be mildly elevated for the first 2 to 3 days after transplant.

        a)   This elevation could be related to the handling of the organ prior to transplant or ischemic injury prior to procurement and may not be clinically significant.[18-26]

        b)   Patients should be monitored closely as pancreatitis can be an early sign of acute rejection.

        c)   Patients who experience late pancreatitis could have a stricture of their anastomosis.[18]

c.   Leaks

    i.   Leaks can be one of the more serious complications postoperatively.

    ii.   Anastomotic leak

        a)   Anastomotic leaks are common after pancreas transplantation, especially in the first 3 months.

        b)   Patients with an anastomotic leak may present with:

            1)   Fever

            2)   Increased white blood cell counts

            3)   Abdominal pain

            4)   Elevated serum amylase

            5)   Elevated serum creatinine

        c)   Anastomotic leaks are the most frequent postoperative complication.

        d)   Leaks are treated based on size, with either surgical re-exploration or stenting if the leak is small.[18]

    iii.   Urine leaks

        a)   A urine leak is one of the most serious complications of a bladder drained pancreas transplant.

        b)   This type of leak can occur early or late after pancreas transplant.

        c)   Urine leaks usually originate from the deterioration of the duodenal segment.[10]

        d)   Patients experiencing urine leaks can present with:

            1)   Lower abdominal pain

            2)   Fever

            3)   Elevated serum amylase

        e)   Symptoms are not unlike those seen with rejection or pancreatitis.

        f)   Timely diagnosis and surgical intervention are usually required in combination with computed tomography (CT) scans and other imaging technology to confirm diagnosis.[10]

d.   Infection/sepsis

    i.   Both infection and sepsis are common post pancreas transplant.

    ii.   Some typical infections include:

        a)   Urinary tract infections

        b)   Wound infections

        c)   Opportunistic infections

        d)   Sepsis

      e) Cystitis

iii. Urinary tract infection

    a) Pancreas transplant recipients, like many other postsurgical patients, are at risk for urinary tract infection by presence of a Foley catheter postoperatively.

    b) Pancreas transplant recipients are also at risk secondary to neurogenic bladder related to diabetes mellitus (DM) or retained foreign bodies.[26]

    c) In recipients of bladder drained pancreas transplants, these infections can become quite serious leading to cystitis.

iv. Opportunistic infections

    a) Opportunistic infections, particularly CMV, are troublesome in all immunosuppressed patients.

        1) Many transplant programs utilize CMV prophylaxis regimens to address CMV risk.

        2) This virus is common post-transplant; its occurrence is dependent on preoperative serologic status as well as induction therapy used.

        3) Infection of the pancreas transplant recipient with CMV can lead to ulceration, perforation, and leak on the duodenal segment.[26]

v. Deep wound infections

    a) Wound infections post pancreas transplant are often related to the placement of the organ.

    b) In recipients who have a pancreas placed in the retroperitoneum, deep wound infections occur that may require drainage.

    c) Conversely, recipients with a pancreas transplant placed in the intraperitoneum have a decreased chance of deep wound infection.

vi. Sepsis

    a) Sepsis is responsible for the most deaths following pancreas transplantation.[10]

    b) Sepsis is most commonly attributed to the acidic pancreatic enzymes which can lead to an anastomotic erosion and peritonitis.[1]

    c) Treatment of sepsis

        1) Once identified, the pancreas transplant patient with sepsis must be treated urgently and aggressively with intravenous antibiotics and may require exploratory laparotomy.

        2) Routine nursing care.[10]

           i) Strict monitoring of blood glucose levels

           ii) Management of fluid intake and output

           iii) Medical management of any drains that may have been placed

vii. Cystitis

    a) Cystitis can occur in the pancreas transplant recipient who has a bladder drained pancreas, secondary to the effect of pancreatic enzymes on the urinary tract.

          b) Cystitis can be treated with insertion of a Foley catheter or, in extreme cases, the patient may require enteric conversion.[10-26]

  e. Hematuria

      i. Hematuria may occur early after pancreas transplant without clinical significance and may resolve spontaneously without clinical significance.

      ii. The occurrence of hematuria post-transplant could be related to anticoagulation efforts to prevent graft thrombosis.

      iii. Treatment of severe hematuria would be the discontinuation of anticoagulation.

      iv. If hematuria persists, cystoscopy may be necessary.[10-26]

      v. Hematuria cannot be completely disregarded because it may be a symptom of graft rejection.

  f. PTLD: post-transplant lymphoproliferative disorder

      i. The occurrence of malignancy, specifically lymhoproliferative disorder, is increased following organ transplant as a result of immunosuppressive medications.

      ii. Post-transplant lymphoproliferative disorder (PTLD), in particular, is related to both the intensity and duration of immunosuppression.[26]

      iii. Patients and their families should be made aware of this increased risk of malignancy in their pretransplant education/evaluation session.

  g. Rejection

      i. Despite advances in transplant care, rejection remains the second most common cause of pancreas graft loss.

      ii. According to IPTR, acute rejection rates vary between 4%-20% for U.S. recipients.[5]

          a) Rejection frequently occurs 13-24 months post-transplant for SPK.

          b) 25-48 months post-transplant for PAK and PTA

          c) Chronic rejection occurs in 3%-43% of recipients

          d) For SPK, rejection occurred most frequently 25-48 months post-transplant

          e) For PAK, rejection occurred most frequently 13-24 months post-transplant

          f) For PTA, rejection occurred most frequently 7-12 months post-transplant

      iii. Rejection is sometimes difficult to detect.

          a) Pancreas graft rejection should be considered if patients experience:

              1) Pain at the graft site

              2) Increased serum amylase or lipase

              3) If it is a bladder drained graft, decreased urine amylase[10-18]

          b) Hyperglycemia is not an early sign of pancreas transplant rejection; in fact, in the initial stages glucose levels remain normal.

              1) Hyperglycemia is a much later sign when damage has occurred to islet cells.

                  i) It usually signifies an irreversible situation.[10-18]

     ii) Patients with symptoms suspicious of graft rejection should have a pancreas biopsy if possible.

     iii) Diagnosis of pancreas transplant rejection is confirmed by biopsy.[10-18]

  h. Postbiopsy nursing care

    i. Patients undergoing pancreas transplant biopsies must remain on bed rest for observation after the procedure.

    ii. Patients should be monitored for external bleeding at biopsy puncture site, hematoma, changes in vital signs, and pain.

 i. Rejection treatment options

   i. Pancreas transplant rejection treatment is directed by the severity of rejection.

   ii. The occurrence of pancreas transplant rejection is now lower with the development and use of newer immunosuppressive agents.

   iii. Patients and their families and/or caregivers should be educated about rejection treatment options including:

    a) The possibility of being hospitalized for treatment of rejection

    b) Needing intravenous medications

    c) Potentially altering their oral immunosuppressive regimen

   iv. Common rejection treatment regimens include intravenous pulse steroids and antilymphocyte preparations.

X. Summary

 A. Pancreas transplant has become widely accepted as an effective therapeutic treatment for certain patients.

  1. It is not without complications.

  2. As discussed, vascular thrombosis, pancreatitis, leaks, infections/sepsis, cystitis, pancreatitis hematuria, rejection and PTLD are all common complications of which to be cognizant.

  3. The increased use of enteric drainage instead of bladder drainage techniques has decreased some of the urologic and metabolic complications.[1]

   a. It is important to realize the extreme negative impact the postoperative complications can have on morbidity and mortality.

   b. Transplant practitioners must continue aggressive efforts in prophylactic care as well as stringent postoperative management in order to prevent complications and improve the overall quality of life in the post pancreas transplant patient.

REFERENCES

1. International Diabetes Federation. Diabetes Atlas. Available at: http://www.eatlas.idf.org/Types_of_diabetes#Type2diabetes. Accessed August 10, 2005.

2. National Diabetes Information Clearinghouse, National Diabetes Statistics Available at: http://diabetes.niddk.nih.gov/dm/pubs/statistics/#7. Accessed August 10, 2005.

3. Onkano P, Vaananen S, Karvonen M, Toumilehto J. Worldwide increase in incidence of type 1 diabetes – the analysis of the data on published incidence trends. *Diabetologia,* 1999; 42: 12: 1395-1403.

4. American Diabetes Association, Diabetes Statistics. Available at: http://www.diabetes.org/diabetes-statistics.jsp. Accessed August 10, 2005.

5. International Pancreas Transplant Registry. 2003 Annual Data Report, Pancreas Transplants by Category. Available at: http://www.iptr.umn.edu/ar_2003/2003_page2.htm. Accessed August 10, 2005.

6. United Network for Organ Sharing, Donation and Transplantation: About Transplantation: History. Available at: http://www.optn.org/about/transplantation/history.asp. Accessed August 3, 2005.

7. Atkinson M, Maclaren N. The pathogenesis of insulin-dependent diabetes mellitus. *N Engl J Med,* 1994; 331: 1428-1436.

8. Cowan PA, Wicks MN, Rutland TC, Ammons J, et al. Pancreas Transplantation. From Organ transplantation: Concepts, issues, practice, and outcomes. Medscape from WebMD. 2002. Available at: http://www.medscape.com/viewarticle/436542. Accessed July 17, 2005 and August 16, 2005.

9. Makowka L, Sher L. *Ortho Biotech Handbook of Organ Transplantation.* Austin: Landes Bioscience Publishers, 1995. 297-303.

10. Kaufman DB. Pancreas transplantation. In Stuart FP, Abecassis MM, Kaufman DB. *Organ Transplantation,* 2nd ed. Georgetown, TX: Landes Bioscience, 2003. 155-176.

11. Pirsh JD, Sollinger HW. Kidney and kidney-pancreas transplantation in diabetic patients. In Danovitch GM. *Handbook of Kidney Transplantation,* 3rd ed. Philadelphia: Lippincott Williams & Wilkins, 2001. 164, 317.

12. Robertson PR. Patient selection for and immunologic issues relating to kidney-pancreas transplantation in diabetes mellitus. UpToDate Online version 13.2, 2005. Available at: http://www.uptodateonline.com/application/topic.asp?file=renltran/12278&type=A&selectedTitle=3~6. Accessed July 17, 2005.

13. Professional Handbook of Diagnostic Tests. Springhouse, PA: Springhouse Corporation, 1995. 142, 212.

14. Pagana KD, Pagana TJ. *Mosby's Diagnostic and Laboratory Test Reference,* 7th ed. St. Louis: Elsevier, Inc., 2005. 62, 317, 496.

15. Kaufman D, Koffron A. Pancreas transplantation. eMedicine Journal, 2001. Available at: http://www.emedicine.com/med/topic2605.htm. Accessed July 29, 2005.

16. Robertson PR. Benefits and complications associated with kidney-pancreas transplantation in diabetes mellitus. UpToDate Online version 13.2, 2005. Available at: http://www.uptodate.com/application/topic.asp?file=renltran/14457&type=A&selectedTitle=2~6. Accessed July 17, 2005.

17. Keven K, Basu A, Re L, et al. *Clostridium difficile* colitis in patients after kidney and pancreas-kidney transplantation. *Transplant Infect Dis,* 2004; 6: 10-14.

18. Mize JB. Pancreas and simultaneous pancreas-kidney transplantation. In Cupples SA, Ohler L (Eds.). *Transplantation Nursing Secrets.* Phildelphia: Hanley & Belfus; 2003. 143-150.

19. Robertson PR. Pancreas and islet transplantation in diabetes mellitus. UpToDate Online version 13.2, 2005. Available at: http://www.uptodateonline.com/application/topic.asp?file=diabetes/16031&type=A&selectedTitle=1~6. Accessed July 17, 2005.

20. Lustman PJ, Clouse RE. Depression in diabetic patients: The relationship between mood and glycemic control. *J Diabetes Complications,* March-April 2005. 113-122.

21. Crone CC. Treating depression in a renal transplant recipient. Response to ask the experts about general transplantation. Medscape from WebMD, 2005. Available at: http://www.medscape.com/viewarticle/506475. Accessed August 1, 2005.

22. CCTN Candidate Handbook. American Board for Transplant Certification, Inc., 2004.

23. Pirsch J, Simmons W, Sollinger H. *Transplantation Drug Manual,* 4th ed. Austin, TX: Landes Bioscience, 2003.

24. Skidmore-Roth L. *Mosby's 2005 Nursing Drug Reference.* St Louis: Elsevier, Inc., 2005. 313, 713-714, 851, 936, 965.

25. Turkoski BB, Lance BR, Bonfiglio MF. *Drug Information Handbook for Nursing,* 6th ed. Hudson, OH: Lexi-Comp, Inc., 2004. 147, 350.

26. Auchincloss H, Shaffer D. Pancreas transplantation. In Ginns LC, Cosimi AB, Morris PJ (Eds.). *Organ Transplantation.* Blackwell Sciences, 1999. 395-421.

REVIEW QUESTIONS

1. There are two surgical approaches to handling exocrine secretions produced by the transplanted pancreas: enteric drainage and bladder drainage. When drained enterically, the bowel reabsorbs approximately what amount of fluid?
   a. 500 ml
   b. 100 ml
   c. 2 liters
   d. 5 liters

2. The benefit of bladder drainage is that rejection episodes of the pancreas can be detected more readily by measuring which of the following in the urine?
   a. Sodium and potassium
   b. Solutes
   c. Amylase
   d. Glucose

3. Approximately 34% of individuals with type I diabetes develop which of the following within 15 years of the onset of diabetes?
   a. Insulin dependence
   b. End-stage renal disease
   c. Coronary artery disease
   d. Diabetes insipidus

4. Bladder drainage of exocrine secretions may predispose the patient to which of the following complications?
   a. Dehydration
   b. Metabolic acidosis
   c. Volume overload
   d. Cystitis
   e. b, c, d
   f. a, b, d

5. Approximately 15%-20% of BD recipients undergo a surgical procedure called "enteric conversion," which is best described as:
   a. Sterilization of the bowel to minimize risk of post-transplant infections
   b. The development of a postoperative ileus with nausea and vomiting
   c. Damage to the organ during cold ischemia preservation
   d. Movement of the duodenal segment from the bladder to the bowel

6. The central venous pressure should be maintained at what level cm H_2O during the postoperative period following pancreas transplantation?
   a. 4-8
   b. 2-4
   c. 6-10
   d. 10-15

7. Postoperative ileus with nausea and vomiting are not uncommon following pancreas transplantation. These complications are attributed to which of the following pretransplant problems?
   a. Peripheral neuropathy
   b. ESRD
   c. Gastroparesis
   d. All of the above

8. A patient experiencing vascular thrombosis may present with which of the following symptoms?
   a. Elevated blood glucose levels
   b. Elevated serum amylase
   c. Acute abdominal pain
   d. Acute thrombosis of the hepatic artery
   e. b, c, d
   f. a, b, c

9. Patients with an anastomotic leak may present with which of the following symptoms?
   a. Sharp rise in blood glucose levels
   b. Increase in white blood cells
   c. Abdominal pain
   d. Elevated serum creatinine
   e. a and c
   f. b, c, d

10. Nursing management of a pancreas transplant recipient with sepsis includes which of the following interventions?
    a. Strict monitoring of blood glucose levels
    b. Management of drains
    c. Strict intake and output
    d. Strict handwashing techniques
    e. All of the above
    f. a and d only

15 Pediatric Solid Organ Transplantation

BARBARA V. WISE

GRAINNE WALSH

I. Organ transplantation for end-stage disease in children is a viable treatment option.
   A. Longer waiting times for organs is a result of:
      1. Critical shortage of potential donor organs
      2. Expansion of acceptable diagnoses for transplantation
      3. The number of children on the waiting list has doubled in the last 10 years
      4. Exploration of creative surgical techniques for pediatric recipients
   B. Improving graft and patient outcomes has led the transplant community to focus on the quality of life of pediatric recipients
      1. Long-term survivors of transplantation become children with a chronic illness.
II. Pediatric kidney transplantation
   A. Renal failure in children
      1. Causes of renal failure in children are different than those of adulthood.
      2. Incidence is age-dependent.
         a. In the younger child, the cause is more commonly congenital.
         b. In the older child, glomerulonephritis or focal segmental glomerulosclerosis (FSGS) are more frequently the cause.
      3. The most common diagnoses leading to end-stage renal disease include:
         a. Glomerulonephritis
         b. FSGS
         c. Polycystic kidney disease
         d. Pyelonephritis
         e. Rarely, metabolic disease such as cystinosis
         f. Malignancy due to bilateral Wilms' tumor (Table 15-1)
      4. According to the UNOS data[1]:
         a. 585 children 0-17 years old underwent kidney transplantation in 2005 in the United States.
         b. More than 800 children continue to wait for a new kidney on the waiting list.
      5. Timing of kidney transplant

TABLE 15-1

■ **Diagnoses Leading to End-Stage Disease in Children**

Lung Diseases

Alveolar proteinosis
Bronchiectasis
Bronchopulmonary dysplasia
Cystic fibrosis
Interstitial lung disease
Pulmonary hypertension

Liver Diseases

Biliary atresia
Alpha-1 antitrypsin deficiency
Wilson's disease
Alagille's syndrome
Tyrosinemia
Viral hepatitis
Glycogen storage disease

Kidney Diseases

Renal dysplasia/hypoplastic/aplastic
Obstructive uropathy
Focal segmental glomerulosclerosis
Reflux pyelonephritis
Henoch-Schönlein purpura
Bilateral Wilms' tumor

Heart Disease

Hypoplastic left heart syndrome

   a. Transplantation is considered necessary when the glomerular filtration rate (GFR) is approximately 10 ml/min per 1.73 m²
   b. Internationally there are differences in practice:
       i. Some countries promote pre-emptive transplantation
       ii. Others stabilize children on dialysis prior to transplantation.
       iii. Some countries do not promote living donor transplantation
       iv. Others have live donation programs accounting for greater than 50% of their pediatric program.
6. Procedure
   a. Native kidneys usually are not removed prior to renal transplantation
       i. Clinical situations that may involve removing native kidneys in a child include:
           a) Severe or poorly controlled hypertension to prevent damage to the new kidney
           b) Polycystic kidney disease owing to space issues
   b. Children with suspected or confirmed bladder problems need to be investigated prior to transplant.
       i. Poor bladder function can cause kidney damage to the newly transplanted kidney.
       ii. Investigations can include ultrasound, micturating cystourethrogram (MCUG), and urodynamics.
       iii. Bladder function tests need to be carried out with the patient awake because sedatives will affect the bladder and confuse the test results.

    c. Renal failure secondary to reflux nephropathy, obstructive uropathy, or neuropathic bladder may demonstrate abnormalities which affect continence and bladder capacity.

    d. Extent of the problem needs to be identified.

    e. Corrective action may include:

        i.   Double voiding

        ii. Initiating self-catheterization

        iii. Bladder augmentation

        iv. Mitranoff procedure may be required.

            a) Treatment is done prior to transplantation to ensure the bladder is safe.

            b) Occasionally the surgical procedure is performed post-transplantation.

B. Pretransplant evaluation and preparation

    1. Pretransplant preparation is multi-factorial and should be holistic.

        a. The child should be prepared physically, psychologically, and socially with support given to families on the transplant journey.

        b. Specific cultural and religious beliefs need to be identified and addressed on an individual basis and include issues such as:

            i.   Dietary requirements

            ii. Use of blood products

            iii. Beliefs surrounding transplantation

        c. The renal transplant evaluation

            i.   Blood tests:

               a) Blood grouping (ABO typing)

               b) Human lymphocyte antigen typing (HLA typing)

               c) Panel of reactive antibodies (PRA)

                   1) See Chapter 13 for an explanation of HLA typing and PRA.

               d) Biochemical profile

               e) Full blood cell count (CBC)

               f) Urinalysis and urine culture

               g) Lipid profile

               h) Viral screening to include:

                   1) Cytomegalovirus (CMV)

                   2) Epstein-Barr virus (EBV)

                   3) Hepatitis profile

                   4) Tuberculosis (TB) skin test

                   5) Measles, mumps, rubella

                   6) Varicella zoster titers (VZV)

                   7) Some pediatric protocols also include human immunodeficiency virus (HIV).

               i) Thrombophilia screen

                   1) Arterial or venous thrombosis can cause graft failure in the immediate postoperative period, usually within the first 2 to 3 days[2]

                   2) Screening includes[2]

                       i)   Anti-cardiolipin antibodies

                       ii) Factor V Leidin

                       iii) Anti-lupus coagulant

                       iv) Protein C

              v) Protein S

              vi) The genetic component methlyenetetrahydrofolate reductase (MTHFR)

          3) Patients found to have a clotting tendency or genetic predisposition to coagulation are treated with anticoagulants immediately after the operation

             i) Treatment may continue for approximately 6 months thereafter depending on the center protocol.

      j) Dental examinations are an important part of the pretransplant evaluation.

          1) Poor dental hygiene and caries are a potential source of infection in the immunocompromised patient.

          2) It is essential that dental health is optimal prior to transplant.

      k) Potential recipients also may be screened with the following:

          1) Audiologic examination

          2) Bone age films

          3) Ophthomalogic examination

      l) Diagnostic tests

          1) Renal ultrasound

      m) Children should be fully immunized pretransplant.

          1) Significant morbidity and mortality result from preventable diseases.

          2) Many diseases are prevented by using "live" vaccines.

             i) Live vaccines are contraindicated in immunocompromised individuals and thus should be given before transplant.

             ii) If the child has no antibodies to specific diseases appropriate vaccination will be administered during the evaluation period.

             iii) Vaccination protocols depend on a country's or transplant center guidelines[3, 4]

2. Transplant team meeting

    a. Once the evaluation has been completed, the child will be presented to the multidisciplinary team.

    b. If found to be a suitable candidate, the child is placed on call for a deceased donor organ.

    c. Candidates are listed with the national/international service (e.g., UNOS, UK transplant, Eurotransplant, the Australian or Canadian allocation systems).

    d. Children in need of a liver, kidney, or lung transplant may have the option of living donation.

C. Immediate preoperative care

  1. Kidney-specific preoperative considerations

    a. If the child has been dialysis-dependent, a dialysis session may be necessary immediately prior to transplantation.

      i. Ensures optimal biochemistry

      ii.   If the child is receiving peritoneal dialysis, continue passes until 2 hours before surgery.

2. Emotional support is important for families and for children.
   a. This period can be an emotionallt trying, particularly when families have been called in for a transplant from a deceased donor.
      i. Explain procedures
      ii. Provide emotional support
      iii. Allow time for questions from both the child and family
      iv. Provide an explanation of postoperative expectations
3. Vital signs
   a. Measurement of temperature, blood pressure, and heart and respiratory rates will provide a baseline check.
4. Preoperative tests include:
   a. ECG/EKG
   b. Chest x-ray
   c. Blood tests (chemical profile, clotting screen, complete blood count)
   d. Urinalysis and microscopy
   e. Type and cross for two units of blood
5. Calculation of a child's body surface area (BSA) is essential for accurate prescribing and administration of medication.
   a. $BSA = height \times weight / 3600$
   b. Medication should be given as prescribed.
   c. Preoperatively, this will include:
      i. Induction immunosuppressive agents depending on center protocols
      ii. May also include a monoclonal antibody, steroids, calcineurin inhibitors, or antiproliferative agents.

D. Surgical procedure
   1. Ultrasonic angiography carried out during the workup will have determined vessel patency.
   2. The main blood vessels used in this procedure are:
      a. Inferior vena cava (IVC)
      b. Aorta
      c. Iliac arteries and veins
   3. Older children (circa > 3 years) will have their kidney transplanted in an extraperitoneal position.
      a. Donor vessels are anastomosed to the iliac vessels.
   4. Infants or small children have the kidney placed intraperitoneally.
      a. Donor blood vessels are anastomosed directly to the aorta and the IVC.
      b. Following reperfusion, the donor ureter is anastomosed to the bladder.

E. Post-transplant care
   1. In the immediate postoperative period, emphasis will be on patient safety.
      a. Regular clinical recording of vital signs (Table 15-2) will be carried out.
      b. Frequency is determined by center protocols.
      c. Observations include:
         i. Blood pressure

TABLE 15-2
■ Postoperative Observations

	Kidney	Liver	Heart/Lung
General observation	Y	Y	Y
Temperature (core +/- peripheral)	Y	Y	Y
Blood pressure	Y	Y	Y
Heart rate	Y	Y	Y
Respiratory rate	Y	Y	Y
CVP	Y	Y	Y
Pulse oximetry	Y	Y	Y
Pulmonary artery catheter measurement	N	N	Y
Telemetry/epicardial pacemaker	N	N	Y
Fluid balance	Y	Y	Y
Wound site	Y	Y	Y
Daily weights	Y	Y	Y

      ii. Heart and respiratory rates
      iii. Core/ peripheral temperature
      iv. Pulse oximetry
      v. Central venous pressure (CVP) monitoring
   d. Reassurance for the child and family, an essential component of pediatric nursing, should be ongoing.
   e. Perfusion of the kidney will be evaluated immediately postoperatively using Doppler ultrasound or DPTA scan depending on the transplant protocol.
   f. Hemodynamic stability is a priority and is multifactorial in nature.
   g. Fluid balance:
      i. If the child is polyuric, hypovolemia may occur rapidly.
      ii. If the child is oliguric, hypervolemia may develop.
         a) Oliguria is defined as a urine output <1 ml/kg/hr in infants and less than 0.5 ml/kg/hr in children.
         b) Initially the intravenous fluid regimen includes 100% replacement of urine output with 0.45% normal saline.
      iii. If the patient is hyponatremic or has a urinary sodium >100 mmol/L:
         a) Urinary replacement fluid should be alternated between 0.45% and 0.9% normal saline.
         b) Urinary sodium, potassium, and creatinine levels can assist with fluid management and should be assessed regularly.

      iv. Close observation of respiratory rate and effort is necessary to monitor for pulmonary edema especially in the oliguric patient.

      v. Central venous pressure (CVP) measurement is continuous.

        a) Maintain in the region of +4 to +8 cm H_2O with intravenous 4.5% albumin or 0.9% saline.

        b) Low CVP can be indicative of hypovolemia which can lead to poor graft perfusion.

          1) Hypovolemia may be presumed if:

            i) There is a gap of >2° C between the core and peripheral temperature.

            ii) The child is hypertensive and has a low CVP.

        c) Hypovolemia can be corrected by:

          1) Administering 5-10 ml/kg 0.45% albumin over 0.5-1 hour with close monitoring of CVP changes.

          2) Repeating albumin infusion as clinically necessary.

        d) Dopamine may be administered to maintain cardiac output and increase allograft perfusion.

        e) Initially fluid balance is recorded hourly including:

          1) Intravenous infusions

          2) Blood loss from drains and surgical incision

          3) Output via urinary catheter

      vi. Observation for excessive bleeding via the wound site, catheter, or abdominal drain is vital.

        a) Should include observing the patient for pallor, hypotension, and tachycardia

        b) The abdominal drain remains *in situ* for the first few days postoperatively until minimal drainage is observed.

        c) The bladder urinary catheter remains on free drainage for a time period determined by center protocols, but usually for 4 days.

          1) If the patient becomes suddenly oliguric, assess for a blocked catheter.

      vii. Monitor laboratory data at a frequency determined by center protocols

        a) Chemistry profile

        b) Complete blood count and differential

        c) Venous blood gas

        d) Immunosuppressive trough levels

        e) Hypocalcemia may present in the very early postoperative period in children with:

          1) A long history of dialysis therapy

          2) Poorly controlled hyperparathyroidism

  h. Pain management

      i. Assessment should be patient-centered and ongoing and dependent on the child's stage of development.

      ii. Explain all procedures using age-appropriate language.

      iii. Patient controlled analgesia (PCA)

        a) Allows the patient or nurse to administer small doses of opioids in addition to a continuous infusion

        b) Appropriate with guidance from the pain team for the management of postoperative pain.

             iv. Common side effects to observe for when opioids are administered via the epidural/intravenous route include
                 a) Facial pruritus
                 b) Urinary retention
                 c) Nausea and vomiting
                 d) Respiratory depression

- i. Postoperative assessment of infants and toddlers includes
  - i. Monitoring vital signs
  - ii. Change in behavior such as
    - a) Characteristics of the cry
    - b) Body movement
    - c) Facial expression
  - iii. Preschoolers may be able to use a simple Likert scale, FACES scale, indicating 0 (no pain) to 10 (worst pain in their life).
  - iv. School-age children and adolescents can use a self-report visual analog scale in addition to behavior and physiologic indicators of pain.

F. Post-transplant complications

1. Complications after renal transplant can be divided into immediate, early, and late complications.
2. Immediate complications relate to the intraoperative period and include:
   a. Hyperacute rejection
   b. Obstruction
   c. Thrombus
   d. Delayed nonfunction
   e. Acute tubular necrosis (ATN)
      i. Major cause of delayed or primary nonfunction in kidney transplants
      ii. Results from damage to the proximal tubular membranes
      iii. May last for variable periods from hours up to several weeks
      iv. Children with ATN present with oliguria prior to becoming anuric.
         a) Close observation of serum potassium levels is vital as an anuric patient will quickly become hyperkalemic.
         b) Dialysis therapy is required.
      v. During prolonged periods of ATN, serial renal biopsies are performed to assess kidney function and monitor for rejection.
      vi. Long cold ischemic times are considered a predisposing factor for ATN.
      vii. Management of ATN includes avoiding nephrotoxic drugs and conservative fluid replacement to prevent hypervolemia.
3. Early complications often relate to surgical issues
   a. Bleeding
      i. Bleeding can occur at the site of the vascular anastomosis or arterial branches.
      ii. Bleeding is manifested clinically as:
         a) Tachycardia
         b) Hypotension

        c) Falling CVP
        d) Abdominal distension
        e) Pain
        f) Oliguria
    iii. Replacement of blood volume and surgical intervention is necessary to control the bleeding.

b. Thrombus
    i. Children younger than 5 years are at highest risk for vascular thrombosis secondary to low flow states.
    ii. Arterial thrombosis presents with sudden anuria and is often irreversible resulting in graft loss.
        a) A related problem is renal artery stenosis.
            1) Diagnosed when the Doppler ultrasound demonstrates turbulent flow
            2) Clinical symptoms are hypertension that is difficult to control with or without erythocytosis and deteriorating renal function.
    iii. Renal vein thrombosis is more common in young recipients.
        a) Can often be treated with heparin
        b) Presents clinically with:
            1) Gross hematuria
            2) Graft swelling
            3) Deterioration of graft function

c. Wound dehiscence

d. Lymphocele
    i. Lymphoceles are collections of lymph which occur when the lymphatic system is cut intraoperatively.
    ii. Majority are asymptomatic
    iii. Larger lymphoceles can cause obstruction and hydronephrosis.
    iv. Diagnosis is made by Doppler ultrasound or nuclear medicine renal scan examination.
    v. Treatment is dependent on whether the lymphocele is causing obstruction or dysfunction.
    vi. Treatment is by percutaneous aspiration
        a) May be drained by a single occasion
        b) May need to leave an indwelling drainage system *in situ*
        c) Drainage that continues long-term may require surgical fenestration.

e. Infection
    i. Prophylactic antibiotics are administered at the time of surgery.
    ii. Usually prophylactic antibiotics are discontinued after 3 doses.
    iii. Initially broad spectrum coverage is provided for both aerobic and anerobic organisms.
    iv. Once a specific organism is identified, the appropriate agent is ordered (antiviral, antifungal, or antibacterial).
    v. Signs of impaired wound healing include redness, purulent discharge, dehiscence, and pyrexia.

        a) Specific immunosuppressive agents and hypoalbumin-emia are predisposing factors.

        b) Intervention should include taking a swab for micros-copy and culture and sensitivities.

f. Urinary leak

   i. Another source of complication after renal transplant is a urinary leak at the ureterovesical anastomosis.

   ii. Clinical signs include:

        a) Unexplained fever

        b) Abdominal pain

        c) Decreased urinary output

        d) Elevated creatinine

        e) Wound drainage

   iii. Treatment

        a) Urine leaks are treated with long-term indwelling uri-nary catheters for minor leaks or surgical intervention.

g. Obstruction at the anastomotic site can occur any time after transplantation and presents with oliguria.

h. Acute rejection

   i. Children with rejection present with:

        a) Decreased urine output

        b) Increased weight

        c) Hypertension

        d) Increased creatinine levels

        e) Pain over the graft

        f) Other clinical signs of acute rejection include:

            1) Allograft swelling

            2) Proteinuria

            3) Hematuria

   ii. Definitive diagnosis of rejection can only be made by a his-topathologic examination of renal tissue following a biopsy

        a) Indications for biopsy include:

            1) Primary nonfunction of the kidney

            2) A >10% rise over the previous day's creatinine mea-surement

        b) Renal biopsy procedure:

            1) Preparations:

                i) Explanation of procedure to parents and child

                ii) Signed informed consent by parents

                iii) Laboratory tests

                    • A clotting screen

                    • Type and cross of blood

                    • At least one unit of blood should be avail-able in case of bleeding postbiopsy.

            2) Renal biopsy can be performed under general anesthesia, conscious sedation, or local anesthesia depending on the age of the child and center proto-col.

            3) Usually performed under ultrasonic guidance.

        c) Biopsy results may demonstrate any of the following:

            1) Healthy kidney tissue

            2) Resolving acute tubular necrosis (ATN)

3) Calcineurin inhibitor toxicity (CNI)
4) Rejection which can be classified as:
   i) Cellular rejection
   ii) Antibody mediated (humoral)
     • Frequently referred to as vascular rejection
     • Always involves blood vessels
5) Rejection is staged using the Banff criteria.
   i) Grades rejection allowing standardization of the diagnosis.
   ii) See Table 15-3 for specific Banff criteria.[5]
6) Treatment of rejection depends on classification.
   i) Acute cellular rejection is treated with methylprednisolone 600 mg per m² intravenously daily for 3 days if within 6 weeks post-transplant or
   ii) Prednisolone 3 mg/kg orally daily for 3 days if it occurs later than 6 weeks
   iii) Vascular rejection is treated with antibody therapy.
     • The choice of which will depend on center protocol and whether patient had antibody therapy as part of the immunosuppressive induction therapy.

4. Late complications of renal transplantation
  a. Chronic rejection
    i. Characterized by slow and progressive increases in creatinine
    ii. Frequently associated with hypertension and proteinuria
    iii. Usually unresponsive to immunosuppressive agents
    iv. Cause is multifactorial
    v. Associated with recipients who have had multiple episodes of acute rejection

TABLE 15-3

■ **Banff Criteria Grading of Rejection in Renal Transplant Recipients**

Grade	Nomenclature
1	Normal
2	Antibody mediated rejection (coincides with grades 3, 4, 5)
	I. ATN
	II. Capillary
	III. Arterial
3	Borderline changes – mild tubulitis
4	Acute/active cellular rejection (histologic changes graded IA, IB, IIA, IIB, and III – moderate tubulitis to lymphocytic inflammation)
5	Chronic sclerosing allograft nephropathy (grade I-III, mild to severe fibrosis)
6	Other

   a) A change in immunosuppressant agents and close monitoring of patient adherence to medications is an important first step.

   b) As the renal function continues to deteriorate, the child experiences symptoms of chronic renal failure.

    1) May require of phosphate binders, vitamin D administration, and erythropoietin to manage anemia

 G. Summary of kidney transplantation

  1. Kidney transplantation is a treatment rather than a cure.

   a. Life-long medication to suppress the immune system

   b. Long-term clinical follow-up

   c. Internationally accepted as the best option for children with end-stage renal failure[6]

   d. A successful kidney transplant is measured by both patient and graft survival rates.

   e. Current U.S. and U.K. data shows that 1-year patient survival is 95% and graft survival is 92%.[7, 8]

III. Pediatric liver transplantation

 A. Liver transplantation has been an accepted treatment for end-stage liver disease in children since 1983.

  1. According to the UNOS database,[1] 403 children 0-17 years of age underwent liver transplantation in 2005.

  2. More than 800 continue to await transplantation.[1]

  3. Until the mid-1990s, survival rates for children had been limited by the lack of available size-matched donors.

  4. Long waiting periods for an appropriate donor resulted in high rates of mortality while on the transplant waiting list.

  5. Reduced-size liver transplantation using the right lobe, left lobe, or left lateral segment from a deceased donor was recommended:

   a. To address the issues of small intra-abdominal space

   b. To alleviate the high rates of mortality

   c. Initially this procedure was used in critically ill children who required immediate transplantation.

   d. Improved survival rates were demonstrated.

   e. Today multiple procedures exist for transplantation of the smallest recipients including:

    i. Living related donor transplants

    ii. Split liver grafts

    iii. Whole liver grafts

 B. Pretransplant liver evaluation

  1. Children referred for liver transplantation have end-stage liver disease; see Table 15-1.

   a. Child is evaluated by the pediatric hepatologist and pediatric transplant surgeon.

   b. The following laboratory tests are recommended:

    i. ABO compatibility

    ii. PT/PTT/INR

    iii. Liver function tests

    iv. HLA typing

    v. Infectious disease screening:

     a) HSV

     b) CMV

        c) Screens for hepatitis A, B, and C

        d) VZV

        e) EBV

        f) Syphilis

        g) Toxoplasmosis

        h) HIV testing

c. Diagnostic tests

    i. Electrocardiography

    ii. Chest radiograph

    iii. Duplex ultrasound of the liver

    iv. CT or MRI of liver

d. Psychosocial screening is performed by the transplant social worker and or psychologist to identify family or financial problems that may interfere with transplant outcomes.

e. Immunization records should be requested.

f. Potential recipients are listed by blood type and weight on the UNOS list.

g. The pediatric end-stage liver disease (PELD) score was developed simultaneously with the adult model to create an effective system for donor liver allocation in the United States.

    i. PELD score lists children and adults on a single liver waiting list according to the probability of death within 3 months of listing.

    ii. Developed from data derived from a sample of children enrolled in the Studies of Pediatric Liver Transplantation (SPLIT).

        a) Factors included in the model predictive of death or moving to the ICU included:

            1) International Normalized Ratio (INR)

            2) Total bilirubin

            3) Serum albumin

            4) Age <1 year

            5) Height 2 standard deviations (SD) from the mean for age

        b) Other variables maintained for listing criteria include:

            1) No minimum or maximum to the PELD score

                i) Adult cap is 40.

            2) Ongoing status 1 criteria for children with chronic liver disease meeting certain criteria

            3) Pediatric donors maintain priority for allocation to pediatric patients

            4) Regional boards maintain discretion to upgrade patients to status 1 if the PELD score does not reflect the urgency for transplantation.[9]

            5) The current status 1 "by exception" is under review

                i) One-third of children listed in category 1 have a low probability of death in 3 months

                ii) Compete with adults and children who are at high risk for death

h. Nutritional support is required in the pretransplant period.

    i. Similar to requirements of lung transplant candidates

      ii. Cholestasis associated with malabsorption deprives the infant/child of essential fat-soluble vitamins (A, D, E, and K)

      iii. May induce diarrhea

      iv. Other factors that affect caloric intake include:

          a) Anorexia that occurs with chronic disease

          b) Increased abdominal pressures associated with ascites and varices, both resulting in:

              1) Early satiety

              2) Increased incidence of emesis.

      v. Management includes the use of increased caloric density formulas with medium chain triglycerides and nighttime drip feedings via nasogastric or nasojejunal tubes.

    i. Children with end-stage liver disease are at risk for several other problems that require management in the pretransplant period.

      i. Portal hypertension results from:

          a) Decreased blood flow to the liver

          b) Increased flow from collateral circulation from the stomach and spleen.

          c) Management involves assessment or signs of bleeding.

              1) Sclerotherapy may be necessary to temporize bleeding varices.

      ii. Encephalopathy results from elevated ammonia levels, causing:

          a) Altered mental status

          b) Complaints of increased sleeping

          c) Poor school performance

          d) Need for administration of lactulose or neomycin[10]

2. Perioperative management

    a. Once a donor organ is available, the child is brought to the hospital and preoperative laboratory tests are obtained.

    b. The liver transplant procedure takes approximately 8-12 hours.

    c. Procurement of the donor liver occurs according to the standard procedure for whole liver transplantation.

      i. Donor liver is prepared at the back table simultaneously with hepatectomy of the native liver by a second surgical team.

      ii. In a reduced liver transplant, the liver is reduced by a formal lobectomy (right or left) or trisegmentectomy for left lateral segment implants, with ligation of the main vessels and ducts.

      iii. The biliary and vascular structures along the cut edge are ligated and the remaining vascular structures are flushed with preservation solution.

      iv. The child is brought to the operating room.

          a) Intubation is performed with a cuffed tube.

              1) Allows for adjustments in pulmonary compliance during the procedure.[11]

          b) Placement of 1-2 large bore catheters in the upper extremities

3. Surgical procedure

    a. Children who have undergone previous abdominal procedures are at higher risk for bleeding and adhesions.

b. A bilateral subcostal incision is made to visualize major structures.
    i. Known as the Mercedes incision
    ii. May be an extension of the previous incision if the child underwent a Kasai portoenterostomy for management of biliary atresia
c. The vena cava, portal vein, and hepatic artery are crossed clamped prior to hepatectomy.
d. Hemodynamic instability is a risk during the anhepatic phase secondary to:
    i. Decreased intravascular volume
    ii. Ongoing fluid and blood losses
    iii. Decreased venous return to the heart
e. The graft is implanted in the usual orthotopic position.
    i. Vascular anastomoses are performed in the following manner:
        a) Suprahepatic inferior vena cava
        b) Infrahepatic inferior vena cava
        c) Portal vein
        d) Hepatic artery
        e) Reperfusion of the graft occurs after the portal vein anastomosis.
            1) During reperfusion, massive fluid shifts can result in intestinal edema, third spacing, and renal compromise.
            2) Children generally tolerate the caval clamping and reperfusion well because of collateral circulation.
    ii. Low molecular weight dextran and subcutaneous heparin are administered in the immediate postoperative period when coagulation factors are normalizing to prevent thromboses.
    iii. Bile duct reconstruction is performed with an end-to-side roux-en-Y limb of the jejunum.
    iv. Two or three Jackson-Pratt drains are inserted.
    v. Duct to duct biliary reconstruction is often performed in children with an adequate biliary tree (recipients diagnosed with metabolic disorders or fulminant hepatic failure).[12]
f. Other surgical options include the split liver transplant and living related liver transplantation.
    i. Split liver grafts differ from reduced sized grafts in the approach to separating the vascular and biliary structures.
    ii. Produce two viable grafts for separate recipients.
    iii. The goal with this procedure had been to address donor shortages by providing a two-for-one application.
        a) Carries a higher incidence of postoperative complications such as biliary leaks and bleeding
            1) Procedure is a less viable option.
    iv. Studies comparing outcomes in living related donor transplants with reduced size or whole liver transplants indicates improved outcomes with living related liver transplantation.

a) Centers that offer this option must consider ethical dilemmas of subjecting a healthy donor to surgery.

b) The arterial reconstruction necessary in a living donor liver transplant produces a surgical challenge because of the many normal variants found in the hepatic arterial system.

4. Post-transplant management of complications

a. The child is taken to the pediatric intensive care unit (PICU), intubated, and monitored for:

i.   Hypothermia

a) Occurs secondary to exposure of the abdominal viscera during the surgical procedure

b) Can predispose the patient to dysrhythmias, clotting abnormalities, impaired renal function, and delayed wound healing

ii. Hemorrhage

a) May occur as a result of preexisting coagulopathy or bleeding at the anastomoses

b) Frequent monitoring of output from the Jackson-Pratt drains is necessary.

c) Indications of bleeding include:

1) Increasing abdominal girth

2) Oozing from the suture line

d) Managing coagulopathies

1) Fresh frozen plasma is used to correct coagulopathies.

2) Usual goal is to maintain a slightly prolonged PT.

3) Thrombocytopenia may occur if >2 blood volumes are transfused during the procedure, necessitating a platelet transfusion.

e) If the bleeding is unresponsive to other therapies:

1) Cryoprecipitate should be given for low fibrinogen levels

2) Factor VII is given for persistent nonsurgical bleeding.[11]

iii. Fluid and electrolyte balance

a) Hyper- or hypotension may occur in the postoperative period related to altered renal function and volume losses.

b) Fluids are administered at 80% of maintenance.

c) Electrolytes are monitored every 6 hours.

d) Hypocalcaemia, hyperkalemia, and hypomagnesemia are common problems.

e) Decreased urine output <1 ml/kg/hr may indicate early graft dysfunction or nephrotoxicity related to calcineurin inhibitors.

iv. Neurologic status

a) Assessments are performed using a modified Glasgow coma scale depending on the age of the child.

b) Monitor for hepatic coma/encephalopathy

c) Monitor for seizures

1) Seizures are rare except in the most ill child.

2) May be a result of neurotoxicity secondary to immunosuppression

v. GI status

a) A nasogastric tube will remain in place for several days
to decompress the stomach.

b) Removed when the child's diet is advanced.

vi. Hepatic artery thrombosis (HAT)

a) Most common postoperative complication occurring in
4%-6% of pediatric recipients

b) A duplex ultrasound of the liver is obtained in the first
24 hours to assess for vessel patency.

c) Diagnosis of HAT in the first 1-6 days postoperative is
possible with a duplex ultrasound.

d) If collateral vessels have developed, angiography may
be the most definitive test.

e) Clinical signs of HAT:

1) Elevated transaminases and bilirubin

2) Change in mental status

3) Biliary leak

4) Sepsis

f) Management of HAT

1) Thrombectomy to restore blood flow

2) Retransplantation

vii. Portal vein (PV) thrombosis

a) Presents with variceal bleeding or a slowly enlarging
liver or spleen and decreasing platelet counts.

b) Recipients of living related liver transplantation are at
higher risk for developing a PV thrombosis

1) Shorter vessel pedicles from living donors

2) Whole liver grafts from deceased donors

c) Frequent use of cryopreserved vein grafts

1) Usually no intervention is required.

2) Children resolve the ascites and the spleen size
decreases.

3) Occasionally an interventional venoplasty is performed to correct the obstruction.[13]

viii. Biliary leaks

a) Leading cause of morbidity and mortality in children

b) Occur in approximately 14% of living related liver transplants

c) In the immediate postoperative period, a change may be
noted in the color of fluid in the Jackson-Pratt drain.

d) Bacterial contamination is possible if the leak occurs at
the roux-en-Y anastomosis.

e) The risk of HAT increases significantly when a biliary
leak is noted in the immediate postoperative period.

f) Diagnosis is made by ultrasound or percutaneous transhepatic cholangiogram.

g) Treatment involves surgical revision with insertion of a
transhepatic biliary stent and broad spectrum antibiotics.

ix. Rejection

a) Early signs of rejection include:
1) Low-grade fever
2) Increased liver enzymes and bilirubin
3) Pain over the graft, irritability, and ascites.
b) Diagnosis is confirmed with a percutaneous liver biopsy.
1) Performed under conscious sedation with local anesthesia
2) Type and cross the child for one unit of blood
3) Obtain a prothrombin and partial thromboplastin time
4) Following the liver biopsy:
i) Hemoglobin level should be obtained 4-6 hours after the procedure
ii) Child should remain flat in bed for 4-6 hours.
c) Treatment of acute rejection
1) Bolus of steroids
i) Intravenous Solu-Medrol
ii) Oral methylprednisolone
d) Late acute rejection
1) Histologically different from early acute rejection.
2) Biopsies demonstrate centrilobular necrosis.
3) Response to treatment is not as rapid as early acute rejection.
e) Chronic rejection
1) Frequent cause of graft loss
2) Biopsies demonstrate bile duct loss with fibrosis and cirrhosis.
3) Cause is unknown.
i) Likely to be multifactorial including:
• Multiple episodes of acute rejection
• CMV infection
• Inconsistent immunosuppressant levels
f) Treatment of chronic rejection
1) Switching immunosuppressant agents to tacrolimus, mycophenolate mofetil, or rapamycin with variable outcomes[10]
5. Outcomes of liver transplantation
a. Austin et al.[14] reported on patient and graft survival in children transplanted between October 1987 and May 2004
b. Factors impacting on patient and graft survival
i. Improved outcome with living related donor transplant compared to whole or split liver transplantation
ii. Shorter cold and warm ischemic times
iii. Recipients less critically ill at the time of transplantation
a) Fewer incidents of retransplantation
IV. Pediatric cardiac transplantation
A. The first pediatric heart transplant was performed in 1985 at Loma Linda Hospital in an infant suffering from hypoplastic left heart syndrome.
B. The number of children and adolescents undergoing heart transplantations has increased to approximately 300-400 per year.

C. According to the Scientific Registry (SRTR) database, 209 children 0-17 years old underwent heart transplantation in 2005 with 227 awaiting transplantation.[1]
1. Survival rates have steadily increased over the last 20 years with 5-year survival ranging between 70%-80%.[1]
2. Advancement in heart and lung transplantation have occurred as a result of:
   a. Improved distance procurement procedures increasing the number of available donors
   b. Development of a consistent grading system to diagnose rejection
   c. Improved immunosuppressive agents
D. Heart transplant is considered a viable option for children with end-stage heart disease that results from congenital heart defects or cardiomyopathy that is not responsive to either medical or surgical treatment.[15-17]
E. Pretransplant evaluation for pediatric heart transplantation
1. Purpose of pretransplant testing is to:
   a. Determine suitability of the candidate
   b. Evaluate medical or surgical alternatives
2. Diagnostic pretransplant evaluation includes:
   a. Echocardiogram
   b. Cardiac catheterization (as needed)
   c. Chest x-ray
   d. Exercise stress test, if patient is able
   e. Cranial ultrasounds for infants
   f. Abdominal ultrasound
3. Laboratory evaluation includes:
   a. ABO typing
   b. Chemistry panel
   c. Thyroid function tests
   d. Lipid profile
   e. Complete blood cell count (CBC)
   f. Human lymphocyte antigens (HLA)
   g. Panel of reactive antibodies (PRA)
   h. Viral screening
      i. Cytomegalovirus (CMV)
      ii. Epstein-Barr virus (EBV)
      iii. Herpes virus
      iv. Hepatitis A, B, and C
      v. Human immunodeficiency virus (HIV)
      vi. Toxoplasmosis
      vii. Varicella zoster in measles, mumps, rubella
F. Pretransplant evaluation consultants
1. Families and candidates older than 7 years are interviewed by:
   a. Financial counselor
   b. Social worker
   c. Psychiatrist
2. Purpose of these interviews is to identify:
   a. Family coping skills
   b. Stressors
   c. Readiness for transplantation process
   d. Financial needs

G. Contraindications
    1. Absolute contraindications to heart transplantation:
        a. Major CNS abnormalities
        b. Active infection
        c. Active malignancy
        d. Substance abuse
        e. Documented history of noncompliance
        f. Diabetes with microvascular disease[16, 18-20]
H. Listing the patient for transplantation
    1. The team reaches consensus about the child's candidacy.
    2. Child is placed on the United Network for Organ Sharing (UNOS) waiting list.
        a. Listed according to height, weight, and blood type
            i. Donor organ may be 10% below and 30% above the recipient's actual weight.
            ii. Pulmonary vascular resistance is required for listing in some countries.
        b. Organ allocation is determined according to urgency.
            i. Children listed as 1A are the sickest and are in the intensive care unit. Clinical criteria include:
                a) Use of mechanical ventilation
                b) Use of mechanical assist device
                c) Younger than 6 months of age
                    1) Congenital heart disease
                    2) Pulmonary hypertension
                    3) High-dose inotropes
            ii. Status 1B signifies a child who is hospitalized but not in the intensive care unit with the following clinical criteria:
                a) Low-dose inotrope support
                b) Younger than 6 months but without hypertension
                c) Growth failure
            iii. Status 2 patients are waiting at home.[1]
I. Waiting for a heart transplant
    1. Children and families should focus on maintaining the child's normal/ideal weight.
        a. Referral to a nutritionist may be necessary to review caloric intake.
        b. Supplemental feedings are often required to provide for adequate growth.
    2. Monitor height weight and head circumference in children younger than 3 years every 2-3 months.
        a. Children should be scheduled for visits to maintain their immunization status.
        b. Some children may require evaluation by physical therapy.
        c. School-age children and adolescents may need hospital- or home-based educational tutoring by certified teachers.
        d. During hospital visits the transplant team (nurses, nurse practitioners, and physicians) should evaluate:
            i. Child's emotional adjustment to waiting for transplantation
            ii. Progress toward developmental milestones
            iii. Plan for the appropriate intervention such as a consult with psychology, physical or occupational therapy, and nutrition

        iv. Child life specialists play an important role in preparing children for painful or invasive procedures.

J. Perioperative management
1. Special surgical options must be considered in children who have undergone previous fontan procedures, hypoplastic left heart syndrome, transposition of the great vessels, or situs inversus.
2. The transplant procedure replaces diseased or absent vascular structures that have been previously treated surgically.
3. Surgical technique is determined by the underlying congenital anomaly and the size mismatch between the donor and recipient.

K. Surgical procedure
1. A median sternotomy incision is made.
2. Patient is placed on cardiopulmonary bypass.
3. Body temperature is cooled to a nasopharyngeal temperature of 18° C.
4. Circulatory arrest is established.
5. Intercardiac lines are placed for pressure monitoring and vascular access.
6. Cardiectomy is performed.
7. The donor heart is prepared and implanted in an orthotopic position
    a. Technique devised by Lower and Shumway.
    b. Known as the biatrial technique.
    c. The left and right atria are sutured *in situ*.
    d. This is followed by reanastomosis of the aorta and main pulmonary arteries to the respective vessels.
    e. Two modifications have been developed to prevent technical problems with atrial arrhythmias.
        i. Procedure is known as the bicaval technique.
        ii. Heart is implanted in a more anatomical position avoiding enlarged atria.
        iii. Separate end to end anastomoses of the caval veins are performed.
        iv. The bicaval technique has been further refined by the addition of a bipulmonary vein technique.
            a) Common cuffs of the pulmonary veins are left in place.
            b) Allows for adaptation in the event of size mismatch between donor and recipient[21]

L. Management of early graft failure
1. Manifests clinically as pulmonary hypertension
2. Medical management includes:
    a. Initiation of vasodilators prior to weaning bypass
        i. Prostaglandin E1 (20-200 ng/kg/min)
        ii. Prostaglandin E2 (1-20 ng/kg/min)
        iii. Nitrous oxide inhalation (5-30 Ppm)
        iv. Milrinon (0.5-2 μg/kg/min)
        v. Isoproterenol (1-5 μg/kg/min)
        vi. Nitroglycerine (5-15 μg/kg/min)
2. Maintain a systolic pulmonary pressure between 30-40 mm Hg.
3. Patients should remain sedated and on mechanical ventilation until the systolic pulmonary pressure normalizes.

4. Serial measurement of pulmonary pressure with left arterial pressure or pulmonary capillary wedge pressures
   i. Assists in the identification of early graft failure.
   ii. If graft failure is suspected, it may be necessary to intervene with either extracorporeal life support (ECMO) or pulsatile assist devices as a bridge to recovery in the immediate transplant period.
      a) Survival rates in pediatric patients with the use of ECMO or an assist device as a bridge to recovery range from 33%-67%.[17, 22]

M. Postoperative management
1. Invasive lines and temporary pacer lines are maintained according to hospital policy.
2. Mediastinal chest tube is connected to a closed sterile chest tube drainage system.
   a. Maintained at -20 cm H_2O suction.
   b. Mediastinal dressing is removed in 24-48 hours.
   c. Monitor site for signs for infection.
3. Foley catheter is removed as soon as possible to prevent urinary tract infections.
4. Patients are suctioned on an as-needed basis until weaned from mechanical ventilation.
5. Once weaned from mechanical ventilation, use of incentive spirometry is encouraged to prevent pulmonary infection.

N. Potential complications of pediatric heart transplantation include:
1. Hemorrhage
2. Decrease in cardiac output
3. Arrhythmias
4. Infection
5. Rejection
6. Malignancies, especially PTLD (post-transplant lymphoproliferative disease)

O. Rejection
1. The gold standard for diagnosing cellular rejection in the heart transplant patient is endomyocaridal biopsy.
   a. The biopsy is performed through a right internal jugular vein or a right femoral approach.
   b. Most centers perform the endomyocardial biopsy in a cardiac catheterization lab.
   c. Some pediatric centers use ECHO-guided biopsies.
   d. Echocardiogram parameters lack sensitivity and specificity in the prediction of histologic rejection.[23]
   e. Although rare, potential complications of endomyocardial biopsy include:
      i. Cardiac perforation
      ii. Tamponade
      iii. Pneumothorax
      iv. Arrhythmias
      v. Tricuspid valve damage
      vi. Loss of peripheral vascular access[22, 24]
      vii. Scar tissue that does not provide an accurate reading of the state of rejection

2. Surveillance biopsy schedules vary from institution to institution approximating a schedule:
   a. Every 10 days for the first month
   b. Every 2 weeks for 2 months
   c. Every 6 weeks for 2-6 months
   d. Every 2-3 months for 6 months
   e. Biannually thereafter
   f. Some institutions are recommending fewer surveillance biopsies with close clinical follow-up and biopsy for symptomatic patients only.
3. Retrospective reviews of biopsies obtained from patients managed with cyclosporine versus tacrolimus immunosuppression
   a. A marked decrease in the number of positive biopsies >1B in patients managed with tacrolimus[24]
   b. Tacrolimus was approved for use in heart transplantation in April 2006.
4. Signs and symptoms of heart rejection may include:
   a. Arrhythmias
   b. Unexplained persistently elevated resting heart rate
   c. Decreased cardiac output
   d. Fatigue
   e. Elevated central venous pressure
   f. Cool extremities
   g. Tachypnea
   h. Diaphoresis
   i. Decreased ventricular compliance
   j. Hepatosplenomegaly
   k. Presence of a third heart sound
   l. Rejection may also present as fever, irritability, or a change in feeding or sleeping patterns.
   m. Unfortunately, few clinical symptoms have been correlated with the endomyocardial biopsy to determine rejection.
5. Rejection is graded according to the revised ISHLT grading system.
   a. See Table 15-4 for complete ISHLT grading of cardiac rejection.
      i. Noninvasive methods to diagnose acute cellular rejection continue to be explored.
   b. Treatment is recommended for grade 3R.
   c. Treatment for acute cellular rejection includes administration of methylprednisolone 10 mg/kg daily for 3 days.

TABLE 15-4

■ International Society of Heart and Lung Transplantation Standard Grading[25]

Grade	Nomenclature
0R	No rejection
1R	Mild or low-grade rejection
2R	Moderate, intermediate-grade acute rejection
3R	Severe, high-grade acute cellular rejection

      i. Repeat biopsy is planned in 1-2 weeks to ensure resolution of rejection.

      ii. The risk of late acute rejection has been documented in several studies.

         a) It has been observed that cardiac transplant recipients do not tolerate the discontinuation of immunosuppression.

         b) Immunosuppression should be considered a lifelong therapy.

  d. Refractory rejection or recurrent rejection is poorly responsive to conventional immunosuppression.

  e. In a multi-institutional study by Chin et al.,[25] risk factors for recurrent rejection in children and adolescents include:

      i. Race (African-American or Hispanic)

      ii. Number of prior incidences of rejection

      iii. Shorter period of time since last episode of rejection

      iv. There is an increased risk of coronary artery disease with recurrent episodes of acute cellular rejection.

  f. A promising innovative strategy to manage refractory rejection includes total lymphoid irradiation (TLI).

      i. Marked improvement has been reported in rejection rates with TLI.

      ii. However, there is an increased risk of CAD and lymphoproliferative disorders associated with TLI.[26]

6. Concomitant medications post-transplantation include:

  a. Antihypertensive agents to prevent hypertension associated with calcineurin inhibitor medication and denervation of the heart

      i. Calcium blocker

      ii. Angiotensin-converting enzyme inhibitor

      iii. Blood pressure in infants and young children must be monitored with the appropriate size cuff, approximately two-thirds of the length of the child's upper arm.

         a) Consider consultation with nephrology if the blood pressure is consistently >95 mm Hg.

      iv. Systolic pressure for an infant 1 year or younger ranges between 70 and 90 mm Hg.

         a) Toddlers between 2 and 3 years have a systolic pressure of 90 mm Hg.

         b) Preschoolers to late school-age have a systolic pressure that reaches 105 mm Hg by age 12 years.

  b. Other medications include cholesterol-lowering medications to prevent coronary artery disease.

  c. Supplementation with magnesium, as needed.

  d. Anemia may be a temporary problem requiring replacement with iron.

  e. Prophylactic treatment against fungal or opportunistic infections

      i. *Pneumocystis carinii* pneumonia with Bactrim (<0.26 m^2 $- 0.52$ m^2 $- 2.5$ ml BID, > 0.53 m$^2 - 5$ ml BID) are required for 6 months post-transplantation.

          ii.   An alternative for sulfa-sensitive patients is inhaled pentam-adine.[22]

P. Cardiac allograft vasculopathy (CAV)

    1. Diffuse and progressive narrowing of the coronary arteries

    2. Major cause of late mortality following cardiac transplantation

    3. Risk factors associated with the development of CAV include:

        a. Older age

        b. Donor recipient race mismatch

        c. Immunosuppressant regimen

        d. Greater lipid abnormalities associated with cyclosporine which may contribute to CAV

        e. The patient with CAV is usually asymptomatic

            i.   Transplanted heart is denervated and will not present with chest pain.

           ii.   Diagnosis is confirmed by coronary angiography that indicates stenosis of 50% or more.

        f. The routine use of pravastatin (0.2 mg/kg/day) reduces cholesterol levels and the associated risk of CAV.[17]

        g. Statins have an added benefit of potentially suppressing the immune system.

Q. Noncompliance

    1. Incidence varies from 6%-30% following pediatric heart transplant.

        a. Highest in school-age children and adolescents

R. Future directions in thoracic transplantation

    1. As fetal echocardiography becomes more accurate, earlier diagnosis of high-risk cardiac lesions is possible.

    2. A new controversial trend of listing a fetus for cardiac transplantation at 36 weeks' gestation further burdens the problems of supply and demand.

    3. Possible temporary or permanent solutions to the long wait on the UNOS list include strategies such as:

        a. Pediatric totally implantable artificial hearts (currently unavailable)

        b. Xenotransplantation

        c. Stem cell biology

        d. Transplantation across ABO barriers[15]

V. Pediatric lung transplantation

A. Progress in lung transplantation has lagged behind other solid organs because of anatomic differences of the bronchial anastomoses and increased risk for bacterial and viral infections.

B. In 1968, Cooley performed the first heart-lung transplant on a 2-month-old child.

    1. Patient survived for 14 hours.[15]

C. In 1987, the first successful lung transplant was performed on a 16-year-old with familial pulmonary fibrosis.[15]

D. Statistics about lung transplantation

    1. According to the UNOS database (2005) 31 children 0-17 years underwent lung transplantation in 2005 with 173 awaiting transplantation.[1]

    2. Most common indications for lung transplantation are:

        a. Cystic fibrosis (36%)

        b. Primary pulmonary hypertension (14%)

      c. Congenital heart disease (11%)

      d. Pulmonary hypertension (7%)[15, 27]

  3. Approximately 60 procedures are performed yearly in the pediatric age group.

  4. Improved survival is noted in recipients who undergo a double lung procedure compared with single lung transplantation.

  5. The leading causes of death continue to be graft failure and infection.

  6. Bronchiolitis obliterans is the leading cause of death (45%) ≥5 years after transplantation.

E. Pretransplant evaluation

  1. Each child is evaluated by the pediatric pulmonologist.

  2. Diagnostic tests include:

      a. Pulmonary function tests (PFTs)

      b. Arterial blood gas

      c. Chest x-ray

      d. Ventilation perfusion scan

      e. Computed tomography scan of the thoracic cavity

      f. Children with cystic fibrosis also undergo an evaluation of the sinuses.

      g. A cardiology consult is obtained to assess anatomic problems such as a patent foramen ovale.

        i. Possible studies include:

          a) EKG

          b) ECHO

          c) Cardiac catheterization

          d) If a cardiac defect is diagnosed, it will be repaired at the time of transplantation.

        ii. Consults for lung transplantation

          a) Similar to potential cardiac transplant recipients, the child and family are evaluated by the social worker and psychologist/psychiatrist.

          b) Infectious disease specialists are usually consulted as part of a lung transplant evaluation.

        iii. Laboratory tests

          a) ABO

          b) HLA typing

          c) HIV

          d) Hepatitis profile

          e) CMV

          f) EBV

          g) Varicella zoster

          h) Chemistry panel

          i) CBC with differential

          j) Triglycerides

F. Listing a child for lung transplantation

  1. The UNOS lung allocation system (LAS) is based on medical information for children older than 12 years.

      a. Age

      b. Height

      c. Weight

      d. Blood type

      e. Lung disease code

      f. O_2 requirements

      g. FVC

      h. 6-minute walk time results

      i. NY heart association class. Waiting time is only used to break a tie between two candidates with a similar score on the LAS.

          i. Children younger than 12 years are listed according to blood type and distance from the hospital.

          ii. Waiting time on the list continues to play a role in decision making for allocation of an organ.

G. Absolute contraindications for lung transplantation

    1. Severe scoliosis

    2. Chest deformity

    3. Severe tracheomegaly or tracheomalacia

    4. Severe transpleural systemic to bronchial artery collateral arteries

    5. *Burkholderia cepacia* genomovar-3

    6. Lower respiratory infection (carries ~50% mortality)

    7. Active malignancy

    8. Active infection (including HIV)

H. Relative risks in pediatric lung transplant

    1. Pan-resistant organisms

    2. Malnutrition

    3. Symptomatic osteoporosis

    4. Daily systemic corticosteroids

I. Surgical contraindications are center-specific.

    1. Previous chemical pleurodesis

      a. May increase intraoperative time and bleeding risks.

    2. Tracheostomy alone is not a contraindication.

      a. It is expected that patients will be decannulated in the early postoperative period.[28]

J. Waiting for a lung transplant

    1. Nutrition

      a. During the waiting period, nutrition must be maximized to prevent muscle wasting.

      b. Referral to a dietitian may be necessary to provide supplementation.

      c. If patients are unable to consume enough calories orally, tube feedings or insertion of a feeding gastrostomy should be considered.

    2. Physical endurance and respiratory requirements

      a. Patients are also referred to physical therapy for endurance and strength training to optimize oxygenation.

      b. Many children require supplemental oxygen prior to transplant through a nasal cannula or mask.

      c. As the lung disease progresses or during sleep, children may require noninvasive positive pressure ventilation with continuous positive airway pressure.

          i. CPAP

          ii. BiPAP

      d. If the child requires additional assistance with breathing, mechanical ventilation is discussed with the family.

          i. Mechanical ventilation prior to transplantation is associated with a poorer outcome post-transplant.

K. Living lung donation
1. Another option is the living related or unrelated lung donation.
    a. This procedure was first used in patients with cystic fibrosis.
    b. Criteria for living related lobar lung transplant includes:
        i. Rapid progression of disease precluding waiting for deceased donor
        ii. Low priority for deceased donor lung transplantation
        iii. Rare ABO compatibility
        iv. High PRA level
        v. Retransplantation
    c. In living donor transplantation, the recipient undergoes bilateral pneumonectomy.
        i. Receives implantation of lower lobes from two healthy donors.
        ii. Children younger than 6 years are not good candidates as the healthy adult donor lobe is too large.
    d. With two living lung donors and a recipient, three simultaneous surgical procedures are carried out requiring a maximum utilization of resources.[28]
L. Size matching lung donors and recipients
1. Size matching of donor lungs is based on height and weight parameters.
    a. May be an inefficient estimate of intrathoracic volume
    b. Calculating the predicted total donor lung capacity compared to the recipient's predicted and real lung capacity may provide a more accurate estimate of recipient intrathoracic volume.
    c. Size mismatch can lead to complications in the postoperative period including:
        i. Atelectasis
        ii. Altered bronchial anatomy leading to retention of secretions
        iii. Increased risk of infection if the lung is oversized
        iv. Undersized lungs can lead to:
            a) Persistent pneumothorax
            b) Hyperexpansion of the lung resulting in increased work of breathing
            c) Limited exercise tolerance[30]
M. Surgical procedure
1. Lungs are removed en bloc
    a. Perfused with a high-molecular, low-potassium dextran solution and epoprestenol
    b. An isolated bilateral segmental lung transplantation performed through a bilateral anterolateral thoracotomy or bilateral transsternal thoracotomy
        i. The "clam shell" incision made at the fourth intercostal space
        ii. In a small child, a double lumen endotracheal tube may not be an option and thus cardiopulmonary bypass (CPB) is often used.

a) The advantages of CPB include:
1) The ability to deflate the native lungs permitting easier dissection
2) The ability to clamp and cleanse the proximal tracheobronchial airway
b) The disadvantages of CPB are:
c) Associated coagulopathy and capillary leak syndrome.[28]

c. If extracorporeal (ECMO) support is required prior to transplantation, it is maintained intraoperatively instead of bypass.
i. In some institutions, ECMO has replaced the use of cardiopulmonary bypass.
ii. After placing the child on bypass, the lungs are removed and implanted in a sequential manner.
iii. An end to end bronchial anastomosis is performed by connecting the donor bronchus with the recipient's bronchus.
iv. Additional suture lines are found at the pulmonary arterial and venous sites.
v. The recipient is weaned from cardiopulmonary bypass or ECMO at the conclusion of the procedure.
a) If the child is unstable, inotropic support may be required.
b) A transesophageal echocardiogram and bronchoscopy may be performed to ensure adequate vascular and bronchial anastomoses.
c) Anterior and posterior bilateral chest tubes are inserted to evacuate chest secretions and obtain accurate measurement of pleural drainage.

N. Perioperative management
1. Similar to liver transplantation, numerous alternative operative techniques to whole lung transplantation have been developed to meet the increasing need for donor lungs.
a. Downsizing of lungs is achieved by:
i. Split-lung/lobar transplantation
a) Left donor lung is separated at the back table.
b) The choice of lobes is determined by chest x-ray.
c) All lobes are usually suitable for transplantation.
d) Estimates the best match of the size of the inflated donor lung and the recipient's chest cavity.
ii. Peripheral wedge section
a) Performed after implantation and full inflation of the lung.
b) Careful estimation of the amount of lung resection necessary is determined prior to stapling of the suture line.
iii. Use of single lobes is warranted if the recipient chest cavity is small or localized pathology is present in one or multiple lobes.
iv. If necessary, these techniques may be combined at the time of transplantation.[29]

O. Postoperative management of pediatric lung recipients
  1. Postoperative care focuses on maintaining pulmonary function.
  2. The lungs are denervated during surgery.
     a. Absent cough reflex from the suture line downward.
     b. Patient must be assisted to mobilize and expel mucus.
     c. This is accomplished by gentle chest physiotherapy or a bed that provides gentle vibration.
        i. Frequent suctioning is required while patient remains intubated.
        ii. Patients are weaned from ventilatory support as quickly as possible, usually within 72 hours.
        iii. Frequent assessment of chest tube function is necessary to prevent air leaks or pleural effusions.
        iv. Initially the suction is kept at low levels (5-10 mm Hg)
            a) Then increased to prevent hemodynamic instability
            b) Chest tubes are removed when fluid drainage is minimal.
        v. Adjustment in caloric intake may be necessary if a pleural effusion persists.[19]
P. Cystic fibrosis (CF) transplant recipients
  1. May require antipseudomonal antibiotics based on recent cultures.
  2. Antifungal agents are added in patients with a history of aspergillus infection.
Q. Non-CF patients can be treated with a first-generation cephalosporin.
R. CMV
  1. If the recipient or donor is positive for cytomegalovirus, the recipient is treated with:
     a. Intravenous ganciclovir for at least 1 week
     b. Then changed to oral valganciclovir for 2-6 months
  2. Prevention of pneumocystis pneumonia
     a. Trimethoprim-sulfamethoxazole is started postoperative week 1 to prevent pneumocystis pneumonia.
     b. Continued for at least 3 months.
     c. Other recommended prevention therapies include:[28]
        i. Oral nystatin or troches to prevent Candida
        ii. Oral acyclovir to prevent herpes simplex infection
S. Rejection
  1. Symptoms of rejection in the lung transplant recipient are vague, presenting with:
     a. Crackles on auscultation
     b. Tachypnea
     c. Wheezing
     d. Decreased breath sounds
     e. Shortness of breath
     f. Activity intolerance
     g. Decreased oxygenation
     h. Decreased pulmonary functions
        i. Documented by a change of >10 % with the portable spirometer
  2. Diagnosis or rejection is made by transbronchial biopsies.
  3. Chronic rejection in the lung transplant recipient is known as obliterative bronchiolitis (OB).

a. An inflammatory process of the small airways that results in:
    i.   Narrowing
    ii. Distortion
    iii. Plugging with granulation tissue
    iv. Scarring of the bronchioles
b. The child develops decreased lung function, shortness of breath, tachypnea, and cough.
c. Risk factors for developing OB include multiple episodes of acute cellular rejection and one episode of severe acute cellular rejection.
d. Prevention or early diagnosis are crucial in the management of OB.
    i.   Management includes:
         a) Frequent clinic visits
         b) Home monitoring of lung function with a handheld spirometer
         c) Formal pulmonary function tests
         d) High-resolution computed tomography
         e) Ventilation/perfusion scans
         f) Gas exhaled measurements
    ii. Diagnosis is confirmed with bronchoalveolar lavage or transbronchial biopsy (TBB).
         a) TBB is the "gold standard" for diagnosing rejection with high sensitivity (61%-94%) and specificity (90%-100%)
             1) Less sensitive in the diagnosis of OB
             2) TBB is obtained through a flexible bronchoscope.
                 i)   Biopsy forceps are passed through the suction channel.
                 ii) Recently a forcep has been developed that fits through the pediatric suction channel with a volume of 0.5 mm^3.
                 iii) Prior to this innovation, pediatric biopsy was performed through a rigid bronchoscope or as an open procedure.
                 iv) At least five samples are obtained from the lower lobe as recommended by the Lung Rejection Study Group.[31, 32]
                 v)   Potential complications of the procedure include:
                      • Bleeding with a platelet count <50,000 mm^3
                      • Pneumothorax
                      • The highest incidence of pneumothorax is found in children that are mechanically ventilated with high PEEP pressures.
                 vi) Similar to heart transplantation the use of surveillance versus clinical biopsy remains controversial and differs from center to center.
                 vii) In a review of the efficacy of surveillance TBB in 11 studies:
                      • Treatable grade rejection was found 13.6% of the time[33]

- Usually within the first 4-6 months after transplant
- TBB may have a more important role in younger recipients of lung transplantation as they are unable to reliably perform reproducible flow-volume loops.

viii) The significance of subclinical rejection in the lung transplant recipient is unclear.

- The use of pulmonary function tests (PFTs) has been suggested as a noninvasive alternative in the diagnosis of OB.
- Sritippayawan et al.[34] reported that $FEF_{25-75\%}$ was the most reliable early predictor of deterioration in lung function in children diagnosed with OB.

ix) Treatment of acute rejection consists of intravenous methylprednisolone 10 mg/kg for 3 consecutive days.

x) Repeat episodes of acute rejection are managed with an antilymphocyte preparation or methotrexate.

T. Postoperative complications of pediatric lung transplantation
1. Frequent complications following lung transplantation include hypertension (37%) and renal dysfunction.
2. In comparison to heart transplant recipients, few lung transplant patients develop hyperlipidemia.
3. Diabetes is common but is most significant in patients with cystic fibrosis.
4. Rates of hypertension and OB increase as survival is extended to 5 years and beyond.
5. Lung transplant recipients are at increased risk for infection because of lifelong immunosuppression and the absence of a cough reflex.

VI. Small bowel transplantation is covered in Chapter 12.

VII. Immunosuppression after pediatric transplantation
A. The goal of immunosuppressant therapy is to avoid overimmunosuppressing the child.
1. The risk of acute rejection is greatest during the first 1-2 months after transplantation.
2. The approach is slightly different for each organ system; however, most recipients receive a combination of drugs.
3. Initially patients receive triple therapy.[28]
   a. Calcineurin inhibitor designed to block T cell cytokine gene expression
   i. Tacrolimus 0.1-0.3 mg/kg/day BID
      a) Initial tacrolimus levels range from 10-15 ng/ml
   ii. Cyclosporine 5-10 mg/kg/day BID
      a) Initially cyclosporine levels are maintained between 300-400 ng/ml
   iii. In stable patients 6 months post-transplant, tacrolimus levels are commonly 5-7 ng/ml and cyclosporine levels are 100-200 ng/ml.

    b. Corticosteroids (1 mg/kg/day tapered)
       i. Block gene transcription
      ii. Inhibit leukotrienes and prostaglandins as part of the inflammatory process
    c. Cell toxins that inhibit purine biosynthesis
       i. Mycophenolate mofetil ($500mg/m^2$) or azathioprine ($2mg/kg$)[16, 20]
    d. Fifty percent of lung transplant recipients receive induction therapy with antilymphocyte globulin, antithymocyte globulin, or an interleukin-2 receptor.
    e. Several new immunosuppressant management strategies include:
       i. The use of induction therapy with antithymocyte globulin
          a) 1.5 mg/kg for 1 to 2 weeks post-transplant
          b) Dose is dependent on age at transplant and lymphocyte count
      ii. Steroid-free maintenance regimens
          a) The goal is to avoid the morbidity associated with corticosteroids.
          b) Providers must carefully identify high-risk patients that are suited to steroid withdrawal or avoidance.
             1) Leonard et al.[35] reported excellent long-term results with steroid withdrawal by 6 weeks after cardiac transplantation.
                i) Fifteen percent of the recipients had moderate rejection in the first 6 months post-transplant.
          c) Similarly, liver transplant recipients are good candidates for steroid withdrawal; timing to initiate the weaning is controversial, with some centers starting at 3 months post-transplant and others waiting for 1 year.
             1) During weaning, it is essential that children be carefully monitored because acute rejection can occur at any time.
    f. Other maintenance options include:
       i. Sirolimus, an mTOR inhibitor (1-5 mg daily)
          a) Sirolimus is contraindicated in the immediate postoperative period following liver transplantation because of the increased risk of thrombotic events.
             1) Sirolimus has been used effectively as a rescue agent in both abdominal and thoracic transplant recipients.
             2) The major complication has been decrease in hematologic parameters and changes in serum lipids.[36]
             3) Sirolimus is noted to have a long half life, approximately 21.5 hours.
      ii. Daclizumab (1 mg/kg times 5 doses every other week).

VIII. Infections post-transplantation
    A. Infection is a common complication and accounts for high levels of post-transplant morbidity and mortality.
    B. Several factors affect the incidence and timing of infection including:

1. The immunosuppressant regimen (dose, duration, and timing)
2. Drug-related neutropenia
3. Presence of invasive objects (catheters) that affect cutaneous barriers
4. Metabolic abnormalities such as:
   a. Malnutrition
   b. Low albumin levels
   c. Viral exposures pre- and post-transplant
   d. Race (African-Americans have lower risk of infectious complications).
C. In the first 30 days post-transplant, infection is related to:
   1. Organisms not eradicated pretransplant
   2. Organisms acquired from the donor
   3. Infections typically found in a general surgical population (pneumonia, bacterial or fungal surgical wounds, or vascular access)
   4. The major infections observed from 1-6 months post-transplant are the viruses of the herpes group.
   5. Signs/symptoms should always be extensively investigated, particularly if the child has pyrexia.
D. Cytomegalovirus (CMV) is the most commonly occurring infection in the early post-transplant period, particularly in the recipient negative/donor positive group.
   1. All recipients are potentially at risk.
   2. There is an association between CMV infection and rejection.
   3. Surveillance +/− prophylactic therapy is dependent on center protocols.
   4. CMV disease presents as fever, hepatitis, enteritis, pneumonia, or a viral syndrome with neutropenia and thrombocytopenia.
      a. In the liver transplant recipient, CMV:
         i. May contribute to vanishing bile duct syndrome
         ii. May accelerate the development of chronic rejection
         iii. May increase the risk of other serious infections such as pneumocystis pneumonia or aspergillosis
         iv. Primary CMV infection occurs secondary to direct exposure to bodily fluids such as saliva, tears, urine, stool, or breast milk.
         v. The highest rate of active transmission is in children aged 12-24 months.[37]
   5. Treatment of CMV is divided into universal prophylaxis versus preemptive therapy.
      a. Universal prophylaxis involves the administration of antiviral agents with or without an immunologic agent to all transplant recipients regardless of CMV risk.
      b. The use of universal CMV prophylaxis delays the onset of symptoms for several months following solid organ transplant.
         i. There is no consensus among experts regarding the best route of administration of antivirals (oral versus intravenous) or the use of immunoglobulin prophylaxis.
         ii. In contrast, preemptive therapy involves focusing effective treatment only to high-risk recipients for a short course of therapy.

a) Preemptive therapy requires the ability to detect changes in the viral load with tests that demonstrated sufficient sensitivity and specificity to differentiate latent from active replicating virus.

b) PCR tests are sensitive predictors of CMV disease in solid organ transplant recipients.

6. Treatment of CMV

   a. Traditionally with intravenous ganciclovir

   b. Cost and safety of long-term administration of ganciclovir has led to other effective management strategies.

   c. Valganciclovir can be used interchangeably with ganciclovir and is administered orally with minimal resistance.

   d. Foscarnet is comparable to intravenous ganciclovir but significant side effects including nephrotoxicity and neurotoxicity are associated with its administration.[37, 38]

7. Epstein-Barr virus is a common viral infection that can lead to post-transplant lymphoproliferative disease (PTLD).

   a. Risk factors of PTLD include:
      i. Lifelong immunosuppression
      ii. Young age at time of transplantation (increasing the risk in liver transplant recipients)
      iii. Recipient seronegative status
      iv. Thoracic transplant recipients have the highest incidence of PTLD.

   b. The incidence is reported between 5%-15% in pediatric solid organ transplants with a mortality rates ranging between 10%-20%.[39]

   c. PTLD can present with polyclonal features increasing the response to reduction in immunosuppression.

   d. Children who present with monoclonal features with a diffuse large B-cell lymphoma such as a Burkitt's lymphoma have no response to reduction in immunosuppression.

   e. Common sites are the tonsil, adenoids, cervical nodes, lung, and abdomen.

   f. Clinical presentation includes:
      i. Fever
      ii. Malaise
      iii. Sore throat
      iv. Abdominal pain
      v. Diarrhea with protein or blood loss in the stool
      vi. Generalized malaise
      vii. Graft dysfunction or headache.

   g. Management includes:[10, 27]
      i. Reduction or withdrawal of immunosuppression
      ii. Surgery
      iii. Antiviral medications
      iv. Cytotoxic T-lymphocytes
      v. Chemotherapy

   h. Serial monitoring of EBV PCR titers has been proposed as a method to reduce the incidence of PTLD.
      i. Every 2-4 weeks in the first 3 months post-transplant
      ii. 1-3 months in patients

        iii.   >3 months post-transplant

        iv.   Patients with >4000 copies/μg DNA or EBV biopsy proven infection undergo weaning of immunosuppression, radiological monitoring with computed tomography, and ongoing assessment of EBV viral loads.[10, 41]

E.   Danzinger-Isakov et al.[42] reported a 26% incidence of bloodstream infection in the first year after lung transplantation.

    1.   The most commonly occurring organisms were:

        a.   Coagulase negative staphylococcus

        b.   *Pseudomonas aeruginosa*

        c.   Candida species

    2.   Infections occurred in the setting of an indwelling catheter.

    3.   Infections that occurred during the first 30 days post-transplant were more frequently associated with death in the first year after transplant.

IX. Living with a solid organ transplant

    A.   Psychosocial adjustment

    B.   Wray and Radley-Smith[40] reported on the incidence of depression and depressive symptoms in children before and 1 year after heart and heart-lung transplantation.

       1.   Children reported more depressive symptoms than their parents reported for them.

          a.   The low level of agreement on depressive symptoms between parents and children with chronic conditions has been previously reported in the literature.

          b.   After transplant, there was a reduction in the mean scores for all participants.

             i.   Girls had higher scores than boys.

          c.   One proposed explanation was the change in physical appearance related to immunosuppressive agents that continue to lead to lower self-esteem and poor body image.

             i.   The authors also noted a difference in depressive symptoms related to the variability associated with the onset of illness; congenital heart disease or cystic fibrosis versus a more acute (cardiomyopathy) illness.

             ii.   For some subjects this resulted in a more realistic understanding that transplant would not "cure" the illness, compared to others who continued to have difficulty coping with not being "normal."

            iii.   Increased psychological distress can lead to behavior problems and anxiety.

            iv.   Early identification of children and families at risk and referral to a psychologist or psychiatrist may help with adjustment in the post-transplant period.[16]

          d.   Many children have significant problems post-transplant such as poor academic performance, low self-esteem, depression, and anxiety.

          e.   Teens are especially at risk for suicidal thoughts, concerns about fertility, financial security, and the inability to obtain health insurance.

          f.   Critical decisions made by all teens regarding sexual behavior and drug and alcohol use have serious potential consequences.

g. Adëback et al.[43] studied cognitive and emotional outcome after liver transplantation.

    i. Found half the children studied had IQ scores <85, indicating learning difficulties that required additional academic resources.

    ii. When compared to age-matched peers, the most significant differences were found in higher function skills such as abstract thinking, logical analyses, and memory.

C. Encourage children to return to school approximately 3 months after transplantation.

    1. Partnerships should be developed with the school to promote successful return of students.

    2. Children should develop new friendships at school, participate in sports (avoiding aggressive contact sports such as football), extracurricular activities, and plan for a future.

X. Infections in pediatric populations

A. Post-transplant solid organ recipients are at risk for common childhood illnesses.

B. Fever should be completely evaluated with a history and physical examination.

    1. A septic work-up is required if no source of the fever is immediately identified including:

        a. CBC

        b. Blood and urine cultures

        c. Metabolic panel

        d. Acetaminophen is the recommended in the treatment of temperature elevation as nonsteroidal anti-inflammatory medications may impair compromised hepatic/renal function.

C. The "common cold" and gastroenteritis occur frequently in the fall and winter months.

    1. If pneumonia is suspected, a chest radiograph should be obtained.

    2. Symptoms of a cough, cold, and GI illness are likely to "hang on" for longer than those in well siblings.

        a. Patients should avoid the use of over-the-counter cold medications, unless they are cleared for use by the physician or the nurse practitioner.

        b. Only recommend cough suppressants if the cough interferes with sleep.

            i. Supportive care to prevent dehydration and keep secretions thin is important.

            ii. If the child is unable to orally hydrate, intravenous fluids should be provided to prevent abnormally elevated calcineurin levels in the face of dehydration.

            iii. Lung transplant recipients who present with a cough should be referred to the transplant center to evaluate for OB.[20]

            iv. Influenza is an acute illness characterized by:

                a) Coryza

                b) Cough

                c) Fever

                d) Pharyngitis

    e) Headache

    f) Myalgia

    g) Malaise

   v. Transplant recipients are likely to experience more short- and long-term complications related to influenza than the general population.

    a) The immunologic response often results in acute allograft rejection.

  D. Infection prevention

   1. Enhanced by encouraging immunization of all household contacts and health care providers on transplant units.

   2. Further study is needed to prove if organ transplant recipients can mount a protective immune response to the live attenuated influenza vaccine.

    a. Antiviral medications in addition to vaccines may be required to prevent or treat influenza.

    b. Infected transplant patients require isolation or should be cohorted to prevent the transmission of virus.

    c. Bronchiolitis obliterans has been reported as a long-term complication of influenza in lung transplant recipients.[44]

  E. Live virus vaccines are contraindicated after transplantation.

   1. Recipients should avoid oral polio, MMR, and varicella vaccine.

   2. Children do not require revaccination but should resume the previous schedule recommended by the American Academy of Pediatrics.

   3. See Table 15-5 for recommendations for immunizations post-transplant.

  F. Antibiotics[16]

   1. Care should be taken when prescribing antibiotics.

   2. Avoid the use of macrolide antibiotics (erythromycin, biaxin, and zithromax)

    a. Interact with calcineurin inhibitors

    b. Elevate levels of tacrolimus and cyclosporine

   3. Indiscriminate use of antibiotics in the transplant recipient increases the risk of developing a fungal infection.

   4. Instruct families to avoid the use of herbal supplements and over-the-counter medications because of the possibility of interacting with immunosuppressant medications.

XI. Endocrine and bone issues post-transplant

  A. Other side effects of immunosuppression include bone disease.

  B. Pretransplant children with end-stage renal disease are at risk for:

   1. Slipped femoral epiphysis

   2. Rickets

   3. Valgus and vargus deformities of the knee

   4. Avascular necrosis of the femoral head, talus, and humerus

  C. Risk factors include:

TABLE 15-5

■ **Vaccinations Pre- and Post-transplant**

Vaccine	Kidney	Liver	Heart/Lung
Polio (inactivated)	Y	Y	Y
Pertussis	Y	Y	Y
Diphtheria	Y	Y	Y
Tetanus	Y	Y	Y
Meningitis (adolescents or splenectomized patients)	Y	Y	Y
BCG (not administered in U.S.)	Y	Y	N
Haemophilus influenzae type B	Y	Y	N
Measles, mumps, rubella	Y	Y	Y
Hepatitis A (2 doses)	N	Y	Y
Hepatitis B (3 doses)	Y	Y	Y
Pneumococcal (2-23 mos)	N	Y	Y
Influenza (yearly)	Y	Y	Y
Varicella	Y	Y	Y

Children should be encouraged to receive all of their vaccines on time. If the schedule is interrupted for transplantation, resume with immunizations at the first missed dose. It is not necessary to revaccinate with all immunizations. Children younger than 2 years should be considered for pavilizumab. AAP recommends 2 doses of PCV7 followed by a single dose of 23V (pneumococcal).

1. Preexisting osteodystrophy found in liver and kidney recipients
2. Exposure to diuretics that effect calcium reabsorption
3. Immobilization secondary to disease severity before and after transplant impact on osseous complications

D. Daniels el at.[45] reported lower bone mineral density in cardiac transplant recipients compared to the general population and documented spinal fractures after transplantation.
   1. Post-transplant risks include prolonged steroid exposure that is exacerbated by retransplantation or repeat episodes of rejection.
   2. Doses as low as 2.5 mg/day of prednisolone over a 7-month period were associated with increased risk of fracture.
   3. Impaired linear growth and delayed pubertal development with the use of steroids are well-documented.
   4. Growth continues to be suboptimal in children continued on prednisone at doses as low as 0.1-0.15 mg/kg/day.

E. Abnormal growth hormone, gonadotropin, and sex hormone secretion has been found following kidney transplantation but is less well-documented in heart and liver transplant recipients.[46]

F.   A quantitative accurate diagnosis with DEXA in the pediatric population is difficult because age, race, and gender-specific normative data sets have not been established.
  1.   Results should be interpreted with caution.
  2.   Younger children have more severe pretransplant growth delay/failure but experience a period of catch-up growth after transplantation.
G.   In the post-transplant period, careful monitoring of growth and pubertal development is required.
  1.   Reduction, early withdrawal, or alternate-day strategies of steroids should be considered.
  2.   Therapies that may prevent bone loss related to steroids include:
    a.   Combined calcium and vitamin D (400 IU ergocalciferol and 500-1000 mg calcium) in low daily doses
    b.   Age-appropriate physical activity
  3.   Periodic measurement of serum 25-hydroxyvitamin D, 1,25 dihydroxyvitamin D, and PTH may be helpful in monitoring for renal insufficiency in solid organ recipients.
H.   End-stage lung disease frequently results in poor somatic growth and malnutrition.
  1.   After transplant, the use of corticosteroids leads to delay in skeletal growth.
  2.   Administration of growth hormone may be appropriate in some patients.
  3.   Other factors that impact on nutrition for the post-transplant lung recipient include:[28]
    a.   Gastroesophageal reflux found in many infants
    b.   Gastroparesis found in adolescents
    c.   Recipients with CF are at high risk for small bowel obstruction that can compromise the transition to oral medications
    d.   Diabetes mellitus
    e.   Children with end-stage liver disease experience growth retardation related to:
      i.   Cholestasis
      ii.   Malabsorption of fats and essential vitamins
      iii.   Enteropathy due to portal hypertension
    f.   Despite evidence of improved growth, Evans[47] reported that 24% of children lag behind peers in height 7 years after liver transplantation.
    g.   Children younger than 2 years and the shortest at the time of transplantation had the largest height gain after transplantation.[48]
XII.   Nonadherence
  A.   While a transplant can dramatically improve a young person's quality of life, it is not without its own set of challenges.
    1.   Adolescents' strong desire to be normal conflicts with the continued reminder of chronic disease that the taking of regular medication engenders.
    2.   Nonadherence with immunosuppressive therapy is a real and common problem affecting approximately 50% of transplant recipients with reports of up to 60% in adolescence.[6]

a. Noncompliant patients may hide their behavior from parents and providers.

b. The result is multiple episodes of acute rejection or chronic rejection that are difficult to treat.

c. Patients may present with symptoms of end-stage disease representative of organ transplanted:
   i. Jaundice (liver)
   ii. Elevated creatinine (kidney)
   iii. Decreased pulmonary function studies (lung)
   iv. Arrhythmias, poor functional capacity (heart)

d. Shemesh[49] reported preliminary data on a clinical adherence monitoring program.
   i. Subjective ratings of adherence by the patient, caregiver, physician, and nurse were compared along with medication blood levels.
   ii. Findings indicated that clinicians were accurate in identifying the most severe cases of nonadherence, but missed patients who continued to do well medically.
   iii. Psychosocial predictors of nonadherence included the existence of post-traumatic stress symptoms described as anxiety, nightmares, or intrusive thoughts.
      a) Treatment involves consultation with a mental health professional and or social worker along with ongoing education.
      b) Clinicians need to be vigilant in assessing children for risk factors and making timely referrals.

XIII. Conclusion

A. Pediatric solid organ transplant is a viable option for infants, children, and adolescents with end-stage disease.

B. Surgical advances and improving immunosuppressant agents and regimens have increased the number of long-term survivors.

C. Addressing the acute and chronic care needs of the children and their families requires a coordinated effort among all transplant professionals.

D. Nurses play a pivotal role in providing continuity of care for the family from diagnoses through the transplant procedure to living with transplantation.

REFERENCES

1. United Network for Organ Sharing (2005). Available at: http://www.unos.org. Accessed November 13, 2005.

2. Albin Gritsch H, Rosenthal JT. The transplant operation and its surgical complications. In Danovitch G. *Handbook of Kidney Transplantation*, 3rd ed. Philadelphia: Lippincott, Williams & Wilkins, 2003.

3. CDC. Epidemiology and Prevention of Vaccine-Preventable Diseases. *The Pink Book*, 8th Edition, 2005.

4. Department of Health. Immunisation Against Infectious Disease. London: HMSO, 1996.

5. Racusen LC, Colvin RB, Solez K, et al. Antibody mediated rejection criteria – An addition to the Banff '97 classification of renal allograft rejection. *Am J Transplant*, 2003; 3: 708-714.

6. Al-Akash S, Ettenger R. Kidney Transplantation in Children. In Danovitch G. *Handbook of Kidney Transplantation*, 3rd ed. Philadelphia: Lippincott, Williams & Wilkins, 2001.

7. 2005 Annual Report. The U.S. Organ Procurement and Transplantation Network and the Scientific Registry of Transplant Recipients. Transplant data 2003-2004.

8. United Kingdom Transplant. Available at: http://www.uktransplant.org Accessed August 12, 2005.

9. McDiarmid SV, Merion RM, Dykstra DM, Harper AM. Selection of pediatric candidates under the PELD system. *Liver Transplant*, 2004; 10: S23-S30.

10. McDiarmid SV. Management of the pediatric liver transplant patient. *Liver Transplant*, 2001; 7: S77-S86.

11. Yudkowitz FS, Chietero M. Anesthetic issues in pediatric liver transplantation. *Ped Transplant*, 2005; 9: 666-672.

12. Okajima H, Inomata Y, Asonuma K, et al. Duct-to-duct biliary reconstruction in pediatric living related liver transplantation. *Ped Transplant*, 2005; 9: 531-533.

13. Ueda M, Egawa H, Ogawa K, et al. Portal vein complications in the long-term course after pediatric living donor living transplantation. *Transplant Proc*, 2005; 37: 1138-1140.

14. Austin MT, Feurer ID, Chari RS, et al. Survival after pediatric liver transplantation. *Arch Surg*, 2005; 140: 465-471.

15. Mendeloff EN. The history of pediatric heart and lung transplantation. *Ped Transplant*, 2002; 6: 270-279.

16. Gabrys CA. Pediatric cardiac transplants: A clinical update. *J Ped Nurs*, 2005; 20: 139-143.

17. Bauer J, Thul J, Valeske K, et al. Perioperative management in pediatric heart transplantation. *Thorac Cardiov Surg*, 2005; 53, Supple2: S155-S158.

18. Berg AB. Pediatric heart transplantation: A clinical overview. *Crit Care Nurs Q*, 2002; 25: 79-87.

19. Teets JM. Nursing care of the cardiothoracic transplant patient. In Wise B, McKenna C, Garvin G, Harmon BJ (Eds.). *Nursing Care of the General Pediatric Surgical Patient*. Gaithersburg, Md: Aspen Publishers, Inc., 2000.

20. Teets JM, Borisuk MJ. Pediatric thoracic organ transplants: Challenges in primary care. *Ped Nurs*, 2004; 30: 23-30.

21. Schmid C, Tjan TD, Scheld HH. Techniques of pediatric heart transplantation. *Thorac Cardiov Surg*, 2005; 53, Suppl. 2: S141-S145.

22. Luikart H. Pediatric cardiac transplantation: Management issues. *J Ped Nurs*, 2001; 16: 320-331.

23. Kirklin JK. Is biopsy-proven cellular rejection an important clinical consideration in heart transplantation? *Curr Op Cardiol*, 2005; 20: 127-131.

24. Levi DS, DeConde AS, Fishbein MC, et al. The yield of surveillance endomyocardial biopsies as a screen for cellular rejection in pediatric heart transplant patients. *Ped Transplant*, 2004; 8: 22-28.

25. Chin C, Naftel DC, Singh TP, et al. PHTS: Risk factors for recurrent rejection in pediatric heart transplantation: A multicenter experience. *J Heart Lung Transplant*, 2004; 23: 178-175.

26. Russo LM, Webber SA. Pediatric heart transplantation: Immunosuppression and its complications. *Curr Op Cardiol*, 2004; 19: 104-109.

27. Boucek MM, Edwards LB, Keck BM, et al. Registry for the International Society for Heart and Lung Transplantation: Seventh official pediatric report--2004. *J Heart Lung Transplant*, Aug 2004; 23(8): 933-947.

28. Mallory GB, Spray TL. Pediatric lung transplantation. *Euro Respir J*, 2004; 24: 839-845.

29. Aigner C, Mazhar S, Jaksch P, et al. Lobar transplantation, split lung transplantation and periopheral segmental reection – Reliable procedures for downsizing donor lungs. *Eur J Cardiothoracic Surg*, 2004; 25: 179-183.

30. Aigner C, Winkler G, Jaksch P, et al. Size-reduced lung transplantation: An advanced operative strategy to alleviate donor organ shortage. *Transplant Proc*, 2004; 36: 2801-2805.

31. Christie JD, Carby M, Bag R, et al. Report of the ISHLT Working Group on Primary Lung Graft Dysfunction Part II: Definition. A consensus statement of the International Society for Heart and Lung Transplantation. *J Heart Lung Transplant*, Oct 2005; 24(10): 1454-1459.

32. Christie JD, VanRaemdonck D, dePerro M. Report of the ISHLT Working Group on Primary Lung Graft Dysfunction Part I: Introduction and methods. *J Heart Lung Transplant*, Oct 2005; 24(10): 1451-1453.

33. Faro A, Visner G. The use of multiple transbronchial biopsies as the standard approach to evaluate lung allograft rejection. *Ped Transplant*, 2004; 8: 322-328.

34. Sritippayawan S, Keens TG, Horn MV, et al. What are the best pulmonary function test parameters for early detection of post-lung transplant bronchiolitis obliterans syndrome in children? *Ped Transplant*, 2003; 7: 200-203.

35. Leonard H, Hornung T, Parry G, Dark JH. Pediatric cardiac transplant: Results using a steroid free maintenance regimen. *Ped Transplant*, 2003; 7: 59-63.

36. Sindhi R, Seward J, Mazariegos G, et al. Replacing calcineurin inhibitors with mTOR inhibitors in children. *Ped Transplant*, 2005; 9: 391-397.

37. Campbell AL, Herold BC. Strategies for the prevention of cytomegalovirus infection and disease in pediatric liver transplantation recipients. *Ped Transplant*, 2004; 8: 619-627.

38. Prasad SA, Kasiske BL, Curtis JJ, et al. Infectious complications post-transplantation. National Institute of Allergy and Infectious Disease National Institutes of Health, 2005.

39. Smets F, Sokal EM. Epstein-Barr virus related lymphoproliferation in children after liver transplantation: Role of immunity, diagnosis and management. *Ped Transplant*, 2002; 6: 280-287.

40. Wray J, Radley Smith R. Depression in pediatric patients before and 1 year after heart or heart-lung transplantation. *J Heart Lung Transplant*, Sep 2004; 23(9): 1103-1110.

41. Lee TC, Savoldo B, Rooney CM, et al. Quantitative EBV viral loads and immunosuppression alterations can decrease PTLD incidence in pediatric liver transplant recipients. *Am J Transplant*, 2005; 5: 2222-2228.

42. Danzinger-Isakov LA, Sweet S, Delamorena M, et al. Epidemiology of bloodstream infection in the first year after pediatric lung transplantation. *Ped Infect Dis J*, 2005; 24: 324-330.

43. Adëback P, Nemeth A, Fischler B. Cognitive and emotional outcome after pediatric liver transplantation. *Ped Transplant*, 2003; 7: 385-389.

44. Vilchez RA, Fung J, Kusne S. The pathogenesis and management of influenza virus infection in organ transplant recipients. *Transp Infect Dis*, 2002; 4: 177-182.

45. Daniels MW, Wilson DM, Paguntalan HG, et al. Bone mineral density in pediatric transplant recipients. *Transplantation*, 2003; 76: 673-678.

46. Saland JM. Osseous complications of pediatric transplantation. *Ped Transplant*, 2004; 8: 400-415.

47. Evans IVR, Belle SH, Wei Y, et al. Post-transplantation growth among pediatric recipients of liver transplantation. *Ped Transplant*, 2005; 9: 480-485.

48. Alonso G, Duca P, Pasqualini T, et al. Evaluation of catch-up growth after liver transplantation in children with biliary. *Ped Transplant*, 2004; 8: 255-259.

49. Shemesh E. Non-adherence to medications following liver transplantation. *Ped Transplant,* 2004; 8: 600-605.

REVIEW QUESTIONS

1. Signs of rejection following pediatric kidney transplantation may include which of the following symptoms?
   a. Increased heart rate, jaundice, and shortness of breath
   b. Hypertension, pain over graft site, hematuria
   c. Proteinuria, increase in weight
   d. All of the above
   e. b and c

2. You are assigned to care for a 12-year-old recipient of a renal transplant that took place 8 days ago. In evaluating your patient's laboratory work and vital signs, you note that the serum creatinine today is 3.4 but was recorded as 1.8, 2.0, and 2.1 on previous days. Which of the following tests would be most important today to evaluate for rejection?
   a. Urine for electrolytes
   b. Renal ultrasound
   c. Spiral CT scan
   d. Renal biopsy
   e. Urine culture for BK viral inclusion cells

3. You are assigned to a 4-year-old female heart transplant recipient. Her transplant was performed 4 days ago and she has been quite unstable with variable vital signs, fever, and alterations in hemodynamics. In your initial assessment of the child, you find her cardiac output to be 2.4, central venous pressure to be 14. She is slightly febrile with a temperature of 38.1° C at 8 AM. Her heart rate is 124 and blood pressure is 88/60. You report your findings to the intensivist and deduce from your knowledge of transplantation that this child may have which of the following problems?

   a. Hyperacute rejection
   b. Chronic rejection
   c. Acute rejection
   d. Bacterial endocarditis

4. In evaluating a child for heart rejection, the most accurate determination of rejection is:
   a. An elevation in the amplitude of the EKG tracing
   b. An endomyocardial biopsy
   c. An echocardiogram to assess left and right ventricular ejection fractions
   d. A MUGA scan to assess LV ejection fraction

5. Your assignment today includes a 6-year-old child who had a liver transplant 3 days ago. She has been reported to be responsive to verbal commands. On your morning assessment, the child is somnolent and difficult to arouse. You check her bilirubin and note a rise from yesterday's findings. Her transaminase is also three times greater than yesterday. She is febrile. You know that these signs are most likely indicative of:
   a. Hyperacute liver rejection
   b. Portal vein thrombosis
   c. Hepatic artery thrombosis
   d. Post-transplant sepsis

6. A liver biopsy has been ordered on a 2-year-old recipient of a living liver transplant from her mother. In preparing the child for a liver biopsy, which of the following tests would be most important?
   a. Liver enzymes
   b. PT/PTT
   c. Hemoglobin level
   d. Protein S

7. In the immediate postoperative care of a child with a lung transplant, you know that suctioning is important due to which of the following?
   a. Lungs are denervated after transplantation.
   b. Lung recipients lack a cough reflex below the site of anastomosis.
   c. Secretions can lead to a severe pulmonary infection.
   d. b and c
   e. All of the above

8. Post lung transplantation, an inflammatory process of the small airways that results in narrowing and scarring of the bronchioles is called:
   a. Hyperacute rejection
   b. Acute rejection
   c. Bronchiolitis obliterans or obliterative bronchitis
   d. Cellular rejection of the alveoli

9. Infections are a major cause of morbidity and mortality in transplant recipients. Factors associated with the development of infections in the immediate postoperative period include which of the following?
   a. Neutropenia secondary to immunosuppression
   b. Invasive monitoring
   c. Malnutrition
   d. All of the above
   e. b and c

10. Post-transplant lymphoproliferative disorder (PTLD) is most commonly diagnosed in children following thoracic transplants. Risk factors for the development of PTLD include which of the following?
    a. Young age at the time of transplantation
    b. Higher doses of immunosuppression
    c. Recipient is EBV negative at the time of transplant
    d. b and c
    e. All of the above

Correct answers:

1. e
2. d
3. c
4. b
5. c
6. b
7. e
8. c
9. d
10. e

16 Psychosocial Issues in Transplantation

KAY KENDALL

MAUREEN I. O'DELL

INTRODUCTION

I. Psychosocial assessments have been an integral component of evaluations of patients for solid organ transplantation since the inception of these programs over 20 years ago.
   A. Despite evolution of the medical and psychosocial criteria for listing patients for transplant, no universal criteria have been adopted across programs; and substantial variability remains, especially with respect to contraindications to transplant.
   B. Research has identified factors that predict survival and quality of life post-transplant.
      1. These findings can help to determine which patients stand to benefit most from this scarce resource.
      2. Transplant programs do not consistently apply existing knowledge in making decisions regarding individual candidates.
      3. Programs are challenged with the need to balance this knowledge with ethical considerations and a desire to serve patients in immediate need.
   C. Evaluation of patients' psychosocial status is part of this decision-making process and is critical in caring for patients and families pre- and post-transplant.
   D. Literature will be reviewed on psychosocial contraindications to listing and predictors of patient outcomes, and describes the difficulties patients and families face before and after transplant and strategies that are useful in promoting better medical management and coping.
II. Psychosocial evaluation and issues: Rationale for psychosocial evaluation
   A. Transplant centers across North America require that patients undergoing transplant evaluations complete psychosocial interviews with qualified social workers.
   B. In some circumstances, other mental health professionals, such as psychologists or psychiatrists may be consulted.[1]
      1. Exceptions to this requirement at some centers are related to large patient volume, inadequate staffing, and approach to care.

2. Even in these instances, there is usually an opportunity for referral of patients for assessment by social workers, psychiatrists, or psychologists if concerns are noted.

C. In the United States, an interview with a social worker is required by Medicare and many state Medicaid programs.

1. Private insurance companies may request information from such an interview before they will approve coverage for transplantation.

2. Although the timing, format, manner of obtaining the information, and its use varies among programs and across centers, the content of the interview is fairly uniform.[2-7]

D. The pretransplant psychosocial evaluation generally takes the form of a structured assessment conducted primarily to provide the team with information to assist them in distinguishing those patients likely to benefit from transplant from those whose risk levels may be too high.

1. Alerts the care-giving team to those eligible candidates most likely to experience individual or family problems during the course of the transplant process.

2. Reveals needs for intervention by other members of the transplant team as they work to prepare the individual for listing, eventual surgery, and reintegration into society.[6]

3. Permits the opportunity for the provision of education and counseling related to the transplant process.

4. This initial interview between patient and social worker serves to establish what may be an ongoing relationship.

   a. The detailed information gathered in this interview is helpful as these patients may be followed for many years by the same clinician and transplant team.

   b. Psychosocial evaluation of potential organ recipients helps to ensure that candidate selection is appropriate, that patients are fully prepared for transplantation, and that the team is addressing the patient's psychosocial needs.[3]

E. During the post-transplant period, psychosocial assessment may be less structured.

1. Tends to focus on the patient's adjustment to transplant or needs during a particular phase of care.

2. Attention is primarily to specific, presenting concerns and appropriate treatments and interventions.

3. Conducted to evaluate the patient's overall functioning and perceived quality of life, which are viewed as primary indicators of successful transplantation.[1]

IV. Process

A. Formal pretransplant psychosocial assessments may vary but generally occur in tandem with the medical work-up.

1. Follows an outline specific to the requirements and preferences of the particular assessor and program.

2. The clinician typically meets with the patient for 1 to 2 hours.

   a. Some programs may require that a support person be present for all or part of the session.[7]

   b. Professional translators are recommended for interviews with patients not proficient in English, as patient responses may not be accurately conveyed by family members.

3. The interview is recorded in a structured format using an outline.

a.   Findings may be shared with the team verbally during formal or informal assessment meetings or by means of the written report.

b.   A copy of the evaluation is placed in the medical chart or in an electronic chart.[8]

4.   Post-transplant psychosocial assessments usually focus on a specific area of patient need disclosed by the patient or identified during a hospital admission or an outpatient clinic visit or may be initiated by the patient.

5.   Findings are discussed with the team; intervention is instituted; and outcomes are recorded as previously described.

V.   Components of the pretransplant psychosocial assessment

A.   The content of the evaluation is rooted in the literature.[1-7] Basic elements are described below:

1.   Demographic data:

a.   Information on the patient's identity and background is obtained early in the assessment interview.

i.   More sensitive areas such as education level may be addressed towards the end of the session when the patient is more comfortable with the interviewer.

ii.   Because information must be understandable to patients and presented at an appropriate level of complexity, the level of attained education and English language proficiency is ascertained.

b.   Name, address, telephone number, and medical record number provide contact information.

c.   Marital status, age, and gender are included as factual information.

d.   Faith is recorded for those indicating that religious involvement represents an important aspect of life, and any beliefs affecting care are noted.

2.   Social history

a.   A family/relationship history gives a snapshot of the patient's family of origin, current family and living arrangements, friendships, and community and religious networks.

b.   This history includes information regarding family members and friends who are positive factors in the patient's life, as well as persons with whom the patient has conflicts or from whom the patient receives little support.

c.   Awareness of any difficult or unstable relationships is useful to the team, as these relationships could create concerns for the patient or become barriers to medical care or patient compliance.

d.   Patients may discuss important past events, quality of relationships or histories of abuse and losses, all of which are significant to the team in helping them understand patient concerns and stressors.

e.   For patients with dependent children or dependent adults, plans for the children/adults should be discussed and families counseled regarding the needs of the children for emotional support, planning, and resources.

3.   Support systems

    a. One important assessment goal is to identify specific individuals or organizations that will be able to offer emotional support and practical help such as:

        i. In-home support and transportation

        ii. Their intended roles

        iii. Any gaps in the plan that could become barriers to pre- or post-transplant care.

            a) Where there is insufficient support, the social worker helps the patient to assess the available alternatives and advocates with government authorities and community agencies.

            b) The social worker counsels patients about these options as they prepare for surgery.

    b. Names and contact information for the next of kin and any designated substitute decision-maker are essential to document.

    c. Patients are also advised to discuss their wishes for life support and decisions related to end of life care in the event of a poor transplant outcome and their inability to make their own health care choices.

4. Motivation for transplant and expectations

    a. Patient motivation and readiness to go forward with the transplant process must be understood.

        i. In some cases, patients may perceive that their current health status does not yet warrant transplantation.

        ii. Others may be having difficulty in resolving conflicting feelings, beliefs, or values.

        iii. They may be responding to pressure from others or be extremely fearful.

    b. Where motivation appears to be low, the reasons need to be determined and a plan formulated.

    c. Patients' understanding of transplant risks and possible complications must be determined.

        i. Patients must have realistic expectations of transplantation.

            a) Transplant teams must ensure that potential recipients fully understand the risks of transplantation.

            b) Transplant recipients need to be aware that the organ they receive may not function optimally or insure them a determined period of survival.

            c) Surgical and medical risk factors must be discussed, as well as the possible side effects of immunosuppressive medications.

        ii. A finding that a patient's expectations of transplantation are not realistic indicates the need for intervention and additional education.

        iii. Patient ambivalence requires further assessment.

5. Coping/response to illness

    a. Patients' past and current adherence to medical regimens and response to their current illness is assessed.[9]

    b. The appropriateness of their efforts to seek medical assistance in the past and to follow through with medical advice may give some indication of their ability to comply with essential future care.

    c.   Understanding how patients view their illness, their sources of emotional and psychological strength, and areas of perceived vulnerability help guide team interventions.

6. Mental and psychiatric history and current status

    a.   Information regarding past and current mental and psychiatric status is needed to assist the team in determining suitability for organ transplantation.

        i.   Identifies areas of concern requiring immediate or possible future intervention.

        ii. Determines if the patient is fully oriented, has appropriate insight, and displays sound judgment.

    b.   Mental status affects patients' ability to understand the transplant process, appreciate their own responsibilities for self-care, and give informed consent.

    c.   Cognitive status may be affected by such factors as the presence of end-stage liver or heart disease or may be a result of pre-existing conditions.

        i.   Impaired cognitive function requires further assessment.

    d.   A psychiatric history should include the presence of mood or anxiety disorders, evidence of personality disorder, suicide attempts or suicidal ideation, psychotic episodes, history of mental health hospitalizations, and willingness to adhere to treatment.

    e.   Patients experiencing such common somatic complaints as panic attacks, depression, or serious sleep disturbances will require further evaluation and possible treatment by psychiatry in preparation for the stresses of the transplant process.

    f.   Those with serious psychological instability or dysfunction may be considered too high risk for transplantation.

7. Substance use history and current status

    a.   A history is taken of the patient's past and current use of alcohol, tobacco, holistic or over-the-counter drugs, prescription medications, and illegal drugs.

        i.   Abuse or dependence on substances may be a contraindication to transplant in some programs, as it may have caused or contributed to the organ failure or may become a source of potential damage to the transplanted organ.[2]

        ii. Many lung and heart transplant programs require patients to be abstinent from smoking for a specified time prior to listing for transplant.

        iii. Heart, liver, and lung transplant programs may defer listing patients until they have ceased alcohol consumption for a prescribed time and completed a treatment program.[10]

8. Resource information

    a.   Questions regarding employment status, income level, and source may reveal areas of potential financial concern.

    b.   Insurance coverage for medication, oxygen, hospital admissions and clinic visits, and surgical and medical expenses must be determined, and any additional financial needs clarified prior to transplantation.

         i.   Patients are advised about procedures for obtaining these necessary resources.

    c.   Social workers are able to advocate on their behalf with institutions and community agencies when requested do so by patients.

    d.   Additional expenses faced by patients may include some cost for relocation, loss of income for patient and family members, travel, parking, meals away from home, and care for dependent members of the family.

    e.   Patients and their families need to be aware of the financial implications of the transplant process so they are able to plan appropriately.

9.   The ultimate outcome of the pretransplant psychosocial evaluation is to permit the team to enter into informed decision-making regarding patient selection.

    a.   Identification of potential patient vulnerabilities allows monitoring and/or intervention by the team throughout the complex and demanding transplant process.

    b.   Identification of any gaps in the individual's plan enables the team to assist in overcoming potential barriers to treatment.

VI. Assessment instruments

  A. When solid organ transplant programs began in the early 1980s, a variety of assessment methods were used to evaluate patients' psychosocial status.

    1.   An interview was completed by a social worker and a psychiatrist.[11]

    2.   It was not unusual for patients to be evaluated by a psychologist or a neuropsychologist, or to undergo an evaluation with a chemical dependency counselor.

    3.   As teams gained more experience with the evaluation process, the assessment process was streamlined to avoid redundancies or unneeded services.

  B. Today at most North American transplant centers, a social worker completes an initial interview and then determines what other professionals need to be consulted to complete the assessment process.

    1.   All patients may not need a chemical dependency evaluation, nor do all patients require a battery of psychological/neuropsychological tests.

    2.   Standardized assessments of psychosocial status are useful in evaluating some patients and in conducting research on quality of life and outcomes pre- and post-transplant.

  C. Standardizing psychosocial evaluations

    1.   Mary Ellen Olbrisch, PhD, and James Levenson, MD, of the Medical College of Virginia, developed the Psychosocial Assessment of Candidates for Transplantation (PACT) in the late 1980s with the goal of standardizing psychosocial criteria.[12]

    a.   The measure was developed to identify psychosocial criteria and to assess how centers viewed the importance of these criteria in the selection process.

    b.   The PACT scale has also been used as a way of rating strengths of candidates in pre- and post-transplant quality of life studies.

      c. The tool has been used by a number of centers to study the clinical decision-making process and to help with consistent interpretation of criteria.[13]

          i. This measure consists of eight items with an initial rating and a final rating score.

          ii. The initial and final ratings are on a scale of 0-4 with the lower number showing the more problematic or concerning behavior.

              a) The information to rate candidates is obtained in the psychosocial evaluation.

              b) After the interview is complete, one general rating is made before considering each of the individual ratings and then there is a final rating.

          iii. The eight items measure aspects of psychosocial functioning including support, lifestyle factors, compliance, psychological health, and substance abuse.

          iv. The scale has been shown to have a high degree of inter-rater reliability.

2. Another standardized measure used to assess psychosocial status is the Transplant Evaluation Rating Scale (TERS).[14]

      a. Developed in the early 1990s, the TERS consists of 10 items, rated 1-3.

      b. Like the PACT scale, the items pertain to psychiatric history, substance abuse, and compliance and health behaviors; and the score is the sum of the item ratings.

3. Several other measures are also frequently used to evaluate patients prior to transplant and to assess post-transplant outcomes.

      a. The Beck Depression Inventory is a self-rating instrument used widely in both medical and psychiatric settings.[15]

      b. The Millon Behavioral Health Inventory (MBHI) is another self-report instrument designed to assess psychological adjustment and has been used to predict post-transplant outcome.[16]

      c. The Health Status Questionnaire (HSQ) is a measure of physical health and of the impact of the patient's physical condition in the areas of social functioning, mental health, fatigue, and pain.[17]

      d. The Psychosocial Adjustment to Illness Scale (PAIS) rates patients' orientation to health care, functioning at work and home, and sexual and social functioning.[17]

      e. The Short Form 36 (SF-36) is another widely used instrument designed to evaluate health-related quality of life.[18]

          i. This self-administered assessment of health status measures several health-related domains, such as physical status, social functioning, pain, and role limitations due to physical problems.

      f. Three other commonly used psychiatric diagnostic measures are:

          i. Structured Clinical Interview for DSMIV (SCID)[19] which measures the patient's response to recent life events and three categories of post-traumatic stress disorder (PTSD)

          ii. Impact of Event Scale (IES-R),[20] which measures the patient's response to recent life events and three categories of PTSD

           iii. Symptoms Checklist 90 (SCL-90),[21] a self-report instrument that assesses multiple types of psychological distress

VII. Contraindications to transplant and factors associated with poor outcome
- A. Psychosocial assessments have been a component of transplant evaluations since the inception of solid organ transplant programs.[22]
  1. Initially, transplant team members were unclear how the information obtained from these assessments would be applied to the decision-making process and how the assessment findings could impact post-transplant survival.
  2. Teams felt that it was important to know about patients' support systems, how they coped and took care of themselves, and about past or present behaviors that might lead to medical management problems after transplant.
  3. However, the assessments also raised ethical dilemmas such as:
     a. Concerns that transplant programs were making judgments about individual worth.
     b. Inconsistencies among programs.[22]
     c. Variable views on contraindications to transplant
        i. Variations in experiences in following patients after transplant have led to differing perspectives on candidacy.
     d. Denying transplant on the basis of psychosocial concerns alone.
        i. Most transplant teams have been uncomfortable with denying a physiological need based on psychosocial concerns.
        ii. Clinical experience supports the need to consider some patients as being at high risk for complications or death following transplant, though few studies have formally researched the criteria used to make these judgments.
        iii. As morbidity and mortality rates have changed over the years, medical and psychosocial criteria for denying transplants to some patients have evolved.
  4. In commenting on the responsibility to fairly evaluate patients and to predict outcome, Olbrisch and Levenson[22] noted that "the science of prediction cannot be divorced from philosophical questions" (p. 239).
     a. Olbrisch and Levenson[23] began researching the psychosocial evaluation process in the early 1980s.
     b. They noted that psychosocial screening was a component of patient evaluation at most transplant centers, but that criteria for determining candidacy for transplant were informal, unpublished, and likely varied from center to center.
     c. In the early 1990s, they surveyed the evaluation methods used at 204 heart transplant programs.[23]
        i. They asked the centers to list psychosocial criteria and to rate each criterion as a relative or absolute contraindication to transplantation.
        ii. Examples of the psychosocial criteria listed by the centers were a psychiatric diagnosis, smoking, substance use, obesity, and noncompliance with medical recommendations.
        iii. The study found agreement between the centers on several *absolute contraindications* including:
           a) Active schizophrenia
           b) Current suicidal ideation

        c) History of multiple suicide attempts

        d) Dementia

        e) Current substance abuse

    iv. The centers disagreed with respect to the use of criteria such as smoking, controlled schizophrenia, or affective disorders.

5. In a second study, Olbrisch and Levenson[11] expanded the groups surveyed to include liver and kidney transplant teams along with heart programs.

    a. This study found that heart transplant programs applied the most stringent psychosocial selection criteria and that kidney programs were the least restrictive.

    b. Significant variations were found across programs.

6. As the number of solid organ transplants performed increased in the 1980s, researchers began to investigate pretransplant behaviors as predictors of post-transplant outcomes.

    a. Would a patient who did not take medications and follow through with a doctors' recommendations pretransplant do the same post-transplant?

    b. Would the lack of a support system affect a patient's survival and would a certain psychiatric diagnosis lead to more medical management problems post-transplant?

7. In one earlier study at the Oregon Health Sciences University, researchers failed to find an association between pretransplantation psychological distress and mortality, graft rejection, or infections.[24]

    a. This study followed patients 3 months post-transplant.

    b. Pretransplant coping factors were based on the results of the SCL-90.

8. Other studies, however, have demonstrated that some patients are at higher risk for poor outcomes than others.

    a. A study completed at Columbia Presbyterian Medical Center in New York City prospectively reviewed psychosocial evaluation data from 125 adult patients who underwent cardiac transplantation from 1992-1994.[25]

        i. They examined a number of variables such as compliance, substance history, and global psychosocial risk.

        ii. They correlated these factors with post-transplant survival outcomes, compliance, and episodes of rejection and infection.

        iii. Psychosocial factors predicted the severity of compliance problems post-transplant:

            a) Number of rejection episodes.

            b) Early development of coronary lesions in the transplanted heart.

        iv. Associated psychosocial factors were not associated with the number of post-transplant infections or survival.

        v. The strongest factor contribution to "global assessment of risk" was a history of substance abuse.

            a) Patients with known substance histories who had short remission periods and had only stopped using substances when their condition declined were especially high risk for poor compliance.

b.   A second study documenting pretransplant risk factors was conducted at the Oklahoma Transplantation Institute Baptist Medical Center in Oklahoma City, Oklahoma.[26]
   i.   This study examined pre- and post-transplant characteristics in 53 patients.
   ii.   Patient data were obtained from audits of charts, physician assessment, and psychosocial evaluations completed by the social worker.
   iii.   Phone interviews were conducted post-transplant by the social worker to assess patient's psychosocial status.
   iv.   The researchers concluded that psychosocial difficulties prior to heart transplantation were likely to continue post-transplant.
      a)   During the first year post-transplant, the only association observed was between pretransplant psychiatric problems and post-transplant infection rates.
      b)   In the second year post-transplant, the study found that both noncompliance and psychiatric problems present prior to transplant were associated with increased morbidity.

c.   A further investigation by Chacko et al.[17] examined the correlation between pretransplant Axis I and II diagnoses and post-transplant outcomes.
   i.   The study sample was comprised of 311 organ transplant candidates at Methodist Hospital in Houston, Texas.
      a)   47% candidates for heart transplantation
      b)   35% candidates for kidney transplantation
      c)   7% candidates for liver transplantation
      d)   10% candidates for lungs or heart/lung transplantation
   ii.   The patients completed in-depth pretransplant psychosocial evaluation and psychometric testing.
      a)   Sixty percent of the patients met criteria for an Axis I diagnosis and 31% met criteria for an Axis II diagnosis.
      b)   The Axis I diagnosis of past or current substance abuse and problematic alcohol use was associated with noncompliance, while the Axis II diagnosis of personality disorder was related to both global noncompliance and lack of adherence to recommendations regarding diet, smoking, and medication management.
      c)   Psychosocial adjustment and health status measures were related to Axis I disorders, while Axis II diagnosis of personality disorders were associated with measures of behavioral noncompliance.
      d)   The researchers did not conclude that patients with certain psychiatric diagnoses shouldn't be transplanted, but focused instead on the need for pretransplant interventions with these high-risk groups.

d.   Mary Amanda Dew, PhD, an epidemiologist in the Department of Psychiatry at the University of Pittsburgh Medical Center, has conducted extensive research on the psychosocial status of patients pre- and post-transplant.

    i.   This research has included quality of life post-transplant and as well as pre- and post-transplant psychiatric disorders.

    ii.   In a prospective study of 154 individuals who underwent heart transplantation between 1989-1994, Dew and colleagues[27] investigated rates and predictors of depression and anxiety during the first year after heart transplant.

        a)   They conducted interviews with post-transplant patients three times in the first year after transplant.

        b)   Diagnoses included major generalized anxiety disorder, adjustment disorder with depressed and/or anxious mood, and PTSD.

        c)   They identified three potential risk factors for psychiatric disorder after transplant:

            1)   Psychiatric history

            2)   Quality of social supports

            3)   Coping strategies and self-image

        d)   Major depressive disorder was the most frequent psychiatric diagnosis in the post-transplant group.

        e)   The rate of PTSD was also high.

        f)   Patients with post-transplant depression were more likely than those with no psychiatric diagnosis to have a pretransplant psychiatric history.

        g)   The researchers summarized literature suggesting that medically ill patients with psychiatric disorders have higher rates of economic expenditures and long-term noncompliance than patients without these disorders.

e.   In another study by the Pittsburgh group, Dew and colleagues[28] examined psychiatric status as a predictor of long-term medical outcomes.

    i.   In this study, 145 individuals who underwent cardiac transplant between 1989 and 1994 were interviewed three times in the first year after transplant.

    ii.   Close attention was paid to compliance with medical recommendations in the first year after transplant.

    iii.   Medical morbidity and mortality were then tracked via chart reviews for 3 years after transplant.

        a)   The results showed that patients with persistently elevated levels of depression, anger, and hostility were four to eight times more likely to develop coronary artery disease (CAD) during the follow-up period.

        b)   Patients who met criteria for PTSD were over 13 times more likely to have died by 3 years after transplant.

        c)   Failure to take medications as prescribed predicted graft rejection and coronary artery disease (CAD).

        d)   Morbid obesity increased the risk of CAD seven-fold.

        e)   In summary, findings revealed that specific areas of medical noncompliance and specific types of psychiatric problems during the first year after transplant were associated with graft rejection and CAD 1-3 years after transplant.

  f. Despite progress in identifying psychosocial factors that may impact post-transplant quality of life and survival, centers continue to vary in the medical and psychosocial criteria they apply to determine candidacy for transplantation.[29]

   i. This cross-sight variation likely reflects the philosophy of the director and members of the team, the number of transplants, survival rates, and recent problematic cases.

   ii. Factors previously considered absolute contraindications may no longer be viewed in that manner.

    a) Body mass index may be ignored if the program has been successful in transplanting obese patients.

    b) A program that has transplanted a number of individuals with histories of recurrent depression may alter this practice if post-transplant outcomes are poor in these patients.

    c) Allocation of transplants to patients who stand to benefit most from these scarce resources remains a fundamental responsibility of the transplant team.

VIII. Patient and family stressors and psychosocial responses to transplantation

  A. Although transplant patients must cope with the waiting period, surgery, and post-transplant recovery, the lives of their families and supports are also significantly disrupted.

  B. Patients often comment that they feel transplantation is more difficult for their families than for themselves.

  C. Each phase of the transplant process presents unique challenges to patients and their support persons.

   1. During the evaluation phase, patients wonder if transplantation will be the recommended treatment or if they will have to make end of life decisions.[30]

    a. Patients report relief after treatment plans have been determined, but then face new uncertainties.

    b. While awaiting transplant, patients may experience:

     i. Deterioration of health

     ii. Increasing disabilities

     iii. Feelings of being a burden

     iv. Worries over finances[31]

     v. Fear of dying

     vi. Distress from seeing fellow patients suffer

     vii. Disappointment from missed opportunities for transplant

     viii. Guilt relating to knowing that someone must die for the patient to receive a suitable organ[32]

    c. Patients are called upon to cope with the prospect of dying while hoping and fighting for extended life.

   2. Spouses and other support persons are required to provide ongoing emotional and physical care to a slowly dying loved one, often with little help or respite.[33]

    a. They are called upon to put their own lives on hold and to ignore personal needs.

    b. These people typically cannot go forward with their lives until the transplant takes place.

    c. Spousal support has a beneficial effect on health and quality of life.[34]

d. Spousal relationships can be a stabilizing factor for pre- and post-transplant patients.[35]

3. The strength of a relationship may be tested as couples have to deal with time apart and the lack of privacy and intimacy afforded by the hospital setting.
   a. As the patient's condition worsens, family responsibilities shift.
   b. A spouse may be required to return to work and children may have to shoulder more household duties.[31, 36]
   c. Patients question their role in the family and their ability to contribute meaningfully to family well-being.
   d. For this reason, the transplant team monitors family coping throughout the transplant process.

4. Most solid organ transplant candidates wait at home for transplant until they are notified of an appropriate donor.

5. There are times when cardiac transplant patients wait in the hospital for transplant.
   a. Hospitalized patients are typically treated with intravenous medications such as milrinone or dobutamine.
   b. Waiting periods for heart transplants vary from days to weeks and months.
   c. Pre-heart-transplant patients in North America who are supported on certain mechanical assist devices may have the option to wait at home for their transplant if they are stable or are staying in a housing area near the hospital campus.
   d. Those patients waiting for kidney, liver, or lung transplants typically wait at home, but may be hospitalized for episodic treatment.
   e. The hospital setting can become a second home for cardiac patients who await transplant in the hospital.

6. The Cleveland Clinic Foundation (CCF) in Cleveland, Ohio has a well-established transplant center.
   a. The cardiac transplant program has performed over 1,100 heart transplants since 1984.
   b. This center hospitalizes inotrope-dependent heart transplant patients in the Transplant Special Care Unit, a 34-bed nursing area providing care to pre- and post- heart, liver, lung, kidney, and kidney/pancreas patients.
   c. At any given time, 5-15 patients remain in this unit awaiting transplant.
      i. They must cope with the many stresses of the hospital environment such as noise, lack of privacy, and interrupted sleep.
      ii. They develop relationships with other transplant patients and become important supports for one another.
      iii. The patients in this unit take on many aspects of their own care, such as taking medications, daily recording of weight, and intake and output of fluids.
      iv. They participate in a cardiac rehabilitation program and dress in street clothes.
      v. Because many of these patients do not live in the Cleveland area, family members and other support people may visit infrequently.

       a) Their families may be with them during the evaluation phase, but most families must return home during the waiting period.

       b) The first trip home for the family is especially difficult, as family members may feel that they are deserting their loved ones.

    vi. Typically, after the first 2 to 3 weeks in the hospital, patients and families adapt to the hospital routine and their separations from family and friends.

       a) Patients receive support from other patients, the nursing staff, the transplant team, and hospital volunteers.

       b) The unit provides a weekly education class on the nursing unit for pretransplant patients, those recently transplanted, and their families.

       c) A monthly dinner is organized off the nursing floor for these patients, as well as for post-transplant patients still in the hospital or living in the area.

D. The immediate post-transplant phase is highly variable in duration.

  1. During this phase, patients receive complex, highly technical care in an unfamiliar hospital unit.

  2. Despite the relief of receiving a transplant, patients and their families remain apprehensive and may wonder when they can feel assured that the transplant has been successful.[37]

  3. Patients experience discomfort in the early postoperative period related to incision pain, complications and side effects from post-transplant medications, and the consequences of confinement in the intensive care unit.

  4. Support people can do little at this time, as the transplant team manages acute care issues.

  5. Uncertainty with regard to the patient's recovery may be especially difficult in programs where treatments, such as dialysis, are not available should transplant fail.

  6. However, in the United States, hospitals may not perform kidney transplants or other solid organ transplants if dialysis is not available at their center.

  7. Concerns related to provision of critical care and to infection and organ rejection are common during the early postsurgical period.

  8. As activity increases and pain decreases, patients are moved to a regular nursing floor.

  9. The days preparing for hospital discharge are filled with activities related to medical management, building the patient's strength, and educating patients and family members on procedures for home care.

  10. Patients often note mood lability in response to treatment with steroids.

    a. This problem that can be manifest in tearfulness, irritability, increased anxiety, and sleep disturbance.[38]

    b. Severe reactions such as a steroid induced psychosis are rare.

  11. The goal for the solid organ transplant patient at hospital discharge is for patients to be medically stable, ambulating, and knowledgeable about their medications and self-care responsibilities.

E. During the early post-transplant phase (0-3 months), patients are adapting both physically and psychologically to having a new and functioning organ.
   1. Concerns arise related to:
      a. The origin and condition of the organ
      b. The possibility of rejection and infection
      c. New medical regimens
      d. The physical and emotional side effects of immunosuppressive medications
      e. An altered body image
      f. Changes in family and personal relationships.[39]
   2. The return home from the hospital will be quite different for patients who waited at home for transplant than for those who had long hospital stays.
      a. Adjustment to the home setting is also impacted by post-transplant length of stay.
      b. Patients hospitalized for extended periods may feel heightened anxiety as they contemplate leaving the security of the hospital environment.
      c. The next phase of post-transplantation recovery begins with the patient's return home.
         i. As a patient's family stated, "We got used to him not being home, now we have to figure out what to do when he is back."
         ii. How do the patient and family re-establish a "normal" life?
         iii. Patients are no longer sick in the way they were pretransplant, but are now required to manage a chronic medical condition.[37]
      d. Routine follow-up visits with the transplant team facilitate patient adjustment.
         i. Monitoring how the patient and family are coping at home is an important component of these visits.
         ii. Ongoing transplant support groups may also be beneficial for the patient and family.
            a) Families and patients are sometimes surprised that day-to-day issues and problems resurface as post-transplant life becomes more routine.[40]
               1) These problems may have seemed unimportant while the patient was awaiting transplant, but they come to the forefront again when the patient returns home.[37]
               2) Spouses or other family members may have harbored hopes that transplantation would transform patients' personality or adjustment; hence the resurgence of prior conflicts can be discouraging.
               3) Spouses may express frustration that patients are not as grateful as would be expected about their transplants, or spouses may be concerned about how patients are caring for themselves.
      e. Frequent post-transplant follow-up visits are scheduled immediately after discharge from the hospital.

          i.   Although some patients resent continuing to have to spend so much time at the hospital, frequent contacts with the treatment team can also be comforting, and these visits gradually decline in frequency.

    f.   Hospital readmissions are a common occurrence after transplant for patients who receive solid organs.

        i.   Patients may delay reporting symptoms to the treatment team because they are afraid of being readmitted to the hospital.

        ii.   They may worry about ever returning home if rehospitalized for serious complications.

    g.   In the first year following transplantation, 17.3% of patients in one study experienced mood disorder, 13.7% showed evidence of PTSD, and 10% had adjustment disorders.[41]

        i.   Because of the high risk of these psychosocial outcomes, the health care team provides post-transplant patients with the opportunity to share their feelings and concerns.

        ii.   Timely supportive interventions can then be offered to enhance patient adjustment.

    h.   As they progress through the first post-transplant year, many patients are required to return to work.[42]

        i.   Concerns for returning to work include:

            a)   Physical demands of the job

            b)   Risk for infections from exposure to groups of people

            c)   Inability to perform job as they did prior to becoming ill.

        ii.   Other patients relish their return to work and view it as a sign of good post-transplant recovery.

        iii.   These patients may welcome the opportunity to begin contributing again to the financial well-being of their families.

        iv.   Some may require job retraining and struggle to reenter the job market.

            a)   Job reentry is often easiest for individuals who have been unemployed for only a brief time pretransplant and are able to return to previously held positions.

            b)   A concern frequently mentioned by post-transplant patients is the potential of returning to work and losing disability insurance, and for U.S. citizens and legal permanent residents the possible loss of disability insurance and Medicare and Medicaid benefits.

3.   Patients describe recovery from transplant as a multi-stage process, with dramatic improvements 4-6 weeks post-transplant, and then again 3, 6, 9, and 12 months after transplant.

    a.   Many patients state that it is a full year before the worst is behind them and they have attained their recovery goals.

4.   Outcomes for patients who survive the first year vary widely with some patients experiencing an excellent quality of life and others hampered by ongoing problems.[43]

    a.   Although transplantation extends life and offers the possibility of improved functional ability, caring for a transplanted organ can be a burdensome task.

        b. Patients and families must learn to handle ongoing psychological stress and face continuing uncertainty about health outcomes.[44]

        c. There are many practical obstacles to providing optimal psychosocial care to transplant patients and their support persons.

           i. Staffing is limited.

           ii. Waiting lists in some programs are very large.

           iii. Patients often wait for extended periods of time.

           iv. Team members may have limited access to patients who live far from the transplant center.

           v. Meeting patient needs may involve: developing support groups that allow for concurrent monitoring of patients, creating mentoring programs that offer local assistance, and establishing a network of health care professionals with transplant experience in the patients' own communities can all help to meet patient needs.

           vi. Data indicate that ignoring pretransplant candidates' psychosocial requirements leaves them in distress and poses risks for noncompliance and graft loss after transplant.[45]

IX. Psychosocial support programs: Importance of social support in the transplantation process

    A. Social support plays a vital role in facilitating patient functioning and coping pre- and post-transplant.[31, 33, 37, 46]

    B. The availability of social support is thoroughly explored as part of the pretransplant psychosocial evaluation.

    C. Support is needed with practical aspects of care, such as transportation to and from appointments and assistance with household tasks.

    D. Patients also require ongoing emotional support.

        1. Pre- and post-transplant patients ideally receive support from various sources.

        2. When asked about sources of support, patients most frequently list their families, but also include friends, church members, and neighbors.

        3. Patients' sources of support expand as they begin the evaluation process.

        4. Their team of doctors, nurses, and social workers becomes an integral part of the lives.

        5. If hospitalized during the evaluation phase or while awaiting transplant, patients gain support from the floor nurses and fellow patients.

        6. A bond often forms among patients that can lead to life-long friendships.

        7. The availability of professionals with previous experience counseling transplant patients is particularly valued, as are multiple sources of emotional support from both the transplant team and network of family and friends.

    E. An international support group, Transplant Recipient International Organization, has chapters in many communities.

        1. Volunteers from this group often visit pre- and post-transplant patients in the hospital.

        2. Group members also invite patients and family members to regular meetings in the community.

      3. Patients frequently find it helpful to speak to persons who have had transplants.

   F. Patients also benefit from reading educational materials on transplantation and from attending formal, instructional sessions.

X. Support groups

   A. Several transplant centers have found support groups useful in meeting patients' needs.[47, 48]

   B. At Toronto General Hospital, all pretransplant lung patients and their support persons are encouraged to attend the ongoing Lung Support and Education group, which has met weekly for the past 15 years.

      1. The group is facilitated by the team's social worker and psychiatric nurse.

      2. Patients generally attend the group until 3 months after surgery, but are welcome to return whenever they wish after this period.

      3. The meetings alternate between a planned speaker and sessions devoted to general discussion.

      4. All members of the lung transplant team attend the group on a rotating basis to offer education and to become acquainted with patients in the program.

      5. The group allows time for conversation, sharing of experiences, and mutually supportive interactions among attendees.

      6. At times, the group is divided into two smaller groups, with patients separated from support persons.

         a. Provides the opportunity for participants to share feelings, experiences, insights, and concerns with one another.

      7. Clinical observation indicates that participants attending the support group are generally better educated about transplantation and more prepared psychologically for the transplant experience than those who are not able to participate.

         a. This finding is also reported in the literature.[49]

      8. Group attendees are able to develop strong support networks within the group, as many may join in for several months during the waiting period.

      9. Patient support may also be provided by multi-organ groups designed for stress management and facilitated by a therapist, or by groups held for persons experiencing severe anxiety as part of critical care in an ICU.

         a. The latter groups may be facilitated by such staff as the ICU social worker, clinical nurse specialist, or program chaplain.

         b. Consultation with social workers in transplant programs across North America indicate that many have developed their own support groups based on patient or program needs.

XI. Mentoring programs

   A. The mentoring program has been applied recently in some transplant programs.[39]

      1. Its primary goals are the provision of social and emotional support and increased or improved education and understanding of the transplant process.[50]

      2. Providing a mentor to pretransplant patients gives them the chance to discuss the prospect of transplant with someone who has already coped successfully with it.

3. Because transplantation is a relatively uncommon medical treatment and one which may seem overwhelming, many candidates have little of the background knowledge required to make informed treatment decisions.
4. Conversations with mentors can help them prepare for what often proves to be a complicated, highly demanding, and stressful process.
5. Currently, many transplant centers are making use of mentoring programs, both formally and informally, to enhance patient care.

XII. Resources
A. The cost of transplantation is covered by most private insurance programs in the U.S. and by Medicare and state Medicaid programs.
B. An estimate of the medical costs for a heart transplant patient who has been waiting at home for a transplant, has an unremarkable hospital course, and is discharged 2 weeks after transplant ranges from $150,000 to $175,000 (U.S.).[51]
C. Costs can mount to $500,000 for a patient with an extended pre- or post-transplant period.
D. Frequent out-patient follow-up visits and ongoing medications result in additional costs.
   1. These expenses will diminish as follow-up visits become less frequent and fewer medications are needed.
E. Maintenance medications given post-transplant can easily cost in excess of $2,000 a month.
F. Insurance coverage for transplant charges may vary over time post-transplant.
   1. Private insurance may be discontinued and a patient may no longer qualify for disability or Medicare benefits after having recovered and being able to return to work.
   2. Individuals, however, can continue to receive Social Security Disability benefits and Medicare and earn a monthly income.
      a. Annual guidelines determine the monthly allowed income.
   3. Many state Medicaid programs have work incentive plans that encourage individuals with disabilities to return to work.
      a. These programs allow individuals to earn defined amounts of income and continue Medicaid benefits.
      b. Patients can apply for grants from some states to pay for medications.
      c. State Medicaid programs typically cover all prescriptions at 100%, but some programs now have a small patient co-pay.
   4. For eligible patients, Medicare covers 80% of costs for the antirejection medications.[51]
      a. Individuals qualify for Medicare if they are over age 65 or if they have been receiving Social Security Disability benefits for two years.
      b. Individuals diagnosed with end-stage renal disease are eligible for Medicare at the time of their kidney transplant or at the initiation of peritoneal dialysis or 3 months after initiating hemodialysis, regardless of age.
   5. Most private U.S. health insurances require patient co-pay.

    a.   With increases in these co-pays over the last 5 years, total patient co-pay responsibility may be several hundred dollars a month.

6.   Most pharmaceutical companies have drug assistance programs to help defray medication expenses.

    a.   Eligibility for these programs is typically need-based.

    b.   However, many of these programs will not offer assistance if patients have private insurance, Medicaid, or Medicare.

    c.   For the Medicare patient, drug assistance programs will not typically assist with the 20% cost of medications not covered by Medicare.

    d.   The post-transplant coordinator and social worker assist patients in applying for these programs.

    e.   With the increased use of the Internet, patients are able to research assistance programs more independently.

    f.   As the transplant team emphasizes the importance of having an uninterrupted supply of medications, patients are urged to let their coordinator or social worker know if they are not able to obtain medication or if they are aware of a change in their coverage.

7.   There are several U.S.-based fund-raising foundations for transplant patients.

    a.   The Children's Organ Transplant Association (COTA) was founded in 1986 and primarily assists children in need of transplantation and their families.[51]

    b.   Funded over 20 years ago, the National Transplant Assistance Fund (NTAF) and the National Foundation for Transplants provides similar assistance to adults.[51]

    c.   The funds raised by these programs help offset the cost of transplantation and related expenses for medications and travel not by covered by the patient's insurance.

8.   In Canada, a universal health-care system is paid for by income tax and administered by the individual provinces.

    a.   This system provides coverage to all qualified residents for hospital costs, and physicians' and surgeons' fees.

    b.   Costs for other treatments, such as for transplant medications and oxygen, may be covered through individuals' private insurance or through public programs available in some provinces.

    c.   Government programs will also cover these services for patients receiving social assistance.

9.   Table 16-1 summarizes coverage of medical costs for patients undergoing solid organ transplantation in the U.S. and Canada.

10. In addition to medical expenses, patients requiring transplant are faced with other associated expenses, including:

    a.   Additional housing costs when relocation is required

    b.   Loss of income both for patients and support persons

    c.   Transportation

    d.   Costly equipment such as microspirometer for lung transplant patients (Table 16-2).

    e.   In Canada, there is little public assistance to offset the cost of relocation.

TABLE 16-1

■ **Medical Costs and Benefits**

	Hospital	Surgical/medical	Medication	Oxygen
U.S.	Medicaid	Medicaid	Medicaid	Medicaid
	Medicare	Medicare	Medicare (antirejection mediations at 80%)	Medicare
	Private insurance (may require patient co-pay)	Private insurance (may require patient co-pay)		Private insurance
			Private insurance (usually requires patient co-pay)	
Canada	Universal coverage	Universal coverage	Private insurance	Private insurance
			Universal programs (some provinces)	Universal programs (some provinces)
			Social assistance	Social assistance

TABLE 16-2

■ **Associated Costs and Benefits**

	Loss of patient income	Relocation	Transportation	Equipment	Loss of caregiver income
U.S.	State and federal (Social Security) disability benefits	Partial benefits with some private insurance plans	Some state Medicaid programs	Medicaid	12-week unpaid leave for family member under Family Medical Leave Act
	Employer disability benefits through employer	Medicaid may provide travel/subsistence assistance if center far from home	Travel, food, and lodging benefits with some private insurance plans	Medicare	
				Private insurance	
Canada	Variable via work benefits	Subsidized only by Newfoundland	Social assistance	Private insurance	8 week compassionate care leave
	15 weeks government illness benefits			Social assistance	15-week stress leave

f. Patients who have worked in organizations with comprehensive benefit packages may receive disability incomes for the duration of their illness.

g. Canadian patients who have paid into the government-run Employment Insurance Program through their employers are entitled to a maximum of 15 weeks illness leave.

   i. Qualified support persons may become entitled to this illness benefit.

   ii. Support persons may also be eligible for income benefits for an additional 8 weeks under entitlements for caretakers of persons with critical illness.

iii. Unemployed individuals will not be eligible for government-sponsored income assistance unless they meet the criteria for social assistance eligibility.

XIII. Noncompliance
   A. Noncompliant behaviors have life-threatening consequences for transplant patients.
   B. The goal of transplant is for patients to preserve their transplanted organ so that their lives can be extended and their quality of life improved.[52]
   C. Noncompliance for a transplant patient includes failure to take medications as prescribed, keep follow-up appointments, and adhere to recommendations regarding cigarette, alcohol, and substance use, and diet.[53]
   D. The psychosocial assessment gathers information about patients' follow-through with medical recommendations, such as keeping doctor appointments, taking medications as prescribed, following through with dietary recommendations, and reporting symptoms and concerns.
      1. Family members' impressions regarding compliance and feedback from other health care professionals who have cared for the patient are also useful in assessing compliance.[54, 55]
      2. The team has a special opportunity to evaluate compliance in patients who are hospitalized at the time of the pretransplant evaluation, through monitoring of patients' response to instruction and their follow-through with recommendations.
   E. Noncompliance may be viewed by health care professionals as irrational, delusional, and willful self-destructive behavior.[36, 53]
      1. Team members attempt to determine reasons for noncompliance as well as to predict the patients at highest risk for this problem.[52]
      2. Numerous studies document that substance abuse history and diagnosis of personality disorder are associated with noncompliance.[53]
      3. Other factors related to noncompliance include the patient's psychological makeup, life experience, and interactions with physicians.[54, 56]
      4. Patients revert to past coping strategies when confronted with a new illness or a change in treatment plans.
         a. Patients' insights into these coping techniques may be limited.
         b. Information about how patients and their families have coped with earlier stresses or life events can be obtained in the psychosocial evaluation and may be useful in determining reasons for noncompliance and in encouraging greater patient cooperation.
      5. Well-intentioned comments, especially those that may evoke a guilt response in the recipient, can backfire by precipitating combative or resistive behaviors.
      6. Determining the best way to assist a patient is the task of the social worker and team coordinators.
   F. Risks for noncompliance with pre- and post-transplant care may be especially high in some age groups.
      1. In the mid-1980s, most transplant programs did not transplant individuals over 50 years of age.
         a. The upper age limit for solid organ transplant in North America is currently 65 years, though a small number of programs no longer consider age as a factor in listing patients for transplant.
         b. Over the past several years, the Cleveland Clinic Foundation has performed heart transplants on 17 patients aged 70-75 years.

    c. All but two of these patients are surviving, and these survivors report a positive quality of life.

    d. Grady et al.[57] note that this over-65 age group may have fewer life stresses than younger patients, in part because their careers and parental responsibilities are largely fulfilled.

    e. Older patients may also have a greater tolerance for medication side effects, less concern about changes in body image, and less frustration with frequent follow-up visits.[46]

    f. Although some findings suggest that survival may be lower in patients transplanted after 55 years of age,[57] other studies have failed to observe age differences in survival.[57, 58]

    g. The results of these studies fail to suggest any special problems with compliance in older patients.

2. Patients aged 18-25 years are also of special concern, as this age group has the lowest survival rate post-heart transplant.[59]

    a. For both newly diagnosed patients and those with onset of symptoms in childhood, the young adult years are a time to begin an occupation, separate from the family of origin, and form a new family system.

    b. Persons in this phase of life may find it challenging to take medications as prescribed, keep follow-up appointments, and cope with body image changes resulting from side effects of medications.[53]

    c. Even those young adults who have previously coped with a chronic illness or congenital health condition may become defiant or feel impervious to medical risks at this stage of their adult development.

3. Similarly, transplant teams view adolescent patients as being at particularly high risk for noncompliance.[53]

4. Although adherence to a medication regimen is imperative to a successful post-transplant course, studies show that patients take only 50% to 90% of their prescribed medications, with an overall compliance rate of 76%.[60]

    a. Patients are more likely to miss doses of medications than to take too many doses.

    b. Noncompliance worsens with increases in the dosing schedule.[60]

        i. As one study concluded, "the simpler the prescription, the better the compliance."[61 (p. 305)]

        ii. An electronic monitoring system reported 87% compliance with once a day dosing and only 39% compliance when medications were taken four times a day.[60]

    c. In a patient self-report study completed with members of a national transplant support group, only 75% of patients surveyed reported that they had never missed doses of medications.

        i. The reasons cited for missing medications were forgetfulness, running out of medications, and avoidance of medication side effects.[62]

        ii. Instructions regarding self-care and the transplant process need to be clear and tailored to patients' individual needs.

    iii. Strategies that improve compliance are education, planning dosing regimens, clinic appointments, and communication with team members.[60]

        a) When providing education, the team considers patient interest in this information.[60]

        b) Typically, the team provides patients with a transplant notebook that describes pre- and post-transplant care.

        c) This may be sufficient for some patients, but others may request additional information or may wish to meet with another post-transplant patient or attend a transplant support group.

        d) The patient and family members may also have different educational needs.

        e) The patient may be content with basic information, but a spouse may request additional materials.

        f) One useful educational approach is to ask patients to summarize the information they read to reiterate verbal instructions.[60]

        g) The team member cannot assume that patients have absorbed or will recall all information presented to them.[61]

        h) Efforts to understand how patients learn and to identify possible learning difficulties may reveal the need for additional instruction or alternative approaches, such as a written outline of procedures or step-by-step listings of medication requirements.

        i) Critically ill pretransplant patients may have difficulty understanding and retaining instructions, though their abilities may improve significantly post-transplant.

        j) Neuropsychological testing is helpful in evaluating concerns about cognitive abilities, as well as in delineating problems that could hinder patients' abilities to care for themselves independently post-transplant.

        k) The psychosocial evaluation is an effective means to identify patients in need of these evaluations.

        l) Another helpful technique to enhance patient compliance is to assist patients in finding ways to cue self-administration of medications.[60]

            1) For example, patients may be counseled to take their medications after showering or brushing their teeth, or at mealtimes or bedtime.

            2) Scheduling specific times for medications and establishing regimens that involve as few dosings as possible facilitate compliance.

      m) Other useful methods are to ask patients about medication compliance at their post-transplant visits, and to institute self-medication programs for patients when they are hospitalized pre- and post-transplant.[61]

1) Self-medication programs can help patients become more comfortable with their medication routines, work out their own cueing systems, and learn how to manage problematic dosing times before discharge home.
2) A special advantage of self-management is that it discourages reliance on family members and health care staff and provides patients an opportunity to demonstrate independence with this task.
3) Assessment of the patients' ability to independently administer medications is an important component of the pretransplant psychosocial evaluation.

n) Patients' relationships with the transplant team may also affect their compliance.[53]
1) Establishing effective communications between patients and all team members is important in establishing patient trust.
2) One of the challenges in working with patients is to encourage input from them and a feeling of being part of treatment planning while also conveying the importance of accepting decisions and recommendations made by health care providers.
3) Maintaining professional boundaries is essential, but can be difficult with patients who have been followed for years post-transplant by the same team members.

XIV. Preparation for end of life issues
  A. Mortality is always of acute concern, even for patients who receive successful transplants.
    1. Most centers require transplant candidates to confront the possibility that their transplant might fail, in which case they would die.
    2. Patients' acknowledgement of this possibility is required as part of the process of obtaining informed consent to insure patients are aware of potential risks.
    3. Thus, the assessment period is a critical time for most individuals and their families, many of them who are learning for the first time about the uncertainties and limitations of transplantation.
    4. The extent to which individuals are able to prepare themselves for dying is highly variable and is related to such factors as personal philosophies and experience, religious beliefs, individual fear of death, age, and the involvement of dependents and other loved ones.[45]
    5. Because transplantation offers the possibility of extended life, many patients and their families focus on a positive outcome, an outlook that can be viewed as a successful coping strategy.[51]
       a. In some cases, however, there is also a conscious or unconscious decision to avoid contemplating mortality issues, which are considered too painful and frightening.
       b. Furthermore, individuals' ages and stage in the life cycle may affect their ability to consider or come to terms with the possible end of life.[45]

   c. For the very young, having to face death often seems both untimely and unimaginable to them and their families.

   d. The inability to come to terms with one's mortality when in the midst of a dying process may lead to increased anxiety and stress levels for patients and families.[45]

   e. Older patients, who have themselves experienced losses, may more readily accept their own vulnerability.

   f. From the time of the initial assessment, the social worker and other care providers have the responsibility to broach issues of mortality at appropriate times with all patients and their families and to help prepare them for this possibility.

 B. On a practical level, patients must choose a substitute decision-maker with whom they can discuss their wishes in the event of their death.

  1. Patients are advised to prepare wills and make any other arrangements to transfer assets to others and to insure that their wishes are fulfilled should they become incapacitated.

  2. The need for such arrangements is especially acute when the patient is also the parent of dependent children.[63]

   a. Integral to the parental role is the responsibility to be present in a nurturing capacity and to protect the child until the child becomes independent.[64]

   b. Facing possible death inevitably plunges parents into projections about a future in which they no longer exist.

   c. Providing emotional support for the child and disclosing the truth about the parent's illness is often problematic for the family.

   d. Many patients seek to protect family members by misleading them or by failing to fully disclose the risks.

   e. If parents have to be separated from their children for lengthy periods to obtain medical care, patients may have concerns about the children's present situation and the possibility of not being with them at the end of life.[65]

   f. Parents frequently express concerns about not being able to meet role expectations, fear and panic about the future, and guilt related to letting their children down.

   g. The team needs to be cognizant of the fact that separated parents may be forced to envision uncomfortable, stressful scenarios with their spouses or other family members.

   h. Single parents may be especially vulnerable to these concerns, at least without a strong extended family.

   9. At the initial contact, the transplant social worker collects information on family supports and ascertains and documents what has been planned for the children in the event of the patient's death.

   j. The plan for the future of the children is discussed, including the children's feelings about the plan.

   k. Parents are encouraged to tell children that they are loved and valued and that the ill parent wants very much to be with them.

   l. Often, parents benefit greatly from counseling with regard to children's coping.

   m. The first step in this process is for the patient to be forthright with the children.[63]

n.   Including children in an age-appropriate manner reduces feeling of isolation and anger.

o.   Parents can be supported by strategizing ways to minimize the children's confusion or pain.

p.   Children have an important role to play in working with patients both pre- and post-transplant.

   i.   If parents die, the children become principal mourners.

   ii.   Excluding them denies them the status they deserve as important and integral members of the family.

q.   Even quite ill or disabled patients can be caring and capable parents.

r.   Children can be assured that the care team will do all it can to help the patient but that even if things do not work out, they will be looked after.

s.   Children also need to know that the patient's health problem has nothing to do with them.

t.   Helping patients who are parents deal effectively with planning for their dependent children and being available to the children are ways in which members of the health care team can provide invaluable assistance to the most vulnerable members of the family.

3.   Post-transplant patients face the prospect of death due to organ failure at any time postsurgery.

a.   Patients with spiritual or religious backgrounds may gain psychological and emotional support from their beliefs and religious communities.

b.   The availability of chaplains and other spiritual advisors, as well as persons familiar with therapies such as meditation, visualization, and Reiki, can offer unique assistance during hospitalization and upon return home.[45]

c.   Expert palliative care is essential when death is imminent.[45]

d.   Patients frequently express worry about potential suffering through the dying process.

   i.   They need reassurance that care will be provided in accordance with their wishes, using all available treatments to relieve discomfort and anxiety.

   ii.   Families of dying patients also require support.

   iii.   Patients and family members are aware that there are uncertainties post-transplant.

   iv.   With the assistance of social workers and team members, they are able to focus on maximizing quality of life.

XV.   Conclusion

A.   Survival rates following solid organ transplantation have improved dramatically in the last 20 years.

1.   We have more information now about how persons who have been transplanted cope with the changes in their lives and the types of adjustment and compliance problems they can encounter.

2.   We know more about the types of information that are most critical in evaluating candidacy for transplant and about patients' quality of life pre- and post-transplant.

B. Further studies are needed to better understand ways to prepare patients for transplant and to promote successful adaptation to life after transplant.
   1. There is substantial consensus about the importance of assessing psychosocial factors and the contents of the evaluation.
   2. We also have learned that successful outcomes depend both on patient characteristics and supports provided by health care professionals and the patient's support system.

REFERENCES

1. Dew MA, Switzer GE, DiMartini AF, Matukaitis J, et al. Psychosocial assessments and outcomes in organ transplantation. *Prog Transplant*, 2000; 10: 239.
2. Dobbels F, De Geest S, Cleemput L, et al. Psychosocial and behavioral selection criteria for solid organ transplantation. *Prog Transplant*, 2001; 11: 121-132.
3. Olbrisch ME, Benedict SM, Ashe K, Levenson, JL. Psychological assessment and care of organ transplant patients. *J Consult Clin Psychol*, 2002; 70: 771-83.
4. Hillerman WL, Russell CL, Barry D, et al. Evaluation guidelines for adult and pediatric kidney transplant programs: The Missouri experience. *Prog Transplant*, 2002; 12: 30-35.
5. Phipps L. Psychiatric evaluation and outcomes in candidates for heart transplantation. *Clin Invest Med*, 1997; 20: 388-395.
6. Favaloro RR, Perrone SV, Moscoloni SE, et al. Value of pre-heart-transplant psychological evaluation. Long-term follow up. *Transplant Proc*, 1993; 31: 3000-3001.
7. Bright MJ, Craven JL, Paul JK, Toronto Lung Transplant Group. Assessment and management of psychological stress in lung transplant candidate. *Health Social Work*, 1990: 125-131.
8. O'Dell MI, Wright L. An electronic psychosocial assessment tool: Use in a living donor organ transplant program. *Prog Transplant*, 2003; 12: 97-104.
9. Burker EJ, Evon DM, Sedway JA, Egan T. Appraisal and coping as predictors of psychological distress and self-reported physical disability before lung transplantation. *Prog Transplant*, 2004; 14: 222-234.
10. Tringali RA, Trzepacz PT, DiMartine A, Dew MA. Assessment and follow-up of alcohol-dependent liver transplantation patients. *Gen Hosp Psychiatry*, 1996; 18: 70S-77S.
11. Levenson JA, Olbrisch ME. Psychosocial evaluation of organ transplant candidates. A comparative survey of process, criteria, and outcomes in heart, liver, and kidney transplantation. *Psychosomatic*, 1993; 34(4): 314-323.
12. Olbrisch ME, Levenson JL, Hamer R. The PACT: A rating scale for the study of clinical decision-making in psychosocial screening of organ transplant candidates. *Clinical Transplantation*, 1989; 3: 164-169.
13. Skotzko CE, Rudis R, Kobashigawa JA, Laks H. Psychiatric disorders and outcome following cardiac transplantation. *J Heart Lung Transplant*, 1999; 18: 952-956.
14. Presberg BA, Levenson JL, Olbrisch ME, Best AM. Rating scales for psychosocial evaluation of organ transplant candidates. Comparison of the PACT and TERS with bone marrow transplant patients. *Psychosomatics*, 1995; 36: 458-446
15. Beck AT, Ward CH, Mendelson M, Mock J, et al. An inventory for measuring depression. *Arch Gen Psychiatry*, 1961; 4: 561-571.
16. Bradwin M, Coffman KL. The Millon Behavioral Health Inventory Life Threat Reactivity Scale as a predictor of mortality in patients awaiting heart transplantation. *Psychosomatics*, 1999; 40: 44-49.
17. Chacko RC, Harper RG, Kunik M, Young J. Relationship of psychiatric morbidity and psychosocial factors in organ transplant candidates. *Psychosomatics*, 1996; 37: 100-107.
18. Rector TS, Ormaza SM, Kubo SH. Health status of heart transplant recipients versus patients awaiting heart transplantation: A preliminary evaluation of the SF-36 Questionnaire. *J Heart Lung Transplant*, 1993; 12: 983-986.
19. Spitzer RL, Williams JBW. Structured clinical interview for DSM-III-R (non-patient version and personality disorders). Biometrics Research, NY State Psychiatric Institute, NY, 1985.
20. Maercker A, Schutzwohl M. Assessment of post-traumatic stress reactions. *Diagnostica*, 1998; 44:130.
21. Deragotis LF. SCL-90 administration, scoring and procedures manual-II—Revised. Baltimore: Clinical Psychometric Research, 1983.
22. Olbrisch ME, Levenson JL. Psychosocial assessment of organ transplant candidates. Current status of methodological and philosophical issues. *Psychosomatics*, 1995; 36: 236-243.

23. Olbrisch ME, Levenson JL. Psychosocial evaluation of heart transplant candidates: An international survey of process, criteria and outcomes. *J Heart Lung Transplant*, 1991; 948-955.

24. Maricle RA, Hosenpud JD, Norman DJ, Ontely GA, et al. The lack of predictive value of pre-operative psychologic distress for post-operative medical outcome in heart transplant recipients. *J Heart Lung Transplant*, 1991; 10: 942-947.

25. Shapiro PA, Williams DL, Foray AT, Gelman IS, et al. Psychosocial evaluation and prediction of compliance problems and morbidity after heart transplantation. *Transplantation*, 1995; 60(10): 1462-1466.

26. Paris W, Muchmore J, Pribil A, Zuhdi N, et al. Study of the relative incidences of psychosocial factors before and after heart transplantation and the influence of post-transplantation psychosocial factors on heart transplantation outcome. *J Heart Lung Transplant*, 1999; 13: 424-432.

27. Dew MA, Roth LH, Schulberg HC, Simmons RG, et al. Prevalence and predictors of depression and anxiety-related disorders during the year after heart transplantation. *Gen Hospital Psychiatry*, 1996; 18: 48S-61S.

28. Dew MA, Kormos RL, Roth LH, Murali S, et al. Early post-transplant medical compliance and mental health predict physical morbidity and mortality one to three years after heart transplantation. *J Heart Lung Transplant*, 1999; 549-562.

29. Cimato TR, Jessup M. Recipient selection in cardiac transplantation: Contraindications and risk factors for mortality. *J Heart Lung Transplant*, 2002; 22: 1161-1173.

30. Deshields TL, McDonough EM, Mannen K, Miller LW. Psychological and cognitive status before and after heart transplantation. *Gen Hosp Psychiatry*, 1996; 8: 62S-69S.

31. Buse McS, Pieper B. Impact of cardiac transplantation on the spouse's life. *J Heart Lung Transplant*, 1990; 16(6): 641-648.

32. Dew MA, Roth LH, Schulberg HC, et al. Prevalence and predictors of depression and anxiety-related disorders during the year after transplantation. *Gen Hosp Psychiatry*, 1996; 18(suppl 6): 48S-61S.

33. Rogers KR. Nature of spousal supportive behaviors that influence heart transplant patient compliance. *J Heart Lung Transplant*, 1987; 6(2): 90-95.

34. Nolan MT, Cupples SA, Brown MM, et al. Perceived stress and coping strategies among families of cardiac transplant candidates during the organ waiting period. *J Heart Lung Transplant*, 1992; 21(6): 540-547.

35. Gier MD, Levick MD, Blazina PJ. Stress reduction with heart transplant patients and their families: A multidisciplinary approach. *J Heart Lung Transplant*, 1988; 7: 342-347.

36. Sharp LA. A medical anthropologist's view on post-transplant compliance: The underground economy of medical survival. *Transplant Proc*, 1999; 31 (Suppl 4A): 31S-33S.

37. Mishel MH, Murdaugh CL. Family adjustment to heart transplantation: Redesigning the dream. *Nursing Research*, 1987; 36(6): 332-338.

38. Shapiro PA, Kornfeld DS. Psychiatric outcome of heart transplantation. *Gen Hosp Psychiatry*, 1989; 11: 352-357.

39. Gardner A. Mentoring in the 1990s: A new look at an old idea. *Maturity*, 1993; 13(5): 6-8.

40. Campbell B, Etringer G. Post-transplant quality of life issues: Depression-related noncompliance in cardiac transplant patients. *Transplant Proc*, 1999; 31(Suppl 4A): 59S-60S.

41. Phipps L. Psychiatric evaluation and outcomes in candidates for heart transplantation. *Clin Invest Med*, 1997; 20: 338-395.

42. Bohachick P, Anton BB, Wooldridge, RL, Kormos, JM. Psychosocial outcome six months after heart transplant surgery: A preliminary report. *Res Nurs Health*, 1992; 15: 165-173.

43. Grady KL, Jalowiec A, White-Williams C. Predictors of quality of life in patients at one year after heart transplantation. *J Heart Lung Transplant*, 1999; 18: 202-210.

44. Skotzko CE, Stowe JA, Wright C, Kendall K, et al. Approaching a consensus: Psychosocial support services for solid organ transplant programs. *Prog Transplant*, 2001; 11: 163-168.

45. Roberson H. Meeting Death: In Hospital, Hospice, and at Home. Toronto: McLeeland & Stewart Ltd., 2000.

46. Barr ML, Schenkel FA, Van Kirk A, et al. Determinants of quality of life changes among long-term cardiac transplant survivors: Results from longitudinal data. *J Heart Lung Transplant*, 2003; 22: 1157-1167.

47. Suszycki LH. Psychosocial aspects of heart transplantation. *Soc Wk*, 1988; 33: 205-209.

48. Suszycki LH. Social work groups in a heart transplant program. *Heart Transplant*, 1988; 5: 66-170.

49. Wright L. Mentorship programs for transplant patients. *Prog Transplant*, 2000; 10: 267-272.

50. Levinson JL, Olbrisch ME. Shortage of donor organ and long waits. *Psychosomatics*, 1987; 28: 399-403.

51. UNOS. Financing transplantation—What every patient needs to know. *Chronic Med Pharmacy*, 2003.

52. Littlefield C, Abbey S, Fiducia D, et al. Quality of life following transplantation of the heart, liver and lungs. *Gen Hosp Psychiatry*, 1996; 18: 36S-47S.

53. Sherry DC, Simmons B, Wung SF, Zerwic, JJ. Noncompliance in heart transplantation: A role for the advanced practice nurse. *Prog Cardiovasc Nurs*, 2003; 18: 141.

54. Hathaway DK, Combs C, De Geest S, Stergachis A, et al. Patient compliance in transplantation: A report on the perceptions of transplant clinicians. *Transplant Proc*, 1991; 31(Suppl 4A): 10S-13S.

55. Collins, DC, Wicks MN, Hathaway DK. Health-care professional perceptions of compliance behaviors in the pre-renal and post-renal transplant patient. *Transplant Proc*, 1999; 31(Suppl 4A): 16S-17S.

56. Pumilia CV. Psychological impact of the physician-patient relationship on compliance: a case study and clinical strategies. *Prog Transplant*, 2002; 12: 10-16.

57. Grady KL. When to transplant: Recipient selection for heart transplantation. *J Cardiovascular Nurs*, 1996; 10(13): 58.

58. Hunt SA. Who and when to consider for heart transplantation. Division of Cardiovascular Medicine, Stanford University School of Medicine. 2001; 9(1): 18.

59. Papajcik D, Mastroianni B, Goormastic M, Flechner SM. A tool to identify risk factors for noncompliance in the adult renal transplant recipient. *Transplant Proc*, 1999; 31(Suppl 4A): 84S-86S.

60. Cramer JA. Practical issues in medication compliance. *Transplant Proc*, 1999; 31(Suppl 4A): 7S-9S.

61. Robbins ML. Medication adherence and the transplant recipient helping patients at each stage of change. *Transplant Proc*, 1999; 31(supp 14A): 29S-30S.

62. Kory L. Non-adherence to immunosuppressive medications: A pilot survey of members of the transplant recipients international organization. *Transplant Proc*, 1999; 31(Suppl 4A): 14S-15S.

63. Muirhead J, Meyerowitz BE, Leedham B, Eastburn TE, et al. Quality of life and coping in patients awaiting heart transplantation. *J Heart Lung Transplant*, 1992; 11: 265-272.

64. Harris M. The Loss That Is Forever: The Lifelong Impact of the Early Death of a Mother or Father. New York: Plume, 1996.

65. Silverman PR. Never Too Young to Know: Death in Children's Lives. New York: Oxford University Press, 2000.

REVIEW QUESTIONS

1. A psychosocial evaluation should include questions pertaining to the patient's history of psychiatric disturbances. This should include problems such as which of the following?
   a. Serious sleep disorders
   b. Suicide attempts
   c. History of hospitalizations for mental health reasons
   d. Panic attacks
   e. All of the above
   f. b and c

2. The ultimate goals of the psychosocial evaluation are which of the following?
   a. Provide education to the patient on pain management related to post-transplant care
   b. Provide the transplant team with information on the candidate's support system
   c. Identify gaps in the patient's insurance plan
   d. Identify potential compliance issues
   e. All of the above
   f. b, c, d

3. Once the social worker has assessed a patient for transplantation, the determination may be made for referral to which of the following services?
   a. Chemical dependency consult
   b. Neuropsychiatry
   c. Endocrinology
   d. Cardiac surgery
   e. All of the above
   f. a and b

4. Research on post heart transplant recipients has demonstrated that individuals with consistently elevated levels of depression, anger, and hostility have a 4-8 times greater likelihood for developing which of the following?
   a. Primary graft failure
   b. Alcoholism
   c. Coronary artery disease
   d. Chronic graft rejection
   e. Chronic renal failure

5. Research has demonstrated that patients with post traumatic stress disorders (PTSD) were 13 times more likely to:
   a. Have chronic rejection episodes
   b. Die within 3 years post transplantation
   c. Require a retransplant within 3 years
   d. Develop chronic renal failure

6. While awaiting transplantation, patients have reported concerns about which of the following?
   a. Becoming a burden to friends and family
   b. Financial issues
   c. Dying while awaiting a suitable donor organ
   d. All of the above
   e. a and c

7. Family burden may increase as the patient's health deteriorates while awaiting a suitable organ for transplantation. Spouses may experience which of the following during the waiting period?
   a. Anxiety related to separation from the individual hospitalized while awaiting transplantation
   b. A need to return to work to support the family
   c. Difficulty coping with added responsibilities that were once shared
   d. All of the above

8. Heart transplant candidates may often be hospitalized while awaiting a suitable donor heart. Social workers and nurses help to create a supportive environment with interventions such as which of the following?
   a. Educational programs for patients and families
   b. Support groups with other patients awaiting transplantation
   c. Weekly dinners together with other patients on the unit
   d. Weekly excursions to the shopping mall with their IV inotropes
   e. All of the above
   f. a, b, c

9. Patients who are hospitalized for several months pre- and post-transplant may experience which of the following upon discharge from the hospital?
   a. Heightened anxiety about leaving the hospital environment
   b. Insecurity related to fear of complications
   c. Fear about changes in personal relationships with family members during the extended absence
   d. Role confusion
   e. All of the above
   f. a, b, d

10. Upon returning to a routine home environment, patients and families are often surprised to find which of the following?
    a. Day to day pretransplant problems resurface and begin to cause conflict
    b. The excitement of a new life overcomes all fears
    c. Transplantation has fixed all the pretransplant family problems
    d. The personality change in the recipient has made life more tolerable

Correct answers:

1. e
2. f
3. f
4. c
5. b
6. d
7. d
8. f
9. e
10. a

Appendix A

Electrolyte Imbalances in Adults: Abnormal Findings, Pathophysiology/Potential Etiology, Clinical Manifestations, Potential Treatment Options, and Monitoring

Electrolyte Imbalance	Potential Abnormal Findings	Pathophysiology/ Potential Etiology	Clinical Manifestations	Potential Treatment Options (Depend on Etiology)	Monitoring
Hyponatremia *Normal* serum sodium level: 135-146 mEq/L (SI units: 135-146 mmol/L) Hyponatremia = serum sodium level < 135 mEq/L (SI units: < 135 mmol/L)	Serum osmolality < 280 mOsm/kg ↑ hematocrit ↑ plasma protein level Urine specific gravity < 1.101 (except in patients with SIADH who have ↑ urine specific gravity)	Inadequate sodium intake Sodium loss Water gain Hypovolemic hyponatremia: Vomiting, diarrhea, gastric suctioning; excessive diaphoresis, burns, wound drainage; glucose-induced diuresis, osmotic diuresis, cystic fibrosis, adrenal insufficiency, diuretic therapy Hypervolemic hyponatremia: Heart or liver failure; nephritic syndrome, hyperaldosteronism, excessive use of hypotonic IV fluids Isovolemic hyponatremia: Glucocorticoid deficiency, hypothyroidism, renal failure, SIADH Medications: Certain loop and thiazide diuretics; certain immunosuppressants (e.g., cyclophosphamide); certain antihyperglycemic agents (e.g., chlorpropamide); certain sedatives (e.g., barbiturates; morphine); certain anticonvulsants (e.g., carbamazepine); certain antineoplastic agents (e.g., vincristine)	Acute onset with serum sodium levels between 115-120 mEq/L: Nausea Vomiting Anorexia Neurologic symptoms: Headache Irritability Disorientation Muscle twitching Weakness Tremors Changes in LOC (↓ attention span, lethargy, confusion) Abdominal cramps Serum sodium levels < 110 mEq/L: stupor, delirium, psychosis, ataxia, seizures, coma Concurrent hypovolemia: Poor skin turgor Dry mucous membranes Weak, rapid pulse Orthostatic hypotension ↓ Blood pressure ↓ CVP ↓ PAWP ↓ PAP Concurrent hypervolemia: Edema ↑ blood pressure Weight gain Rapid, bounding pulse ↑ CVP ↑ PAP	Mild hyponatremia with iso- or hypervolemia (dilutional hyponatremia): Fluid restriction Oral sodium supplements Mild hyponatremia with hypovolemia: Isotonic IV fluids (e.g., NS solution) High-sodium foods Severe hyponatremia (< 120 mEq/L) in setting of seizures or coma: Hypertonic saline solution* (e.g., 3% or 5% saline) infused slowly with concurrent administration of diuretic *Note: hypervolemic patients should not be given hypertonic sodium chloride solutions Discontinue medications that → loss of sodium Treatment of underlying disorders	Neurologic status Vital signs Serum sodium level Serum chloride level Urine specific gravity Urine osmolality Daily weight Intake and output Skin turgor Patient's response to therapy: Signs/symptoms of hypovolemia: Orthostatic hypotension Tachycardia Signs/symptoms of hypervolemia: Dyspnea Crackles Distended neck veins

Electrolyte Imbalance	Potential Abnormal Findings	Pathophysiology/ Potential Etiology	Clinical Manifestations	Potential Treatment Options (Depend on Etiology)	Monitoring
Hypernatremia *Normal* serum sodium level: 135-146 mEq/L (SI units: 135-146 mmol/L) Hypernatremia = serum sodium level > 145 mEq/L (SI units: > 146 mmol/L)	Serum osmolality > 295 mOsm/L Urine specific gravity > 1.030 (except in the setting of diabetes insipidus) Urine osmolality 800-1400 mOsm/L ↑ Hematocrit associated with volume depletion	↑ ECF: sodium and water are retained ↓ ECF: sodium retained; water not retained Hypovolemia Diabetes insipidus (central or nephrogenic) Impaired renal function: Potassium depletion → inability of kidney to concentrate urine → polyuria Hypercalcemia → polyuria, dehydration Excessive use of IV sodium solutions; gastric or enteral tube feedings Excessive oral sodium intake (salt tablets, foods high in sodium, certain medications) Certain medications: e.g., certain antibiotics; osmotic diuretics; laxatives; mineralcorticoids; antacids with sodium bicarbonate; sodium polystyrene sulfonate [Kayexalate®]) Uncontrolled DM with osmotic diuresis secondary to hyperglycemia	Early: Restlessness, agitation Anorexia, nausea, vomiting General: Excessive weight gain Intense thirst Low-grade fever Oliguria Dry mucous membranes Flushed skin Neuromuscular: Twitching, tremors Hyperreflexia Ataxia Weakness, lethargy Confusion Seizures Stupor, coma GU: Dehydration: Oliguria or anuria Osmotic diuresis, polyuria Pulmonary: Dyspnea due to pulmonary edema Hypernatremia due to sodium gain: Hypertension Bounding pulse Dyspnea Hypernatremia due to water loss: Dry mucus membranes Oliguria Orthostatic hypotension CV: ↑ ECF: Weak, thready pulse Hypertension CV: ↓ ECF: Hypotension Tachycardia that may → bradycardia	In setting of hypovolemia: Gradual oral fluid replacement Gradual IV fluid replacement (salt-free solutions until serum sodium level normalizes and then half-NS solution) Sodium restriction Diuretic therapy with fluid replacement to promote sodium loss In setting of diabetes insipidus: Vasopressin Hypotonic IV fluids Thiazide diuretics Note: corticosteroids ↑ reabsorption of sodium and excretion of potassium Treatment of underlying disorders	Vital signs Intake and output Daily weight Serum sodium level Urine specific gravity Urine osmolality Skin, mucous membranes Patient's response to therapy: Neurologic status Volume status

Electrolyte Imbalance	Potential Abnormal Findings	Pathophysiology/ Potential Etiology	Clinical Manifestations	Potential Treatment Options (Depend on Etiology)	Monitoring

Hypokalemia
 	
Normal serum potassium level = 3.5-5.3 mEq/L (SI units: 3.5-5.3 mmol/L)
 	
Hypokalemia: Serum potassium level < 3.5 mEq/L (SI units: < 3.5 mmol/L)
 	
Moderate hypokalemia: Serum potassium level 2.5 – 3.0 mEq/L (SI units: 2.5-3.0 mmol/L)
 	
Severe hypokalemia: Serum potassium level < 2.5 mEq/L (SI units: < 2.5 mmol/L)
	↑ pH and bicarbonate levels
	
	↓ serum magnesium level
	
	↑ (slightly) serum glucose level
	
	↑ 24-hour urine potassium level
		Inadequate potassium intake (oral intake, total parenteral nutrition with insufficient potassium supplement, potassium-deficient IV fluids)
		
		Excessive output of potassium (GI fluid losses associated with suctioning or prolonged vomiting; diarrhea; severe diaphoresis)
		
		Alkalosis or severe stress: potassium shifts into cell
		
		↑ Adrenal corticosteroid secretion
		
		Liver disease
		
		Medications (certain diuretics [thiazides, furosemide], antimicrobial agents [amphotericin B, gentamicin], corticosteroids, insulin, excessive use of laxatives)
			Skeletal muscle weakness
			
			Paresthesia
			
			Leg cramps, pain (calf muscle)
			
			Hyporeflexia
			
			Pulmonary:
			  Respiratory muscle weakness: tachypnea or slow, shallow respirations
			
			CNS:
			  Drowsiness → coma
			  Malaise
			  Confusion
			
			GI:
			  Nausea, vomiting
			  ↓ bowel sounds
			  Constipation
			  Paralytic ileus
			
			GU: Polyuria
			
			CV:
			  Weak, irregular pulse
			  Orthostatic hypotension
			  Palpitations
			  Dysrhythmias: PAT, PVCs, bradycardia, AV blocks, AV tachycardia; VT
			
			ECG changes:
			  Flat or inverted T wave
			  ST segment depression
			  U wave
			  Ventricular dysrhythmias
			  Ectopy
			  Bradycardia
			  Tachycardia
			  Cardiac arrest
			
			For patients on digoxin: digoxin toxicity
				High potassium diet (foods high in potassium: orange juice, raisins, milk, green vegetables, etc.)
				
				High sodium diet
				
				Oral or IV potassium supplements
				
				If diuretic therapy is needed: potassium-sparing diuretic
				
				Treatment of underlying disorders
					Serum potassium level
					
					Vital signs
					
					ECG
					
					Respiratory rate, pattern
					
					Intake and output
					
					Patient's response to therapy

Electrolyte Imbalance	Potential Abnormal Findings	Pathophysiology/ Potential Etiology	Clinical Manifestations	Potential Treatment Options (Depend on Etiology)	Monitoring
Hyperkalemia *Normal* serum potassium level = 3.5-5.3 mEq/L (SI units: 3.5-5.3 mmol/L) Hyperkalemia: Serum potassium level > 5.3-5.5 mEq/L (SI units: > 5.3-5.5 mmol/L) Moderate hyperkalemia: Serum potassium level 6.1-7.0 mEq/L (SI units: 6.1-7.0 mmol/L) Severe hyperkalemia: Serum potassium level > 7.0 mEq/L (SI units: > 7.0 mmol/L)	Most significant electrolyte imbalance; Metabolic acidosis	Metabolic acidosis Increased intake of potassium (↑ dietary intake of potassium; excessive use of salt substitutes; oral or IV potassium supplements) ↓ potassium excretion (renal failure) Movement of potassium out of cells (severe infection, rhabdomyolysis, insulin deficiency) Medications: ACE inhibitors, certain antibiotics (e.g., penicillin G potassium, pentamidine, trimethoprim); β-blockers; digoxin; heparin, potassium-sparing diuretics; NSAIDS; cyclosporine, tacrolimus, chemotherapeutic agents Donated blood that is close to the expiration date (serum potassium level ↑ with amount of time blood is stored)	Neuromuscular: Skeletal muscle weakness (may spread from legs to trunk to muscles of respiration) Flaccid paralysis Fatigue ↓ deep tendon reflexes GI: Nausea, vomiting Abdominal cramps Diarrhea CNS: Lethargy Apathy Confusion CV: Irregular pulse ↓ CO Hypotension Pulmonary: Rapid, deep respirations (in setting of acidosis) Shallow respirations (in setting of muscle paralysis) GU: Oliguria ECG changes: Tall peaked T waves (classic sign) Flat P wave Prolonged PR interval Bundle branch blocks Wide QRS interval Depressed ST segment Dysrhythmias: Bradycardia Heart block Ventricular dysrhythmias Asystole	Mild or moderate hyperkalemia: Loop diuretic to ↑ potassium loss or reverse acidosis Dietary potassium restriction (e.g., avoid orange juice, colas, bananas) Adjust dose of or discontinue medications associated with hyperkalemia Medications: Sorbitol Sodium polystyrene sulfonate (Kayexalate) Moderate to severe hyperkalemia: Hemodialysis Severe hyperkalemia: 10% calcium gluconate* or 10% calcium chloride* In setting of severe metabolic acidosis: IV sodium bicarbonate Note: Regular insulin (IV) will also move potassium into the cells (typically given with hypertonic (10% - 50%) dextrose solution) Treatment of underlying disorders *Contraindicated in patients on digoxin	Neurologic status Vital signs Serum sodium level Serum chloride level Intake and output Skin turgor Patient's response to therapy: Signs/symptoms of hypovolemia: Orthostatic hypotension Tachycardia Signs/symptoms of hypervolemia: Dyspnea Crackles Distended neck veins Urine specific gravity Urine osmolality Weight

Electrolyte Imbalance	Other Abnormal Findings	Pathophysiology/Potential Etiology	Clinical Manifestations	Potential Treatment Options (Depend on Etiology)	Monitoring
Hypomagnesemia *Normal* serum magnesium level: 1.8 to 2.5 mEq/L (SI units: 0.9 to 1.25 mmol/L) Hypomagnesemia: Serum magnesium level < 1.8 mEq/L (SI units: < 0.9 mmol/L)	Hypocalcemia Hypokalemia Can lead to myocardial irritability Dysrhythmias may occur, particularly after cardiac surgery and in patients with concurrent magnesium and potassium imbalances Digoxin toxicity (if taking digoxin): Bradycardia Anorexia Nausea, vomiting Yellow-tinged vision	Inadequate intake of magnesium: lack of adequate magnesium supplementation with IV fluids, TPN, or enteral feedings Poor renal absorption of magnesium Poor absorption of magnesium in GI tract (with, for example, Crohn's disease, ulcerative colitis, steatorrhea) Excessive loss of magnesium from GI tract: diarrhea, NG tube drainage Excessive loss of magnesium from urinary tract that can occur with: Primary aldosteronism Hyperparathyroidism Hypoparathyroidism Osmotic diuresis associated with diabetes mellitus Acute pancreatitis Electrolyte imbalances: Hypokalemia Hypocalcemia Medications: cyclosporine, amphotericin B, loop or thiazide diuretics, aminoglycoside antibiotics (tobramycin, gentamicin) Other: hemodialysis, sepsis, hypercalcemia, hypothermia, SIADH, sepsis, wounds that require debridement, ↑ calcium or sodium in urine, alcohol abuse (results in ↑ urinary secretion of magnesium and poor absorption of magnesium)	Typically develop when serum magnesium level is < 1.0 mEq/L CNS: ↑ deep tendon reflexes Weakness; skeletal muscle weakness Muscle cramping (foot, leg) Paresthesia Tremor Tetany Vertigo Ataxia Insomnia Mental status changes: confusion, emotional lability, depression Seizures, coma Pulmonary: Laryngeal stridor Respiratory muscle weakness/paralysis GI: Anorexia Nausea, vomiting Dysphagia CV: Tachycardia Dysrhythmias: Atrial fibrillation Heart block Torsades de pointes PAT, PVCs, SVT, VT, VF ECG changes: Prolonged PR interval Wide QRS complex Prolonged QT interval Depressed ST segment U wave Flat T wave Signs and symptoms of hypocalcemia	Magnesium supplementation (oral, IV, or IM) Magnesium-rich diet (e.g., seafood, green vegetables, whole grains, nuts) Treatment of underlying disorder	Serum magnesium level Serum calcium level Serum potassium level Mental status Neuromuscular status Ability to swallow Respiratory status Vital signs Hemodynamic status ECG Urine output Signs and symptoms of digitalis toxicity if on digoxin Patient's response to therapy

Electrolyte Imbalance	Potential Abnormal Findings	Pathophysiology/ Potential Etiology	Clinical Manifestations	Potential Treatment Options (Depend on Etiology)	Monitoring
Hypermagnesemia *Normal* serum magnesium level: 1.8 to 2.5 mEq/L (SI units: 0.9 to 1.25 mmol/L) Hypermagnesemia: Serum magnesium > 2.5 mEq/L (SI units: > 1.25 mmol/L)	Symptoms of renal dysfunction or failure Hypothyroidism Severe DKA	Typically uncommon; kidneys can generally rapidly excrete excess magnesium Excessive magnesium intake: Overuse of magnesium supplements Overuse of antacids or laxatives that contain magnesium TPN with excessive magnesium Hemodialysis with dialysate that is rich in magnesium Impaired magnesium excretion: Renal failure Adrenal insufficiency	In order of increasing serum magnesium levels: Vasodilation: Warm feeling and flushed appearance Mild hypotension Nausea, vomiting Facial paresthesia ↓ deep tendon reflexes Muscle weakness Drowsiness ECG changes (see below) Bradycardia Moderate hypotension Loss of deep tendon reflexes Respiratory compromise Heart block Coma Respiratory arrest Cardiac arrest ECG changes: Prolonged PR interval Wide QRS complex Tall T wave	In setting of normal renal function: oral or IV fluids; loop diuretic In setting of severe renal failure: peritoneal dialysis or hemodialysis with magnesium-free dialysate Temporary pacemaker for bradydysrhythmias Avoidance of medications that contain magnesium Restriction of foods that contain magnesium Toxic magnesium levels: Calcium gluconate Mechanical ventilation Treatment of underlying disorder	Serum magnesium levels Serum calcium levels BUN Serum creatinine Urine output Vital signs Respiratory status Neuromuscular status Mental status ECG Skin (flushing, warmth) Signs and symptoms of fluid overload Patient's response to therapy

Electrolyte Imbalance	Potential Abnormal Findings	Pathophysiology/ Potential Etiology	Clinical Manifestations	Potential Treatment Options (Depend on Etiology)	Monitoring

Hypocalcemia
 	
Normal serum calcium level: 8.6 to 10.0 mg/dL (SI units: 2.15 to 2.50 mmol/L)
 	
Hypocalcemia: Total serum calcium level < 8.6 mg/dL (SI units: < 2.15 mmol/L)
 	
Normal ionized calcium level: 4.5-5.1 mg/dL
 	
Low ionized calcium level: < 4.5 mg/dL
	Hypoalbuminemia
	Hyperphosphatemia
	Hypomagnesemia
	Hypoparathyroidism
	Alkalosis
		Excessive loss of calcium: diarrhea, diuretic therapy, ↑ lipoproteins, acute pancreatitis
		
		Hypoalbuminemia (major etiology)
		
		↓ calcium intake (diet low in calcium)
		
		Inadequate absorption of calcium: diarrhea, laxative abuse; lack of vitamin D, gastric acidity, pancreatic insufficiency
		
		↓ PTH secretion due to thyroid surgery, parathyroidectomy, disease of parathyroid gland
		
		Malignancy
		
		Hyperphosphatemia
		
		Medications: loop diuretics; certain anticonvulsants (phenytoin, phenobarbital); calcitonin; mithramycin, gentamicin, phosphates
		
		Massive blood transfusions: citrate in stored blood binds with calcium and ↓ ionized calcium levels
		
		Reduced activity or inactivity
			CNS:
			    Anxiety, confusion, irritability
			    ↑ deep tendon reflexes
			    Seizures
			
			Neuromuscular:
			    Paresthesia (toes, face, area around mouth)
			    Muscle twitching, tremors, cramps, spasms
			    Tetany
			    Twitching
			    Chvostek's sign: facial twitching when facial nerve is tapped
			    Trousseau's sign: carpal spasm with compression of upper arm
			
			GI:
			    Diarrhea
			    Paralytic ileus
			    Constipation
			
			Pulmonary:
			    Labored breathing
			    Wheezing
			    Laryngospasm
			    bronchospasm
			
			GU:
			    Oliguria; anuria
			
			CV:
			    ↓ CO
			    ↓ myocardial contractility
			    Angina
			    Hypotension
			    HF
			    Dysrhythmias
			    Irregular pulse
			
			ECG changes:
			    Prolonged ST segment
			    Long QT interval
			    Torsades de points
			    ↓ response to digoxin
				IV calcium gluconate
				IV calcium chloride
				Magnesium replacement
				
				For chronic hypocalcemia:
				    Calcium supplements
				    Vitamin D supplements
				
				In setting of hyperphosphatemia, aluminum hydroxide antacids to bind phosphorous
				
				Diet adequate in intake of calcium, vitamin D, protein
				
				Ionized calcium levels after every 4 units of blood
				
				Treatment of underlying disorder
					Serum calcium levels
					Serum albumin levels
					Serum phosphate levels
					Serum magnesium levels
					pH
					Vital signs
					Respiratory status
					Heart rate
					ECG
					Intake and output
					Patient's response to therapy

Electrolyte Imbalance	Potential Abnormal Findings	Pathophysiology/ Potential Etiology	Clinical Manifestations	Potential Treatment Options (Depend on Etiology)	Monitoring
Hypercalcemia *Normal* serum calcium level: 8.6 to 10.0 mg/dL (SI units: 2.15 to 2.50 mmol/L) Hypercalcemia: Serum calcium level > 10.0 mg/dL (SI units: > 2.50 mmol/L) *Normal* ionized calcium level: 4.5-5.1 mg/dL High ionized calcium level: > 5.1 mg/dL	Hypophosphatemia Metabolic acidosis	Primary etiologies: Hyperparathyroidism (leads to ↑ resorption of calcium from bone and kidneys; ↑ absorption from intestines) Carcinoma particularly squamous cell carcinoma of lung, myeloma, breast cancer, Hodgkin's lymphoma, renal cell carcinoma Hyperthyroidism Multiple fractures can cause ↑ in calcium release from bone ↑ absorption of calcium from GI tract ↓ excretion of calcium by kidneys Altered renal reabsorption of calcium Renal tubular acidosis Prolonged immobilization: can cause ↑ in calcium release from bone Alkalosis: ↑ calcium binding to protein Medications (abuse of calcium-containing antacids; thiazide diuretics; lithium, excessive amount of vitamin A or vitamin D)	Fatigue Mental status changes Confusion Personality changes Lethargy; coma Neuromuscular: Muscle weakness Hyporeflexia ↓ muscle tone CV: Hypertension Dysrhythmias: Bradycardia Heart block ECG changes: Short QT interval Prolonged PR interval Flat T waves Heart block GI: Anorexia Nausea, vomiting ↓ bowel sounds Constipation Pain (abdominal, flank) Paralytic ileus GU: Polyuria (may lead to dehydration) Kidney stones Flank pain Pathologic bone fractures Digoxin toxicity	↓ calcium intake (oral, IV) Promote diuresis by hydrating patient (e.g, with NS solution) Loop diuretics to ↑ calcium excretion Severe hypercalcemia: Hemodialysis Peritoneal dialysis In setting of malignancy: Biphosphonates to inhibit bone resorption of calcium Asymptomatic hypercalcemia: ↑ calcium excretion ↓ bone resorption of calcium Dialysis for renal failure Treatment of underlying disorder	Serum calcium level Serum phosphorous level Vital signs ECG Intake and output Fluid volume status Neurologic status Neuromuscular status Renal function If on Digoxin: Serum digitalis level Symptoms of digitalis toxicity (nausea, vomiting, anorexia, irregular HR) Patient's response to therapy

Electrolyte Imbalance	Potential Abnormal Findings	Pathophysiology/ Potential Etiology	Clinical Manifestations	Potential Treatment Options (Depend on Etiology)	Monitoring

Hypophosphatemia
 	
Normal serum phosphorous level: 2.3 to 4.5 mg/dL (SI units: 0.74 to 1.45 mmol/L)
 	
Hypophosphatemia: Serum phosphorus level < 2.3 mg/dL (SI units: < 0.74 mmol/L)
	Hyperparathyroidism
	
	Hypercalcemia
	
	Hypomagnesemia
	
	↑ creatine kinase: in setting of rhabdomyolysis
		Phosphorous shift from extracellular to intracellular fluid (respiratory alkalosis, hyperglycemia, insufficient phosphorous supplementation with enteral feedings or TPN)
		
		↓ absorption of phosphorous (vitamin D deficiency, prolonged use of phosphorous-binding antacids or laxatives, diarrhea)
		
		Medications (thiazide or loop diuretics, insulin)
		
		↑ loss of phosphorous (osmotic diuresis secondary to in DKA)
		
		Hyperparathyroidism
			Diplopia (double vision)
			
			Malaise
			
			Anorexia
			
			Slurred speech
			
			Dysphagia
			
			Muscular:
			  Muscle weakness
			  Myalgia
			  Rhabdomyolysis
			
			CNS:
			  Paresthesia
			  Irritability
			  Anxiety
			  Memory loss
			  Confusion
			  Seizures
			  Coma
			
			CV:
			  Hypotension
			  ↓ CO
			  Cyanosis
			
			Hematologic:
			  Hemolytic anemia
			  ↓ WBCs
			
			GI:
			  Bleeding
			
			Pulmonary:
			  Shallow respirations
				Phosphorous replacement:
				  Dietary supplements
				  IV:
				    Potassium phosphate
				    Sodium phosphate
				
				Vitamin D to ↑ absorption of phosphorous
				
				In setting of hypercalcemia: calcium-restricted diet
				
				Treatment of underlying disorder
					Serum phosphorous level
					
					Serum calcium level
					
					Serum magnesium level
					
					WBC count
					
					Vital signs
					
					Neuromuscular status:
					  LOC
					  Muscle strength
					
					Cardiovascular status
					
					Pulmonary status:
					  ABG
					  Pulse oximetry
					
					Intake and output
					
					Signs and symptoms of infection (hypophosphatemia may predispose patient to infection because ↓ ATP in WBCs impairs functioning of leukocytes)
					
					Bruising, bleeding (hypophosphatemia may affect platelet function)
					
					Patient's response to therapy

Electrolyte Imbalance	Potential Abnormal Findings	Pathophysiology/ Potential Etiology	Clinical Manifestations	Potential Treatment Options (Depend on Etiology)	Monitoring
Hyperphosphatemia *Normal* serum phosphorous level: 2.3 to 4.5 mg/dL (SI units: 0.74–1.45 mmol/L) Hyperphosphatemia: Serum phosphorous level > 4.5 mg/dL (SI units: > 1.45 mmol/L)	Hypocalcemia (serum calcium level < 8.5 mg/dL) ↑ BUN ↑ serum creatinine Respiratory acidosis	Impaired renal excretion of phosphorous (renal failure; especially when GFR < 30 ml/minute) Conditions associated with a shift of phosphorous from intracellular to extracellular fluid: for example, respiratory acidosis; DKA, trauma, rhabdomyolysis; infection Excessive phosphorous intake (diet, laxative abuse or medications) Medications (phosphorous- or phosphate-containing laxatives; oral or parenteral phosphorus supplements; excessive vitamin D supplements) Excess administration of IV or oral phosphates Hypoparathyroidism (typically after thyroid or parathyroid surgery)	Note: Hyperphosphatemia may cause hypocalcemia; clinical manifestations of hyperphosphatemia generally are the result of hypocalcemia Neuromuscular: Paresthesia: fingertips, mouth area; may spread to arms and face Muscle spasm, cramps, pain, weakness Hyperreflexia: + Trousseau's sign + Chvostek's sign CNS: ↓ mental status Delirium Seizures ECG changes: Prolonged QT interval Prolonged ST segment Cardiac: Hypotension Heart failure GI: Anorexia Nausea, vomiting Skeletal: Bone abnormalities Chronic hyperphosphatemia: Formation of calcium phosphate may cause: Dysrhythmias Dyspnea Irregular HR ↓ urine output Corneal haziness Conjunctivitis Cataracts Visual impairment Papular eruptions on skin	Limiting phosphorous intake to 0.6 to 0.9 grams/day Correcting hypocalcemia Stopping use of phosphorous-based laxatives and enemas Medications to ↓ absorption of phosphorous: Aluminum gel Magnesium gel Calcium gel Phosphate-binding antacids Calcium salts Polymeric phosphate binders Severe hyperphosphatemia: IV saline solution to ↑ renal excretion of phosphorous Proximal diuretics Hemodialysis Peritoneal dialysis Treat underlying disorder	Serum phosphorous levels Serum calcium levels Serum creatinine BUN pH Vital signs Intake and output Signs/symptoms of hypocalcemia Patient's response to therapy

Electrolyte Imbalance	Potential Abnormal Findings	Pathophysiology/ Potential Etiology	Clinical Manifestations	Potential Treatment Options (Depend on Etiology)	Monitoring

Hypochloremia
Normal serum chloride level: 97 to 107 mEq/L (SI units: 97 to 107 mmol/L)
 	
Hypochloremia: Serum chloride level < 97 mEq/L
	Hyponatremia (serum sodium level < 135 mEq/L)
	
	Hypokalemia
	
	Metabolic alkalosis: pH > 7.45 and serum bicarbonate level > 26 mEq/L
		↓ chloride intake (salt-restricted diet; IV fluids without electrolyte supplements)
		
		↓ chloride absorption (prolonged vomiting, diarrhea, severe diaphoresis, GI tube drainage)
		
		↑ chloride loss via gastric suctioning, GI losses, diuretic therapy
		
		Medications: corticosteroids, theophylline, bicarbonate, loop or thiazide diuretics, laxatives, osmotic diuretics (e.g., mannitol)
		
		Sodium deficiency
		
		Potassium deficiency
		
		Changes in acid-base balance
		
		Retention of fluid associated with heart failure
			Pulmonary:
			  Shallow, slow respirations
			  Respiratory arrest
			
			Neuromuscular:
			  Tetany
			  ↑ deep tendon reflexes
			  Hypertonicity
			  Muscle cramps
			  Muscle twitching
			  Muscle weakness
			
			CNS:
			  Irritability
			  Seizures
			  Coma
			
			CV:
			  Dysrhythmias (may be associated with concurrent hypokalemia)
				↑ chloride intake:
				  Diet
				  Supplements
				  IV fluids (e.g., normal saline solution)
				  Medications (e.g., potassium chloride)
				
				Treat metabolic alkalosis
				
				Treat underlying disorders
					Serum chloride levels
					Serum sodium levels
					Serum potassium levels
					Serum calcium levels
					Serum bicarbonate levels
					pH
					Vital signs (especially respiratory rate, pattern)
					ECG (particularly in setting of concurrent hypokalemia)
					Arterial blood gases (particularly for acid-base balance)
					LOC
					Neuromuscular status
					Cardiovascular status
					Respiratory status
					Intake and output
					Patient's response to therapy

Electrolyte Imbalance	Potential Abnormal Findings	Pathophysiology/ Potential Etiology	Clinical Manifestations	Potential Treatment Options (Depend on Etiology)	Monitoring

Hyperchloremia
Normal serum chloride level:
97 to 107 mEq/L
(SI units: 97 to 107 mmol/L)
 	
Hyperchloremia:
Serum chloride level > 107 mEq/L
(SI units: > 107 mmol/L)
	Hypernatremia
	↓ bicarbonate level
	Fluid retention
	Metabolic acidosis: pH < 7.35 and bicarbonate < 22 mEq/L)
		↑ chloride intake
		↑ chloride absorption
		Renal retention of chloride
		Metabolic acidosis (due to dehydration, renal failure, respiratory alkalosis, hypernatremia)
		Medications: acetazolamide [Diamox], sodium polystyrene sulfonate [Kayexalate], triamterene, ammonium chloride
			Majority of signs and symptoms are related to metabolic acidosis:
			  Tachypnea
			  Lethargy
			  Weakness
			  Cognitive impairment
			  Kussmaul's respirations (rapid, deep respirations)
			Untreated metabolic acidosis:
			  Dysrhythmias
			  ↓ CO
			  ↓ LOC
			  Coma
			Signs and symptoms associated with hypervolemia and hypernatremia:
			  Fluid retention
			  Agitation
			  Dyspnea
			  Tachycardia
			  Hypertension
			  Pitting edema
				Restore fluid and electrolyte balance:
				  IV fluids to dilute chloride and ↑ renal excretion of chloride
				  Restrict intake of chloride and sodium
				  Restore acid-base balance
				In setting of adequate liver function: IV lactated Ringer's solution (converts lactate to bicarbonate, thus ↑ base bicarbonate level and reversing acidosis)
				Severe hyperchloremia: IV sodium bicarbonate
				Diuretic therapy to ↑ excretion of chloride
				Treating underlying disorders
					Serum chloride levels
					Serum bicarbonate levels
					Serum sodium levels
					Serum potassium levels
					Vital signs
					Intake and output
					ECG
					ABGs
					Mental status
					Cardiovascular status
					Respiratory status
					Neuromuscular status
					Fluid status
					Acid-base balance
					If patient is receiving sodium bicarbonate: Observe patient for compensatory metabolic alkalosis and hypokalemia
					Patient's response to therapy

Data from Brady CL. *Fluids and Electrolytes Made Easy*, 3rd ed. Philadelphia: Lippincott Williams & Wilkins, 2005; Stark JL. The renal system. In Alspach JG (Ed.). *Core Curriculum for Critical Care Nursing*, 6th ed. St. Louis: Elsevier, 2006, pp. 525-610.

ABG = arterial blood gases; ACE = angiotensin-converting enzyme; AV = atrioventricular; BUN = blood urea nitrogen; CNS = central nervous system; CO = cardiac output; CVP = central venous pressure; CV = cardiovascular; DKA = diabetic ketoacidosis; DM = diabetes mellitus; ECF = extracellular fluid; ECG = electrocardiogram; GFR = glomerular filtration rate; GI = gastrointestinal; GU = genitourinary; HR = heart rate; IM = intramuscular; IV = intravenous; LOC = level of consciousness; mEq/L = milliequivalent per liter; mOsm/kg = milliosmoles per kilogram; NG = nasogastric; NS = normal saline; NSAIDS = nonsteroidal antiinflammatory drugs; PAP = pulmonary artery pressure; PAT = paroxysmal atrial tachycardia; PAWP = pulmonary artery wedge pressure; PVCs = premature ventricular contractions; SIADH = syndrome of inappropriate antidiuretic hormone; SVT = supraventricular tachycardia; TPN = total parenteral nutrition; VF = ventricular fibrillation; VT = ventricular tachycardia; WBCs = white blood cells.

Appendix B
Basic Adult Laboratory Values

Test	Conventional Units	System of International Units (SI Units)
Alanine aminotransferase (ALT) (Component of Hepatic Function Panel)	Females: 4-19 U/L or 10-30 Karmen units/mL Males: 7-30 U/L or 14-50 Karmen units/mL	4-19 U/L or 317 nKat/L 7-30 U/L or 500 nKat/L
Albumin (serum) (Component of Hepatic Function Panel)	3.5-5.0 g/dL	35-50 g/L
Alkaline phosphatase (ALP) (total; serum) (Component of Hepatic Function Panel)	20-125 U/L	20-125 U/L or 0.33-2.08 µKat/L
Ammonia (plasma)	15-45 µg/dL	11-32 µmol/L
Amylase (serum)	50-180 U/dL	92-330 U/L (Somogyi method) 20-125 U/L (Beckman method) 0.50-2.83 µkat/L
Aspartate aminotransferase (AST) (Component of Hepatic Function Panel)	Females: 8-26 U/L or 10-40 Karmen units/mL Males: 8-20 U/L or 10-40 Karmen units/mL	8-26 U/L or 0.14-0.44 µkat/L 8-20 U/L or 0.14-0.34 µkat/L
Bilirubin (serum) (Component of Hepatic Function Panel)		
Direct	0.0-0.3 mg/dL	1.7-5.1 µmol/L
Indirect	0.1-1.0 mg/dL	1.7-17.1 µmol/L
Total	<1.5 mg/dL	1.7-20.5 µmol/L
Brain natriuretic peptide (see Natriuretic Peptides)		
Calcium (total; serum)	8.6-10.0 mg/dL	2.15-2.50 mmol/L
Carbon dioxide (total content, blood)	22-30 mEq/L Panic levels: <15 mEq/L >50 mEq/L	22-30 mmol/L Panic levels: <15 mmol/L >50 mmol/L

Test	Conventional Units	System of International Units (SI Units)
Carcinoembryonic antigen (CEA)	<3.0 ng/mL (non-smoker)	<3.0 mg/L
	<5.0 ng/mL (smoker)	<5.0 mg/L
Chloride (serum)	97-107 mEq/L	97-107 mmol/L
Clotting Times		
Partial thromboplastin time (PTT) activated	Vary with type of activator used; typically <35 seconds	Vary with type of activator used; typically <35 seconds
	Panic level: >70 seconds	Panic level: >70 seconds
Prothrombin time (PT)	10-15 seconds	10-15 seconds
	Anticoagulated condition: >3 × the laboratory control	Anticoagulated condition: >3 × the laboratory control
International Normalized Ratio (INR): low-intensity therapy	≤2.5: to decrease risk of bleeding during endoscopic procedures	
	2.0 (range 1.6-2.5): to prevent stroke in patients >75 years with atrial fibrillation	
	2.5 (range: 2.0-3.0): to prevent stroke in patients <75 years with atrial fibrillation	
	2.0-3.0: deep vein thrombosis; prevention of systemic emboli; prosthetic mitral and aortic tissue valves	
INR: high-intensity therapy	2.5-3.5: recent acute myocardial infarction; bi-leaflet or tilting mechanical heart valves; left-sided prosthetic valve thrombosis; recurrent systemic emboli; prophylaxis for high-risk surgery	

Test	Conventional Units	System of International Units (SI Units)
Complete Blood Cell Count (CBC)		
Hemoglobin	Females: 12-16 g/dL	Females: 120-160 g/L or 7.45-9.9 mmol/L
	Males: 14-18 g/dL	Males: 140-180 g/L or 8.7-11.2 mmol/L
	Panic levels: <5 g/dL >18 g/dL	Panic levels: <50 g/L or <3.10 mmol/L >180 g/L or >11.2 mmol/L
Hematocrit (whole blood)	Female: 35-47%	Female: 0.35-0.47
	Male: 37-51%	Male: 0.37-0.51
Red blood cell count	4.0-6.2 million/μL	$4.0-6.2 \times 10^{12}$/L
Platelet count	150,000-400,000/μL or mm³	$150-400 \times 10^9$/L
	Panic levels: < 30,000/μL or mm³ > 1,000,000/μL or mm³	Panic levels: $<30 \times 10^9$/L $>1000 \times 10^9$/L
White blood cell count (WBC)	4500-11,000/μL	$4.5-11.0 \times 10^9$/L
Neutrophils (segmented)	54%-62% 3800 /μL or mm³	0.54-0.62 3800×10^6/L
Neutrophils (bands)	3%-5% 620/μL or mm³	0.03-0.05 620×10^6/L
Eosinophils	1%-3% 200/μL or mm³	0.01-0.03 200×10^6/L

Test	Conventional Units	System of International Units (SI Units)
Basophils	0%-0.75%	0-0.0075
	40/μL or mm³	40 × 10⁶/L
Lymphocytes	25%-33%	0.25-0.33
	2500/μL or mm³	2500 × 10⁶/L
Monocytes	3%-7%	0.03-0.07
	300/μL or mm³	300 × 10⁶/L
C-Reactive protein (CRP) (serum)	68-8200 ng/mL or	68-8200 μg/L
	20 mg/dL or	
	<8 μg/mL	
Creatine kinase (CK) (serum) (Total) Ambulatory patient	Females: 10-70 U/L	10-70 U/L or 0.17-1.16 μKat/L
	Males: 25-90 U/L	25-90 U/L or 0.42-1.5 μKat/L
Creatine kinase isoenzymes	CK-MM (muscle): 90%-97% of total CK	CK-MM: 0.90-0.97 fraction of total CK
	CK-MB (heart): 0-6 % of total CK	CK-MB: 0-0.06 fraction of total CK
	CK-BB (brain): 0-3% of total CK	CK-BB: 0-0.03 fraction of total CK
Creatinine (serum)	≤1.2 mg/dL	≤105 μmol/L
Creatinine clearance	Female: 90-126 mL/min	Female: 1.5-21 mL/sec
	Male: 96-126 mL/min	Male: 1.60-21 mL/sec
Digoxin (serum)	Therapeutic level (trough)	Therapeutic level (trough)
	0.5-2.0 ng/mL	0.6-2.6 nmol/L
	Panic level:	Panic level:
	>2.4 ng/mL	> 3.2 nmol/L
Erythrocyte sedimentation rate (ESR) (blood)	Female: 20-42 mm/hr	Female: 20-42 mm/hr
	Male: 15-30 mm/hr	Male: 15-30 mm/hr
Ferritin	Females:	Females:
	≤ 40 years: 11-122 ng/mL	≤ 40 years: 24.7-274 pmol/L or 11-122 μg/L
	> 40 years: 12-263 ng/mL	> 40 years: 26.9-590 pmol/L or 12-263 μg/L
	Males: 15-200 ng/mL	Males: 33.7-449 pmol/L or 15-200 μg/L
Folic acid (serum)	≤60 years: 1.8-9 ng/mL	≤60 years: 4.1-20.4 nmol/L
	>60 years: 1.2-12 ng/L	>60 years: 4.1-27.2 nmol/L
Glucose-6-Phosphate Dehydrogenase (G6PD) Quantitative (blood)	Vary with test method:	
	140-280 U/billion cells	
	125-280 U/dL packed red blood cells	
	8.6-18.6 U/g hemoglobin	
	4.5-10.8 U/g hemoglobin	
	Zinkham method:	Zinkham method:
	5.5-9.3 U/g hemoglobin	0.35-0.60 U/mol hemoglobin
	160-270 U/10¹² Ercs	0.16-0.27 U/L Ercs
	1.87-3.16 U/mL Ercs	1.87-3.16 kU/L Ercs
Glucose		
Fasting (whole blood)	60-89 mg/dL	3.3-4.9 mmol/L
Fasting (serum)	70-105 mg/dL	3.9-5.8 mmol/L
Random (serum)	70-125 mg/dL	3.9-6.9 mmol/L
	Panic levels:	Panic levels:
	<40 mg/dL or >700 mg/dL	<2.2 mmol/L or >38.6 mmol/L

Test	Conventional Units	System of International Units (SI Units)
Glucose: 2-hour postprandial (serum)	18-50 years: 65-140 mg/dL 50-60 years: 65-150 mg/dL >60 years: 65-160 mg/dL	18-50 years: 3.6-7.7 mmol/L 50-60 years: 3.6-8.3 mmol/L >60 years: 3.6-8.8 mmol/L
ADA diagnosis of diabetes (following 75 g glucose load)	>200 mg/dL	>11 mmol/L
Glycosylated hemoglobin (HgbA$_{1c}$)	<6% of total hemoglobin	<0.06 of total hemoglobin
Haptoglobin	40-240 mg/dL	4-24 µmol/L or 0.4-2.4 g/L
Homocysteine (plasma; fasting)	6.1-17.0 µmol/L	6.1-17.0 µmol/L
Iron (serum)	Females: 40-150 µg/dL Males: 50-160 µg/dL	Females: 7.2-26.9 µmol/L Males: 8.9-28.7 µmol/L
Iron-binding capacity, total (TIBC)	250-400 µg/dL	44.8-71.6 µmol/L
Lactic acid (blood)	Venous: 4.5-19.8 mg/dL or 0.5-2.2. mEq/L Arterial: 4.5-14.4 mg/dL or 0.5-1.6 mEq/L	Venous: 0.5-2.2 mmol/L Arterial: 0.5-1.6 mmol/L
Lactate dehydrogenase (LDH or LD) (Component of Hepatic Function Panel)	Wróblewski method 30° C 150-450 U/L Enzymatic colorimetry: ≤4.5 µkat/L ≤60 years: 45-90 U/L >60 years 55-102 U/L	Wróblewski method 30° C 72-217 IU/L Enzymatic colorimetry: ≤270 U/L ≤60 years: 45-90 U/L >60 years 55-102 U/L
Lipase (serum)	13-141 U/L	13-141 U/L or 0.22-2.40 µkat/L
Lipid Panel (American Heart Association Guidelines)		
Total cholesterol	Desirable: <200 mg/dL Borderline high: 200-239 mg/dL High: ≥240 mg/dL	Desirable: <5.17 mmol/L Borderline high: 5.17-6.18 mmol/L High: ≥6.21 mmol/L
Low density lipoprotein (LDL)	Desirable: <100 mg/dL Borderline-high: 130-159mg/dL High: ≥160-189mg/dL Very high: ≥190 mg/dL	Desirable: <2.58 mmol/L Borderline-high: 3.36-4.11 mmol/L High: ≥4.14 mmol/L Very high: ≥4.9 mmol/L
High density lipoprotein	Female: low ≤50 mg/dL Male: low ≤40 mg/dL	Female: low ≤1.29 mmol/L Male low ≤1.03 mmol/L
Triglycerides	Normal: <150 mg/dL Borderline-high: 150-199 mg/dL High: 200-499 mg/dL Very high: ≥500 mg/dL	Normal: < 3.87 mmol/L Borderline-high: 3.87-5.13 mmol/L High: 5.16-12.87 mmol/L Very high: ≥12.9 mmol/L
Magnesium	1.8–2.5 mEq/L	0.9–1.25 mmol/L

Test	Conventional Units	System of International Units (SI Units)
Natriuretic Peptides		
Atrial	20-77 pg/mL	20-77 ng/L
Brain	Females:	Females:
Note: Brain natriuretic peptide (BNP) increases with age and, at certain ages, is higher in women than men. Research has shown that BNP may be related to a number of other factors such as weight, kidney function, and indicators of cardiovascular damage such as hypertension, previous myocardial infarction or stroke, angina, and diabetes mellitus. Serum BNP levels may parallel the severity of heart failure (HF); however, at this time there is insufficient clinical evidence to warrant the use of BNP levels as targets for the adjustment of therapy in individual patients. Patients on optimal HF medications may have markedly increased BNP levels and patients with advanced HF may have normal BNP levels. Further clinical trials are need to determine the role of BNP measurement in diagnosing and managing HF.*	<74 years: <96 pg/mL ≥75 years: <181 pg/mL Males: <74 years: <64 pg/mL ≥75 years: <79 mg/mL	<74 years: <96 ng/L ≥75 years: <181 ng/L Males: <74 years: <64 ng/L ≥75 years: <79 ng/L
Phosphorus (serum)	2.3-4.5 mg/dL	0.74-1.45 mmol/L
Potassium	3.5-5.3 mEq/L Panic levels: <2.5 mEq/L >6.6 mEq/L	3.5-5.3 mmol/L Panic levels: <2.5 mmol/L >6.6 mmol/L
Prealbumin (transthyretin) (serum)	10-40 mg/dL	100-400 mg/L
Prostate-specific antigen (PSA) (serum)	<2.5 ng/mL	<2.5 µg/L
Protein, total (serum)	6.0-8.0 g/dL	60-80 g/L
Reticulocyte count (blood)	1%-2% of red blood cells	1%-2% of red blood cells
Sodium (plasma or serum)	135-146 mEq/L	135-146 mmol/L
Thyroid Test: T_3 (triiodothyronine)	80-230 ng/dL	1.2-3.5 nmol/L
Thyroid Test: Thyroxine Free (FT4)	0.58-1.64 ng/dL	7.48-18.06 pmol/L

Test	Conventional Units	System of International Units (SI Units)
Thyroid Test: Thyroid Stimulating Hormone (TSH)	0.4-4.2 μU/mL	0.4-4.2 mU/L
Testosterone, total	Females: 30-95 ng/dL	Females: 1.0-3.3 nmol/L
	Males: 300-1200 ng/dL	Males: 10.4-41.6 nmol/ L
Testosterone, free	Females: 1.0-8.5 pg/mL	Females: 3.5-29.5 pmol/L
	Males: 50-210 pg/mL	Males: 174-729 pmol/L
Transferrin	200-400 mg/dL	2.0-4.0 g/L
Uric acid	Females: 2.4 – 6.0 mg/dL	Females: 143-357 μmol/L
	Males: 3.4-7.0 mg/dL	Males: 202-416 μmol/L
Urinalysis, complete	Appearance: clear, yellow	
	Specific gravity: 1.003-1.030	
	pH: 4.5-8.0	
	Albumin: negative	
	Protein: negative	
	Glucose: negative	
	Ketones: negative	
	Bilirubin: negative	
	Occult blood: negative	
	Leukocyte esterase: negative	
	Nitrite: negative	
	WBC: ≤4 cells/high-power field	
	RBC: ≤3 cells/high-power field	
	Squamous epithelial cells: none or few/high-power field	
	Casts: none	
	Crystals: small amount	
	Bacteria: none or <1000/mL	
	Yeast: none or <1000/mL	

Arterial Blood Gases

Test	Conventional Units	System of International Units (SI Units)
pH	7.35-7.45	7.35-7.45
	Panic levels:	Panic levels:
	≤7.2 or >7.6	≤7.2 or >7.6
Bicarbonate (HCO_3)	22-26 mEq/L	22-26 mEq/L or 22-26 mmol/L
	Panic levels:	Panic levels:
	≤10 mEq/L or >40 mEq/L	<10 mmol/L or >40 mmol/L
Partial pressure of arterial CO_2 ($PaCO_2$)	35-45 mm Hg	35-45 mm Hg or 4.7-6.0 kPa
	Panic levels:	Panic levels:
	≤20 mm Hg or >70 mm Hg	≤20 mm Hg or >70 mm Hg
		≤2.7 kPa or >9.4 kPa
Partial pressure of arterial O_2 (PaO_2)	75-100 mm Hg	75-100 mm Hg or 10.3-13.3 kPa
	Panic level:	Panic level:
	≤40 mm Hg	≤40 mm Hg or <5.3 kPa
Oxygen saturation	96%-100%	0.96-1.0
	Panic level:	Panic level:
	<60%	<0.60

Data from *ACC/AHA 2005 Guideline Update for the Diagnosis and Management of Chronic Heart Failure in the Adult: available at http://content.onlinejacc.org/cgi/reprint/46/6/e1; American Heart Association: available at: www.americanheart.org; Chernecky CC, Berger BJ. *Laboratory and Diagnostic Procedures*, 4th ed. Philadelphia: Saunders, 2004; *Merck Manual of Diagnosis and Therapy*: available at: www.merck.com/mrkshared/mmanual/home.jsp.

Abbreviations:

dL = deciliter; Ercs = electronic counters; g = gram; g/dL = grams/deciliter; g/L = grams/liter; Hg = mercury; IU/L = international units per liter; kU/L = kilounits/liter; kPa = kilopascal; L = liter; mEq = mille-equivalent; mEq/L = mille-equivalent per liter; mg = milligram; mg/dL = milligrams per deciliter; mg/L = milligrams per liter; mL = milliliter; mL/min = milliliters per minute; mL/sec = milliliters per second; mm = millimeter; mm^3 = cubic millimeters; mm Hg = millimeters of mercury; mol = mole; mmol/L = millimole per liter; mOsm = milliosmole; mU = milliunits; mIU/L = milli-International Units per Liter; ng = nanograms; ng//L = nanograms per liter; ng/mL = nanograms per milliliter; nkat/L = nanokatal per liter; nmol/L = nanomoles per liter; pg = picogram; pg/mL = picograms per milliliter; pmol/L = picomole per liter; μg = microgram; μg/L = micrograms per liter; μg/mL = micrograms per milliliter; μkat/L = microkatal per liter; μL = microliter; μmol = micromole; μmol/L = micromole per liter; μU/mL = microunits per milliliter; U = units; U/dL = units per deciliter; U/g = units per gram; U/L = units per liter; U/mL = units per milliliter; U/mol = units per mole.

Index

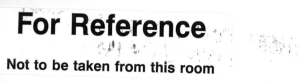